An
American
Physical
Therapy
Association
Anthology

CEREBRAL PALSY

Case Reports, Orthotics and Devices, Measurement and Assessment, and Schools and Education

VOL. 3

This anthology is a compilation of articles originally published in issues of *PT Review* and *Physical Therapy*, from 1931 through 1994.

ISBN # 1-887759-06-9

For more information about this and other APTA publications, contact the American Physical Therapy Association, 1111 North Fairfax Street, Alexandria, VA 22314-1488.

[Order No. P-125]

Table of Contents

Foreword

For three quarters of a century, *Physical Therapy* has been publishing the ideas and research of therapists and others. In that time, we have seen many articles on many topics, and interest in these topics has often waned. But interest in cerebral palsy (CP) has been consistent and strong since we began. As a result, few tasks have been as daunting for me as preparing this anthology series on cerebral palsy. Our literature on this clinical condition is not only vast but also remarkably diverse. This volume reflects the diversity.

First, we offer all the case reports that have been published—and there are many. The second section contains articles on orthotics and devices. The thinking on this topic has changed time and again; the ebb and flow of ideas and approaches is clear in this section. We also see how important measurement and assessment were to clinicians. In Volume 2 of this anthology series, we included articles on research on measurement. In this volume, we include articles dealing with measurement in general or offering clinical suggestions.

The last section in this volume includes articles on schools and education. Today, we consider mainstreaming as a modern concept, but as you can see from what follows, the role of schools and mechanisms for providing services in school settings have been discussed since 1931.

There are multiple purposes for an anthology such as this. One purpose is to present all of the material on the topic published in our journal, *Physical Therapy*. This can facilitate the reader's ability to see all that has been published on a topic by one journal, and it provides a historical perspective not just for a body of knowledge but also for a profession. But I would be remiss as an editor if I did not encourage the reader to also pause and ponder other issues. Although, on the one hand, we can be impressed by the remarkable programmatic publication efforts of some of our authors and the great effort that many authors made years ago in contributing to our body of knowledge, we should also be impressed by our growth. The articles reflect not just the growth of knowledge but also the growth in sophistication in the way physical therapists examine issues. This is not to suggest that what is new is always better than what is old, but the observation should serve as a warning to readers to look cautiously at all that lies within the pages of this volume.

Our views often change over time. For example, readers will be shocked by the use of such terms as "spastic" and "cripple" in many of the articles we included. These are words that we now see as pejorative but that were once used freely and consistently throughout society. We can take solace that growth has led to sensitivity and that stereotypic language has been replaced with words that put the emphasis on the person—not the disease, impairment, or disability.

With time, just as the enthusiasm for a topic may change, so might standards for acceptable scholarship, research, and documentation. We have made no effort to alter the historical record by re-editing or re-reviewing papers. All articles relating to CP have been published in one of the three anthologies, regardless of whether they would meet the standards of the Journal today. The compendium therefore is rich in content and diverse in quality. It is as if we have presented before the interested reader a rather extensive smorgasbord, of regional cuisine. Some of the offerings you may like better, and some you may not like at all, but only by offering the array can we represent the cuisine as it is, rather than as we would like it to be. Like any smorgasbord, there can be many schemes for the organization of the presentation. In this volume, articles have been placed in four sections based on content and then organized within those sections based on chronology.

On behalf of the Journal, I encourage you to read what lies between the covers and to appreciate those authors whose work has increased our understanding. Few areas of patient care have garnered so much attention as CP, and the efforts of so many people to publish and elucidate can be an example for us all. This anthology series not only provides information, it is also a reminder of the debt we owe to all those who care enough to take pen to paper in order to expand the horizons of their colleagues. These authors are worthy of our respect and appreciation because they contributed to a profession and its efforts on behalf of patients. History may have been unkind to their concepts or, by today's standards, their scholarship may appear lacking, but that is irrelevant, because in their time and in their day they did what too few people do. We salute them not only by including their works here, but also by recognizing that they helped build the foundation on which we now stand, a foundation all the more secure because of their publications.

Jules M Rothstein, PhD, PT, FAPTA
Editor, *Physical Therapy*
December 1995

Part I: Case Reports

Case Reports

Red Shoes: A Case Study

Steps in the Rehabilitation of an Adult Cerebral Palsied Patient

F. A. Hellebrandt, M.D., C. Etta Walters, Ph.D., and Harriet Styche, B.A.

M.A., a 39 year old white female with a chief complaint of difficulty in walking and in the use of the hands, was admitted to the Outpatient Clinics of the Research and Educational Hospitals in February of 1953. Her disability was diagnosed as a moderately severe quadriplegic athetosis, exaggerated by lability in the responsiveness of the neuromuscular system to sensory stimuli and affective states. She did not walk until she was 9. She had received an elementary education in a special school and limited tutorial instruction on the high school level. She had led a restricted life largely because her father "was afraid" to let her leave the confines of the home. Upon his death, at a time when the patient had already reached adulthood, she forced herself to go out alone and to use public transportation. The latter achievement had an almost symbolic connotation which continued to exert a dynamogenic effect. When first seen M.A. expressed three well defined objectives: to use her hands better, to walk without crutches, and to seek employment.

The history and physical findings were typical and require no special comment. Muscular development was good. Voluntary motion was essentially normal. There was considerable reduction in the speed of movement, however, and a characteristic secondary incoordination due to involuntary athetotic movements which were worse in the upper than the lower extremities, and relatively mild in the head and neck region. There were no deformities. Hand and arm function were poor, especially when the patient was excited. Communicative ability was adequate. There was minimal grimacing and no drooling. When first seen, M.A. was indifferent to personal appearance. She was cheerful, loquacious, cooperative, and eager to enter upon a rehabilitation program.

To begin with the gait was wide-based, ungainly, and sidling. Ambulation without crutches was barely possible (Fig. 1) and M.A. reported that if she found it necessary to get out of bed at night, she could not walk without first putting on her shoes. She wore old-fashioned, black kid laced shoes with pointed toes and small, moderately high heels.

M.A. made appreciable progress under the usual training program for the treatment of athetosis. This began with instruction in relaxation, and table exercises for the execution of controlled normal range movements. She was provided with heavy soled steel shank high-top shoes with broad flat heels and rounded toes. The gait improved in rhythm and stability. Timed treadmill walking was instituted for endurance training and to assist in establishing a more symmetric ambulation pattern. Table exercises were gradually replaced by more generalized activity against increasing resistance. Improvement in general health and physical fitness followed in due course. Selected muscle groups of the upper extremities were subjected to a strenuous program of ergographic exercise. The Minnesota Rate of Manipulation Test and routine occupational therapy activities were used to augment manual dexterity and to improve facility in ordinary hand skills. Under sympathetic guidance M.A. showed considerable growth in social maturity. She participated also in a grooming program instituted by the Occupational Therapy Department.

In the spring of 1955 two events occurred which led to the primary observations herein reported. The first was the development and standardization by one of us (C.E.W.) of a simple obstacle course designed to train the athetotic person to make quick changes in ambulatory progression. Figure 2 shows the patient running the course which was approximately 13 feet long and 4 feet wide. Three obstacles were circumvented in successive clockwise counterclockwise half-circles. M.A. was instructed to traverse the course as rapidly as she could, and in any manner short of crawling. If she fell, she was to get up as fast as possible, and continue the run. In her regular physical therapy program she had already been taught how to fall safely and regain standing balance, but she had had virtually no previous experience in running. All runs were timed with a stopwatch; from 12 to 18 were attempted per practice session with a brief rest pause between trials. This program was followed two to four times per week for one month. The moving pictures from which the illustrations were drawn (Fig. 2 and 3) were made three weeks later, after

Dr. Hellebrandt, RFD #3, Cable Lane, Athens, Ohio; Dr. Walters, Department of Physical Education for Women, The Florida State University, Tallahassee, Florida; and Miss Styche, formerly occupational therapist at the Research and Educational Hospitals of the University of Illinois. The observations reported were made in the Disability Evaluation Laboratory of the Department of Physical Medicine and Rehabilitation, University of Illinois, Chicago. This study was supported in part by United Cerebral Palsy of Chicago.

the patient had returned from a fortnight at camp during which activity was much curtailed. It was a rule of the camp that inability to ambulate without falling would confine the camper to a wheel chair.

The objective of the obstacle course was to determine whether progressively increasing speed and competitive stress would augment or disrupt the neuromuscular coordination of an athetotic patient. Traditional methods of treatment call for training by deliberate and meticulously controlled movement from a carefully relaxed starting position. The deviation in approach was part of a broad general study of the overload principle, its physiological and therapeutic implications. *A priori* reasoning suggested that a volatile and excitable patient might gain more control by attempting to execute a familiar task in a progressively more stressful situation, than by the repetition of the endeavor in an environment devoid of stimulation and challenge. The procedure was aimed also at probing some of the many uncertainties that surround empirical methods of treating the cerebral palsied.

The second event leading to the observations herein recorded grew out of the occupational therapy grooming program. Newly conscious of self and factors affecting personal appearance, M.A. developed a distaste for the heavy high-top shoes thought to be obligatory for effective ambulation. Heretofore they had been accepted as a necessary assistive device. Without consultation M.A. purchased a pair of light sandals. She could neither stand nor walk in these, but wore them at home when inactive, "because they looked so nice." At the same time she entered into the obstacle course training program enthusiastically, in the secret expectation that this might improve her gait sufficiently to enable her to walk on the streets of the city wearing inconspicuous low shoes. When her obsession with this objective became known, its feasibility was studied systematically. Further observation suggested that M.A.'s major disability stemmed from lack of control over the musculature activating the proximal appendicular joints. Was distal support, therefore, indicated?

The effect of removing all footgear is illustrated in the top row of figure 3. The frames reproduced show M.A. walking the obstacle course barefooted. This was an unexpectedly difficult feat to perform. Standing was precariously unstable. Preliminary training was necessary before the obstacle course could be attempted. When M.A. was permitted to stand in a sandpile, she learned quickly how to grip the supporting surface with her bare feet. She progressed rapidly then to walking in sand, on thick turf, and finally, on the smooth asphalt tile floor of the laboratory.

When walking barefooted, M.A. invariably assumed the crouching posture illustrated in the top row of figure 3. This carriage augments stability autonomously by lowering the center of gravity of

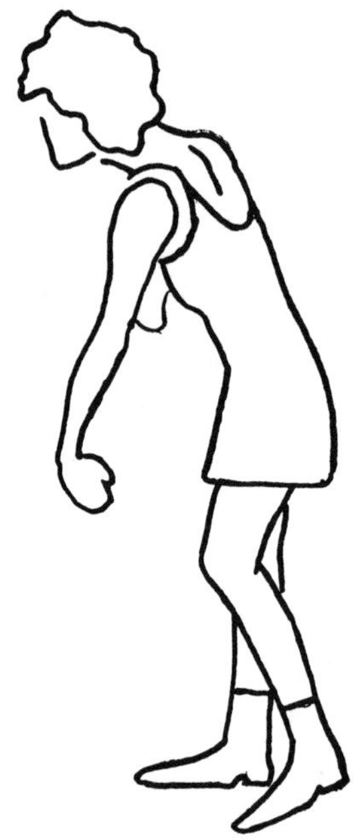

Figure 1. Free walking of M.A. (quadriplegic athetosis) in 1953 prior to the onset of training.

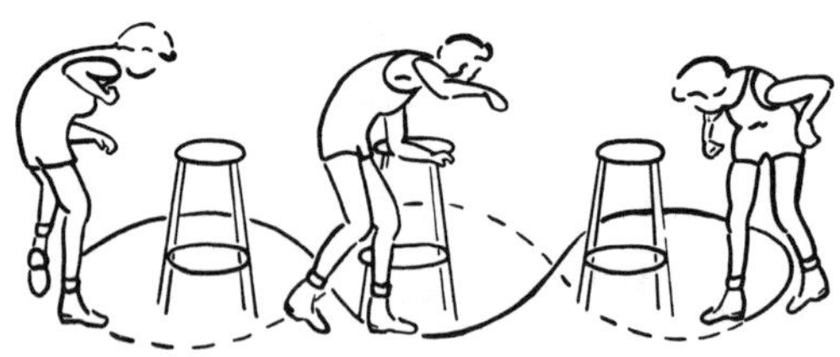

Figure 2. Three frames from a moving picture film showing a quadriplegic athetoid patient running a simple obstacle course. Note that the head always turns spontaneously toward the leg that is extending and away from the leg that is flexing.

the body as a whole. It is expedited further, by a tendency to hyperextend the cervical spine, which in turn evokes one of the general attitudinal reflexes of Mangus and de Kleijn. The forward thrust of the chin is clearly evident in the fourth figure from the left (top row, Fig. 3). The forelimbs are extended stiffly while the vertebral column and lower extremities sag by virtue of reflex differential variations in the tonus of the antigravity muscles. Maximal instability occurred at the hip joint.

The application of a many-tailed scultetus binder had an immediately salutary effect on the postural alinement assumed while walking the obstacle course barefooted (2nd row, Fig. 3). With the

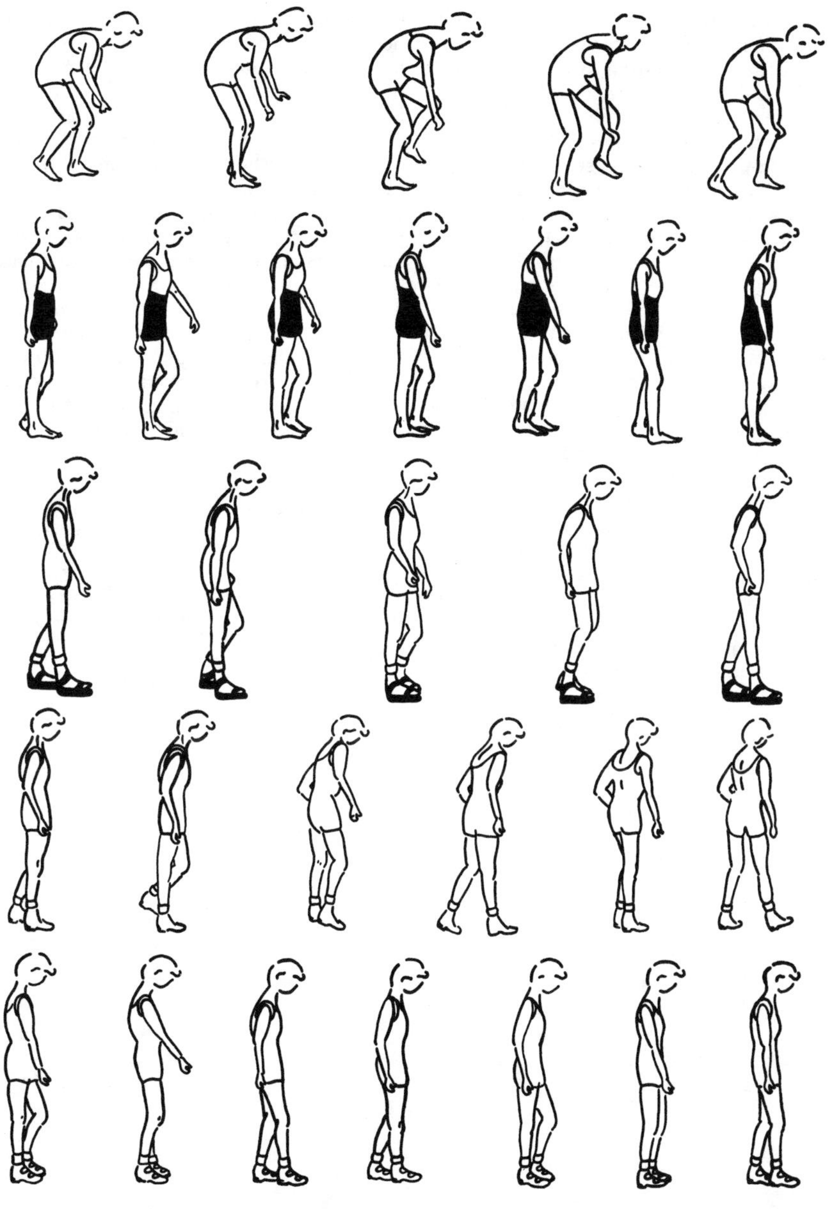

Figure 3. Selected sequential frames from a moving picture film showing a quadriplegic athetoid patient walking a simple obstacle course as rapidly as possible while maintaining the best attainable gait and posture. Succeeding rows from top to bottom: 1) barefooted; 2) barefooted with a scultetus binder; 3) Houtz-Sharon boots (weighted); 4) heavy high-top shoes; 5) weighted red slippers.

binder removed, reasonably stable walking in an unexpectedly good upright posture was also possible when heavily weighted boots were strapped to the feet (3rd row, Fig. 3). Both devices improve hip joint control, one mechanically and the other reflexly. Muscles operate in functionally related units. The proprioceptive feedback from the heavily loaded distal joint influences the reactivity of proximal fixators and the number and extent of involuntary movements are much reduced.

M.A. had practiced running the obstacle course at maximal speed in her heavy high-top shoes. It is not surprising that she could now walk the same path with considerable grace and ease (4th row,

Fig. 3). In all three procedures there was strong involuntary ventroflexion of the cervical spine. This reflexly increases the equilibrating tension exerted by the antigravity extensors, and accounts in large measure for the great improvement in postural alinement. There is nothing new in those observations. They are interesting primarily because of the fundamental nature of the phenomena demonstrated, the automaticity of the responses, and the remarkable degree to which they can be mobilized to help the disabled person meet his ambulatory problems.

The evidence suggested that stabilization of the ankle joint was not the key to M.A.'s rehabilitation as far as locomotion was concerned. A much improved gait was attainable with and without ankle support. Accordingly steps were taken to provide M.A. with a much desired low shoe, modified if necessary, but suitable for street wear. In the first visit ever made to a large department store, M.A. selected a pair of red slippers with one strap across the instep. The welt sole was opened and three and one-half pounds of lead was put in each shoe, distributed approximately 2:1 between the region of the sole and the heel. The sole was then resewn and covered with a Perlstein corrugated rubber treading which gives a good gripping surface. An additional strap that passed around the ankle held the heel of the slipper more securely to the foot.

The bottom row of figure 3 shows M.A. walking the obstacle course with dignity, stability, and poise, wearing her red shoes. No amount of speculation can throw light on the degree to which hard physical training contributed to the progress made by this adult cerebral palsied patient. The motivational drive fired by the grooming program of the occupational therapy department was an indispensable factor. Nothing can surpass the efficacy of practical, meaningful goals. The excitement of pitting each day's performance against past achievement was as dynamogenic to this patient as it is to the normal person. Emotional stress was not a disrupter of skill when the effort demanded was increased progressively in the course of systematic training. The cerebral palsied subject appears to mobilize reserves of residual ability in response to the same stimuli which augment the functional capacity of the normal person.

REFERENCES

Hellebrandt, F. A., and Sara Jane Houtz: Mechanisms of muscle training in man; experimental demonstration of the overload principle. Phys. Ther. Rev., 36:371-383, June, 1956.

Magnus, Rudolph: Croonian lecture—animal posture. Proc. Roy. Soc. London, 98(B): 339-353, August, 1925.

Sherrington, Charles: Problems of muscular receptivity. Nature, 13:892-894, June 21, 1924; 929-932, June 28, 1924.

Walters, C. Etta: The application of the overload principle to the learning of a motor skill. Am. J. Occup. Ther., 10:1-6, January-February, 1956.

A Cerebral Palsied Infant Under Treatment

Edna M. Blumenthal, B.S., and Katharine M. Banham, Ph.D.

The purpose of this paper is to point out the effects of early physical therapy in the preambulatory cerebral palsied patient. In the young infant only gradual and minute degrees of improvement can be anticipated. Ranges of motion and repeated correct joint positioning are stressed. By such efforts mild contractures can be eliminated and more severe ones avoided. When a child is not under treatment overstretched muscles are protected in a position of mechanical and physiological advantage by molded casts, splints and/or braces. Careful muscle reeducation is used to prevent gross muscle substitution. Through early treatment even a retarded baby with an apparently useless upper extremity may develop a good assisting hand.

Case history

This 12 month old female child, product of a term pregnancy and normal delivery, referred by her pediatrician, was seen Jan. 13, 1957. She was reported to have held her head up at one month and to have sat alone at six months. The parents first noted at the age of 3 months that the patient did not use her left arm and hand. At age 1 year she could not stand, walk, or feed herself. The conclusions of the psychologist at this hospital after examination were: "This pleasant and charming 1 year old appears to be average in her social and mental growth."

Physical findings

This well developed, emotionally secure child could not use the left arm but had grasp and release in the left hand. On attempted passive internal rotation, forward flexion, or abduction there was blocking at the shoulder. Resistance was present on passive flexion of elbow due to moderate spasticity of the elbow extensors. The thumb was held in the palm. The first metacarpophalangeal joint tended to sublux. The left lower extremity was in equino valgus with spastic peroneals. DIAGNOSIS: Infantile Cerebral Palsy with Left Spastic Hemiplegia. A short leg brace with outside bar and inside pullover strap with 90 degree stop (for day and night wear) and a molded thumb splint were prescribed along with left tendo achilles stretching and hand work in physical therapy.

First physical therapy visit

This friendly and cooperative child, whose mother was tense and apprehensive, was started on a very simple daily home program. The mother was taught to apply gentle "relaxed stretching" to the thumb (very slow passive movement to achieve relaxation of tight adductors and flexors of thumb) with emphasis on extension-abduction. To motivate the baby and hold her attention it was suggested to the mother that she kiss the baby's palm each time the hand was fully opened. Since rapport with mother, child, and therapist was being established no formal exercises were started.

Second week

A less tense mother volunteered the information, "She opens her hand more than last week and keeps thumb out of palm oftener." The mother had made a game out of the relaxed stretching exercise and the baby chortled as the mother demonstrated the "treatment." Further investigation revealed that the child, if held by the right hand, would attempt to walk. She would not creep because the left upper extremity could not support her weight. Left hand was clutched. With the left elbow supported and the hand opened and placed by the physical therapist the child attempted to creep. The mother was instructed to encourage the baby to reach overhead for her favorite toys.

Third week

It was noted that the child brought the left thumb out of her palm many times. Good rapport was now well established and a formal program was begun. The mother was instructed and given written exercises with songs for forward

Edna M. Blumenthal, Director of Rehabilitation, The North Carolina Cerebral Palsy Hospital, Durham; Katharine M. Banham, Associate Professor of Psychology, Duke University, Durham, North Carolina.

flexion, extension, abduction, adduction, and rotation of left shoulder. In addition, slow relaxed stretching for tight tendo achilles was started. These exercises were to be done once a day, six days a week. With elbow supported and fingers opened by the therapist the baby moved forward with normal movements in a four-point creeping position. She was fascinated when the thumb splint was molded in occupational therapy.

Fifth week

The mother stated that the child now kept her thumb out of her palm most of the time. During her treatment period she opened her hand voluntarily with thumb extended. The thumb splint, molded to maintain abduction and opposition, was fitted. The splint was worn only at night as the child used her hand during the day.

Seventh week

The child could now support her own weight in the four-point kneeling position without assistance to left elbow. Thumb to finger opposition (with song) was started by the physical therapist (the mother observed execution of this exercise for two sessions before adding it to her program). There was no resistance of the thumb adductors to passive exercise. The baby, wearing short leg brace and with slight assistance, was beginning to walk.

Eighth week

Mother stated that child was pulling up in her play pen with *both hands* and would let go and walk across the pen unaided. She would walk from one piece of furniture to another. With her right hand held she would run across the room but if the left hand was held she walked with caution. The thumb splint was adjusted. Passive exercises for supination and pronation of forearm and extension and flexion of wrist were started by the physical therapist but not added to the home program.

Ninth-tenth weeks

The child, according to the mother, frequently used a four-point kneeling position at home and pulled up at a chair with her left arm. At the hospital she reached with left upper extremity for objects on a high chair when encouraged to do so, and grasped a lollipop (awkwardly) overhead. With short leg brace the child stood alone with feet and knees in good alinement and, by following a wall, walked unassisted.

Eleventh-thirteenth weeks

The child, at this time, walked independently with the left leg brace. However, it was noted when barefooted she still pronated the left ankle. The patient was ill and kept only one appointment in three weeks. She was very fussy. The mother stated that the baby screamed at night and bit and pulled on the thumb splint, but when splint was removed she slept well.

Fourteenth week

Seen in diagnostic clinic. A soft leather thumb splint was ordered and the comment was made that this child had a good gait for a 15 month old. Outpatient treatments were re-ordered.

Fifteenth week

Mother stated child could now support her weight on left arm, place right foot on the floor, and come to a standing position unassisted. This was demonstrated at the hospital. It was obvious that both mother and child were ill and treatment was cancelled.

Sixteenth-seventeenth weeks

The child had had immunizations and was cutting four teeth which necessitated temporary discontinuance of outpatient treatments. The mother continued treatment at home as she insisted that the child was cooperating perfectly in the home environment.

Twenty-sixth–twenty-seventh weeks

The child returned for treatment after a two month summer holiday. She walked with an excellent gait and ran without difficulty, wearing left leg brace. The mother stated that the child now places her fully opened left hand on her high chair tray when eating. At this time she demonstrated a fully opened left hand when creeping. She was as happy and inquisitive as on her initial treatment visit. The therapist watched the mother give the exercises and made no changes as reestablishing rapport was considered of more vital importance. Exercises were well demonstrated by the mother. The child again worked well the next week. The physical therapist helped dress the child and on departure the baby waved good-bye with her left upper extremity.

Twenty-eighth week

On her most recent visit the mother stated that the child opened her fingers more frequently and picked objects up with left hand, but had a weak grasp. It was noted that her thumb stayed out of the palm during most of the treatment. In creeping the child had to be reminded to open her left hand. She needed assistance to do this particularly when she crept rapidly. Using her short leg brace she walked and ran without stumbling or falling. Child was in a gay mood and the therapist resumed the exercises which were started in July. These will be added to the mother's home program after the child has become accustomed to them in her hospital visits.

SUMMARY

It is obvious that maturation played a definite role in this young child's physical development; however, some important points should be stressed:

1. Limitation of motion on passive internal rotation, forward flexion and abduction of shoulder had been materially reduced.
2. Resistance to passive elbow flexion was also maaterially reduced.
3. Within three weeks after initial treatment child brought thumb out of palm many times.
4. Seven weeks after initial treatment child supported weight on left upper extremity in four-point kneeling position.
5. Nine weeks after initial treatment child reached overhead with left upper extremity and grasped (awkwardly) lollipop.
6. Fifteen weeks after first treatment child could get up from sitting position on the floor using left upper extremity to support her weight.
7. A rest period from hospital treatment, due to illness, had no adverse effects. The child walked and ran independently wearing her left leg brace, had no marked contractures and, according to the mother, was beginning to pick things up with her left hand. She was happy and worked well.

CONCLUSION

It is felt by this therapist that early physical therapy in the cerebral palsied infant prevents contractures, promotes psychological as well as physical awareness of correct joint position and motion, and prepares the extremity for voluntary functional use as the infant matures. The use of casts, splints and/or braces to maintain normal joint position removes already involved muscles from an overstretched condition and so reduces abnormal stresses and strains on forming bones.

The fact that the child has learned to modify movements as a result of treatment procedures offers hope that the impairment of form sense and two-point discrimination, so frequently found in older spastic hemiplegics, will be considerably reduced by early treatment of the cerebral palsied infant.

Psychological Aspects

Following is a brief summary of psychological benefits which were noted during observation of this case and further benefits which might result from the rehabilitation program for cerebral palsied children begun within the first or second year of life.

BENEFITS FOR THE PARENT

During treatment the mother's attitude towards the child's handicap was a constantly reinforced hopeful one. She probably identified herself to some extent with the child and she experienced pleasure from each step in her child's control of movements.

The regular program of exercises brought the mother and child closer together in affectionate attachment, to the mutual satisfaction of both.

Weekly visits to the hospital to report progress and give the child exercises under supervision helped the mother to keep actively cooperative in the rehabilitation program. She received encouragement from the therapist which increased her self confidence and motivated her to continue the program prescribed.

Keeping the child at home during the outpatient treatment period, with the thought of possibly avoiding the necessity of hospitalization for the child later, was comforting to the mother and father alike.

BENEFITS FOR THE CHILD

The gratifying rewards of the mother's personal attention during the exercises, the rhythmic tunes that she sang to accompany the movements, and the caresses received on their completion apparently made the rehabilitation process an enjoyable one for the child. Rewarding experiences of this kind are likely to facilitate the learning of all behaviors, including social cooperation, active exploration and use of limbs, vocalization and the development of language.

The early use of specific muscle groups, for example those used in grasping or lifting objects, would facilitate the child's general mental development. These simple actions are the raw material required for the later development of specific skills, such as dressing and undressing, writing, or typing.

The rhythmic exercises and the smiling, friendly attention of the physical therapist in the hospital played a positive role in the child's social development and adjustment. They provided happy associations with the hospital and at the same time reinforced the child's attention to specific movements that she needed to learn to make and control.

The regular repetition of the rehabilitation exercises, moreover, may have the effect of increasing the child's sensitivity to movement and of developing the kinesthetic sensations and perception necessary for voluntary control of movement. Laboratory studies showing the summation effect of subliminal stimuli in the sensory areas of vision and hearing suggest that repetition of barely conscious, passive movements may help to increase a child's awareness of those movements.

It would appear that much valuable time may be wasted if rehabilitation is delayed until the child is able to cooperate voluntarily in the exercises, say at the age of 3 or 4 years. Learning will be harder after spasticity has become habitual and taken for granted. A 4 year old child with cerebral palsy might have been able to gain voluntary control of his movements at an earlier age if he had been helped by passive exercises to develop a sense of movement.

A child's general mental ability grows with his skill in controlling all kinds of movements, including those involved in speech. Delay in the development of motor skills interferes with every phase of psychological development, in intelligent behavior, emotional expression and control, language, and thought. Similarly, absence of loving care and attention has been shown to warp a child's personality, whereas the presence of kindly personal attention helps a child to develop into an alert, happy, socially outgoing youngster. It seems likely that the rehabilitation program for very young children with cerebral palsy, through its beneficial effect on the growth of their total personalities, could be of lasting significance throughout their lives.

REFERENCES

Hohman, Leslie B., Baker, Lenox D., Reed, Ruth: Sensory Disturbances in Children With Infantile Hemiplegia, Triplegia and Quadriplegia. Read before the American Academy for Cerebral Palsy, Memphis, Tenn., 1955.

Murphy, Gardner: Personality. A Biosocial Approach to Origins and Structure (particularly Parts I and II) Harper, 1947.

Mussen, Paul Henry and Conger, John Janeway: Child Development and Personality, Harper, 1956.

Case Reports

Teaching a Blind Cerebral Palsied Child to Walk

Ruth P. Rigg, M.S.

Yvonne is a 9 year old sightless cerebral palsied child of the spastic paraplegic type. She is left handed. At age 5 years, 10 months, her psychological test showed, "she was friendly, but her responses were poor, included much perseveration, and it was hard to hold her attention. Speech indistinct." On the Intermin Hayes-Benet scale for the blind her performance ranked her well below average in ability for school work.

At this age the child was sent to the Cerebral Palsy Center, but was unable to attend regularly because her family could not provide transportation for her. Reports from the C. P. Center stated that, "Yvonne is a happy, appealing and cooperative blind child whose arm and hand activities are limited by lack of vision. She sits well, creeps, but has no standing balance and needs complete assistance to walk."

Yvonne was enrolled at Condon School in September 1956. She wore bilateral control braces with pelvic band. The prescription requested walking and balance training with supplemental stretching of knee and hip structures and achilles tendon. The child was extremely apprehensive upon admission to the physical therapy department, crying if the therapist could not work with her immediately. She had no sense of balance or reciprocation for a walking pattern. She sat with her head drooped, arms flexed, and trunk relaxed.

Standing balance was practiced in standing tables while in the physical therapy department and the classroom. Walking sense was encouraged by manually moving Yvonne's lower extremities as she attempted walking between parallel bars and during use of "stabilizers." These stabilizers have supporting strap iron up to the knees and the child's feet are fastened to the base, but the feet are separated so the child can move them as skiis. The child feels the security of stabilizers and can at the same time simulate the walking pattern by the use of skiis.

It was found that Yvonne had no feeling of extension of her back, neck, or elbows. Standing and sitting tall and elbow extension exercises were emphasized. A spring steel back extension brace was incorporated with her leg braces. After several weeks a weighted chair was procured for the child to push. She constantly pulled it to her. After following this pattern of performance twice a week for four months, Yvonne grasped the sensation of pushing the chair ahead of her with straight elbows. In an attempt to make her independent of her physical therapist a wide supporting strap was fastened to the chair, at buttocks level, so that she could maintain the "pushing position."

Physical Therapist, Condon School, Cincinnati, Ohio.

In September, 1957, a second physical therapist found that the child habitually slumped while sitting, but she could sit tall and hold her head up if reminded to do so. Table exercises were again started for hip, knee, and elbow extension against resistance in the supine position. In prone position pushups to the hand-knee position were emphasized. This activity was extremely difficult for Yvonne to grasp. She could assume an elbow-knee position, but it was very difficult for her to proceed to bearing her weight upon her hands. She also stood beside the table and practiced pushing herself away. She did pushups in the walking bars.

In January, 1958, the Braille teacher said Yvonne needed more strength in her fingers and hands. Crutches were introduced to her, first by merely trying to get her to push and lift her body weight. Following this the physical therapist would swing the crutches forward then assist Yvonne to lift and push her body through in a small step. Gradually by May 1958, Yvonne is learning the feel of crutch position necessary for even support when she pushes her body through. She likes to hear the crutches tap the floor, and if complimented is apt to swing and push too vigorously. With concentration, she can now place her crutches correctly and use a swing-through gait for a distance of 300 feet. If disturbed by others, she easily loses the rhythm.

There is still much to be done to improve Yvonne's elbow and back extension. It is hoped that by the next school year she will have gained enough to begin work on the 4 point and 2 point crutch walking. Thus, with guidance, she will be able to move around limited areas independently.

Each year the mother is called in to Condon School to learn what Yvonne is doing so that she and the family can continue the work at home. They are interested and love their child, but have a large family.

This report has been compiled from the records of two physical therapists. Mrs. Doris B. Hall, the first year, and Ruth E. Pratt, the second. I feel that since this is a school and the classroom teacher is important to the child's program, Frances Stoelting can add comments of her work as follows:

"Yvonne entered the special class for cerebral palsied children at Condon School in September of 1956. She liked to play with toys and manipulate materials, but she wanted a great deal of attention from the teacher, constantly asking 'Now what are you doing?' "

To prepare for Braille she was taught to discriminate between various materials, paper, cloth, leaves, nuts, buttons, and seeds as well as toys. At first she was presented with things that had gross difference then gradually finer and finer distinctions were required.

Concepts of up and down, right and left, under and over were strengthened. Number experiences were planned beginning with a concept of 2. Gradually it increased. The shapes of the circle, triangle and square were introduced and compared.

Meanwhile any plan Yvonne expressed was carried out cooperatively. She made houses, baskets, paper dolls, and books. Gradually she learned to use one hand assistively, often as the "watching" hand, as the other one reached for more material.

Cards with the Braille symbols enlarged were introduced much as a seeing child plays with ABC's. She found likeness and difference in these. Toward spring Yvonne was introduced to the Braille symbols. She was shown her name, the names of friends, a word for each beginning sound. Not only did she match them, she began to show she could recall them. In the last months of the year she could begin a pre-primer in Braille writing.

This year a special Braille teacher has come to give Yvonne assistance with reading. She will soon be ready to read a primer. Her progress is not rapid, but it seems to be steady.

She is still eager to work with her hands. She likes to be busy all the time, but she is less demanding of the teacher's attention. Now she can amuse herself for as long as 30 minutes at a time.

A Cerebral Palsied Child with a Secondary Cerebellar Tumor

Alex Geller, M.S.

Michael D. was first seen at the Cerebral Palsy Clinic of Long Island College Hospital, on Nov. 10, 1953, for diagnostic evaluation. At that time he was 19 months of age.

The history revealed that the child's birth was uneventful. He was a full term baby whose mother was in labor for 10 hours. Presentation was vertex and low forceps was employed. His birth weight was 6 pounds 14 ounces.

The maturation status was normal until about the tenth month when the parents noticed that the child would stiffen his legs in walking and that he appeared to have lost interest in his environment. The parents attributed this regression to a fall down a flight of stairs. After this the child became fearful and never tried to walk alone again.

The orthopedic examination of Nov. 10, 1953, showed that a mildly exaggerated stretch reflex was present in the wrist pronators, elbow flexors, and shoulder adductors bilaterally. Function appeared normal. The lower extremities showed a severely exaggerated stretch reflex in the heel cords and toe extensors. The knee extensors and hip adductors showed a moderately increased stretch reflex. He could not stand alone but with manual support he was able to stand in a position of marked equinus and back knee. The deep tendon reflexes were positive and clonus was elicited.

Senior Physical Therapist, Cerebral Palsy Clinic, Long Island College Hospital, Brooklyn, New York.

A diagnosis of spastic quadriplegia with maximal involvement of the lower extremities was given. Etiological factor was thought to have been the fall at 10 months of age.

Physical therapy was instituted twice weekly and consisted of therapeutic exercises for the knee flexors, hip abductors, and ankle dorsiflexors. Passive stretching of the heel cords was prescribed as well as reciprocal conditioning of the lower extremity movements.

A psychological examination in March, 1954, showed the child to be functioning at the lower level of the average range of intellectual development.

Progress in overcoming hyperactive stretch reflexes and in increasing strength was steady but slow. Early in June and throughout July, 1954, the child exhibited signs of petit mal seizures, (staring vacantly and falling asleep) during therapy sessions. He was examined by the pediatrician, who ordered an electroencephalogram but no definite signs of seizures were noted. Physical therapy was continued under observation. In October, 1954, the therapist noted that the child offered extreme resistance to movement, as though he were in pain, and there was a questionable enlargement of the skull. These observations were reported to the pediatrician who requested that X rays of the child's skull be made. In November, 1954, X rays of the skull revealed a hydrocephalic condition. The child was referred to the neurology department where the neurologist gave a diagnosis of internal hydrocephalus due to a posterior fossa tumor. On Jan. 17, 1955, a craniectomy was performed and a cyst was removed below the cerebellum. Postoperative course was uneventful and he was discharged after 23 days.

By May, 1955, he was back on the schedule for physical, functional, and occupational therapy.

Speech was normal. In June, 1955, he was fitted for long leg braces with a pelvic band. The braces had slip locks at the hips and knees with 90 degree posterior stops at the ankles. The braces were prescribed to facilitate the teaching of ambulation.

The child showed marked behavioral and motor improvement. He was more alert and was able to stand and walk within the parallel bars. By March. 1956, Michael had begun to master the tripod training canes in conjunction with his long leg braces and was walking, using the 4 point gait, with a fair amount of control and confidence. In October. 1956, he was transferred to the cerebral palsy class of Public School 67 where he is making further progress in independent ambulation.

The *Review* invites case reports from physical therapists who have followed an interesting course of treatment with or an unusual response to treatment by patients having one of the conditions listed below.

Diabetic neuropathy
Paralysis agitans—postchemopallidectomy
Volkmann's ischemic contracture
Dupuytren's contracture
Osteoarthritis
Coronary thrombosis
Cerebral palsy with sensory disturbance
Postmastectomy lymphedema

NOTE: Suggestions for preparation of case reports were published in the October 1957 issue of the *Review*, pages 666-667. Reprints of the suggestions may be requested by writing to the *Physical Therapy Review*.

The Influence of Athetoid Cerebral Palsy on the Execution of Sport Skills: Bowling

A Study of One Case

F. A. Hellebrandt, M.D., Joan C. Waterland, M.S., and C. Etta Walters, Ph.D.*

Even the severely disabled cerebral palsied patient can execute selected sport skills. An adult subject suffering from quadriplegic athetosis was permitted to perform a basic movement associated with four different athletic activities. The resultant behavior patterns were studied. Bowling was the first sport skill analyzed.

Throwing a bowling ball suppressed all overt manifestations of involuntary motion on the ipsilateral side. The movement cycle looked surprisingly smooth and efficient. Such athetosis as could be seen was limited to the distal parts of the contralateral appendages. It was more evident in the upper extremity than in the lower. A primary finding was the strong operation of the attitudinal reflexes.

The purpose of this case report is to present a cinematographic and electromyographic analysis of the bowling throw as executed by a cerebral palsied patient and to compare this with normal performance.

Methods

Subjects of the Investigation

Two adult females, both in the early fifth decade of life, participated in the experiment herein reported. M. A. had a moderately severe athetoid cerebral palsy of congenital origin, quadriplegic in distribution and more marked in the upper than in the lower extremities. The disability was worse in the right than in the left hand. The left upper extremity was therefore chosen for training. The subject could ambulate with Canadian crutches. There was consistently more athetosis in the left than in the right lower extremity. Balance was too precarious to permit bowling from the standing position. The act was therefore performed from a comfortable sitting posture on a sturdy stool provided with a smoothly revolving seat. The height of the stool was adjusted to allow the bowling ball to clear the floor at the lowest point in the arc of the anteroposterior swing.

The control subject was a professional physical educator with bowling experience, both as a performer and a teacher. She supervised the training of two pathological subjects, one of whom was the athetoid subject reported here. The other was a cerebral palsied patient with spastic hemiplegia upon whom observations also were made.

The Bowling Throw

The cerebral palsied patient and the normal control subject executed the act with opposite arms. Instead of holding the ball in front of the chest at the starting position and steadying it with the opposite hand, which is customary, the volitional aspect of the act was simplified for the cerebral palsied subjects by limiting motion to humeral advancement and retraction. The ball was placed on the floor approximately in the mid-coronal plane, to the right or left side of the subject, depending on the handedness. It could be grasped easily by bending forward

From the Motor Learning Research Laboratory, Medical School and School of Education, University of Wisconsin (310 Lathrop Hall), Madison, Wisconsin. Supported by the Easter Seal Research Foundation, National Society for Crippled Children and Adults, Inc., and the University Research Committee, the Graduate School, University of Wisconsin.

*Department of Physical Education for Women, Florida State University, Tallahassee, Florida.

slightly and leaning to the side. A bowling ball is held by the thumb and the third and fourth fingers. To throw a "straight ball" the forearm must be supinated and the wrist hyperextended. The subjects were instructed to bring the ball forward in a preparatory swing, then let it drop back, and finally, to drive it forward again in the power stroke. There were no pauses between the forward-backward-forward phases of the cycle. The ball was released shortly after the arm had swung through the perpendicular position on the "beat" or power stroke. The follow-through and recovery segments of the movement pattern also were studied.

The Training Program

Bowling not only requires the use of many muscles in appropriate sequence, but also the development of sufficient power to impart enough velocity to the ball for it to traverse the alley and disperse the pins. M. A., the cerebral palsied patient, needed training in both elements of the act: skill and strength. To expedite motor learning the throwing pattern was first practiced on the shoulder ergograph. This device restricts motion to virtually pure flexion and extension at the glenohumeral joint. To augment the strength constituent, resistance, speed, and range of motion could be increased progressively. As soon as the "idea" and "feel" of the throw had been grasped, M. A. extended her learning experience to manipulation of a bowling ball fitted to her individual left-handed grasp. A ten-pound ball was selected. This is lighter than the ball used by the average female bowler. Strength and endurance were gained by increasing systematically the number of throws per diem, assuring that the range of the preparatory forward and back swings was always the maximal attainable. Eventually, as many as one hundred throws could be made in a single practice session. These were divided into bouts of ten in which the hemiplegic and the athetoid subjects threw the ball in alternation. Competition proved to be an excellent motivational device. The subjects practiced three times a week. Approximately one month of training was required before the act had been sufficiently well learned to warrant cinematographic and electromyographic observations.

Photographing the Movement Pattern

Both M. A. and the normal control subject were photographed on the same day. To prevent fatigue, one performer and then the other threw the ball in each of four positions: *first*, in profile with the throwing arm facing the camera; *second*, in profile from the contralateral side; *third*, directly facing the camera; and *fourth*, from the rear view. Two consecutive trials were allowed in every position. Thus, each subject threw the ball eight different times. Motion pictures were made at the normal speed of sixteen frames per second. To expedite frame-by-frame analysis of the movement patterns, the cinematograms were enlarged to 3.5 inches by 5 inches and were recorded on direct positive paper in sequential strips of consecutive exposures. Each throwing cycle was then compressed into a short frieze which could be encompassed in a single glance. The series usually contained eight exposures. The first depicted the subject fitting the hand to the ball in preparation for the throw. There then followed in succession the posture assumed at the instant the ball began to move forward, the end of the forward swing, the point in the back swing when the arm is approximately perpendicular to the floor, the end of the back swing, that point in the power or "beat" stroke when the ball is released, the end of the follow-through movement of the throwing arm, and finally, recovery from the throw. Approximately equivalent points were identified in all four views. By looking at the friezes horizontally the observer could reconstruct the movement cycle as visualized in any one of the four orientation planes. The friezes could then be aligned vertically to permit examination of each key phase, as though being viewed concurrently from the front, back, right, and left sides. Patterning on repeated throws was sufficiently similar to make vertical alignment of approximately identical phases of each movement cycle a worthwhile analytical procedure.

Electromyography

Action potentials were recorded by an eight-channel ink-writing oscillograph, using bipolar surface electrodes. Various combinations of the following muscles were sampled: anterior, middle and posterior deltoid; biceps; triceps; pectoralis major; latissimus dorsi; upper, middle, and lower trapezius; teres major or minor; infraspinatus; wrist flexor; wrist extensor; and right and left sternocleidomastoids. Major observations were confined to the ipsilateral or throwing side. More limited recordings were obtained from selected muscle groups of the opposite side, especially the deltoid, biceps, triceps, and wrist muscles.

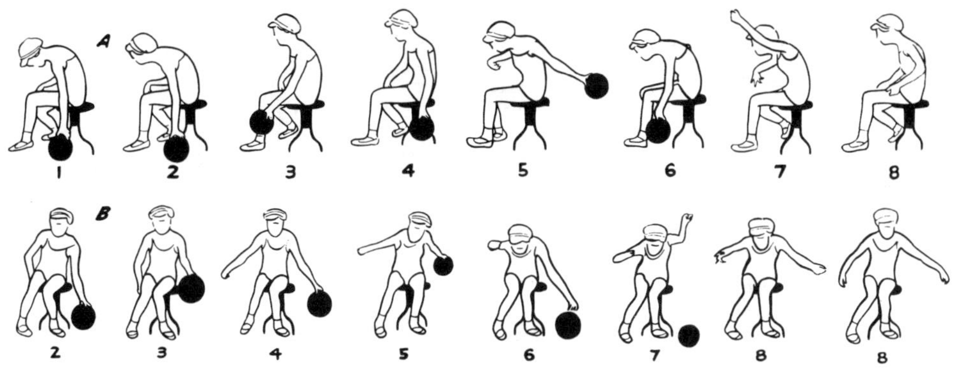

FIG. 1. Key positions in the bowling throw of an adult athetoid cerebral palsied subject: (1) preliminary placement of hand, (2) first discernible movement of the ball forward, (3) end of preparatory forward swing, (4) point in back stroke where arm is approximately perpendicular, (5) end of back swing, (6) point of release in power stroke, (7) follow-through, and (8) recovery.

RESULTS AND THEIR DISCUSSION

The photographic data consisted of eight bowling throws by each of two subjects, one pathologic and one normal, yielding 823 and 601 frames, respectively. Of these, 1093 were enlarged photographically to facilitate detailed study. The main features of the response of the athetoid cerebral palsied subject are illustrated in Figure 1.

Kinesiological Analysis from Photographic Observations

Onset of the Preparatory Forward Swing. The first frame in Figure 1-A shows the position spontaneously assumed in grasping the bowling ball preparatory to throwing. The arm used is approximately perpendicular to the floor. The head is turned to the left side, so as to bring the ball into view. The cerebral palsied patient uses vision to assist in the placement of the fingers in the holes provided in the bowling ball. The left foot rests firmly on the floor. Except for the positioning of the right arm and leg, the pose is comparatively natural and graceful.

Frames 2 to 8 on the profile and front view of Figure 1 are roughly equivalent points in the movement cycle. By the time the first discernible movement of the ball forward in the sagittal plane can be detected, the head has swung to a position of hypertension. This probably facilitates the stiffening of the forelimb engaged in the throwing act. The head usually appears also to have rotated slightly away from the active side, as though to facilitate the anticipated flexor movement. The opposite arm is abducted to help counteract the influence of the ball on the center of gravity of the body as a whole.

Forward Swing. The preparatory swing, per se, is characterized by a straightening of the vertebral column as the ball comes forward. The head is less extended than previously. Before the end of the swing has been reached, the head turns toward the moving side in anticipation of the backstroke. This interesting phenomenon of a symmetric head positioning was most clearly defined in the contralateral profile and the front views, in both of which the right sternocleidomastoid was visibly contracted. In the side view the whole belly of the muscle could be traced. The thighs, already adducted in the starting position, continue moving inward until the knees come almost into contact. In general, the forward swing appears to put little stress on the neuromuscular machinery. The task seems to be accomplished easily and smoothly.

Backstroke. Humeral advancement reverses without any apparent break in the prescribed throwing cycle. The ball drops easily, aided by gravity. The vertebral column begins to flex again and the head moves into more marked extension. Athetosis of the contralateral arm usually augments at this time. That the stress mounts during the terminal phase of the backstroke is easily seen. By the end of the swing which precedes the power stroke, the thoracic spine has flexed sharply and hyperextension at the atlanto-occipital joint is extreme. The head has rotated away from the throwing arm in anticipation of the shoulder joint flexion which is to follow. The left sternocleidomastoid stands out as a well-defined band in the ipsilateral profile view. The right wrist is flexed. The fingers of the right hand are extended and the thumb is

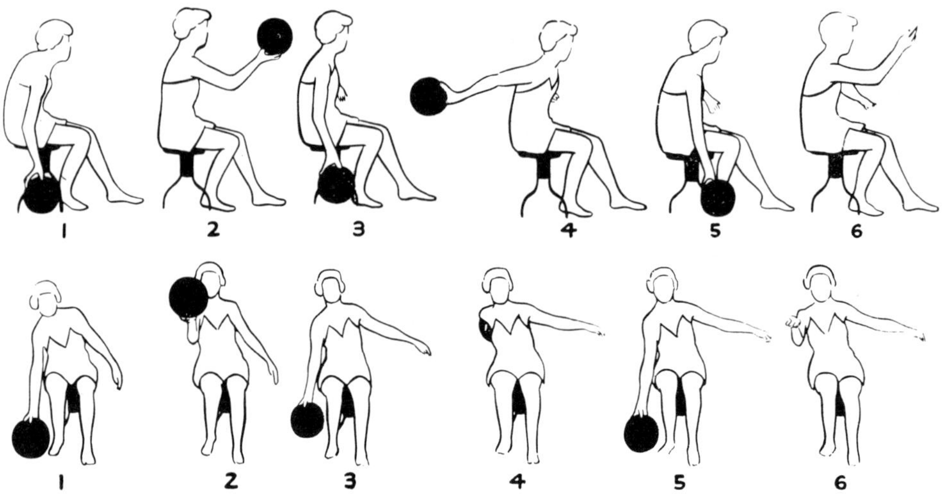

FIG. 2. Key positions in the bowling throw of the normal control subject.

sharply adducted. This is a typical athetotic hand posture, similar to those described by Herz[1] in his moving-picture analysis of involuntary movements. The thighs, which had started to abduct at the beginning of the backstroke, are now widely separated. The mobilization of available muscle power for supreme effort is depicted in every line of the pose caught and frozen by the camera.

The position of the right upper extremity is the reciprocal of the left during the backstroke, except that abduction at the shoulder joint dominates rather than flexion. This compensates for gravitational stresses introduced by the weight of the ball being swung at the end of a long lever. Lateral stability is less secure than anteroposterior in the sitting posture. The thighs are widely separated and the right foot is inverted, as though to increase coronal plane security.

Power Stroke. The ball is released after the arm has passed ten or fifteen degrees beyond the vertical. Back flexion and neck hyperextension reach their maximum at this point. The head is usually still turned away from the throwing arm to facilitate the flexion that drives the limb forward. The thighs, which had been abducted, come together again. Involuntary movement of the right hand reaches its peak during the interval of maximal stress and immediately thereafter.

Follow-Through and Recovery. Once the ball is released, the throwing arm continues to swing forward and then returns to the side. The pattern appears to be smoothly controlled and harmonious. The right arm recovers more slowly than the left. It relaxes gradually and derotates after the throwing arm has recovered.

The most striking feature in every throw made by M. A. is the comparative normality of the behavior of the throwing arm. No involuntary motions obtrude to distort the pattern of that extremity. The contralateral limb, which played no direct role in bowling, showed some dyskinesia. Thus, unilateral exercise, while carrying a considerable load at comparatively high speed in a competitive atmosphere, did not disrupt coordination. Rather, it appears to have suppressed discordant movements and/or mobilized reserves of strength and control, normalizing neuromuscular behavior.

No attempt was made to determine whether a cerebral palsied patient as disabled as M. A. could acquire sufficient strength and skill to participate effectively in the sport of bowling. The experience was astonishingly dynamogenic. The use for therapeutic purposes of a type of exercise enjoyed by normal men and women had a profound psychological effect.

It would be a mistake to give the impression that the performance of this athetoid cerebral palsied patient is classifiable as normal because the pattern of activity of the throwing arm appears to be so agreeably consonant with expected behavior. The frank abnormality in the total response can be seen by comparing Figure 1 with Figure 2. The performance of the pathological subject now looks labored. The magnitude of the effort required to achieve what the normal subject does with graceful ease is self-evident.

The most biologically significant difference in the response of the normal and pathological subject is the degree to which attitudinal reflexes are operative in the latter. These are tonic reactions evoked by head movements, in consequence of which ". . . the whole body musculature is integrated for a combined and highly adapted function."[2] Thus, Magnus points out that good pictures and statues are satisfying and give the impression of being natural if the disposition of the body parts is in accord with the laws of the attitudinal reflexes.

Much of the posturing of the pathological subject seems to be tied to head positioning. Hyperextension of the upper cervical spine fluctuates directly with the severity of the effort demanded during the different phases of the throwing cycle. To achieve this and yet keep the line of sight focussed on the target at the end of the alley, the vertebral column flexes strongly; the spine curls, but the head retains its normal poise. The resultant atlanto-occipital and upper cervical spine movement is extreme indeed.

In 1951, McCouch, Deering, and Ling[3] localized the receptors for the tonic neck reflexes in the upper joints of the neck, especially the atlanto-axial and atlanto-occipital. In the quadruped, dorsiflexion of the head stiffens the forelimbs and causes the hind quarters to sink to the ground. It is well known that remnants of this archaic response emerge at the least provocation in the individual with brain damage. Presumably the attitudinal reflexes reinforce a distribution of tonus which is obligatory to the successful performance of the bowling act.

Rotatory movements of the head were less conspicuous than the dorsiflexion described, but they could be picked up in the frame-by-frame examination of the cinematograms. It was of considerable interest to note that they invariably precede the movement known to be facilitated by the head turning, observed as though anticipating what is to come. The shifts in tonus that result are like those known to occur during ballistic movement.[4]

Close and careful inspection of the head position of the control subject indicated that it remained virtually unchanged during the execution of the bowling throw as modified to expedite performance by the disabled. No sagittal plane variations in flexion or extension occurred. Rotatory movements were detected but these were rare, and when observed, were always minute.[1] Those identified were invariably in a direction consonant with the operation of the attitudinal reflexes.

Work done previously by Hellebrandt, *et al.*[5] yielded unequivocal evidence that head positioning, contrary to archaic quadrupedal patterning, inhibits the mobilization of the muscular resources of the normal subject. Volitional head turning, in harmony with the tonic neck reflexes, was facilitating. The head and the limbs appear to be yoked together irrevocably. The head leads and the limbs follow in an invariable manner. In the disabled individual, plagued by weakness incidental to deficits in neuromuscular training and experience, dependance on these built-in augmenters to step-up performance is to be expected. To suppress these ancient facilitatory devices may deprive the handicapped individual of benefits accruing from the spontaneous operation of a compensatory type of behavior.

Mechanical analysis of the bowling swing executed by the normal and pathological subjects revealed a number of significant differences. One of the most marked and persistent was the extent to which M. A. kept the throwing arm abducted. The shoulder joint abductors were probably stronger than the muscles which advance or depress the humerus. Certainly they operate continuously during ambulation, to assist in the maintenance of a precarious balance.

The normal subject moved the ball forward on the preparatory swing by flexing the forearm first and then advancing the humerus. Apparently the athetoid cerebral palsied patient could accomplish this only by stiffening the appendage at the elbow joint and then advancing the limb in toto. The range of motion, both forward and back, was also grossly limited in M. A. This is due probably to weakness. The lower backswing means a slower momentum and a less effective "beat" stroke.

Electromyographic Kinesiology of the Bowling Throw

Each subject threw the bowling ball between 35 and 40 times for electromyographic purposes. Because of limitations in space, and the risk of damage to the copper screening of the electromyographic cage, it was necessary to reduce the power of the "beat" stroke. This should be remembered when the electromyograms are examined.

The main features of the patterned action of the muscles used to actuate the throwing arm are illustrated in Figure 3. Unlike the throws executed by the control subject for photographic purposes, this multiple lead electromyogram illustrates a completely normal, so-called "straight

Vol. 41, No. 2 THE PHYSICAL THERAPY REVIEW 111

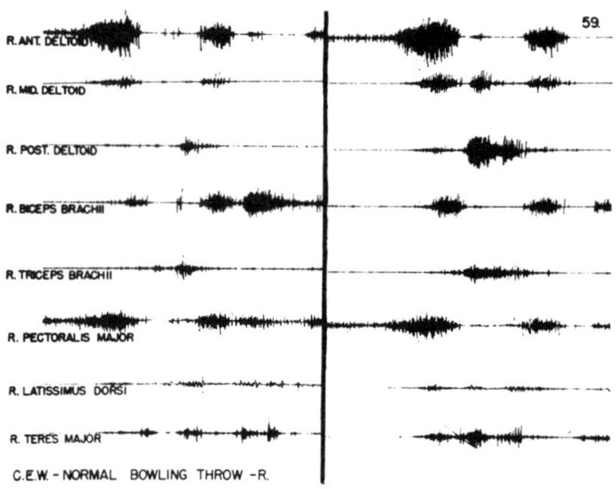

FIG. 3. Electromyograms of two normal bowling throws made by the control subject in the usual standing position with a four-step approach.

ball," executed in the standing posture with a traditional four-step approach. The ball is held in front of the chest in the starting position and is steadied by the fingers of the left hand. There is considerable tension in the anterior deltoid and the pectoralis major during the readiness interval. At the onset of the throw, the arm swings forward under the influence of activity by the anterior deltoid and the pectoralis major. The biceps participates late in this phase of the cycle. The antagonists to humeral advancement offer a slight modulating action. Vigorous contraction of the posterior deltoid, triceps, and teres major activate the backstroke. The latissimus dorsi contributes relatively little to the pattern as executed by this subject. A return of activity to the muscles which advance the humerus marks the onset of the power stroke. The middle deltoid shows a discrete burst of activity in all three phases of the movement cycle to keep the arm sufficiently abducted for the ball to clear the body in its sweep through the sagittal plane. Once the ball has picked up momentum, it seems that less muscular effort is required to direct its course through the path prescribed than to initiate the movement, but this is without doubt an artifact, due to volitional reduction in the force of the "beat" stroke, for the reasons already cited.

Figure 4 illustrates the sequential action of the same muscle groups when the athetoid cerebral palsied patient bowls from the sitting posture. The action potentials are, first and foremost, appreciably larger in amplitude than those manifest by the control subject, and the pattern has lost some of its discreetness. The middle deltoid, biceps, triceps, pectoralis major, and latissimus dorsi fire erratically in anticipation of the preparatory swing. The athetotic subject is struggling to keeping the throwing arm extended and away from the body. Turner, Perlstein, and Elam[6] found that it was difficult or impossible to get electromyographic silence at rest in the athetoid patient.

The bowling pattern can be identified without difficulty in every multiple lead electromyogram obtained on M. A. The anterior deltoid, biceps, and pectoralis major advance the humerus. It is depressed by the posterior deltoid, triceps, and latissimus dorsi. As in the normal subject, the power or "beat" stroke is characterized by an unexpectedly small barrage of activity in the shoulder joint flexors, due to volitional suppression. The middle deltoid dominates the picture in M. A. It fires strongly and continuously during all three phases of the throwing cycle. This confirms what is seen in the cinematograms of the athetoid cerebral palsied patient. One of the most characteristic and constant abnormalities manifest was the degree of abduction maintained throughout the throw.

The teres minor helps to keep the humerus laterally rotated. In electromyograms sampling the infraspinatus, this muscle functioned strongly and synchronously with the teres minor to help keep the throwing arm moving straight forward without rotation. Subject M. A. had great difficulty achieving the purity of motion demanded to throw a "straight ball." She tended persis-

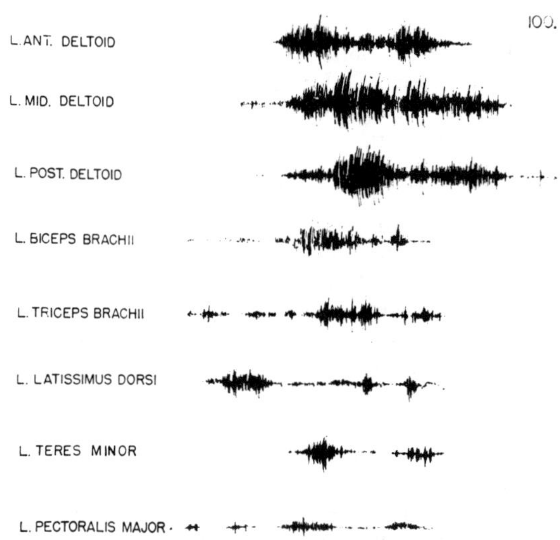

FIG. 4. Electromyograms of "straight ball" thrown from the sitting position by a patient with athetoid cerebral palsy.

tently to pronate the forearm and medially rotate the arm as the extremity swung forward.

Activity was consistently greatest in the lowest division of the three parts of the trapezius. This was strongly active during all phases of the cycle, presumably to stabilize the scapula. The upper trapezius fired more discretely, usually when the humerus advanced in preparation for the throw, and especially on the "beat" stroke. It could be seen bulging in many of the front view cinematograms.

An example of imbalance in the activity of the sternocleidomastoids is illustrated in Figure 5. The ipsilateral wrist extensors showed continuous strong contraction, reasonably well maintained. Co-contraction of the wrist flexors was present invariably.

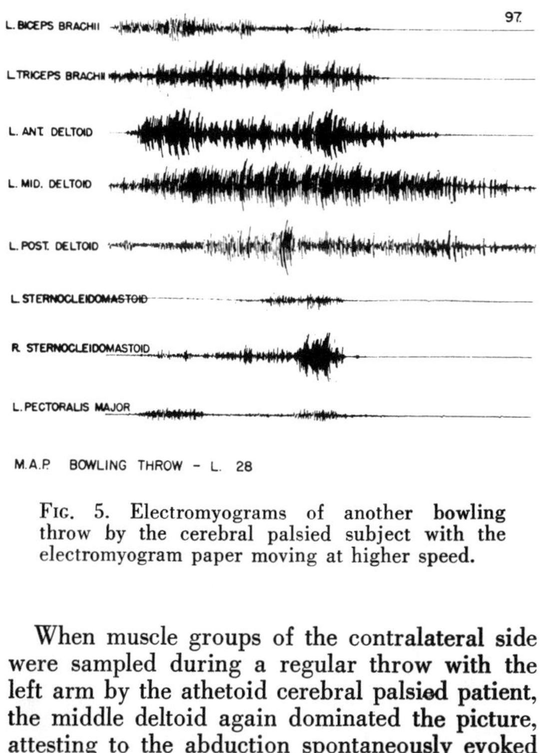

FIG. 5. Electromyograms of another bowling throw by the cerebral palsied subject with the electromyogram paper moving at higher speed.

When muscle groups of the contralateral side were sampled during a regular throw with the left arm by the athetoid cerebral palsied patient, the middle deltoid again dominated the picture, attesting to the abduction spontaneously evoked to equilibrate gravitational stresses and to maintain balance. Wrist flexion was also consistently present as the reciprocal of the strong extension demanded on the throwing side by the manner in which a bowling ball is held.

Agonists and antagonists fire simultaneously in virtually all phases of the throwing cycle as executed by the athetotic subject. The amplitude of the action potentials fluctuates, mounting in one member of the pair as it subsides in the other, only to reverse at the instant the movement changes direction. This does not appear to be abnormal, except perhaps for the degree of co-contraction. No muscle can act strongly without collateral effects on other muscles. Many years ago, Duchenne[7] emphasized that in order to move a part, all the musculature belonging to it must cooperate, including the antagonists. Subsequently, Beevor[8] expressed the same view. Thus the co-contraction of antagonists characteristic of athetoid cerebral palsy may be no more than an exaggeration of normal behavior.

SUMMARY

One adult female patient, suffering from a moderately severe athetoid cerebral palsy of congenital origin, was systematically trained to throw a bowling ball from a comfortable sitting posture. The shoulder ergograph was used to expedite the learning of the basic throwing pattern. After kinesthetic awareness had been aroused, training and experience were extended to include the throwing of a ten-pound bowling ball fitted to the left-handed grasp of the disabled subject. After approximately one month of practice, skill, strength, and endurance had developed sufficiently to warrant cinematographic and electromyographic study of the bowling throw. Control observations were made on one normal adult female. Kinesiological analysis was based on a frame-by-frame study of motion pictures taken from the front, back, right, and left sides. To aid in the identification of key cue positions, more than 1,000 consecutive motion-picture frames were enlarged to 3.5 inches by 5 inches. An eight-channel ink-writing oscillograph was used to record action potentials from various combinations of the neck, shoulder, elbow, and wrist joint muscles of the throwing or the contralateral side, using surface electrodes. The evidence suggests that:

1. A bowling ball may be thrown by a patient suffering from athetoid cerebral palsy of moderate severity.

2. No involuntary motions distort the movement pattern of the throwing arm.

3. Exercise stress evokes attitudinal reflexes which appear to facilitate performance.

4. Similarities in the neuromuscular patterning of the normal and the cerebral palsied subject are more conspicuous than abnormalities in behavior.

ACKNOWLEDGMENTS: The data analyzed were collected in the Department of Physical Medicine and Rehabilitation of the Research and Educational Hospitals of the University of Illinois. The technical assistance of Miriam J. Partridge is greatly appreciated.

REFERENCES

1. Herz, E.: Die amyostatischen Unruheerscheinungen, Klinisch-kinematographische Analyse ihrer Kennzeichen und Begleiterscheinungen. J. Psychologie und Neurologie, 43:3-182, 1931.
2. Magnus, R.: Cameron prize lectures on some results of studies in the physiology of posture. Lancet, 2:531-536, September 11, 1926.
3. McCouch, G. P., Deering, I. D., and Ling, T. H.: Location of receptors for tonic neck reflexes. J. Neurophysiol., 14:191-195, May, 1951.
4. Hellebrandt, F. A., Houtz, S. J., Partridge, M. J., and Walters, C. E.: The Chandler table: analysis of its relationale in the mobilization of the shoulder joint. Phys. Ther. Rev., 35:545-556, October, 1955.
5. Hellebrandt, F. A., Houtz, S. J., Partridge, M. J., and Walters, C. E.: Tonic neck reflexes in exercises of stress in man. Am. J. Phys. Med., 35:144-159, June, 1956.
6. Turner, M., Perlstein, M. A., and Elam, H.: Electromyographic studies in cerebral palsy. Am. J. Phys. Med., 37:302-326, December, 1958.
7. Duchenne, G. B.: Physiology of Motion. (Translated and edited by Emanuel B. Kaplan.) Philadelphia, W. B. Saunders, 1959.
8. Beevor, C.: The Croonian Lectures on Muscular Movements. London, Macmillan Co., 1903.

Vol. 41, No. 4 THE PHYSICAL THERAPY REVIEW 257

The Influence of Athetoid Cerebral Palsy on the Execution of Sport Skills: Tennis and Golf*

A Study of One Case

F. A. Hellebrandt, M.D. and Joan C. Waterland, M.S.

The defective neural mechanism of the athetoid cerebral palsied adult has a greater influence on the autonomous components of a purposive act than on the movement willed. This observation came from analysis of the performance of a quadriplegic athetoid patient attempting to execute selected sport skills. Her response to the throwing of a "straight ball" in bowling has already been described.[1] This report is limited to a discussion of the way in which she performed a basic stroke in tennis (the forehand drive) and the drive in golf.

The swinging of a tennis racket or golf club suppressed all overt manifestations of athetosis in the appendages directly implicated in the performance. No unwanted activity marred the primary movement pattern in either the preparatory or the power phase of the drive. The volitional component of the total response looked surprisingly smooth, as it had in the bowling throw. Close frame by frame inspection of cinematograms revealed that gross abnormalities were confined to exaggeration of postural adjustments, prominence of the tonic neck reflexes (TNR), and variable degrees of unsteadiness before getting the willed act under way or after its completion.

It is well known that the involuntary movements of the athetoid cerebral palsied patient are augmented by emotional stress, excessive sensory stimulation, and muscular activity. Classical treatment emphasizes voluntary relaxation, meticulously controlled movement, diminution of the volume and scope of the afferent input, and avoidance of strain. Attention is focussed on circumventing the disability by operating within limits that bear little relation to the exigencies of real life. Neglect of intact functions is virtually inevitable. The consequence may be a neuromuscularly unfit cerebral palsied patient who has been denied many opportunities for the exploitation of his residual capacities.

The normal person acquires tolerance to physical and emotional stress through training and experience. During the period of growth and development he finds himself often in emotionally charged or competitive situations. Motor exploration is encouraged. The maturing individual gradually becomes inured to symptoms summoned forth by stress and strain. Eventually these are accepted as the natural concomitants of daily living and are coped with accordingly. It seemed to us that something of value might be learned by observing how the adult athetoid cerebral palsied patient responds to the same kind of neuromuscular training. The details of this program have already been reported.[2] The purpose of this aspect of the same case study is to demonstrate how the stress associated with the execution of wholly unfamiliar motor acts may be used further to reveal the built-in automatisms that safeguard neuromuscular performance.

MATERIALS AND METHODS

Subject of the Investigations. M. A., a woman in the early fifth decade of life, was studied. Her chief complaint was difficulty in walking and in the use of the hands. Her disability was diagnosed as athetoid cerebral palsy of congenital origin, rotary in type, and worse in the upper than the lower extremities. She had been under treatment in the Outpatient Physical Medicine and Occupational Therapy Departments of the Research and Educational Hospitals of the University of Illinois for approximately one and a half years when the observations reported herein were made.

Procedure. The subject was essentially untrained in the two activities analyzed. Instructions were given by an experienced teacher of physical education who demonstrated the skills to be performed and served as a control subject. Motion pictures were made at the normal speed of sixteen frames per second. The prescribed activities were performed left-handedly because

* From the Motor Learning Research Laboratory, Medical School and School of Education, University of Wisconsin (310 Lathrop Hall), Madison, Wisconsin. Supported by the Easter Seal Research Foundation; National Society for Crippled Children and Adults, Inc.; and the University Research Committee, the Graduate School, University of Wisconsin.

the functional capacity of the patient's left upper extremity was significantly better than the right. The tennis racket and the Number 5 Iron used in the golf drive weighed approximately twelve to fifteen ounces.

Frame by frame enlargements were made of the motion pictures. This is the same procedure followed in the bowling study. The technique developed is described elsewhere.[3] Examination of sequential frames, printed in long strips to retain the sense of movement, was supplemented by viewing the motion picture film at normal and reduced speeds, using a Bell and Howell time and motion study projector. A Recordak microfilm reader was used to expedite the making of sketches from frames selected for illustrative purposes. This enlarges the figure to about ten inches, or approximately twenty-three times. At this magnification the bulging of superficial muscles during contraction is clearly visible on the opaque screen.

Observations were limited primarily to inspectional examination of the 1,384 single frame enlargements available for study. The sample included ten tennis strokes and nine golf drives. Eleven of these were performed by the disabled subject. Comparisons with the normal were used only as guides to help in the identification of abnormal motor behavior. Little attention was given to the strokes *per se*. These are obviously poor when judged from the view point of the individual interested in sport proficiency.

RESULTS

The ability of the athetoid cerebral palsied subject to conceive the end result desired appeared to be unimpaired. Nor was there any evidence of disturbance in the ability to initiate the movement conceived. The patient swung the racket and the golf club in much the same way as any novice. Once the movement got under way it was executed without disruption. This was true of the bowling throw, tennis stroke and the golf drive. They may not have been very effective in the pursuit of the sports represented, but the movements *per se* appeared to be perfectly co-ordinated.

The dyskinesia of athetoid cerebral palsy is commonly referred to as an involuntary, slow and writhing movement, most evident in the distal segments of the limbs. Strange postures are assumed, supposedly because of the simultaneous contraction of antagonists. Crothers and Paine[4] describe the movements as chaotic. Turner, Perlstein and Elam[5] found the electromyographic response of the athetoid patient to standardized stimuli irregular in pattern and variable in amplitude, frequency and duration. However, the action potentials observed were channeled consistently towards those muscle groups which demonstrated sudden outbursts of activity at rest.

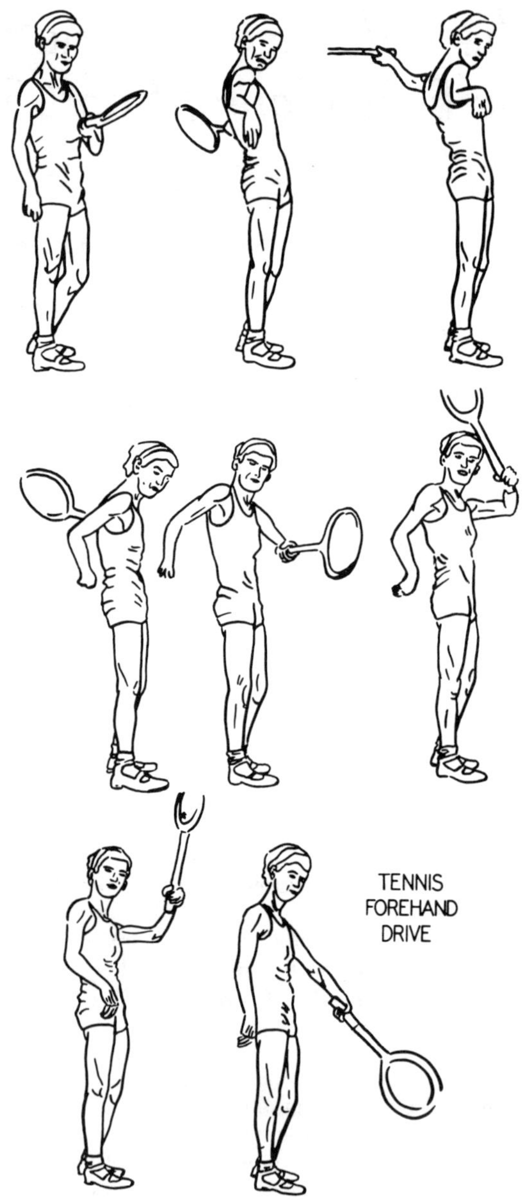

FIG. 1. Forehand drive performed by an athetoid cerebral palsied patient: top row, the preparatory backswing; middle row, the power stroke and the follow through; bottom row, the recovery from the voluntary act.

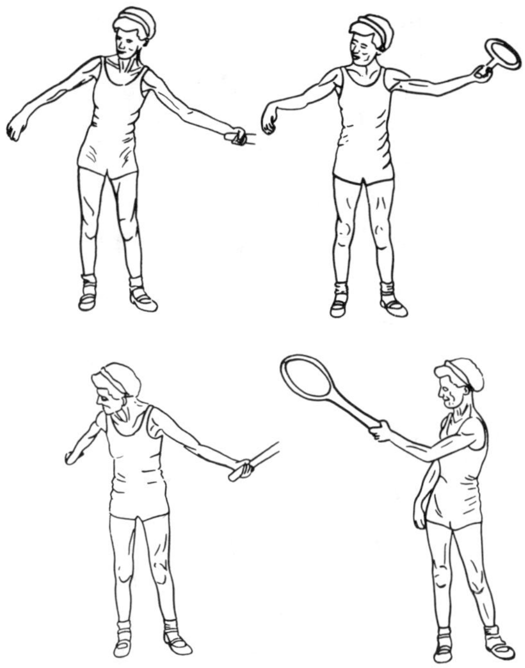

FIG. 2. The two upper figures show the racket moving backward. Note persistence of the TNR to the right and the reluctance to shift the weight to the left leg. The racket is moving forward in the lower left figure.

We had expected, therefore, to see purposeless, wormlike, irrelevant and disabling movements superimposed upon the act willed. This never occurred. Athetosis was clearly demonstrable but it invariably was present in anatomic parts not directly concerned with the execution of the voluntary act. This may be seen in all of the movement sequences illustrated.

Figure 1 shows the left forehand drive photographed from the right side. The backswing looks constrained mainly because the head positioning is opposed to that dictated by the law of the attitudinal reflexes.[6] The head moved to the left reluctantly but never crossed the midline during the tennis stroke. Before the preparatory backswing was completed, the head position invariably reversed and then continued rotating strongly to the right as though to facilitate the onset of the power phase of the stroke. Once the drive got under way the postural alignment appeared to be quite natural and graceful. The head and the appendages now move as predicted by operation of the tonic neck reflexes.

Athetosis was consistently evident in the balancing arm during the tennis stroke. The limb was relaxed in the initial stages of the preparatory backswing but began to rotate medially before the stroke reversed. Rotary athetosis reached its peak in the power phase of the forehand drive and then subsided during the follow through. The balancing arm relaxed again with recovery from the stroke. A much less conspicuous rotary athetosis could be detected in the reciprocal leg. Lower extremity involuntary movement was more marked in the golf drive which gives rise to serious balance problems because one arm is no longer free to serve an equilibrial function. These spontaneous movements appear to be well co-ordinated. They may be purposeless but they are by no means random motions. Frame by frame inspection of cinematograms suggests that they are grossly repetitious in both their spatial and temporal components. Furthermore, when a normal individual attempts to simulate the athetosis, the pattern of the response is indistinguishable from that exhibited by the cerebral palsied patient. Thus the rotary athetosis of the free arm looks like unwanted but normal medial rotation at the shoulder joint associated with radioulnar pronation. Strong volar flexion of the wrist accompanies the arm athetosis. This is, in part at least, the reciprocal of the pattern demonstrable in the homologous limb performing the volitional act. The manipulation of the racket required a firm grasping motion of the left hand. Beevor[7] has pointed out that this evokes a synergic action of the wrist extensors. The contralateral wrist flexors contract spontaneously. We have observed this repeatedly on normal subjects during wrist extension ergography, and interpret it to be a natural manifestation of automatic cord level patterning, revealed during exercise stress.

The sagittal plane movements of the balancing limb appear to be entirely normal. This arm moves anteriorly as the racket is swung back and reverses itself in precise reciprocal synchrony as soon as the racket begins to come forward (Fig. 2). Instability in balance is indicated by two signs: (1) the degree of arm abduction (Fig. 2), and (2) the persistent ventroflexion of the head (Fig. 1). The latter is seen commonly in the cerebral palsied; it probably reinforces extensor tonus in the lower extremities and thus stabilizes the stance. Ventroflexion of the head was especially evident at the beginning of the power phase of the forehand tennis drive.

Persistence of a right tonic neck reflex in this patient is suggested by her reluctance to turn the head to the left as previously mentioned, and by the tendency of the opposite leg to remain slightly flexed. The left leg never bears its full

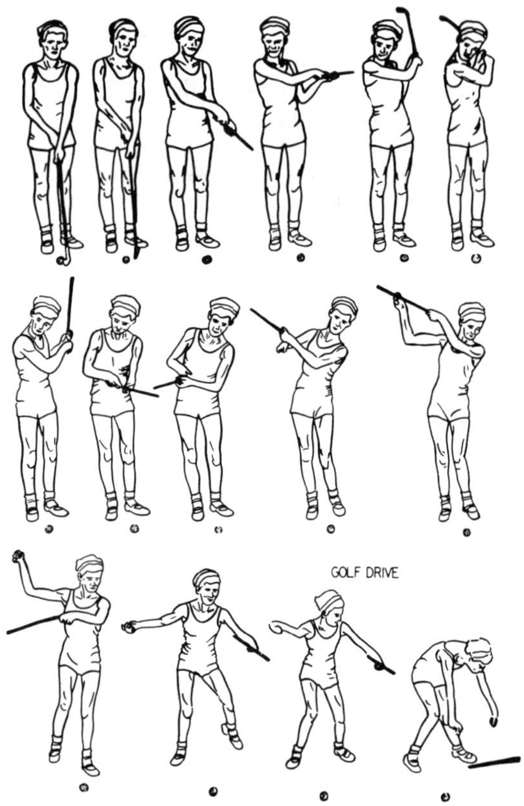

FIG. 3. Top row, preparatory phase of a golf drive performed by the same adult athetoid cerebral palsied patient; middle row, power stroke and follow through. Involuntary movements disturb balance in the recovery phase of the golf drive.

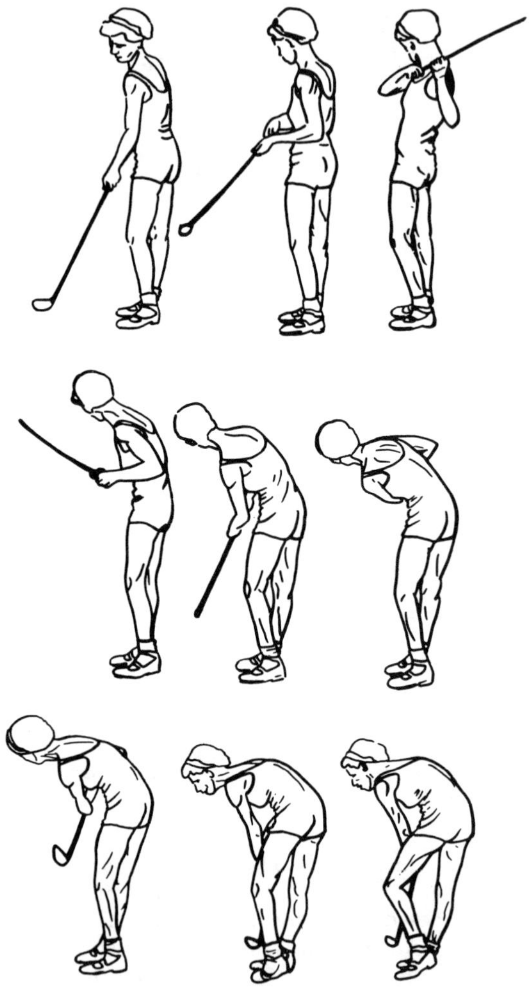

FIG. 4. Preparatory, power and recovery phases of another attempt to execute the golf drive.

share of the superimposed load. Instead of shifting the weight to the left leg during the backswing of the forehand drive, which is the expected response, the end result desired is simulated by trunk rotation.

Figure 3 illustrates the patient's first golf drive. She never swung the club with such abandon again, having promptly sensed the importance to equilibrium of restraining the extent of the stroke. The necessity of using both hands on the club greatly augments instability. The main abnormalities in motor behavior discussed in the analysis of the tennis stroke are present also in the golf drive. One additional feature appears. During the recovery phase of the golf stroke the head rotates to the left and dorsiflexes. This seems to trigger athetosis of the left leg. Figures 3 and 4 both illustrate that the major difficulty arises after the volitional act has been completed and not during its execution. The power phase of the drive again looks quite natural and graceful. Strange postures are assumed only after equilibrium is threatened by involuntary movement in one of the weight bearing limbs. This promptly evokes a compensatory maneuver which may look bizarre but which nonetheless is effective. It keeps the subject from falling to the ground.

DISCUSSION

Jung and Hassler[8] credit Lewandowsky with characterizing athetosis as the "disease of associated movements." According to Walsh[9] the latter are concerned with equilibrium, readjustments of the center of gravity, and with fixation of the limb girdles and the proximal segments of the appendages. Lewandowsky's phrase aptly describes the behavior of the patient under study. The features which mark her performance as abnormal are (1) the exaggeration of the tonic neck reflexes, and (2) the magnitude of the equilibrating adjustment to the gravitational stresses imposed by swinging (with considerable speed) a comparatively heavy elongated object grasped at the end of a long lever. How much of the automatic posturing is the result of a lesion in subcortical centers implicated in the organization of voluntary movement, how much to compensation for involuntary athetosis, and how much to muscle weakness is open to speculation. The latter is operative to a degree at least. The handling of a bowling ball, tennis racket, or golf club places extraordinarily severe demands on the relatively untrained neuromuscular apparatus of the chronically disabled individual. The spreading of an initially discrete movement pattern to incorporate an expanding galaxy of total limb synergies is the way in which a normal individual responds to hard work. Hence, the exaggerated associated movements evident during the execution of unfamiliar sport skills by the athetoid cerebral palsied subject may be in part a compensatory device mobilized spontaneously to meet the exigencies of the situation imposed.

Jung and Hassler have also presented a model of teleokinetic and ereismatic motility, drawn from an unpublished motion picture made by Hess, which further clarifies the basic motor difficulty of the patient under study. Hess's concept of statokinetic regulation differentiates the voluntary or teleokinetic phase of motion from what we have referred to as its autonomous component. Hess calls the latter ereismatic or supportive, and pictures this as a "dynamic support", governed by vestibular and proprioceptive mechanisms. Thus voluntary movements are superimposed upon a mobile substrate which must be tuned accurately to the continuously changing conditions associated with the execution of willed acts. Jung and Hassler point out that to be effective an anticipatory activation of the proprioceptive control of supporting action is necessary. They postulate that the mechanism subserving this function probably involves regulation of the gamma motoneuron system by supraspinal extrapyramidal structures. The latter constitute that portion of the motor control complex thought to be defective in the individual suffering from athetosis.[10] The four illustrations presented demonstrate how a reasonably adequate voluntary movement pattern may be rendered ineffective when supportive reactions are disproportionately augmented, either for want of central inhibition, because of the magnitude of the volitional effort required, or the necessity of compensating for unwanted involuntary movements. Reasoning from first principles suggests that the disruptive effect of a disturbed ereismatic component may be minimized as the teleokinetic phase of movement is strengthened.

SUMMARY AND CONCLUSIONS

Cinematographic recordings were made of the performance of an adult athetoid cerebral palsied patient when attempting to execute two wholly unfamiliar sport skills, the forehand drive in tennis and the golf drive. The activities selected were used as a means of placing easily elicited stress on a neuromuscular system known to have a defect in the subcortical neural mechanisms implicated in the control of movement. The response of a well trained normal subject, experienced in both sports, was used as a guide to identification of abnormal motor behavior. To expedite movement analysis more than 1,000 consecutive motion picture frames were enlarged. Study of these was supplemented by observation of the filmed movement cycles at normal and reduced speeds and by detailed inspection of single frames magnified twenty-three times. The evidence suggests that as far as this particular patient with athetoid cerebral palsy is concerned:

1. The will to perform the activity prescribed is unimpaired.
2. The act itself is conceived adequately.
3. The volitional component of the response is as effective as that of the average novice.
4. No involuntary movements mar the execution of the primary movement pattern.
5. Athetosis is limited to parts not employed in the sport skill performed. If parts implicated in the execution of the primary movement pattern are involved, the athetosis appears either before, or more usually, after the power phase of the stroke and the follow through have been completed.
6. The athetotic movements recorded cinematographically appear to be orderly manifestations of rotation, although irrelevant and purposeless as far as the act willed is concerned.
7. The most conspicuous abnormality in motor behavior is exaggeration of associated movements which in themselves also appear to be well co-ordinated.
8. The associated movements subserve easily recognizable compensatory functions and thus demonstrate how built-in automatisms safeguard neuromuscular performance.

ACKNOWLEDGMENT: Dr. C. Etta Walters, now affiliated with the Florida State University, Tallahassee, Florida, instructed the patient in the physical education activities analyzed and herself served as a normal control subject.

REFERENCES

1. Hellebrandt, F. A., Waterland, J. C., and Walters, C. E.: The influence of athetoid cerebral palsy on the execution of sport skills: bowling, Phys. Ther. Rev., 41:106, 1961.
2. Hellebrandt, F. A., Walters, C. E., and Styche, H.: Red Shoes: A case study. Steps in the rehabilitation of an adult cerebral palsied patient, Phys. Ther. Rev., 38:104-107, (February) 1958.
3. Hellebrandt, F. A., Hellebrandt, E. T., and White, C. H.: Methods of recording movement. An appraisal of photographic techniques for the study of motor performance and learning, Am. J. Phys. Med., 39:178-183, (October) 1960.
4. Crothers, B., and Paine, R. S.: The Natural History of Cerebral Palsy. Cambridge, Mass., Harvard University Press, 1959.
5. Turner, M., Perlstein, M. A., and Elam, H.: Electromyographic studies in cerebral palsy, Am. J. Phys. Med., 37:302-326, (December) 1958.
6. Magnus, R.: Cameron prize lectures on some results of studies in the physiology of posture, Lancet 2: 531-536, (September 11) 1926.
7. Beevor, C.: The Croonian Lectures on Muscular Movements. London, Macmillan Co., 1903.
8. Jung, R., and Hassler, R.: The extrapyramidal motor system. In: Handbook of Physiology, Chap. 35, Vol. 2. Edited by Field, J., Magoun, H. W., and Hall, V. E. Washington, D. C., American Physiological Society, 1960.
9. Walsh, E. G., and Marshall, J.: Physiology of the Nervous System. London, Longmans, Green & Co., 1957.
10. Bucy, P. C.: Relation to abnormal involuntary movements. In: The Precentral Motor Cortex, Chap. 15. Edited by Bucy, P. C. Urbana, Illinois, University of Illinois Press, 1949.

case report

Treating a Hyperactive Child

BARBARA S. SMITH, B.S., and
ELIZABETH H. PHILLIPS, R.N.

A four-year-old hyperactive retarded child with a mental age of seven months was treated by reduction of external sensory stimuli except touch. After an initial treatment period of six weeks, the child exhibited higher-level motor skills, better eye contact, less irritability, better manipulative skills, and self-feeding. The treatment which followed gradually became less structured, with consistently good results. One and one-half years after the initial period of highly structured treatment, the child shows a higher level of motor skills, continues to feed herself, has a vocabulary of at least ten words, and is making progress in a school program.

This paper describes the treatment of a mentally retarded, hyperactive child by the reduction of sensory stimuli. The patient was uncoordinated, uncontrolled, uninhibited, and erratic, as described by Strauss and Kephart.[1]

The patient was admitted to Central Wisconsin Colony and Training School in December 1966 at the age of forty-nine months. Her mental age, assessed on the Cattell Infant Intelligence Scale shortly after admission, was seven months. Her preadmission screening records showed that the patient could not talk or understand speech; could not learn in nursery school; was restless, excitable, nervous, fearful; was generally considered to have poor motor coordination; derived satisfaction from internal stimuli; and found objects more comforting than people.

A physical therapy program with goals of kneeling, standing balance, and independent ambulation began shortly after the patient's admission. When not in treatment, her behavior consisted of moving her head in all directions, gritting her teeth, and flopping her legs randomly while sitting. She waved her hands in the air, and threw or mouthed toys. When approached, she whined, bit her lips, or tried to pull the approacher's hair. She seemed compelled to concentrate on everything at once.

Ward personnel noted that the child seldom sat still for meals. When she attempted to feed herself, the spoon had to be taped to her hand to prevent her from throwing it. Eating was

Mrs. Smith is Staff Physical Therapist, Central Wisconsin Colony and Training School, Madison, Wisconsin 53704.

Miss Phillips is Head Nurse, Central Wisconsin Colony and Training School, Madison, Wisconsin 53704.

slow. Each attempt to toilet train her resulted in a fit of crying.

Motor skills, using the Kiwanis Children's Center Form Adapted from the Gesell Developmental Scale, include rolling in all directions, assuming sitting posture independently, and assuming the four-point kneeling position but not creeping. The child moved backward on her buttocks, using her hands to push herself. With bilateral support, she walked with stiff legs. She would not hold the therapist's hands. When using a walker, she moved her legs simultaneously, moving the walker without direction or purpose. In three months of preambulatory and ambulatory activities in physical therapy, no progress was noted. The staff decided to present her case to the orthopedist, with a recommendation to discontinue treatment.

REVIEW OF THE LITERATURE

Prior to the staff discussion of the patient's status, the supervisor of the Physical Therapy Department evaluated her program and suggested a new treatment plan which concentrated on the patient's problem of hyperactivity and distractability. A review of the literature revealed few suggestions on how to deal with these types of problems in the severely retarded.

Strauss and Lehtinen discussed the general principles of education of the brain-injured child.[2] They stated that efforts must extend in two directions: manipulation and control of the external, overstimulating environment; and education of the child to exercise voluntary control. They further stated that most brain-injured children require an environment especially suited to their particular needs, and that the environment must be planned initially to counteract general organic disturbances of behavior and attention. As the child gains knowledge, the area of successful performance is enlarged. The direction of the child's behavior should eventually be effected from within himself rather than from externally regulated conditions.

Moore stated that the nervous system is dependent initially and entirely upon purposeful stimuli (input) to help its development and to promote early learning.[3] The stimulus must be meaningful in order for the system to respond and to remember the stimulus. Use of abnormal input or deprivation of stimuli produces abnormal output, and eventually nervous system degeneration.

Bobath referred to hyperkinetic children as "motor-driven children."[4] In his treatment principles, he stressed the need to keep the child as quiet as possible, with a minimum of stimulation and distraction. To increase the child's attention span, Bobath suggested that he be kept in one place by using a reflex-inhibiting pattern while stories are told or soft music is played. Routine must also be emphasized.

Manaster used "controlled illumination" in the treatment of brain-damaged adults with hemiplegia to aid reintegration of perceptual processes.[5] The suggestion was made that this technique might be helpful in working with extremely agitated patients or hyperactive children. By reducing the degree of environmental stimulation and distraction, combined with individual contact in therapy, an increase may occur in the subject's psychological control and attention span, and a reduction in motor activity may result.

GENERAL TECHNIQUE

The general technique described here was used originally at an outpatient center with a patient with spastic hemiplegia with seizures who demonstrated behavior similar to that of the patient described in this paper.[6] The environment chosen for the child was a room kept as free as possible of noise, light, and odors. A mat was placed on the floor. No reward was given. Only tactile stimulation was considered in the actual treatment. The reflex-inhibiting pattern consisted of passive rolling. Once reduction of hyperactivity occurred, purposeful motor and manipulative skills became desirable. The immediate goals were constructive play, consistency in moving from sitting to four-point kneeling, maintenance of this position, and assistive creeping.

Treatment for one-half hour daily began April 24, 1967, and ended June 12, 1967, omitting the week of May 5 because of patient illness. The first five treatments consisted only of passive rolling on a mat with one person managing the legs and one the arms. When taken into the room, the patient cried. After two treatments, she ceased to cry. After using rolling as a preliminary activity for the sixth treatment period, work began on assistive grasp, release, and placement in long sitting position. The patient put blocks in a bucket. In the dimly lighted room, her eye contact was good, as measured by her head movements. These movements were necessary because of the placement of the bucket in front of her between her legs. She also had to reach over her leg and one of the therapists' legs to pick up or place the block on the mat. In successive treatments, no rolling was necessary before working on motor and manipulative skills. During the seventh treatment, the attempt at maintenance of four-point kneeling position resulted in the patient sitting on her heels.

Approximately two weeks after treatment had started, the child began to smile in apparent recognition of the persons treating her. During the third week of treatment, she began raising her arms to be picked up, and her smile became more evident and eager. Apparently she was absorbing more of the activities about her; she looked at ward personnel for longer periods of time and followed their movements with her eyes rather than using the quick, fleeting glances which had been characteristic.

The following week, illness confined the patient to bed. She sat in her bed holding a doll and moving its extremities. She was much quieter, and did not grit her teeth or whine. During the first treatment after her illness, she maintained the four-point kneeling position without falling when placed in this posture. Her attention to constructive play with blocks did not diminish, although some light was let in under the door. Noise obviously distracted her more than light, because the next day the same activity lost her attention when noise was made outside the door, although more light did not bother her. After this incident, light was let in from under the door.

As the patient became more manageable in treatment, assistive creeping began by passively moving her hands and feet in a reciprocal pattern when she maintained the four-point position. Kneeling, half-kneeling, and standing were also facilitated from this position. She stood by having one person hold her hands while the other applied pressure downward through her legs from the crests of the ilia. At the end of the third week of treatment, the patient crept a few paces on the mat in the physical therapy room. The same hand skills with blocks continued, while she was helped to maintain the kneeling position at a small table. Eye contact remained good for the same play activities in this new posture. She took blocks out of the bucket and placed them on the mat independently and consistently when sitting.

To increase her level of constructive play, transfer activities in the same posture became part of her program at the beginning of the fourth week of treatment. She grasped this new skill quickly, and after one week consistently transferred blocks from one hand to the other. For this activity the bucket was placed on one side of the patient and the blocks on the other side.

Because of her rapid gains during the first four weeks, she was introduced to dressing skills. Although she had been considered totally dependent in dressing skills at the beginning of the program, she now helped put her arms in and out of the sleeves once her hands were placed in the holes. In the next two weeks, she learned to put her arms through the sleeves independently and needed less help to get her arms out. She was also able to pull her shirt up over her head once her arms were out of the shirt.

At the end of the fifth week, the patient consistently held the therapist's hands when walking with bilateral support. At the end of the sixth week of treatment, the child assumed a standing position with assistance and took hesitant steps with unilateral support. She stood briefly without support. Her eye contact remained good when in the semidarkened room, and with the door open she continued independent constructive play as long as the noise level remained low.

Ward personnel who had frequent contact with the child noticed changes in her behavior during this treatment period. Approximately two weeks after her structured therapy began, one staff member began to play "pat-a-cake" with her immediately after her treatment. She smiled and seemed to enjoy this game as she watched the staff member move her hands for her. Feeding skills progressed with less throwing of the spoon.

At the end of the fourth week, the patient visited her home. A short questionnaire was sent to her parents regarding her behavior during this weekend. Although her parents did not know of the patient's progress, they did know that a new approach to treatment was being used. The parents reported that she was much quieter, played purposefully with toys, and concentrated more on feeding herself.

By the end of the sixth week, the spoon no longer had to be taped to her hand for feeding, but only placed in her hand. Her rate of eating increased. Her concentration on this activity was at a higher level than at the beginning of the six-week program.

Playing "pat-a-cake" continued after every treatment with the same staff member, and the patient learned how to clap her hands together at the appropriate time. At the end of the six-week treatment program, she went through the entire "pat-a-cake" rhyme with appropriate gestures. She sat for longer periods of time watching ward activities, and seemed content while on the toilet. When a familiar staff member entered the ward one morning and passed the toilet area, the patient gave her a long searching look, then a broad smile, and said "Hi!"

Following this six-week trial period, treatment continued to stress structured activities in the small room, but with direct light. She began to respond to verbal commands to pick up a block, and she tried unsuccessfully to stack two blocks. She removed rings from a stacking toy and replaced them independently and consistently. Her attention span for an activity lasted up to ten minutes when noise was at a minimum. She continued at a task when a new person was in the room with the therapist. Creeping instead of moving on her buttocks became her method of locomotion. She showed a fear of falling when walking with bilateral support—a fear which had not been present at the onset of treatment. Her gait was still much like a wooden soldier's and genu recurvatum was present.

Because of her excellent progress, the patient was transferred to the Rehabilitation Unit on January 12, 1968. The purpose of this unit is to involve all required disciplines in the best interest of the children. From here they may return home or be transferred to another ward within the colony to function with higher-level skills.

The patient seemed to adjust well to the situation. Since this was a new environment for her, the physical therapy program resumed for two weeks in a semidarkened room in order to reduce distractions. Therapy continued for the perfection of skills of ring removal and placement for eye-hand coordination improvement. When the bucket overturned, she placed it upright and put blocks in it. When blocks and rings were mixed, she threw the rings out. Pulling to standing by holding onto the therapist's hands became more automatic. When a familiar person extended his hands to her, she grabbed them and pulled herself from sitting by first kneeling, then half-kneeling, and then standing. When placed in a position so that she could hold onto furniture, and coaxed by the therapist, she took a few steps with minimal support at the hips. She continued feeding herself and assisting in dressing.

A full treatment program started in February 1968 in a quiet area, but with the lights on. The child continued at the same level of constructive play. To develop a pincer grasp, small beads and a cup were substituted for blocks and the bucket. She had difficulty picking up these small objects in the usual way and used a modified lateral pincer grasp.

In May 1968, the patient's motor skills level remained the same as three months prior, except that she occasionally "cruised" around furniture on the ward if she was placed near the bed. At this time, staff of all disciplines working with her believed that her rate of improvement was no longer changing. When transferred to her former ward, she continued in the physical therapy program, and made a rapid readjustment to her old surroundings.

SCHOOL PROGRAM

The patient started a school program in October 1968. The immediate goals of the program were improvement of eye-hand coordination, increased attention span, and language development. When first enrolled, she could not put four clothespins in a bottle in thirty minutes. Now she does this in two minutes and asks for the activity by saying "bottle." She no longer throws toys, and does less mouthing of objects. Since mid-November, 1968, the patient has worked on a form box. She has mastered circles and works to put the square in the box. At first, when the square would not go in, she refused to continue. Her general progress includes a longer attention span and increased cooperation.

She remained in the physical therapy program with goals of independent ambulation and constructive play without an actual structured environment until November 1968. Since then, her mode of locomotion has varied between moving on her buttocks and creeping. She has taken steps readily when placed by furniture, has pushed a chair, and has walked with unilateral support. She has demonstrated a high-steppage gait, and severe genu recurvatum has necessitated discontinuing walking practice on the ward.

Ward personnel report the patient continues to feed herself and helps with dressing. Her vocabulary includes "come on," "let's go," "hand," and "morning" (for "good morning"). All these words are used appropriately. She is still placed on the toilet, but neither toilet regulation nor training have yet been accomplished. Her constructive play with toys is limited but she no longer throws them. She prefers to observe certain children rather than to interact with them.

CONCLUSION

The success of this approach to treatment with this child has led to planning of similar programs for other children who have comparable motor and behavioral characteristics. The first goal is to provide these children with some structure in their environment. When the results achieved in treatment are seen on the ward, the daily care of the child is easier, the continuance of skills development is possible, and the child's reaction to external stimuli is better controlled.

The results of the treatment described above have led the staff to believe that this technique has promise. Further research should be undertaken so that an evaluation can be made of the potential of the treatment in the rehabilitation of the hyperactive child regardless of his intelligence.

REFERENCES

1. Strauss, Alfred A., and Newell C. Kephart. Behavior differences in mentally retarded children measured by a new behavior rating scale. Amer. J. Psychiat. 96:1117–1123, March 1940.
2. Strauss, Alfred A., and Laura A. Lehtinen. Psychopathology and Education of the Brain Injured Child. New York: Grune & Stratton, Inc., 1947.
3. Moore, Josephine C. A new look at the nervous system in relation to rehabilitation techniques. Amer. J. Occup. Ther. 22:489–501, November–December 1968.
4. Bobath, Karl, and Berta Bobath. Unpublished data.
5. Manaster, A. Perceptual retaining in brain damage through use of controlled illumination. Chicago Med. Sch. Quart. 26:56–63, Summer 1966.
6. Green, Leila H. Treatment suggestion: the hyperkinetic child. Int. Bobath Alumni Ass. Newsletter 3:2–3, Summer 1968.

the authors

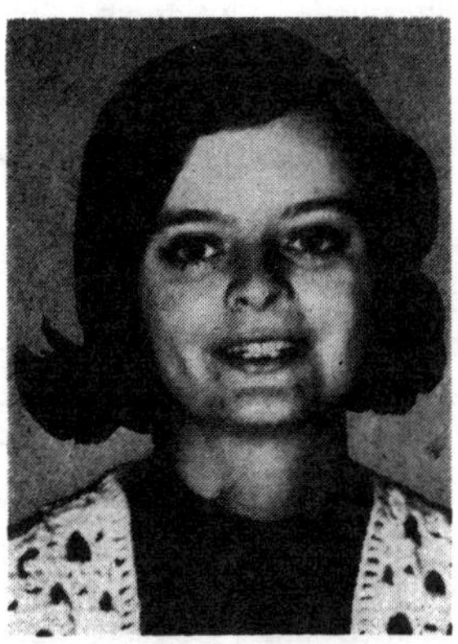

Barbara S. Smith, a staff physical therapist at Central Wisconsin Colony and Training School in Madison, holds a B.S. degree and a certificate in physical therapy from the University of Wisconsin. She is an associate member of the American Association on Mental Deficiency, and a member of the Wisconsin Chapter of the APTA and of the International Bobath Alumni Association.

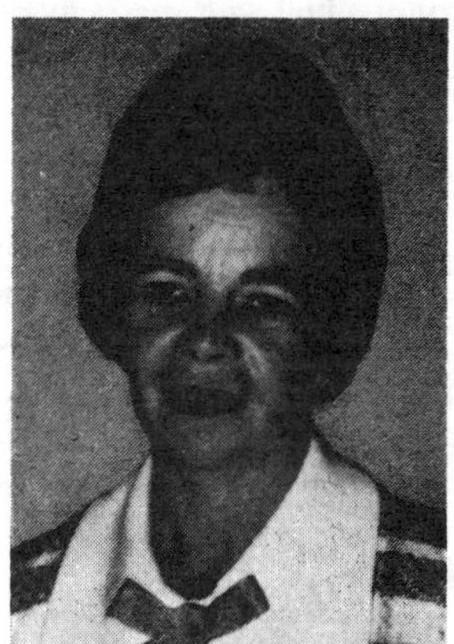

Elizabeth H. Phillips is head nurse at the Central Wisconsin Colony and Training School. She earned her R.N. diploma from the School of Nursing of St. Mary's Hospital. Like Mrs. Smith, she is a certified Bobath (neurodevelopmental treatment) therapist.

EMG Biofeedback Training for a Mentally Retarded Individual with Cerebral Palsy

HIDEO ASATO, PhD,
DENNIS G. TWIGGS, PhD,
and SHELLEY ELLISON, BS

Electromyographic biofeedback training was used to facilitate finger and wrist extension movements in a mentally retarded individual with spastic hemiplegia. The client was a 29-year-old woman with profound mental retardation and cerebral palsy as a result of postnatal meningitis. During treatment, the client demonstrated a short attention span, lack of motivation, low frustration tolerance, and increased spasticity in her left hand. The client was able to hyperextend her fingers following finger extension training, although goniometric measurements showed a marked degree of wrist flexion and wrist ulnar deviation. Therefore, training was implemented to develop wrist extension movements. Biofeedback therapy resulted in a substantial increase in active wrist extension and a marked reduction in wrist ulnar deviation.

Key Words: *Biofeedback, Mental retardation, Cerebral palsy, Electromyography.*

Uses of muscle biofeedback in the treatment of individuals with various neurological disorders are just beginning to be explored.[1] The major thrust of neuromuscular reeducation has emphasized inhibition of spasticity, recruitment of motor unit activity, and muscle relaxation.[2] For instance, EMG biofeedback has been used to develop inhibitory control of spastic gastrocnemius muscles,[3] recruit tibialis anterior muscle activity in paralytic foot-drop,[4, 5] and relax sternocleidomastoid muscle in spasmodic torticollis.[6, 7] Electromyographic biofeedback training has also been used to inhibit abnormal muscle synergy and restore normal synergy.[8] This article reports the results of a study to determine the effectiveness of electromyographic biofeedback in facilitating finger and wrist extension movements in a mentally retarded individual with spasticity of wrist flexor muscles.

METHOD

The client was a 29-year-old woman who functioned in the profound range of mental retardation. Her mental retardation and cerebral palsy (spastic left hemiparesis) was the result of postnatal meningitis. Her mental age was 2.7 years with an IQ of 13 and she functioned at Level III on the Adaptive Behavior Scale. The client's expressive communication skills consisted of two- and three-word utterances (noun-verb combinations). Language receptive skills included performance of appropriate action following a simple verbal request, responding correctly and nonverbally to questions concerning physical condition (eg, "Are you tired?"), and demonstrating an awareness of positional concepts (eg, "up-down," "in-out," "under-over").

The physical therapy assessment results indicated the left upper extremity position was characterized by shoulder adduction and internal rotation, elbow hyperextension, forearm pronation, wrist and finger flexion, and wrist ulnar deviation. Goniometric measurements indicated 84 degrees wrist flexion, 66 degrees of wrist ulnar deviation, and full finger flexion. The thumb was "indwelling." Weakness and spasticity were present in the left upper extremity: weakness was characterized by muscular atrophy in the hand and forearm, and spasticity was indicated by an essentially nonfunctional clubbed hand. Calluses were also noted over the proximal interphalangeal joints of her left hand. These calluses were self-inflicted wounds we thought occurred because of the client's frustration and inability to use the affected limb. The only functional use of the left hand was giving occasional assistance to the right extremity.

The client received daily physical therapy at this institution for 35 weeks before biofeedback training. Goals of treatment were 1) to strengthen and increase

Dr. Asato is Clinical Psychologist, Department of Psychology, San Antonio State Hospital/School, Box 23310, Highland Hills Station, San Antonio, TX 78223 (USA).

Dr. Twiggs is Director, Rehabilitation Therapies, San Antonio State Hospital/School.

Ms. Ellison is Director of Physical Therapy, Rehabilitation Therapies, San Antonio State Hospital/School.

This article was submitted June 11, 1980, and accepted March 22, 1981.

functional ability of left upper and left lower extremities and 2) to improve gait posture. The various therapeutic techniques implemented to initiate functional nonsynergistic movements included 1) stimulation of cutaneous receptors by light stroking and brushing, 2) encouragement of spontaneous exploratory movements of a relaxed extremity in relation to various objects situated around the individual, 3) passive exercise, and 4) active assistive exercise.

As a result of the client's short attention span, lack of motivation, and low frustration tolerance during physical therapy, spasticity in her left hand increased during treatment, and no functional improvement was observed after 35 weeks of therapy. Biofeedback therapy was initiated to circumvent the motivational problems encountered in physical therapy and to provide a method of restoring upper extremity function. Although the client was profoundly mentally retarded, she possessed a modicum of cognitive abilities that made it possible for biofeedback training to be implemented in conjunction with regular physical therapy programing.

Treatment of motor system dysfunction is guided by the principle that distal motor development follows proximal motor development.[9] Application of the proximodistal principle for an individual exhibiting weakness and spasticity in the hand means initiating wrist extension training before finger extension training. We found that an alternative method of treatment was indicated in our case, however, because of several factors: 1) a significant amount (66°) of wrist ulnar deviation, 2) a profound level of mental retardation, and 3) a noticeable increase in motivational level of the client after finger extension during the initial session of biofeedback training.

Biofeedback Training: Finger Extension

A 30-minute baseline session was conducted to determine whether the client could exhibit finger or wrist extensor movements without the occurrence of abnormal, synergistic movements. The following sequence of synergistic movements typically preceded finger extension: shoulder abduction, elbow flexion, shoulder external rotation, forearm supination, and elbow hyperextension. To facilitate extensor movements, a pillow was placed on the client's lap with her hands resting on top of the pillow and with open palms facing down. At the beginning of the baseline session, the client was given verbal instructions for performing extensor movements ("Raise your hand") and was also provided with a model of the appropriate response.

After this baseline session, training sessions were conducted to determine the efficacy of biofeedback therapy in facilitating hand extensor movements. There were 13 training sessions with an average of 2 sessions a week. Each session lasted about 30 minutes.

During the initial training session, the function of the biofeedback device was explained to the client by stating that music would be turned on if she displayed extension movements of her left hand. Verbal instructions were accompanied by passive extension of the client's wrist and fingers in order to 1) demonstrate the biofeedback principle and 2) serve as a procedure for shaping the desired response. The therapist also provided a model of the appropriate response by demonstrating wrist-finger extension. The procedure of passively extending the client's wrist and fingers was not repeated after the initial training session because she demonstrated an understanding of the feedback principle: she was able to exhibit an extension response (of her fingers) after the verbal instruction ("Turn the music on!") and modeling cues were given. A motor response that occurred immediately after passive extension of the client's hand was not defined as an extension response initiated by the client. Although the client's interest and motivation were quite noticeable, she was not able to demonstrate any wrist extension movements during the initial training session. The client's inability to demonstrate any wrist extension responses may have been due to a marked degree of wrist ulnar deviation. Therefore, the remaining therapy sessions incorporated finger, and not wrist, extension training.

In the remaining sessions (2–13) for finger extensor training, the client was given a verbal cue ("Turn the music on!") and a modeling cue (therapist performing wrist-finger extensor response) as the method of initiating the appropriate response. There was a total of 15 trials for each training session. If finger extension occurred without any cues (verbal or modeling), it was defined as a "spontaneous finger extensor response."

Biofeedback Apparatus

Surface silver/silver chloride pregelled electrodes* were placed over the extensor digitorum communis muscle. (Skin-electrode impedance was measured 10 minutes after electrode application and found to be about 10k Ω.) Muscle activity was monitored by a Model S75-01 Bioamplifier† operated in the EMG mode. Myoelectric potentials were detected, amplified, filtered (90 to 1,000 Hz), rectified, and integrated.

A threshold feedback program was devised by having integrated muscle signals fed into a potentiometer. The potentiometer was used to detect the presence of signals above a predetermined voltage. Whenever a signal was above threshold, the potentiometer activated a timer that determined the duration that an AC switch (optically isolated between system and

* Vermont Medical Inc, Rockingham Rd, Bellows Falls, VT 05101.

† Coulbourn Instruments, Box 194, Laramie, WY 82070.

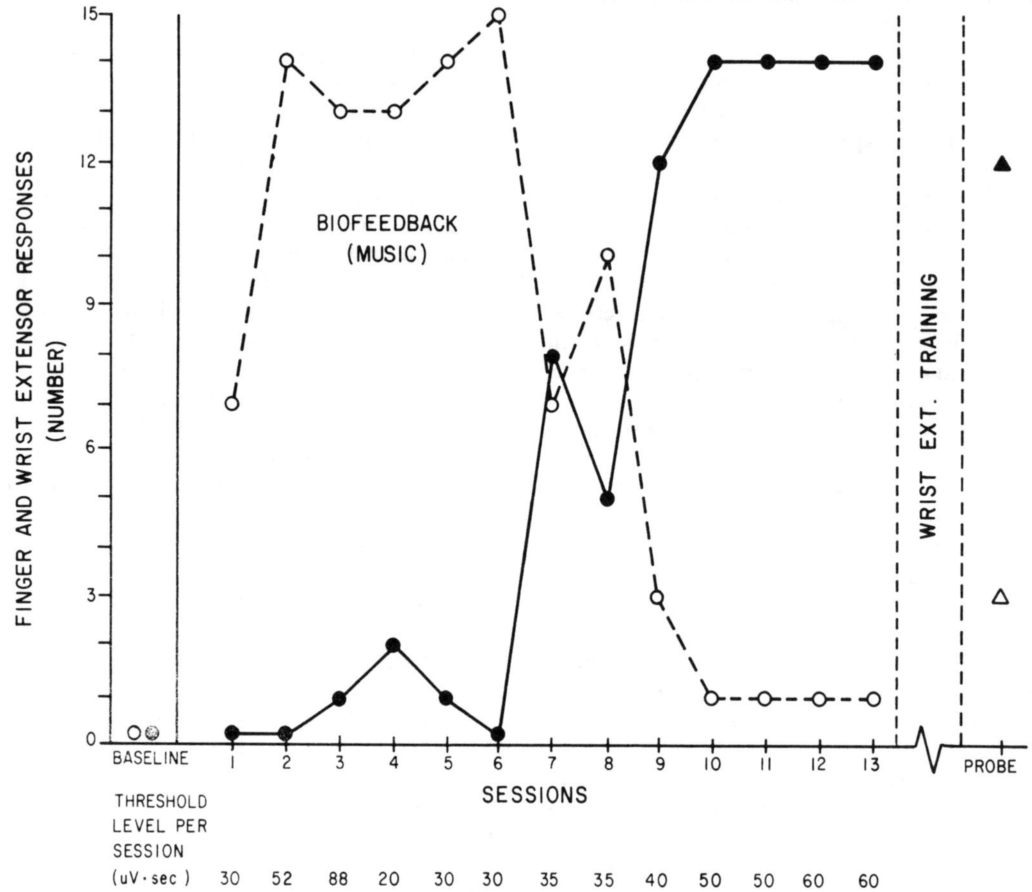

Figure. Development of finger and wrist extensor responses as a function of neuromuscular reeducation in a hemiplegic mentally retarded individual. (●——● = finger extension; ○- - -○ = finger extension—verbal/modeling cues; ▲ = wrist and finger extension; and △ = wrist flexion and finger extension.)

load) supplied an external device (eg, FM radio) with 110 V alternating current (VAC). Thus, a training program for coordinating EMG activity and feedback (music) was implemented by having an AC control provide an FM radio with 110 VAC. A timer determined the duration of feedback whenever muscle activity was above threshold. For example, if the feedback timer was set for 10 seconds, any EMG potentials above the preset threshold level (on the potentiometer) for 1,000 msec activated the timer and led to presentation of feedback for 10 seconds. Whenever muscle activity was above threshold during the feedback period, the timer automatically reset itself and feedback continued for 10 more seconds. If EMG activity remained above threshold level, the feedback recycled continuously for 10 second intervals.

Results: Finger Extension Training

A baseline session was conducted to determine the frequency of wrist or finger extensor movements initiated by the client without the occurrence of synergistic movements. No wrist or finger extensor responses were observed during the baseline session.

At the beginning of biofeedback training, threshold for EMG activity was set at approximately 30 μV·sec so that minimal extensor movements could initiate the feedback process. As training progressed and as finger extension improved sufficiently, the threshold for feedback was increased (about 5 to 10 μV·sec a session) so that a stronger extension response was required to initiate feedback. If a training session began where the level of the extensor response was below the threshold level set for the previous session, the threshold for EMG activity on the potentiometer was lowered to a point about 5 to 10 μV·sec above the resting EMG. This procedure increased the probability of a weaker extensor response initiating feedback (FM music) and thus strengthened the response itself. However, during most of the training sessions, threshold for EMG activity was slowly increased as the client showed progressively greater improvement in extensor motor responses (Figure).

By the end of the sixth session, the client was able to hyperextend (15°) the metacarpophalangeal joints of her fingers on cue for all 15 trials without initiating any abnormal synergistic movements (Figure). Prior to therapy, the resting position of her metacarpophalangeal joints was 95 degrees. The thumb remained indwelling throughout therapy. After 10 sessions, the client was able to perform this extensor response without cues on 90 percent of the trials.

At the termination of finger extension training, goniometric measurements showed that hyperextension of the fingers was accompanied by 52 degrees of wrist flexion and 47 degrees of wrist ulnar deviation. This indicated a net increase in the client's ability to extend her wrist 32 degrees actively.

Wrist Extension Training

At the end of finger extension training, extensor movements were accompanied by a marked degree of wrist flexion. To alleviate this condition, training was implemented to develop wrist extensor movements. The schedule was similar to the one implemented for finger extension training (two sessions a week). The client's hands were placed on top of a pillow with open palms facing down. Verbal instructions were given to the client ("Turn the music on!") along with passive extension of the wrist to demonstrate the appropriate response. A therapist also modeled the appropriate response for the client.

During the initial training session, the client exhibited a great deal of confusion as a result of the change in the desired response (ie, wrist extension as opposed to finger extension). In order to maintain the biofeedback setting as a pleasant and therapeutic environment, the remaining sessions were conducted without the new response demand (wrist extension) placed on the client. The only instruction given to the client was "Turn the music on!" Whenever an extensor response occurred with wrist flexion, the therapist brought the wrist slowly and progressively into extension. This training procedure to reduce wrist flexion was conducted for eight weeks (16 sessions). Electrode placement for recording wrist extensor movements was the same as the placement used for recording finger extensor responses.

Results: Wrist Extension Training

One month after the termination of wrist extension training, a probe (follow-up session) was conducted to determine the efficacy of training. The client was able to initiate extensor movements on all 15 probe trials without any cues (verbal or modeling). In 80 percent of the probe trials (see Probe in Figure), finger hyperextension was accompanied by wrist extension (0 to 10°). On the remaining probe trials, finger hyperextension was accompanied by wrist flexion (52°). Finger extension was observed in all 15 trials: a 10 percent improvement in the response after wrist extension training. At the end of wrist extension training, goniometric measurements showed that finger hyperextension was accompanied by 10 degrees of wrist extension and 45 degrees of wrist ulnar deviation. (Before biofeedback training, goniometric measurements indicated 84 degrees of wrist flexion and 66 degrees of wrist ulnar deviation.) Biofeedback therapy resulted in a net increase of 94 degrees of active wrist extension and a reduction of 21 degrees of wrist ulnar deviation.

During early training sessions the client occasionally complained of soreness in her arm, which apparently reduced her motivation to respond. In later sessions, however, no complaints of soreness were made during biofeedback training. A marked softening of the calluses on her proximal interphalangeal joints was noted and she began to initiate attempts to grasp objects (parallel bars, doors, toys) with her left hand.

One year following biofeedback training, several members of other disciplines have reported that the client has attempted to make extensor hand movements in various settings outside biofeedback therapy. In the dormitory, staff members commented that the client frequently demonstrated finger and wrist extensor responses and appeared quite pleased that she could perform this movement. This same observation was also made by staff in the client's speech therapy class. In physical therapy, the technician reported that the client started placing her extended left hand over the parallel bar (when she walked between them) and over textured surfaces (when she made horizontal movements with the hand). In dance therapy, she started clapping with her left hand to music, held hands with other patients to form a circle, and used her open left hand to pat her thigh. These behaviors were observed frequently by the dance therapist since the initiation of biofeedback therapy.

COMMENTS

Muscle reeducation studies generally use feedback in both auditory and visual modalities. There are attentional deficits in mentally retarded individuals, however, that influence the choice of modality. In a study designed to assess the nature of attentional problems that impair performance, Krupski reported that retarded participants exhibited a greater degree of off-task glancing than nonretarded participants in a visual reaction-time task.[10] On the other hand, Harrison and associates found that an auditory cue (music) facilitated manual dexterity in severely and profoundly retarded individuals.[11] These findings indicate that feedback presentation in the auditory mode may be an initial point of investigation in training the mentally retarded population to process information.

In our study, auditory feedback (FM music) was effective in facilitating the appropriate motor responses. The effectiveness of biofeedback therapy also seemed to be related to the observation that the client was in a setting where she had control of the contingencies: music could be turned on by the client whenever a finger and wrist extensor response (EMG activity) exceeded the preset threshold level. Severely and profoundly retarded individuals typically encounter situations where others take care of their needs and thus develop a history best described as "learned helplessness."[12] In contrast, biofeedback therapy provides a setting in which the contingencies are determined by the individual. The rapid development of extension movements and the observations that improved motor function appeared outside the therapy setting indicate the possibilities of EMG biofeedback in neuromuscular reeducation for mentally retarded individuals.

REFERENCES

1. Baker M, Regenos E, Wolf SL, et al: Developing strategies for biofeedback: Applications in neurologically handicapped patients. Phys Ther 57:402–408, 1977
2. Fernando CK, Basmajian JV: Biofeedback in physical medicine and rehabilitation. Biofeedback Self Regul 3:435–455, 1978
3. Amato A, Hermsmeyer CA, Kleinman KM: Use of electromyographic feedback to increase inhibitory control of spastic muscles. Phys Ther 53:1063–1066, 1973
4. Basmajian JV, Kukulka CG, Narayan MG, et al: Biofeedback treatment of foot-drop after stroke compared with standard rehabilitation technique: Effects on voluntary control and strength. Arch Phys Med Rehabil 56:231–236, 1975
5. Nafpliotis H: Electromyographic feedback to improve ankle dorsiflexion, wrist extension, and hand grasp. Phys Ther 56: 821–825, 1976
6. Brudny J, Grynbaum BB, Korein J: Spasmodic torticollis: Treatment by feedback display of the EMG. Arch Phys Med Rehabil 55:403–408, 1974
7. Korein J, Brudny J, Grynbaum BB, et al: Sensory feedback therapy of spasmodic torticollis and dystonia: Results in treatment of 55 patients. Adv Neurol 14:375–402, 1976
8. Kelly JL, Baker MP, Wolf SL: Procedures for EMG biofeedback training in involved upper extremities of hemiplegic patients. Phys Ther 59:1500–1507, 1979
9. Ayres AJ: Ontogenetic principles in the development of arm and hand functions. AJOT 8:95–99, 1954
10. Krupski A: Role of attention in the reaction-time performance of mentally retarded adolescents. Am J Ment Defic 82:79–83, 1977
11. Harrison W, Lecrone H, Temerlin MK, et al: The effect of music and exercise upon the self-help skills of nonverbal retardates. Am J Ment Defic 71:279–282, 1966
12. Seligman MEP: Helplessness: On Depression, Development, and Death. San Francisco, CA, W. H. Freeman & Co, Publishers, 1975, pp 181–188

Remediation of Toe-walking Behavior with Neutral-position, Serial-inhibitory Casts

A Case Report

LISA SELBY

This report details a case history and outpatient physical therapy management of a 4-year-old boy diagnosed with lower extremity hypertonia secondary to static encephalopathy of unknown etiology. Serial application of neutral-position inhibitory casts is detailed as is definitive orthotic management. A theoretical rationale for the management plan is also presented.

Key Words: *Gait training; Lower extremity, ankle and foot; Orthotics/splints/casts, lower extremity; Pediatrics, treatment; Physical therapy.*

Toe walking has been documented in children and adults with neurological impairments and emotional disturbances and in seemingly "normal" (neurologically unimpaired) children where the toe walking has no known cause.[1] Reasons for toe-walking behavior are varied (eg, hypersensitivity, balance difficulties, hypertonicity), and treatments addressing toe walking are as varied as the hypotheses of why people toe walk. Physical therapy can be aimed either at altering the cause of the problem or at remediating toe walking as a functional impairment. The goal of treatment may be normal gross motor development, improved self-image, improved circulation, or a more efficient gait pattern.[1-3]

Although numerous approaches to remediation of toe walking have been attempted for children with cerebral palsy, the original pattern of ambulation frequently returns.[1,4] Because many researchers theorize that the central nervous system learns what it practices, practice of the desired movement pattern may be the missing link for successful remediation of the toe-walking problem.[5,6] In addition, muscle length and bone formation are affected by the functional demands placed on them.[7,8] This observation supports orthotic management aimed at promoting practice of improved movement patterns. By improving biomechanical alignment, casting and orthotic management provide the physical therapist with a valuable method of promoting practice of a desired gait pattern.[9,10] The purpose of this case report is to present a treatment technique for toe-walking behavior that was applied to a child with hypertonia, muscle contractures, and delayed gross motor development.

L. Selby, MA, PT, is Physical Therapy Site Coordinator, Moss Rehabilitation Hospital, 12th St and Tabor Rd, Philadelphia, PA 19141, and a doctoral candidate, Program in Pediatric Physical Therapy, Hahnemann University, Philadelphia, PA. Address correspondence to 2401 Pennsylvania Ave, Apt 21C46, Philadelphia, PA 19130 (USA).

PATIENT DATA

The patient was a 4-year-old boy diagnosed with lower extremity hypertonia secondary to a static encephalopathy of unknown etiology. He was referred for physical therapy because of parental complaints of consistent toe walking, but he also reportedly had been having problems in school because of clumsiness.

The child's medical history included a visual problem diagnosed as Duane's syndrome that required two eye surgeries to help his left eye to turn outward, one at 25 months of age and the second at 39 months of age. During the period of physical therapy intervention, he received eyeglasses and patching of his right eye to increase his ability to use his left eye actively. In addition, the child was observed by his family and the physical therapist (L.S.) to display some hyperactivity and aggressive and obstinate behaviors at home and during physical therapy. These behaviors had been observed before initiation of physical therapy intervention and during the intervention period. The behaviors were not considered to be related to the intervention and necessitated psychological and later psychiatric intervention. Lastly, the child frequently engaged in stereotypical arm movements involving twirling objects and belts of various textures.

To document the child's developmental status, the Peabody Gross Motor Developmental Test was administered. The child was chronologically 45 months of age at the time of initial testing, and he attained an age-equivalent test score of 28 months with a basal age of 23 to 28 months and a ceiling age of 36 to 41 months. The child's primary difficulties in gross motor skills were climbing and descending stairs, riding a tricycle, standing on one foot, jumping, and running. Physical examination revealed incomplete righting and equilibrium responses to the right side in standing and in all developmental positions.

Evaluation of the child's feet and ankles revealed limitations in range of motion. Specifically, passive ROM measurement revealed a 20-degree ankle plantar-flexion contracture on the right side and a 10-degree ankle plantar-flexion contracture on the left side. When passively moved, particularly into ankle dorsiflexion or foot inversion-eversion, both lower extremities exhibited hypertonicity, with the right side being more resistant to passive motion than the left side. No clonus was evident. The child's gait was characterized by a lack of heel contact during the entire gait cycle; this observation was further substantiated by no signs of wear on the heels of the child's shoes.

PHYSICAL THERAPY PLAN

The physical therapy goals stated that the patient would

1. Ambulate indoors and outdoors for unlimited distances, attaining heel contact for 90% of his steps with orthotic management including heel lifts when necessary. When this goal

was attained with orthotic devices, a new goal was set for attaining heel contact without orthotic devices.

2. Develop age-appropriate gross motor skills, including the ability to stand on one foot, jump, run, ascend and descend stairs in an alternating fashion, and ride a tricycle.

After discussion with the child's physician and parents, I determined that physical therapy intervention should be implemented on a consultation and home program basis. The goals outlined above necessitated lengthening of the gastrocnemius-soleus tendon. Serial casting was suggested by the child's physician to avoid heel-cord lengthening surgery. The physical therapy casting technique chosen combined the goals of serial and inhibitory casting and emphasized stretch of the heel cords, practice of heel contact during gait, and ease of home use. A home program of activities that addressed developmental motor skills was also developed.

The serial application of bivalved casts set in the subtalar neutral (STN) position (see article by Oatis in this issue) was used to gradually lengthen the child's tight tendons while allowing him to practice a heel-toe gait pattern. The STN position was chosen for the following reasons: 1) It reportedly provides maximum congruency of the foot and ankle joints, thereby providing an optimally stable position for weight-bearing; 2) the STN position has been described as a midposition for the foot around which the motions of supination and pronation occur[3]; and 3) I have found that the STN position produces the fewest problems with skin condition during use of casts and orthoses. The child initially was casted in 20 degrees of plantar flexion on the left side and 10 degrees of plantar flexion on the right side while maintaining the STN position bilaterally. When the child extended his knees to stand, the tendons were expected to be stretched because of the two-joint nature of the gastrocnemius muscle. The child was instructed to wear the casts for five hours a day during functional activities including various balance and walking activities.

The casts were applied with the subject in a prone position. The STN position was maintained, and the talocrural (ankle) joint was dorsiflexed as much as was comfortably possible with the knee flexed to 90 degrees. The casting procedure began with the foot and leg being covered by two socks with a lead strip taped on top that bisected the full length of the anterior foot and leg. No padding was used in the cast fabrication other than a double thickness of the sock the child was going to wear with the casts. The lack of additional padding in the casts permitted exact duplication of the casting condition each time the child wore the bivalved casts. Cuttercast® casting tape* was then wrapped circumferentially around the foot and leg, taking care never to pull the material taut. A wet elastic bandage was then applied to assist in the setting of the casting material. When the elastic bandage was removed, the casts were univalved using a stainless steel blade to cut on top of the lead strip.

The casts were then removed from the child's feet, and the univalve sites were matched perfectly. Reinforcing Maxcast® fiberglass casting tape* was then wrapped around each cast proximal to the region of the metatarsal heads, forming an area for toe break to occur during gait. The reinforced casts were then bivalved at sites anterior to the medial malleoli and posterior to the lateral malleoli. The final cast edges were rounded with cloth tape. To permit proper biomechanical positioning of the proximal body parts, provide equal leg length, and facilitate weight-bearing through the subject's heels during the stance phase of gait, the casts were aligned, or *posted*, with a plastic material (Aquaplast®†).[3] Each cast was held in a position that would promote optimal proximal alignment of the leg, and Aquaplast® was inserted between the cast and the horizontal surface. Rubber soles from an old pair of the child's shoes were glued to the bottom of the casts to provide a nonskid, nonstick surface for ambulation. After a short trial walk, the posting and soles were modified to attain optimal biomechanical alignment including heel contact during 90% of the child's steps.

Heel contacts were at first assessed by observation of the child's gait and by calculating the ratio of the number of heel contacts to the number of steps. This method proved fairly difficult and unreliable, so videotapes were taken of the child from a sagittal view with a video camera placed in a fixed position on a tripod. The videotaped portion of the child's 30-ft‡ walk gathered data for between three and four steady-state steps of the entire walk. Samplings from three of the child's walks were recorded for three conditions: 1) barefoot, 2) wearing sneakers, and 3) wearing orthoses and sneakers. To avoid the possibility of the child introducing artificial attempts to attain or not attain heel-strike, attention was not called to the video camera or to the section of the walk recorded on the videotape. The recording of a walk was considered usable if the child was not skipping, running, or performing any other form of play.

RESULTS OF TREATMENT

The posted serial-inhibitory casts were effective in providing the child with a heel-toe gait pattern for at least 90% of his steps as his plantar-flexion contractures were being reduced. Attaining neutral talocrural joint position bilaterally while maintaining the STN position took about four separate pairs of casts and about four months. No skin irritation or redness was noted during the entire casting period. The child's family taught the child to don and doff his casts independently, and he wore his casts about five hours a day throughout the entire eight-month period. The child's functional activities were not curtailed by the casts, and his parents were educated in ways to structure new gross motor opportunities for the child.

Definitive orthoses were fabricated by an orthotist after the eight months of treatment when the child could ambulate with a heel-toe pattern about 70% of the time in sneakers without the casts and demonstrated greater than a neutral amount of passive ankle dorsiflexion. The physical therapist assisted in the casting for these orthoses to ensure STN alignment. The goals of the new intervention were to 1) continue to require a heel-toe gait pattern during 90% of the child's steps and 2) permit dorsiflexion ROM past a neutral talocrural position while blocking plantar-flexion range past a neutral position during gait. A hinged, neutral-position polypropylene molded ankle-foot orthosis with a 90-degree plantar-flexion stop and free dorsiflexion was used. The orthosis permitted free dorsiflexion while preventing ankle plantar flexion or excessive subtalar joint movement deviating from a neutral position. In this way, the heel-toe gait pattern could continue to be practiced with the orthoses, and the toe-walking pattern avoided.

About one year after initiation of

* Johnson & Johnson Orthopaedics, 501 George St, New Brunswick, NJ 08903-2400.

† WFR/Aquaplast Corp, PO Box 635, Wyckoff, NJ 07481.

‡ 1 ft = 0.3048 m.

treatment, the child wore his polypropylene orthosis for five hours a day. He could maintain neutral foot and ankle position with extended knees. He also could stand on one foot, jump, ascend and descend stairs (alternating feet), run, and ride a tricycle. Parental report and videotape analysis documented that the child attained heel contact for 70% of steps observed when wearing sneakers alone and 100% of steps observed during orthosis use. Unfortunately, however, the child exhibited a heel-toe gait pattern for only 50% of observed steps when he was barefoot. Lastly, the child's shoes showed signs of wear in the heel area typical of a heel-toe gait pattern.

DISCUSSION

Many studies have examined the short-term effects of short leg casts on ambulation in persons with neurological deficits. To date, however, no known studies have examined the effects of combined serial and inhibitory casting or the long-term effects of such intervention. In this case study, neutral-position, serial-inhibitory casts resulted in decreased plantar-flexion contractures while simultaneously encouraging practice of the desired heel-toe gait pattern. In addition, some carry-over of the heel-toe gait pattern was suggested by the child's ability to perform a heel-toe pattern during 70% of his steps wearing sneakers without orthoses and 50% of his steps when barefoot. The posting of the casts introduced heel weight-bearing in a gradual fashion so that when full ROM was attained, the patient could tolerate full-heel weight-bearing. I believe that a combination of serial and inhibitory casting, when appropriately used, is more effective than either procedure alone.

The definitive orthosis permits practice of a heel-toe walking pattern using the child's available passive ROM into dorsiflexion while preventing loss of ROM as a result of toe walking. The orthosis also requires repetition of the desired gait pattern and thereby may provide the child with the practice needed to allow true learning of the new gait pattern to occur. Hence, the long-term goal of orthotic management for this child is that the new heel-toe pattern of walking will become his pattern of choice, abolishing his toe-walking pattern. The possibility of achieving this goal and the amount of time it will take will probably depend on how well the toe-walking pattern was initially established, the original cause of the toe-walking behavior, and the effectiveness with which the child practices the heel-toe gait pattern.

Acknowledgments. I thank my patient and his parents for allowing me to publish this case report and Dr. Robert Palisano and H. A. Thubi Kolobe for their editorial assistance.

REFERENCES

1. Furrer F, Deonna T: Persistent toe walking in children: A comprehensive clinical study of 28 cases. Helv Paediatr Acta 37:130–141, 1980
2. Olney SJ, Costigan PA, Hedden DM: Mechanical energy patterns in gait of cerebral palsied children with hemiplegia. Phys Ther 67:1348–1354, 1987
3. Jordon RP: Therapeutic considerations of the feet and lower extremities in the cerebral palsied child. Clin Podiatr 1:547–561, 1984
4. Perry J: Rehabilitation of spasticity. In Feldman RG, et al (eds): Spasticity: Disordered Motor Control. Chicago, IL, Year Book Medical Publishers Inc, 1980, pp 87–100
5. Herdman SJ: Effect of experience on recovery following CNS lesions. Phys Ther 63:51–55, 1983
6. Held JM: Recovery of function after brain damage: Theoretical implications for therapeutic intervention. In Carr JH, et al (eds): Movement Science Foundation for Physical Therapy in Rehabilitation. Rockville, MD, Aspen Publishers Inc, 1987, pp 155–173
7. Gossman MR, Sahrmann SA, Rose SJ: Review of length-associated changes in muscle: Experimental evidence and clinical implications. Phys Ther 62:1799–1808, 1982
8. Rose SJ, Rothstein JM: Muscle mutability: Part I. General concepts and adaptations to altered patterns of use. Phys Ther 62:1773–1787, 1982
9. Carlson SJ: A neurophysiological analysis of inhibitive casting. Physical and Occupational Therapy in Pediatrics 4(4):31–42, 1985
10. Sussman MD, Cusick B: Preliminary report: The role of short leg tone reducing casts as an adjunct to physical therapy of patients with cerebral palsy. Johns Hopkins Medical Journal 145:112–114, 1979

Case Report

Clinical Use of Neuromuscular Electrical Stimulation for Children With Cerebral Palsy, Part 1: Lower Extremity

Judy Carmick

This report, part 1 of a two-part case report on the clinical use of neuromuscular electrical stimulation (NMES) for children with cerebral palsy, documents the functional changes that occurred with the application of NMES to the lower extremity of three male children, 1.6, 6.7, and 10 years of age, all with hemiplegia due to cerebral palsy. Neuromuscular electrical stimulation was used in conjunction with a dynamic-systems, task-oriented model of motor learning. The children tolerated NMES well and at times demonstrated carryover after the removal of NMES. The youngest child showed immediate change in the ability to walk and run symmetrically. The two older boys demonstrated significant improvement in locomotor efficiency in a short time, although they were of an age when this improvement was not expected. One boy's Physiological Cost Index (PCI) measurement (a measure of locomotor efficiency) improved fourfold, and the other boy's PCI measurement improved by a factor of two. The results show preliminary evidence for the usefulness of NMES as an adjunct to the physical therapy program for improving function in children with cerebral palsy. [Carmick J. Clinical use of neuromuscular electrical stimulation for children with cerebral palsy, part 1: lower extremity. Phys Ther. 1993;73:505–513.]

Key Words: *Cerebral palsy, Lower extremity, Motor control, Neuromuscular electrical stimulation, Pediatrics.*

Research showing that electrical stimulation can increase the strength[1] of normally innervated muscle has increased interest in neuromuscular electrical stimulation (NMES). Neuromuscular electrical stimulation has been used to improve range of motion (ROM), temporarily reduce excessive spasticity (hyperreflexia),[2] facilitate motor control and muscle reeducation,[3] and assist in gait training.[4] Most studies have been conducted on adult subjects; very little has been written about electrical stimulation with children.

Leyendecker[5] studied 20 children with cerebral palsy whose mean age was just over 10 years. There was no description of the NMES treatment method or measurements, including which muscles were stimulated or whether the children were required to be active. At the beginning of the study, the 10 children who received NMES with neurodevelopmental therapy (NDT)* progressed faster than the 10 children who received only NDT. At the end of the study, however, the two groups were equal.

J Carmick, PT, is in private practice, 3060 Miranda Ave, Alamo, CA 94507-1611 (USA).

This paper was presented in poster format at the Combined Sections Meeting of the American Physical Therapy Association; February 5-10, 1992; San Francisco, CA.

This article was submitted December 14, 1992, and was accepted March 22, 1993.

*Traditional NDT[6,7] follows a hierarchical and reflex model[8,9] of motor control. Abnormal muscle tone (spasticity) is considered a major problem for treatment and a cause of much of the motor deficit. Patients are advised not to exert excessive effort, which is believed to be a potential for increasing abnormal muscle tone and to result in loss of reciprocal movement activity. Development was expected to progress from proximal to distal, so the hip was expected to develop before the foot. Current NDT assumptions[10] are changing as new knowledge of motor control and motor learning is discovered.

Gracanin et al[11] reported the results of a 6-year study of functional electrical stimulation (FES) given to 120 children with cerebral palsy. The peroneal nerve was stimulated during gait in children with varus deformities of the feet who exhibited hyperreflexia. The FES results had a positive effect in the improvement of walking and posture in mild cases in which the child had a varus forefoot, a hypertonic triceps surae muscle, and no hypotonia. Some of the children showed improvement in walking and posture that lasted after the removal of FES. The positive effects were mainly in the swing phase, including absence or decrease of "hikes" (abnormal elevations) and medial (internal) rotation of the hip joint, decrease of equinovarus, and inadequate dorsiflexion at the ankle joint. In the stance phase, the effects were manifested in the decrease of medial rotation and adduction of the hip joint and in hyperextension of the knee joint. The child was able to touch the floor with the heel, which was not possible before application of FES.

Kieklak and DeVahl[12] and Kieklak[13] discussed using NMES as an adjunct to traditional developmental pediatric therapy. Carryover was not mentioned, other than a decrease in muscle tone that was proportional to the frequency of NMES use.

Dubowitz et al[14] reported on the use of chronic electrical stimulation applied to two 3-year-old girls with hemiplegia secondary to cerebral palsy to determine whether motor performance could be improved. The tibialis anterior muscle of the affected leg received stimulation for 1 hour three times a day while the children were active. Motor performance and gait improved after a few weeks of stimulation. One child also showed signs of equilibrium reactions for the first time.

Atwater and colleagues[15] used electromyography (EMG)-driven NMES with 10 children with cerebral palsy, aged from 5.5 to 16 years. The children received EMG-driven NMES to either the wrist extensors or ankle dorsiflexors and a total-body NDT exercise program three times a week for 8 weeks. The children needed to actively contract and then fully relax their muscles. The youngest child, the only one with athetoid cerebral palsy, dropped out of the study because the child did not like the electrical stimulation. The children who remained in the study showed improvement in general motor function; those receiving wrist stimulation improved more than those receiving ankle dorsiflexor stimulation. Results suggested that children needed to be at least 6 years old in order to actively participate in the treatment procedure.

Nothing was found in the literature that described using NMES as an adjunct to the contemporary task-oriented or systems-based model of physical therapy. This report, part 1 of a two-part case report on the clinical use of neuromuscular electrical stimulation (NMES) for children with cerebral palsy, documents the functional changes that occurred with the application of NMES to the lower extremity of three children, 1.6, 6.7, and 10 years of age, all with hemiplegia due to cerebral palsy.

Neuromuscular Electrical Stimulation Used as an Adjunct to a Task-Oriented Physical Therapy Program

The subjects in the case studies presented in this report received NMES, along with a physical therapy program based on a task-oriented model of motor control.[16-18] It was not necessary for the children to be able to actively contract the stimulated muscle, as in the study by Atwater et al.[15] Thus, a 19-month-old child could participate as well as others who are not physically able to isolate muscle contraction. Various techniques were used, with an emphasis on the task-oriented motor model. The NDT techniques were also used where the principles did not conflict.[10] The NMES was used for muscle education, strengthening, increasing sensory awareness, and evaluation.

The principles of motor learning that were emphasized included having the child play in a task-specific activity or a self-directed, goal-driven activity while in a position in which the stimulated muscle would normally function. Pathological movement patterns were considered to be compensations for central nervous system dysfunction and/or biomechanical mechanisms. Neuromuscular electrical stimulation was used to facilitate muscles or movements that were weak, whether they were considered to be spastic or not. The superficial muscle that was felt not to be working at the proper moment was chosen. A remote-control switch was used to stimulate the muscle at the time it was needed.

The children did not have to be in a perfect position and were given freedom to make and learn from mistakes. They were allowed at times to move unsuccessfully and to independently try to correct the movement. They were often given concrete directions in order to assist in motor learning.[18] After success occurred, the stimulus was given intermittently in a weaning process to increase motor learning.

Neuromuscular Electrical Stimulation Equipment Used

The Respond II unit[†] was used. This unit has two channels that allowed two different muscles to be stimulated at the same time or at alternating times. The portability of the unit allowed the child to move freely.

Reusable, self-adhering, pregelled, carbonized-rubber electrodes[†] were used. The active electrode was placed on the motor point, and the inactive electrode was placed on the same muscle or muscle group a short distance away from the involved extremity. The active electrode was cut to

[†]Medtronic Nortech Division, 10237 Flanders Ct, San Diego, CA 92121.

size, never smaller than a nickel, so that only the desired muscle would be stimulated and thus eliminate or decrease overflow. The suggestions of Baker and Parker[19] and Delitto and Robinson[20] for electrode placements were often used.

The pulse rate was often initially set to about 5 to 7 pulses per second (pps), which gave a tapping sensation and sensory input but not a fused contraction. When this sensation was tolerated by the child, the setting was increased to between 30 and 35 pps to give a fused muscle contraction. The pulse duration was fixed at 300 microseconds.

The output-limit control was set for 50% of the stimulator's maximum amplitude. The amplitude was increased very slowly, to the child's tolerance, and only when the current was on. It was not necessary to have a maximal contraction to increase sensory awareness or the strength of weak muscle[2,21] (see part 2 of this case report in this issue). With a low pulse rate, a higher amplitude is usually comfortable.[3]

The ramp, or rise time, was initially set at the lowest setting (8 seconds) for the most comfort. When the child was accustomed to NMES, the ramp was set for approximately 2 seconds. When a quicker response was needed, as for gait activities, the fastest rise time (0.5 second) was used.

On-off times initially were set for 10 seconds on and 25 seconds off. Once the child was comfortable with electrical stimulation and not showing signs of fatigue, the cycle was set at 15 seconds on and 15 seconds off for a total of 15 to 20 minutes. When the remote-control switch was used, the on time was determined by activation of the switch, which was stimulated at the time the child was seen to need that muscle to function. For example, when the child in case 1 was walking and not flexing the knee, the remote-control switch was used to facilitate the NMES, which was stimulating the medial hamstring muscle. When stimulating the lower extremity and while the child remained standing, not moving out of position, the stimulus control was set to the alternating mode to prevent the muscle from being constantly stimulated or constantly silent.

Introducing Children to Neuromuscular Electrical Stimulation

Initially, NMES was demonstrated on the therapist's arm and then on the parent's arm. This was to give the parent experience with NMES to help eliminate any fear of electrical stimulation that might be transferred to the child.

The patients in cases 1 and 2 were first introduced to a hand-held vibrator, which was called a "tickler." The child in case 3 was 10 years of age, had experience with EMG, and did not need this elementary level of introduction. The NMES was described as being like the "tickler," and the children were told they would feel a tapping sensation. The electrode was then placed on the cleaned body part. The amplitude was increased very slowly until the child indicated that he felt the stimulation or until a trace contraction was felt or seen.

The child was given time to experience and accept the sensation. Letting the child in case 2 turn the unit on and off with the remote-control switch gave him a chance to control what was happening to his body. Once he had a turn at controlling the mechanics of the NMES unit, he was then willing to return to the actual therapy. This took little time as he quickly showed interest in returning to his therapeutic activity. With acceptance and experience, the amplitude was increased as needed and tolerated to improve the muscle function. Acceptance of NMES is expected if the child's needs are respected, the amplitude is kept within the child's tolerance, and the child is given some control over the situation.

Case Studies of Three Children With Cerebral Palsy, Hemiplegic Type

Case 1

The child in case 1 was a 1.6-year-old boy who was diagnosed with left hemiplegia secondary to cerebral palsy following a computerized tomography (CT) scan. The lesion was believed to have occurred prenatally. He began receiving physical therapy at age 7 months. Physical therapy followed the task-oriented model of motor learning and included NDT techniques and various therapeutic techniques to increase sensory awareness. He walked at age 15 months. The child initially received NMES when he was only 19 months of age. He received NMES to both the lower and upper extremities.

Before neuromuscular electrical stimulation. At age 21 months, the child toe-walked on the left foot with excessive lateral (external) rotation of the leg. He stood with a pronated foot. Passive range of motion (PROM) was complete throughout the left leg and left hip. No active dorsiflexion of the left foot was possible. Passive dorsiflexion was 15 degrees with knee extension.

Treatment of the tibialis anterior muscle. Neuromuscular electrical stimulation was used on the motor points of the child's tibialis anterior muscle when he was 21 months of age. This treatment was initially done while the child was in a sitting position. In the second session, NMES was applied while the child was standing and walking. The remote-control switch was used to stimulate the tibialis anterior muscle during the swing phase of gait.

When the child was standing and walking, there was no real gait change. He intermittently used a flat foot, but only slightly more than without NMES. No active dorsiflexion occurred when requested. There was little or no carryover. This treatment was tried intermittently once weekly for 5 months without success. As the

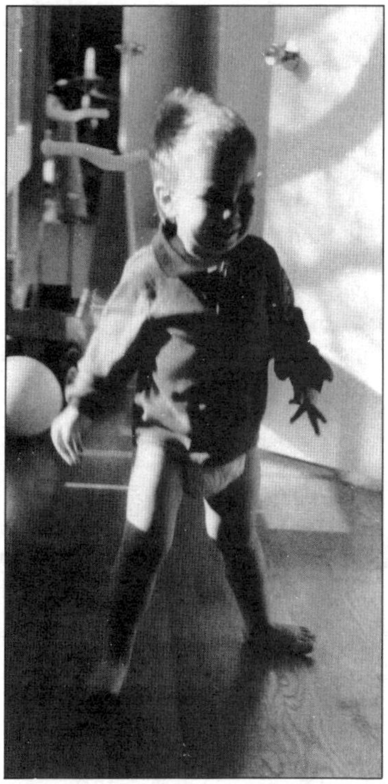

Figure 1. *Child in case 1 photographed at 27 months of age while running before neuromuscular electrical stimulation was used on the medial hamstring muscle. The child's right side is leading; the left side is retracted. His walking gait posture was similar.*

child became heavier and more active, his gait deteriorated. There was less weight shift to the left and more toe-walking, and the child developed genu recurvatum.

Treatment of the triceps surae muscle. At 26 months of age, after 5 months of stimulation of the tibialis anterior muscle, the triceps surae muscle was added to the child's NMES lower-extremity program. The muscles were alternately stimulated while the child was standing and walking with a remote-control switch to achieve the correct timing. It was discovered on the second session that when the NMES was facilitating the gastrocnemius-soleus muscle group, the child's foot was plantigrade. The child's gait had intermittent improvement of foot flat on initial contact, but the improvement did not last after NMES was removed. The program was done for 15 minutes at each of four weekly sessions conducted over a 5-week period. The child's gait improved intermittently, but the ROM of the foot was not improved.

At 29 months of age, when only the triceps surae muscle was stimulated, the child's foot immediately became plantigrade. The NMES to the triceps surae muscle was used for about 5 minutes while the child was standing. The tibialis anterior muscle was then added for alternate stimulation while the child walked and stepped in and out of hoops for a total of 15 minutes with the use of the remote-control switch. The child's gait was not changed, and his foot was plantigrade when NMES stimulated the gastrocnemius-soleus muscle group.

For the next 5 weekly sessions, the triceps surae muscle was stimulated for 15 minutes without stimulation of the tibialis anterior muscle. The child stood plantigrade more frequently, and after 3 weeks, he was walking with foot-flat gait and shifting his weight to the left. Although he was doing well without NMES stimulating the tibialis anterior muscle, that muscle was again stimulated for fear that the muscle was not functioning well enough. After that session, the child returned to toe walking for 2 days.

When only the triceps surae muscle was stimulated, the child's foot immediately became plantigrade during stance and he had a foot-flat gait. Fear of increasing reflex activity in the triceps surae muscle if that muscle was stimulated alone without intermittently stimulating the tibialis anterior muscle led to continued stimulation of the tibialis anterior muscle. A foot-flat gait, however, was not achieved with the alternating stimulation of the tibialis anterior and triceps surae muscles. The foot-flat gait occurred only when the triceps surae muscle was stimulated. The child's PROM improved throughout the foot and ankle. Active dorsiflexion was intermittently improving. There was no increase in reflex activity.

The child's gait improved with triceps surae muscle NMES, and he used a flat foot and occasionally a heel-strike. With NMES, he would spontaneously shift weight to the left side and maintain that weight shift for several minutes while playing at a table. The NMES needed to be repeated each week, as his gait improvements lasted a few days and then decreased. After success with the triceps surae muscle, the gluteus maximus muscle was stimulated to increase strength. When this was done, the child would shift weight to the left side while standing and playing at a table. He did not need verbal direction.

Treatment of the medial hamstring muscle. When the child learned to run, it turned into a gallop because of the excessive retraction of the left side of the body; he led with the right extremities. The photograph shown in Figure 1 was taken while the child was running. His usual body position is shown when walking or running; the left extremities, hip, and shoulder were held and remained behind the right hip and shoulder.

During physical therapy, an attempt was made to correct the compensating trunk rotation and improve symmetry. Two adults each grasped one of the child's hands and rotated his body so that the left extremities would lead. He strongly refused by pulling down on the arms, rotating his body to the right and starting to cry. Continuing with this attempt was unwarranted; the sensation of leading with the left extremities was extremely upsetting to the child. It was decided to try NMES to correct the unwanted rotation.

Electrodes were placed on the child's medial hamstring muscle to balance the excessive use of the lateral hamstring muscle thought to cause the excessive lateral rotation of the left leg. Neuromuscular electrical stimulation was used as the child played while standing at a bench. He showed total acceptance of the stimulus. After a few minutes, he was again encouraged to gallop, with NMES still operat-

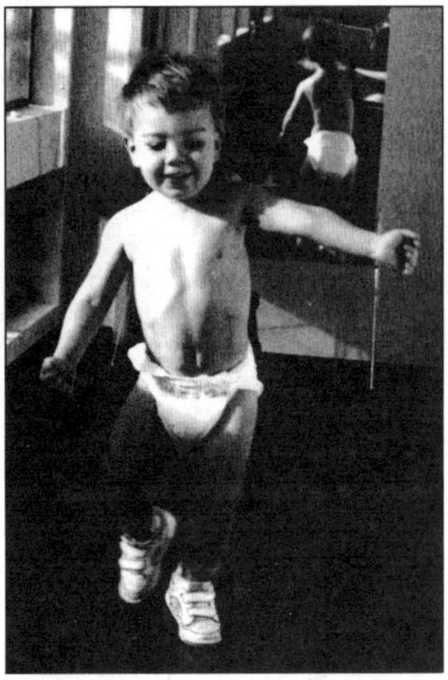

Figure 2. *Child in case 1 photographed at 29 months of age while walking after two sessions of neuromuscular electrical stimulation applied to the medial hamstring muscle. Improved symmetry is shown; the left leg is in an acceptable placement and the left shoulder is no longer retracted. He is wearing supramalleolar foot orthoses.*

ing, leading with the left side as two adults each held one hand.

When NMES was applied, galloping and leading with the left extremities became immediately possible. The child enjoyed the activity and for a few times galloped about 4.6 m (15 ft) at a time. The manual assistance was removed, and he was able to gallop unassisted, leading with the left (involved) side.

The entire time of stimulation to the medial hamstring muscle was 15 minutes. The cycle was set for 15 seconds on and 15 seconds off while the child was galloping. When he walked, the remote-control switch was used to stimulate the medial hamstring muscle in the normal, age-appropriate timing in accordance with Sutherland and colleagues'[22] EMG charts.

Following this treatment, the child's gait improved; the hip moved symmetrically, and the left leg was no longer excessively laterally rotated. Carryover was maintained for 2 days, as reported by his mother. The NMES was given on the return visit in the same manner. The photograph shown in Figure 2 was taken after two sessions of NMES applied to the medial hamstring muscle. It shows improved rotation of the left lower extremity and shoulder while the child was walking. After only two 15-minute sessions, he was able to maintain the improved alignment without further stimulation. He was wearing a supramalleolar foot orthosis.

The extent of carryover is shown in the photograph in Figure 3, which was taken while the child was running, 4 weeks after the last time the medial hamstring muscle was stimulated. Figure 3 shows that he was still able to run while alternating his arms and legs; the left leg and right arm were leading at that moment in the gait cycle. It had not been necessary to repeat the treatment at that time because the child was able to maintain the skill.

Case 2

The child in case 2 was a 6.7-year-old boy when he began receiving NMES to both the upper and lower extremities. He was diagnosed as having cerebral palsy attributable to sporadic oxygen deprivation at birth. A CT scan showed damage in the left hemisphere. At 10 months of age, he began twice-weekly sessions of traditional NDT physical therapy at this clinic and occupational therapy at a local clinic. When he was 5.5 years of age, he moved to a new location where the frequency of his program was decreased to once weekly.

The child in case 2 was beyond the age that physical therapy is expected to be beneficial.[23] In order to document changes, the Physiological Cost Index (PCI)[24] was measured, and pedographs and gait videos were taken. The PCI is a measure of locomotor efficiency, and a reduction in PCI indicates improved efficiency.

At age 6.7 years, when the child returned for a trial of NMES, the right foot had full passive dorsiflexion while the foot was in subtalar neutral position. Active dorsiflexion was limited to 2 or 3 degrees from a plantarflexed position with knee flexion. When standing, the right foot was markedly pronated. The child walked with a right drop foot and tended to use toe touch at initial contact. He wore a right supramalleolar foot orthosis and a left University of California, Berkeley (UCB) orthosis. A Shutrak pedograph paper[‡] evaluation showed that the left, stronger foot was rotated medially 13 degrees, often crossing in front of the right foot.

The child received NMES for both the right arm and leg. During summer vacation, he was treated for 6 weeks, for a total of 10 visits, with a 2-week break in the middle. The NMES was used initially to stimulate the child's tibialis anterior muscle. The triceps surae muscle was also stimulated after the second week. As the child walked, the tibialis anterior muscle was stimulated with the remote-control hand switch during swing. The triceps surae muscle was stimulated with the release of the switch at foot-strike. The normal immature triceps surae muscle gait pattern[23] was used to determine when to stimulate the leg muscles. Neuromuscular electrical stimulation was used during 15 minutes of walking outdoors, where the child chose the pace.

Following treatment with NMES, the child's PCI[24] measurements showed a factor of four reduction (Tab. 1), indicating a large improvement in walking efficiency.

The child demonstrated increased active range of motion (AROM) of the right foot after receiving NMES. He exhibited from 2 to 3 degrees of active dorsiflexion from a plantarflexed position with knee flexion and

‡Autred-Shutrak Inc, PO Box 20189, Reno, NV 89515-0189.

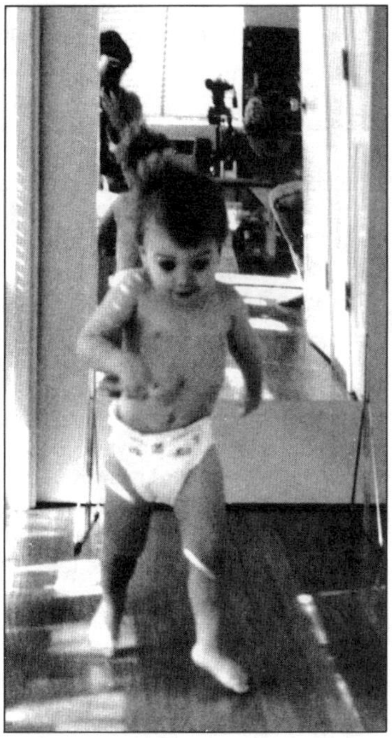

Figure 3. *Carryover is shown as the child in case 1 was photographed while running 4 weeks after the photograph in Figure 2 was taken. Neuromuscular electrical stimulation had not been applied to the medial hamstring muscle for 4 weeks. He is able to alternate his arms and legs.*

from 8 to 10 degrees of active dorsiflexion beyond 90 degrees with or without knee flexion.

Pedographs of the child's left foot showed a change of 13 degrees of medial rotation to 3 degrees of lateral rotation, a 16-degree total change (Tab. 2). Heel-strike occurred at foot contact following treatment with NMES, and the child was able to progress from a right supramalleolar foot orthosis to a UCB orthosis.

The child succeeded in riding a two-wheel bicycle without training wheels. He had tried unsuccessfully to ride a two-wheel bicycle without training wheels for many months before being treated with NMES. According to his parents, he could not balance well enough to stay on the bike to get it moving. After using NMES, he was strong enough to push the pedal with his right foot to get the bike moving. Once it was moving, he could ride and maintain his balance. Increased strength in plantar flexion gave the needed push.

Carryover remained for 1 year after stopping NMES and physical therapy. On return to the school clinic, following the 10 sessions of NMES, his clinic physician discontinued physical therapy. Occupational therapy was continued.

Case 3

The patient in case 3 was a 10-year-old boy at the time NMES was begun. He had left hemiplegia, secondary to cerebral palsy due to prematurity, which affected the lower extremity and trunk more than the upper extremity. His left hand was functional, and no therapy was given to the upper extremity.

The child participated in a brief program of physical therapy during the previous year and was, at the time, on a home program to improve weight shifting to the left side and general strength and coordination. He had also been receiving EMG biofeedback for the tibialis anterior muscle once weekly at another clinic for a year to try to improve active dorsiflexion.

The patient was 10 years of age at the start of the 2-month program with NMES and thus beyond the age that physical therapy is expected to be beneficial.[23] In order to document changes, the child's PCI[24] was measured, and pedographs and gait videos were taken.

Full PROM of the boy's involved foot was present at the beginning of the NMES sessions. Active dorsiflexion was limited to a few degrees from a plantar-flexed position with knee flexion. He was active in sports and attended a regular school program. He wore a left supramalleolar foot orthosis and walked with an obvious vault of the right foot. He had excessive bilateral knee flexion. On initial foot contact, there was approximately 15 degrees of flexion, which increased to 20 to 30 degrees on the loading response. Flexion was more excessive in the right uninvolved knee than in the left involved knee. The child could balance while standing on the right foot with hands on his hips, but he could not do this on the left foot. He was not able to stand on both feet and balance on a large platform swing without strongly holding on with both hands, and his weight shift to the left was inadequate.

On the initial visit, NMES was applied to the motor points of the tibialis anterior and triceps surae muscles reciprocally for a total of 15 minutes while the child was in a sitting position. He was encouraged to actively assist the contractions. When walking, the remote-control switch activated

Table 1. *Physiological Cost Index (PCI)[a] Results[b]*

	Case 2		Case 3	
	Start	End	Start	End
Resting heart rate (beats/min)	98	92	72	71
Walking heart rate (beats/min)	124	100	120	93
Walking speed (m/min)	67.8	81.7	66.5	70.0
PCI (beats/m)	0.38	0.10	0.72	0.31

[a] $PCI=(HR_W-HR_R)/S$, where HR_W=heart rate immediately after walking 100 m, HR_R=resting heart rate, and S=walking speed.

[b] Children walked in their usual orthosis.

Table 2. *Pedograph Results*[a]

	Case 2			Case 3		
	Start	End	Change	Start	End	Change
Left stride (cm)	75.0	82.7	7.7	92.5	85.7	−6.8
Right stride (cm)	74.9	74.6	−0.3	93.8	85.8	−8.0
Left step (cm)	40.5	45.1	4.6	45.7	41.8	−3.9
Right step (cm)	36.3	37.3	1.0	49.0	45.7	−3.3
Step width (cm)	7.8	8.0	0.2	8.5	7.3	−1.2
Angle of toe in/out (°)						
Left	13.5 in	3.0 out	16.5	15.0 out	15.0 out	0.0
Right	2.5 out	5.0 out	2.5	2.3 out	4.0 out	1.7

[a]Values are averaged from footprints made on impression paper.

the tibialis anterior muscle during swing, and when released at heel-strike, the triceps surae muscle was stimulated. Although the child was well over 7 years of age, the immature EMG activity pattern[22] was chosen, as it was felt that he had not experienced this pattern. The time off and on was determined by the timing of the gait. After a return visit to evaluate the home program, the child came once monthly for physical therapy. His mother was instructed in the procedure, and NMES was used at home an average of three times a week for 15 minutes during ambulation. Active dorsiflexion and plantarflexion exercises were also performed over the 2-month treatment period.

Following the 2-month period of treatment, the child's PCI measurements showed a factor of two reduction (Tab. 1), indicating a significant improvement in walking efficiency. Active dorsiflexion improved from 3 degrees of movement in a plantarflexed foot position with a flexed knee to 5 degrees of dorsiflexion beyond 90 degrees with a straight knee in the long-leg sitting position.

The child obtained a smoother gait, with a more symmetrical posture. Vaulting on the right foot was no longer obvious, and the lateral trunk deviation was gone. His balance also improved. He was able to stand on a large mobile four-point swing and tilt it in every direction without holding on with his hands. He was able to put as much weight on the left leg when shifting to the left as he did when shifting to the right side.

The circumference of the boy's left (involved) calf increased 1.3 cm (0.5 in), and that of the right (uninvolved) calf increased 0.6 cm (0.25 in) in the 2-month treatment period. His mother reported a noticeable increase in endurance, as he was able to spend more time in sports. He had an apparent increase in strength in plantar flexion. His improved gait pattern is believed to be due to increased strength of the left leg with increased knee extension.

Physiological Cost Index measurements were taken while the child walked 100 m at a normal pace. The average step length was 58.6 cm/step before NMES and 60.2 cm/step after NMES. His walking speed also increased after NMES (Tab. 1). The cadence was 113 steps/min before NMES and 116 steps/min after NMES.

Pedographs (Tab. 2) show a decrease in stride and step length, perhaps because, as noted at the time, the child slowed down when he reached the starting edge of the paper. Step width narrowed, perhaps due to improved balance. The record also showed slightly improved lateral rotation of the right foot, which could be due to increased strength in the left plantar flexors. Perhaps the increased strength of the left leg allowed time to increase lateral rotation of the right leg.

Discussion

The child in case 1 showed immediate changes, with carryover in his gait, when NMES was used to stimulate the medial hamstring and triceps surae muscles, but NMES did not help when given to the tibialis anterior muscle. Stimulation of the tibialis anterior muscle gave a slight momentary correction to the gait, but this change was not as dramatic as it was when the triceps surae or medial hamstring muscle corrected the gait. After the tibialis anterior muscle was stimulated, the child walked more on the toe than when only the triceps surae muscle was stimulated. Dubowitz et al[14] and Atwater et al[15] also used the tibialis anterior muscle for stimulation without dramatic or immediate results.

Berger and colleagues' EMG studies[25] have shown that the tibialis anterior muscle is active throughout the gait cycle in the immature gait pattern and that the magnitude of the tibialis anterior muscle's EMG activity does not change with the maturation of gait. In nondisabled children, the gastrocnemius muscle's EMG magnitude begins to increase in strength at around 2 years of age and reaches maximal strength at about 4 or 5 years of age. The muscle's EMG magnitude is then about twice as high as that of the tibialis anterior muscle. These EMG studies have also shown that children with cerebral palsy walk with the immature gait pattern of nondisabled 1-year-old children. That is, they walk with a reduced magnitude of gastrocnemius muscle EMG activity, and the tibialis anterior muscle is active throughout the whole step cycle. It may be that lack of coordination and strength of the triceps surae muscle is a significant problem with the walking pattern of children with cerebral palsy and not the lack of tibialis anterior muscle contraction.

The triceps surae muscles of the children in cases 1 through 3 were treated with NMES with no resulting increase in spasticity. Instead, increased ease of PROM of the foot occurred, and the children later learned to actively dorsiflex the foot. In my clinical experience, eight out of eight children with a variety of types of cerebral palsy immediately moved from a plantar-flexed to a plantigrade position with stimulation of the triceps surae muscle.

More time was needed to see improvements in the children in cases 2 and 3. Once the triceps surae muscle of the child in case 1 was stimulated, he immediately became plantigrade. The child in case 2 achieved full dorsiflexion AROM after seven sessions. The child in case 3 achieved full dorsiflexion AROM after 2 months of home sessions conducted three times per week. It appears that the early use of NMES before a pattern becomes too strong a habit makes success much more likely. The older children may have needed more time to build enough strength in the triceps surae muscle to lift their weight. It has been shown that the plantar flexors are normally responsible for two thirds of the total concentric work of gait, whereas the power generation of the ankle plantar flexors in children with cerebral palsy provides only one third.[26]

Another concept concerns stimulating just the triceps surae muscle and not the tibialis anterior muscle. The child in case 1 did not progress with heel-strike or a flat foot until the tibialis anterior muscle was not stimulated. Perhaps the older children would have progressed faster if the triceps surae muscle alone had been stimulated, and then later, if the tibialis anterior muscle was seen to be weak, it could have been stimulated. At the time, the tibialis anterior muscle appeared to be weak in the older children, as the leg appeared somewhat atrophied compared with the uninvolved leg.

It was not expected that the children in cases 2 and 3 would improve in gait due to their age and current skill level. Bleck[23] cites various physicians and researchers who have found that, for children with cerebral palsy, motor gains reached a plateau or ceased between the ages of 6 and 7 years. The child in case 2, at almost 7 years of age, and the child in case 3, at 10 years of age, however, showed significant improvement after a short time with NMES.

The child in case 3 had been treated with biofeedback EMG to the tibialis anterior muscle without significant change. It was only when alternating NMES was applied to the triceps surae and tibialis anterior muscles that complete active dorsiflexion occurred and strength and gait efficiency increased in plantar flexion and dorsiflexion.

The child in case 2 had received 4 years of NDT physical therapy and occupational therapy without NMES. The only change in his program that occurred during the 6-week period was the addition of NMES with the task-oriented model of motor control. I believe that the use of NMES was very important in improving the child's sensory awareness and strength, which resulted in increased coordination.

Summary and Conclusions

Following a program of NMES, three children demonstrated rapid functional changes. The children in cases 2 and 3 showed significant improvement in gait efficiency and balance in a short time even though they were past the age when this improvement was expected. The child in case 2 maintained the improved gait for 1 year after stopping physical therapy. The child in case 1 showed immediate and more rapid results, with greater carryover, than did the older children. It is possible that the abnormal movement strategies were not as habitual in the younger child and biomechanical changes had not yet occurred in the muscles, making change easier to obtain.

Preliminary findings suggest that NMES may be a useful physical therapy tool when used with task-oriented functional activities. Electrical stimulation may enhance muscle contraction and provide sensation so that a child can add a weak response with effective results and assist in improving motor control.

Acknowledgments

I thank Cathleen Pewthers for her initial suggestion to try NMES when biofeedback EMG was unsuccessful; the subjects and their parents for allowing the clinical results to be shared; and Medtronic Nortech Division for the loan of one of the NMES instruments, together with the necessary disposable electrodes, used in this research.

References

1 Delitto A, Snyder-Mackler L. Two theories of muscle strength augmentation using percutaneous electrical stimulation. *Phys Ther.* 1990; 70:158–164.

2 Alfieri V. Electrical treatment of spasticity. *Scand J Rehabil Med.* 1982;14:177–182.

3 DeVahl J. Neuromuscular electrical stimulation in rehabilitation. In: Gersh MR, ed. *Electrotherapy in Rehabilitation.* Philadelphia, Pa: FA Davis Co; 1992:218–268.

4 Carnstam B, Larsson L, Prevec TS. Improvement of gait following functional electrical stimulation. *Scand J Rehabil Med.* 1977;9:7–13.

5 Leyendecker CH. Electrical stimulation therapy and its effect on the general activity of motor-impaired cerebral-palsied children: a comparative study of the Bobath physiotherapy and its combination with the Hufschmidt electrical stimulation therapy. *Rehabilitation.* 1975; 14:150–159.

6 Gorden J. Assumptions underlying physical therapy intervention: theoretical and historical perspectives. In: Carr JH, Shepherd RB, Gorden J, et al, eds. *Movement Science Foundation for Physical Therapy in Rehabilitation.* Rockville, Md: Aspen Publishers Inc; 1987:1–30.

7 Valvano J, Long T. Neurodevelopmental treatment: a review of the writings of the Bobaths. *Pediatric Physical Therapy.* 1991; 3:125–129.

8 Horak FB. Assumptions underlying motor control for neurologic rehabilitation. In: *Contemporary Management of Motor Control Problems: Proceedings of the II Step Conference.* Alexandria, Va: Foundation for Physical Therapy Inc; 1991:11–27.

9 Atwater SW. Should the normal motor developmental sequence be used as a theoretical model in pediatric physical therapy? In: *Contemporary Management of Motor Control Problems: Proceedings of the II Step Conference.* Alexandria, Va: Foundation for Physical Therapy Inc; 1991:89–93.

10 Bly L. A historical and current view basis of NDT. *Pediatric Physical Therapy.* 1991; 3:131–135.

11 Gracanin F, Vrabic M, Vrabic G. Six years of experiences with FES method applied to children. *Europa Medicophysia.* 1976;12:61–68.

12 Kieklak H, DeVahl J. Protocol for pediatric applications. In: *Medtronic Bulletin on Use of the Respond II.* San Diego, Calif: Medtronic Nortech Division; 1986.

13 Kieklak H. Use of neuromuscular electrical stimulation (NMES) for children with neuromuscular disorders. *Tot Line* (publication of the Americal Physical Therapy Association Section on Pediatrics). 1987;13:27.

14 Dubowitz L, Finnie N, Hyde SA, et al. Improvement of muscle performance by chronic electrical stimulation in children with cerebral palsy. *Lancet.* March 12, 1988:587–588. Letter.

15 Atwater SW, Tatarka ME, Kathrein JE, Shapiro S. Electromyography-triggered electrical muscle stimulation for children with cerebral palsy: a pilot study. *Pediatric Physical Therapy.* 1991;3:190–199.

16 Carr JH, Shepherd RB, Gorden J, et al. *Movement Science Foundation for Physical Therapy in Rehabilitation.* Rockville, Md. Aspen Publishers Inc; 1987.

17 Carr JH, Shepherd RB. A motor-learning model for rehabilitation of the movement disabled. Ada L, Canning C, eds. *Key Issues in Neurological Physiotherapy.* Oxford, England: Butterworth-Heinemann Ltd; 1990:1–24.

18 Van der Weel FR, Vandermeer ALH, Lee DN. Effect of task on movement control in cerebral palsy: implication for assessment and therapy. *Dev Med Child Neurol.* 1991; 33:419–426.

19 Baker LL, Parker K. Neuromuscular electrical stimulation of the muscles surrounding the shoulder. *Phys Ther.* 1986;66:1930–1937.

20 Delitto A, Robinson AJ. Electrical stimulation of muscle: techniques and applications. In: Snyder-Mackler L, Robinson AJ, eds. *Clinical Electrophysiology.* Baltimore, Md: Williams & Wilkins; 1989:97–138.

21 Kahanovitz N, Nordin M, Verderame R, et al. Normal trunk muscle strength and endurance in women and the effect of exercises and electrical stimulation, part 2: comparative analysis of electrical stimulation and exercises to increase trunk muscle strength and endurance. *Science.* 1982;216:112–118.

22 Sutherland D, Olshen R, Biden E, Watt M. *The Development of Mature Walking.* Philadelphia, Pa; Mac Keith Press; 1988:158.

23 Bleck E. *Orthopaedic Management in Cerebral Palsy.* Philadelphia, Pa: Mac Keith Press; 1987.

24 Butler P, Engelbrecht M, Major RE, et al. Physiological cost index of walking for normal children and its use as an indicator of physical handicap. *Dev Med Child Neurol.* 1984; 26:607–612.

25 Berger W, Altenmueller E, Dietz V. Normal and impaired development of children's gait. *Human Neurobiology.* 1984;3:163–170.

26 Olney SJ. Work and power in hemiplegic cerebral palsy gait. *Phys Ther.* 1990;70:431–438.

Case Report

Clinical Use of Neuromuscular Electrical Stimulation for Children With Cerebral Palsy, Part 2: Upper Extremity

Judy Carmick

This report, part 2 of a two-part case report on the clinical use of neuromuscular electrical stimulation (NMES) for children with cerebral palsy, documents the functional changes that occurred with the application of NMES to the upper extremity of two children, 1.6 and 6.7 years of age, with hemiplegia due to cerebral palsy. The NMES was used as an adjunct to a dynamic-systems, task-oriented physical therapy program. The youngest child showed immediate improvement in the ability to crawl and use both hands together. The older child demonstrated increased sensory awareness and use of the nonfunctional hand. Preliminary findings suggest that NMES may be a useful physical therapy tool for enhancing muscle strength, increasing sensory awareness, and assisting motor learning and coordination. [Carmick J. Clinical use of neuromuscular electrical stimulation for children with cerebral palsy, part 2: upper extremity. Phys Ther. 1993;73:514–527.]

Key Words: *Cerebral palsy, Motor control, Neuromuscular electrical stimulation, Pediatrics, Upper extremity.*

This report, part 2 of a two-part case report on the clinical use of neuromuscular electrical stimulation (NMES) for children with cerebral palsy, documents the use of NMES for improving the motor control and sensory awareness of the upper extremity of two children with hemiplegic cerebral palsy from birth. The NMES was given as an adjunct to a dynamic-systems or contemporary motor-learning physical therapy program. The principles of motor learning that were emphasized included playing in a task-specific activity in a position in which the stimulated muscle would normally function and allowing the child freedom to make mistakes and learn from them. The children in this report are the same children discussed in cases 1 and 2 in part 1 of the two-part case report.

Neuromuscular Electrical Stimulation Equipment Used

The Respond II unit* was used. This unit has two channels that allowed two different muscles to be stimulated at the same time or at alternating times. Electrical stimulation was always kept within the child's tolerance. The portability of the unit allowed the child to move freely. A remote-control switch was used to stimulate the muscle as needed.

Reuseable, self-adhering, pregelled, carbonized-rubber electrodes* were used. The active electrode was placed on the motor point, and the inactive electrode was placed on the same muscle or muscle group a short distance away from the active electrode. The active electrode was cut to size, never smaller than a nickel, so that only the desired muscle would be stimulated and thus eliminate or decrease overflow. The suggestions of Baker and Parker[1] and Delitto and Robinson[2] for electrode placements were often used.

The pulse rate was often initially set to about 5 to 7 pulses per second (pps), which gave a tapping sensation

J Carmick, PT, is in private practice, 3060 Miranda Ave, Alamo, CA 94507-1611 (USA).

This paper was presented in poster format at the Combined Sections Meeting of the American Physical Therapy Association; February 5-10, 1992; San Francisco, CA.

This article was submitted December 14, 1992, and was accepted March 22, 1993.

*Medtronic Nortech Division, 10237 Flanders Ct, San Diego, CA 92121.

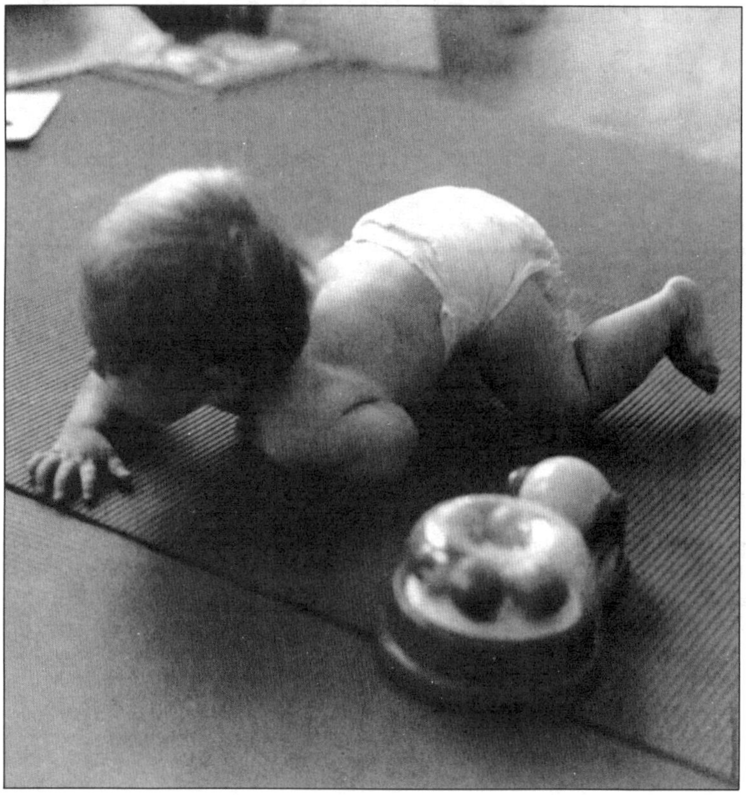

Figure 1. *Child in case 1 at 10 months of age, before neuromuscular electrical stimulation, shown as he was attempting to creep. He continued with this creeping style, with no weight bearing on the left upper extremity unless given assistance, until age 15 months when he could walk. After he learned to walk, he was not interested in creeping.*

and sensory input but not a fused contraction. When this sensation was tolerated by the child, the setting was increased to between 30 and 35 pps to give a fused muscle contraction. The amplitude was slowly increased until a contraction could be felt and kept within the child's tolerance.

The output-limit control was set for 50% of the stimulator's maximum amplitude. The amplitude was increased very slowly, to the child's tolerance, and only when the current was on. As the child became familiar with the simulation, his tolerance increased and the amplitude could be increased to obtain a stronger muscle contraction. It was not necessary to have a maximal contraction to increase sensory awareness or strength of the weak muscle.[3,4] With a low pulse rate, a higher amplitude is tolerated.[5] Thus, the muscle contraction can be more easily seen so that the physical therapist can determine whether the correct muscle is being stimulated before changing the rate to obtain a sustained muscle contraction at a less visible amplitude.

The ramp, or rise time, was initially set at the lowest setting (8 seconds) for the most comfort. When the child was accustomed to NMES, the ramp was set for approximately 2 seconds. When a quicker response was needed, such as during gait, the fastest rise time (0.5 second) was used. On-off times initially were set for 10 seconds on and 25 seconds off. Once the child was comfortable with electrical stimulation and not showing signs of fatigue, the cycle was set at 15 seconds on and 15 seconds off for a total of 15 to 20 minutes. When the remote-control switch was used, the on time was determined by activation of the switch, which was facilitated according to the child's functional needs. For example, when the child was picking up an object to put into a container, the electrodes on the wrist extensors were facilitated with the remote-control switch the entire time he was doing the movement. This could be longer or shorter than 15 seconds. The finger extensors were then stimulated at the time of release until the release was accomplished. All electrodes were then silent when the child returned his arm to pick up another item.

The electrodes could also be used to assist with opening of the hand to grasp an item. When the child was first experiencing wrist extension with NMES, the alternating mode was used as he played with toys on a table. Wrist extension is used for both grasp and release, so the periodic timing of the unit cycling on and off for 15 seconds on the wrist extensors as he played would not have interfered with the acquisition of wrist extension skill. When he was comfortable with NMES and could tolerate a quicker rise time, the remote-control switch was used to stimulate the muscle when he began to reach or to release.

The child was given time to experience and accept the sensation. Letting the child in case 2 turn the unit on and off with the remote-control switch gave him appropriate control initially. He was almost 7 years of age and curious about mechanical items. He was also interested in what was going to happen to him, and he needed to have some control over the situation in order to more easily accept the intrusion. When the child was allowed to use the remote-control switch, he could determine how long or how short the stimulation would be. He was learning what would happen if he left it on. It took only a short time for him to understand the mechanics and to be satisfied that all would be com-

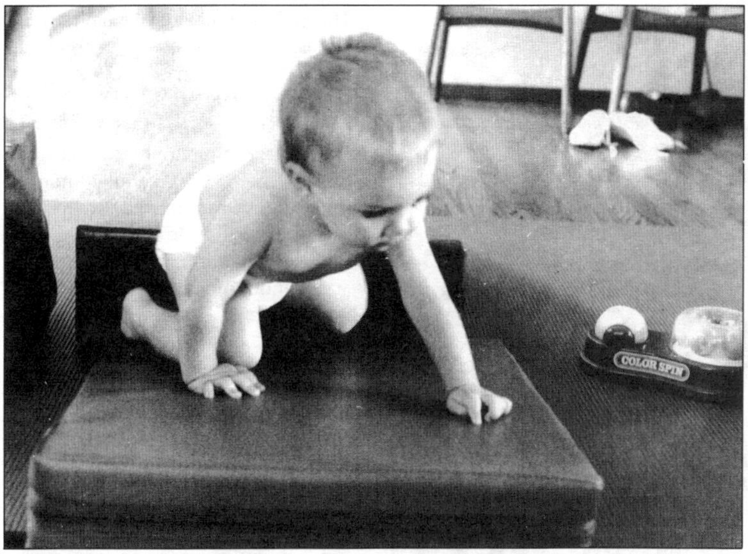

Figure 2. *Child in case 1 shown creeping down from one wedge to another 3 weeks after initial application of neuromuscular electrical stimulation to the triceps brachii muscle. He was 19.5 months of age.*

fortable enough. This took little time, as the child quickly showed interest in returning to his therapeutic activity. With acceptance and experience of the child, the amplitude was increased with the child's approval to improve muscle contraction.

Introducing Children to Neuromuscular Electrical Stimulation

Initially, NMES was demonstrated on the therapist's arm and then on the parent's arm. This was to give the parent experience with NMES to help eliminate any fear of electrical stimulation that might be transferred to the child.

The children in cases 1 and 2 were first introduced to a hand-held vibrator, which was called a "tickler." The NMES was described as being like the "tickler," and the children were told they would feel a tapping sensation. The electrode was then placed on the cleaned body part. The amplitude was initially increased very slowly until the child indicated that he felt the stimulation or until a trace contraction was felt or seen. As the child became accustomed to the stimulus, a higher amplitude was used to obtain a stronger contraction.

Case 1

The child in case 1 was a 19-month-old boy who was diagnosed with left hemiplegia secondary to cerebral palsy following a computerized tomography (CT) scan. The lesion was believed to have occurred prenatally. He began receiving physical therapy at age 7 months. Physical therapy followed the task-oriented model of motor learning and included neurodevelopmental therapy (NDT) techniques and various therapeutic techniques to increase sensory awareness. He walked at age 15 months. The child initially received NMES to his upper extremity when he was only 19 months of age and to the lower extremity when he was 21 months of age.

At age 19 months, the child's upper-extremity function and regard were limited. He did not use the hand, and his arm was usually seen just hanging by his side; he rarely appeared to notice his left upper extremity. He could not creep on his hands and knees or play with the left hand. He often placed the back, not the palm, of the left hand on the supporting surface when he was placed in a quadrupedal position. The child could take some weight on the extended arm if given assistance to maintain elbow extension, but he would resist any assistance to creep. He would collapse and struggle to get out of the

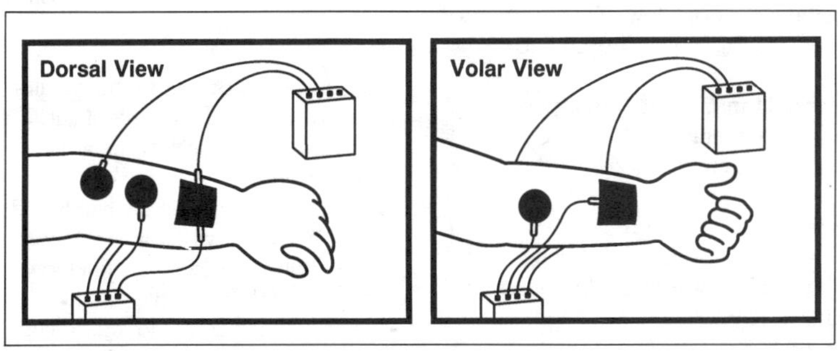

Figure 3. *Drawings show dorsal and volar views of an advanced hookup with two neuromuscular electrical stimulation (NMES) units. Each unit used a remote-control switch (not shown) for independent operation. The NMES unit in the foreground stimulated either the finger extensors or flexors, as determined by the remote-control switch. When the switch was pressed, the finger flexors were stimulated, enabling the child to grasp an object. When the switch was not pressed, the finger extensors were stimulated, enabling the child to release the object. The NMES unit in the background stimulated the wrist extensors when the remote-control switch was pressed.*

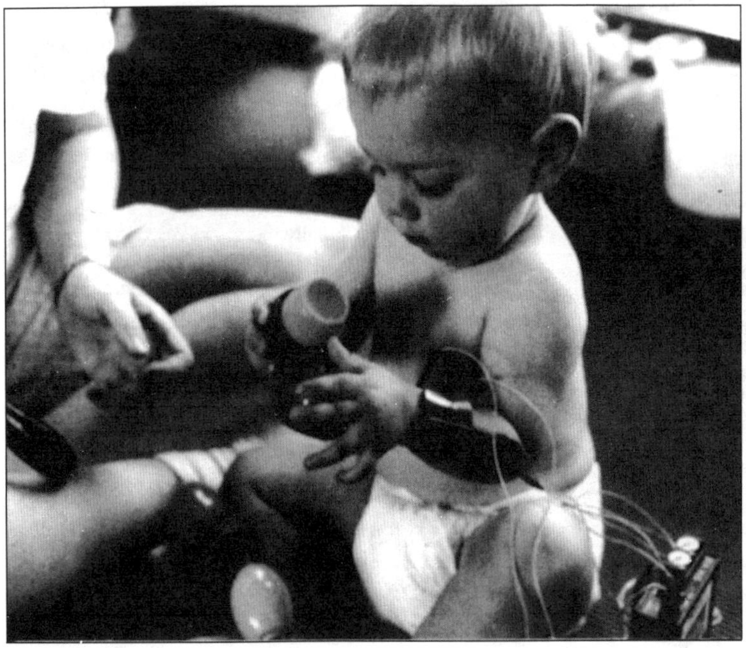

Figure 4. *Photograph taken the first time neuromuscular electrical stimulation was used on the forearm of the child in case 1 for wrist extension and finger flexion. He was taking apart loosely fitted nested barrels. He was 21 months of age.*

position. He learned to walk at 15 months of age, before he could creep.

By age 19 months, the child had learned to push an object into his left hand with his right hand but was unable to release the object due to the tight grasp. He needed to pull it out strongly with the right hand. When walking and carrying an object in the left hand, the hand would open and the toy would fall out. He had never played with both hands together without assistance, nor could he clap his hands. He had just begun to reach with the left arm but lacked full active range of motion of shoulder flexion and elbow and wrist extension. Passive range of motion of all upper-extremity joints was complete.

Various therapeutic techniques were included in the child's program to increase sensory awareness, active weight shifting, and weight bearing to the left side and extremities. A vibrator had been used for the triceps brachii muscle when the child was attempting to creep or rock on his hands and knees. It was used to give sensory input to the muscle and to increase muscle contraction slightly with the tonic vibratory response.[6] The vibrator was helpful, but when removed, the arm would collapse. An inflatable sleeve[7] was also used while creeping, but the splinting of the elbow did not allow elbow flexion for play after creeping over to a toy.

After 11 months of 1 hour-per-week physical therapy and a home program, the child's moderate disuse of his arm continued. Figure 1 shows his creeping style before NMES was used. He was 10 months of age when the photograph was taken, but his creeping style was the same at age 15 months.

At 19 months of age, NMES was used on the child's left triceps brachii muscle to augment muscle contraction and/or awareness. The amplitude was raised slowly until he appeared to notice the sensation. He indicated this by looking at the arm, but he made no attempt to remove the electrodes. The child immediately began to use the arm for the first time in creeping about the room unassisted, except for the use of NMES. He seemed very pleased and continued with creeping and moving to a sitting position and back to creeping for about 10 minutes until NMES was removed. Creeping was unexpected. He had never crept on his hands and knees unassisted and without much protesting when it was attempted. The low-amplitude NMES was able to assist in improving the child's muscle contraction and, probably, his sensory awareness.

Carryover occurred when NMES was removed. During the following week, the child continued to creep 0.3 to 0.6 m (1-2 ft) at home each day. Figure 2 shows his creeping style after only three weekly 15-minute sessions of NMES applied to the triceps brachii muscle. This dramatic improvement may be due to increased sensory awareness and augmented contraction[5,8] of the muscle, as enough strength appeared to be present to permit the activity.

When low-amplitude NMES was added to the child's active weak muscle contraction, the resulting contraction was augmented. As discussed in this report and illustrated by the photographs, with NMES to augment the muscle contraction, the child was immediately able to perform activities that he had not done previously.

The sensory assistance of the vibrator coupled with the therapist's slight physical pressure against the arm would maintain the elbow extension when the child was on his hands and knees. When the vibrator or support was withdrawn, however, the elbow collapsed and the child could not remain on his hands and knees. With NMES augmenting the child's weak triceps brachii muscle contraction, no outside support was needed and the child was able to functionally succeed at creeping on his hands and knees for the first time.

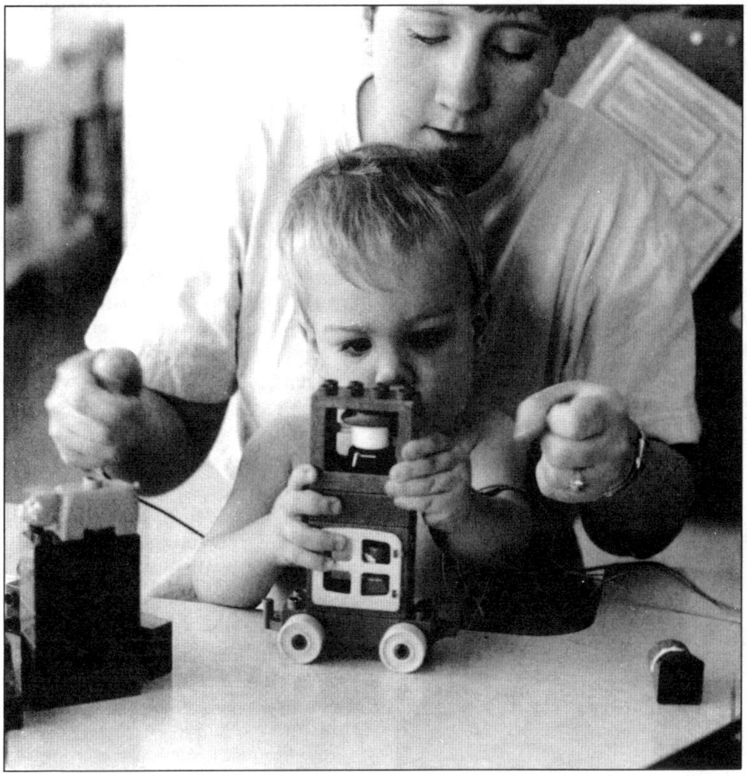

Figure 5. *Photograph of child in case 1 taken 2 months after photograph shown in figure 4. The child is shown building with interlocking toy blocks as neuromuscular electrical stimulation is used to stimulate the finger flexors and elbow extensors. He is using active wrist extension. The remote-control switch in the adult's hand controlled stimulation of the finger flexors. The child was 23 months old.*

The child's hand remained nonfunctional. He could bear weight on it, but when he tried to put something in the hand, the wrist remained flexed and the fingers did not often grasp. He needed to be able to use finger flexion and extension for grasp and release. He needed to use wrist extension to make grasp efficient and strong, as grasp is weak with the wrist held in flexion.

Figure 3 shows how NMES was used for various hand and wrist movement patterns. Initially, one NMES unit was used, with the electrodes on the dorsal surface of the arm stimulating the wrist extensors and those on the volar surface stimulating the finger flexors. Initially, the unit was set in a symmetrical mode so that both the wrist extensors and the finger flexors were stimulated simultaneously when the remote-control switch was used. When the switch was released, no stimulus was felt.

Five weeks after the initial use on the triceps brachii muscle, NMES was used to stimulate hand function. The child had not used wrist extension or both hands together. The electrodes were placed to stimulate the wrist extensors and finger flexors. He was given loosely fitted nesting barrels to play with to encourage him to use both hands together.

With NMES, the child immediately began to use both hands together, as shown by photographs taken during that first session. Figure 4 shows him using both hands together for the first time. With NMES stimulating the wrist extensors and finger flexors, he was able to separate the barrels. The carryover was maintained in the following week. The child appeared more aware of his left hand, and he could be encouraged fairly easily to use both hands together.

In the next 2 months, NMES was used for various movement patterns, depending on need. Observations of the child, combined with the parents' report on the results from the previous physical therapy visit, formed the clinical judgment for which muscle groups needed stimulation that day. Occasionally, when the child did not bring the arm forward, the anterior deltoid or triceps brachii muscle was stimulated. If he still did not use shoulder flexion or bring the arm forward, both muscles were stimulated. The wrist was usually stimulated during each visit, with electrodes added to other areas, depending on success. The wrist extensors and the finger flexors and extensors were often stimulated while the child played with manipulative toys. Two NMES units and two remote-control switches were used to accomplish this assist (Fig. 3). One unit stimulated the wrist extensors only. The other unit alternately stimulated the finger extensors and flexors. Each unit had a separate remote-control switch. As the child played, grasp or release could be facilitated without the therapist's hands constantly interfering with play. With NMES augmenting the muscle contraction, the child had enough muscle output to move the body part without needing assistance. This freedom to move and function gave the child a chance for better motor learning, including developing some anticipatory or feed-forward skills.

The child's functional abilities during the treatment session determined which muscles were facilitated. The setup shown in Figure 3 allows four different muscle groups to be used. The child was observed to determine which muscles he was using and which muscles were not being used. The three leads allow wrist extension

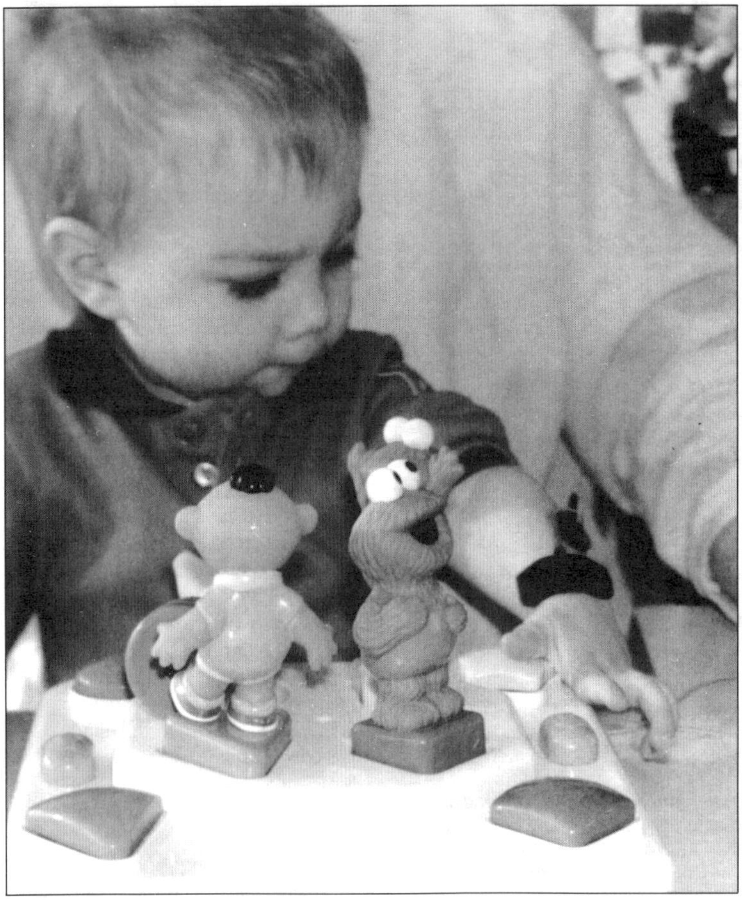

Figure 6. *Child in case 1 demonstrating thumb abduction and extension with neuromuscular electrical stimulation as he pushed buttons on a pop-up toy. He was 28 months of age.*

on one unit with another lead not being used. Sometimes the elbow extensors, shoulder flexors, or thumb abductors were stimulated. The lead on the unit with the lead to the wrist extensors was often used to stimulate the additional muscle. If his reaching was not adequate, the lead assisted the anterior deltoid muscle. If the thumb tended to be held in the palm, the lead stimulated the thumb abductors. The stimulus was given simultaneously with the wrist extensors.

The child in case 1 used the wrist extensors much of the time but was not able to maintain finger flexion to hold on to an object. In Figure 5, he is shown using active wrist extension with NMES to assist in finger flexion and elbow extension while stacking interlocking toy blocks. The amplitude was low, just enough for him to feel the stimulus but not enough for him to be distracted.

Two months after beginning NMES, the child in case 1 extended his involved hand to his mother to wash after eating. This was the first time that he had extended his involved hand to his mother, as he had not previously used that hand when eating. It appeared that NMES was improving the child's sensory awareness. A month later, he was able to hold on to a toy golf club and maintain his grasp as he swung. He was also able to hold a plastic baseball bat with both hands and was sometimes able to maintain the two-handed grip at the end of the swing.

The child's thumb extensors and abductors were stimulated with NMES as he played with toys that motivated thumb movement. Figure 6 shows NMES used to increase extension and abduction of the thumb. The result was easier passive range of motion of the hand and thumb. The child showed good carryover, as he used the thumb intermittently during therapy when playing with and without NMES. The photograph shown in Figure 6 was taken 9 months after the initial use of NMES. Weekly NDT occupational therapy was added to the weekly physical therapy program when he was 24 months of age.

The child's abilities varied from week to week. Carryover from NMES lasted for a few days to an entire week. Task-oriented activities were chosen that were thought to be age-appropriate and of interest to him. Neuromuscular electrical stimulation was used to encourage the movement pattern or muscle group that was not being used.

At 25 months of age, the child made many gains after 6 months of once-weekly physical therapy with NMES. The most significant gain was increased awareness and spontaneous use of the left arm and hand. He was able to creep, climb, and use both hands together. His grasp and release were much improved. Disregard of the left extremity was no longer observed.

Case 2

The child in case 2 was a 6.7-year-old boy when he began receiving NMES to both the upper and lower extremities. He was diagnosed as having cerebral palsy due to sporadic oxygen deprivation at birth. A CT scan showed damage in the left hemisphere. At 10 months of age, he began twice-weekly sessions of tradi-

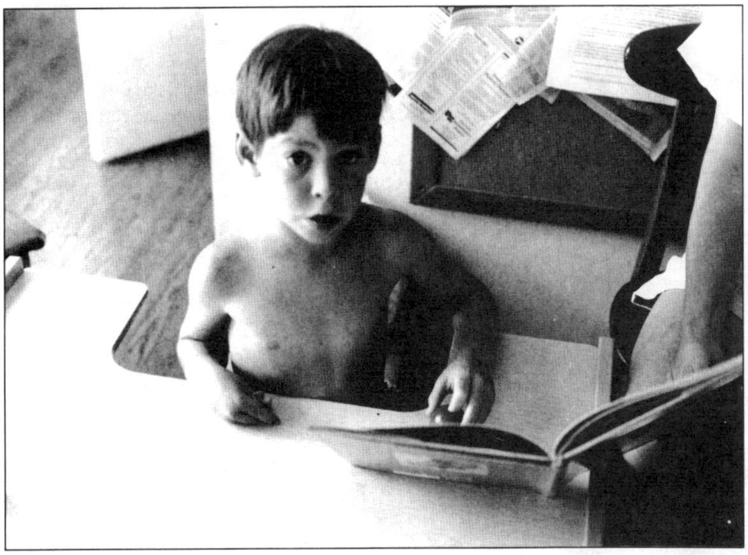

Figure 7. *Child in case 2 before neuromuscular electrical stimulation was used. He was 6.7 years old.*

tional NDT† physical therapy at this clinic and occupational therapy at a local clinic. When he was 5.5 years of age, he moved to a new location where the frequency of his program was decreased to once weekly.

When the child was 5 years of age and receiving twice-weekly physical therapy and occupational therapy, in the clinic he demonstrated minimal ability to use his right hand to assist the left hand. He had slight active dorsiflexion and would use a lateral pinch with his right thumb and index finger to help hold a lightweight object. When he returned to this clinic to receive NMES at almost 7 years of age, his hand was not functional and was infrequently used. There was strong disregard of the upper extremity, and he was not able to contract the wrist extensors. The right arm was noticeably smaller and shorter than the left arm. The forearm and hand appeared atrophied. Figure 7 shows the child before NMES was used.

Evaluation showed that the child was unable to extend the wrist and that he had a poor understanding of how to use the left hand to put an object into the right hand, even when he was requested to do so. Figure 8 shows the child attempting to wind a top by pushing it against the lip of the table. The right wrist was often held in excessive flexion, with the fingers extended with ulnar deviation. The thumb was flexed and adducted in the palm. When the fingers extended, hyperextension occurred at the metacarpophalangeal joint and the wrist remained in excessive flexion. He sometimes used his left hand as a block or post for the right hand. If an object was put into the hand so that the fingers were placed around it, the flexor grasp reflex tended to keep the object in the hand for a short time. The child had to pull the object out of the hand, as release was not possible.

The child at 6.7 years of age received twice-weekly NMES sessions for 6 weeks, for a total of 10 visits, with a 2-week break in the middle. The NMES was given to the elbow extensors, wrist and thumb extensors, thumb abductors, and finger flexors during task-oriented activities. Suggestions for physical therapy activities were taken from Carr and colleagues.[13–15]

Initially, stimulation of the wrist extensors did not demonstrate even a trace contraction. The child did have feeling in the arm and was able to verbalize when the amplitude was high enough. After 2 weeks, a trace contraction was barely felt when NMES was used. Although the wrist did not actively extend except in a mass movement pattern, the child appeared to have more sensation, as shown by his increased use of the hand.

The photograph in Figure 9 was taken after seven sessions with NMES. The child appeared to have more awareness of the hand, and he was able to put the spinning top into the left hand and use both hands together to wind the top and press the button so that it could spin, without the use of NMES.

Spontaneous use of the hand improved. After the sixth session, the child spontaneously took an ice-cream cone in his right hand from his mother. After nine sessions, the photograph in Figure 10 was taken. His hands are on a hoop that he picked up and rolled back and forth before releasing it to send it rolling. As his hand awareness progressed, he continued to use it more for reaching and touching objects that he was passing, such as running his hand along a banister. He learned how to put items into the right hand to hold

†Traditional NDT assumptions[9] follow a hierarchical and reflex model[10,11] of motor control. Abnormal muscle tone (spasticity) is considered a major problem for treatment and a cause of much of the motor deficit. Patients are advised not to exert excessive effort, which is believed to be a potential for increasing abnormal muscle tone and to result in loss of reciprocal movement activity. Normal movement is facilitated, and abnormal movement patterns are inhibited. The child does not have much opportunity to move unassisted and learn to correct his or her own mistakes. Development is expected to progress from proximal to distal, so the shoulder is expected to develop before the hand. Current NDT assumptions[12] and therapy techniques are changing as new knowledge of motor control and motor learning is discovered.

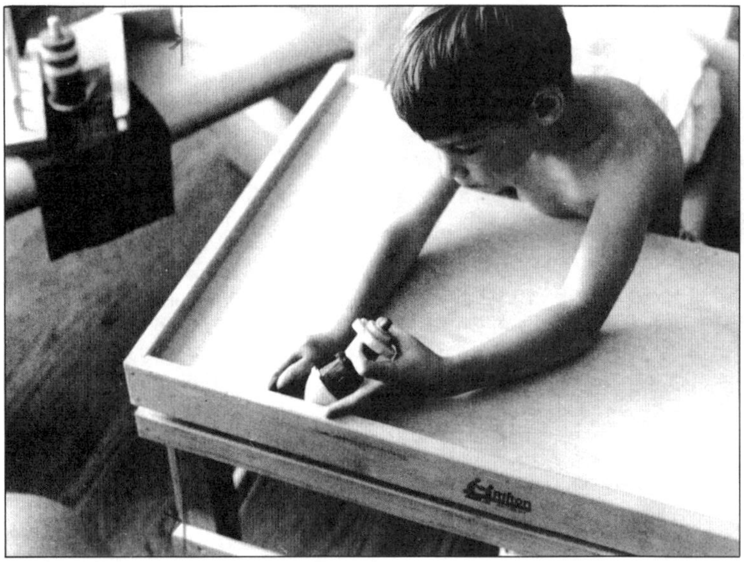

Figure 8. *Child in case 2, before neuromuscular electrical stimulation was used, trying unsuccessfully to push two spinning top pieces together.*

with the left hand and had better understanding of using the hands together. He was able to release objects, although not quickly, without having to pull them from the hand. He maintained hand awareness, including the ability to contract the wrist extensors, although there was only a Trace grade of contraction, for 1 year after discontinuing the program of NMES and physical therapy.

Discussion

Although the younger child (case 1) had 11 months of physical therapy with a systems-model approach, the poor function and awareness of the arm and hand did not change until NMES was added to the program when he was 1.6 years of age. When that happened, he learned to creep and to use both hands together. His functional use of the hand and arm continued to progress with further use of NMES, and disregard of the hand and arm was no longer seen at 2 years of age.

The older child (case 2) had a hierarchical-model (NDT) physical therapy program from age 2 years until he was 6.8 years of age. At that time, he had lost the little skill that he had when he was 5 years of age. His upper extremity was not functioning, his hand appeared atrophied, and the right arm was noticeably smaller than the left arm. He had grown over the almost 2-year period, so it would be expected that biomechanical changes in the involved extremity could have some effect on the loss of function.[16] It took four sessions of electrical stimulation of the wrist extensors before a muscle contraction could clearly be felt. After only 10 sessions of physical therapy with NMES, the child was spontaneously using his right (involved) hand, and occasionally he used the right hand independently to hold items.

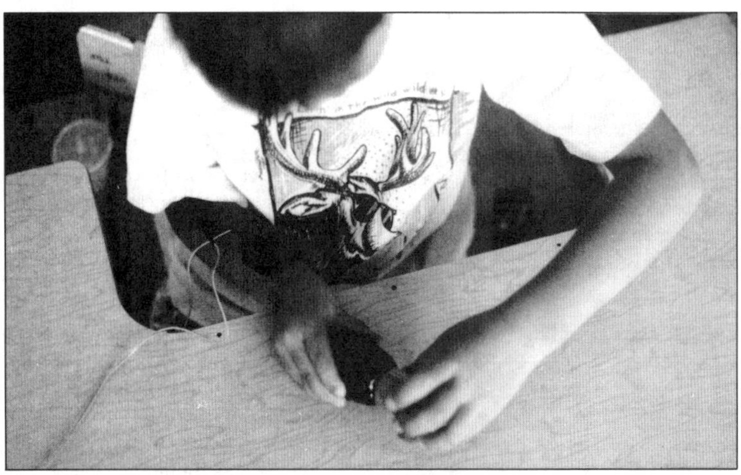

Figure 9. *Child in case 2 after seven treatments with neuromuscular electrical stimulation. He is using both hands together to wind a spinning top.*

Recommendations

The muscles of the hand are small, especially in children. I prefer to use a low pulse rate initially for treating children with cerebral palsy by use of NMES. A low rate, about 5 to 7 pps, is usually more comfortable to the child, and the amplitude can be higher. This produces a more discernable twitch that will allow the therapist to see whether the desired muscle is actually the one being stimulated or whether there is too much overflow.

Lack of coordination or sensory awareness of how to use the hand is often a major problem in a child with cerebral palsy.[17] A low pulse rate may give enough sensory input to assist the child with function. Some children do not like the low rate. It is

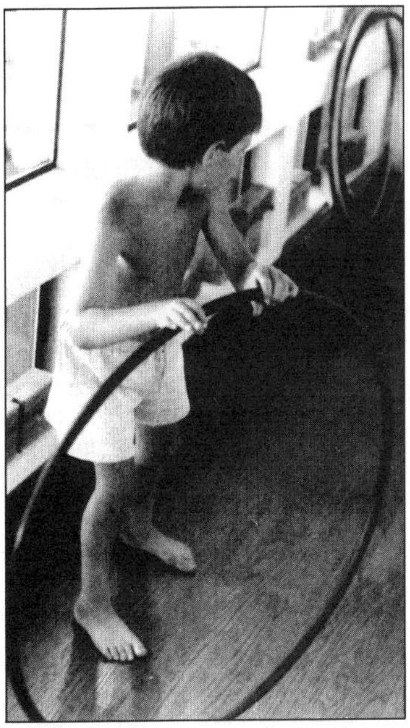

Figure 10. *Child in case 2 photographed as he spontaneously picked up and rolled a hoop back and forth before releasing it to roll down the hall. Photograph was taken after eight sessions of neuromuscular electrical stimulation.*

necessary to experiment to find what works best for each individual.

I believe that NMES should be used in conjunction with a task-oriented model of motor learning. The physical therapist should consider the recent discoveries in motor control and motor learning. Normal development does not progress only from proximal to distal, but in parallel.[9,17] Hand or wrist development may help the shoulder development. I believe that suggestions by Carr and colleagues,[13–15] although for adults, often can apply or be adapted to children.

Summary and Conclusions

Two children, both with hemiplegic cerebral palsy from birth, improved in upper-extremity function and awareness after the addition of NMES to their systems-model physical therapy program. The child in case 1, who began NMES at 1.6 years of age, showed immediate and surprising functional changes in both the upper and lower extremities that were more dramatic and rapid than those seen in the child in case 2 at almost 7 years of age.

The use of NMES demonstrated important functional changes with children with cerebral palsy that warrant further investigation. Preliminary findings suggest that NMES may be a useful physical therapy tool when used with a task-oriented model of motor learning. It would be of interest to learn whether electrical stimulation could enhance motor learning and control enough to increase function so that the biomechanical changes that occur with growth deficiencies would not occur. More studies are needed to determine whether NMES can benefit other children with upper motor neuron lesions.

Acknowledgments

I thank Herb Kieklak for his suggestions, including urging me to use NMES on young children and to consider working with the thumb. I also thank Medtronic Nortech Division for the loan of one of the NMES instruments, together with the necessary disposable electrodes, used in this research.

References

1 Baker LL, Parker K. Neuromuscular electrical stimulation of the muscles surrounding the shoulder. *Phys Ther.* 1986;66:1930–1937.

2 Delitto A, Robinson AJ. Electrical stimulation of muscle: techniques and applications. In: Snyder-Mackler L, Robinson AJ, eds. *Clinical Electrophysiology.* Baltimore, Md: Williams & Wilkins; 1989:97–138.

3 Kahanovitz N, Nordin M, Verderame R, et al. Normal trunk muscle strength and endurance in women and the effect of exercises and electrical stimulation, part 2: comparative analysis of electrical stimulation and exercises to increase trunk muscle strength and endurance. *Science.* 1982;216:112–118.

4 Alfieri V. Electrical treatment of spasticity. *Scand J Rehabil Med.* 1982;14:177–182.

5 DeVahl J. Neuromuscular electrical stimulation in rehabilitation. In: Gersh MR, ed. *Electrotherapy in Rehabilitation.* Philadelphia, Pa: FA Davis Co; 1992:218–268.

6 Bishop B. Vibratory stimulation, part III: possible applications of vibration in treatment of motor dysfunctions. *Phys Ther.* 1975;55: 139–143.

7 Montgomery P. Use of air splints in brachial plexus injuries. *Pediatric Physical Therapy.* 1989;1:85–86.

8 Trimble MH, Enoka RM. Mechanisms underlying the training effects associated with neuromuscular electrical stimulation. *Phys Ther.* 1991;71:273–281.

9 Gorden J. Assumptions underlying physical therapy intervention: theoretical and historical perspectives. In: Carr JH, Shepherd RB, Gorden J, et al, eds. *Movement Science Foundation for Physical Therapy in Rehabilitation.* Rockville, Md: Aspen Publishers Inc; 1987:1–30.

10 Horak FB. Assumptions underlying motor control for neurologic rehabilitation. In: *Contemporary Management of Motor Control Problems: Proceedings of the II Step Conference.* Alexandria, Va: Foundation for Physical Therapy Inc; 1991:11–27.

11 Valvano J, Long T. Neurodevelopmental treatment: a review of the writings of the Bobaths. *Pediatric Physical Therapy.* 1991;3: 125–129.

12 Bly L. A historical and current view basis of NDT. *Pediatric Physical Therapy.* 1991;3: 131–135.

13 Carr JH, Shepherd RB, Gorden J, et al. *Movement Science Foundation for Physical Therapy in Rehabilitation.* Rockville, Md: Aspen Publishers Inc; 1987.

14 Carr JH, Shepherd RB. A motor-learning model for rehabilitation of the movement disabled. Ada L, Canning C, eds. *Key Issues in Neurological Physiotherapy.* Oxford, England: Butterworth-Heinemann Ltd; 1990:1–24.

15 Carr JH, Shepherd RB, Gorden J, et al. *A Motor-Relearning Programme for Stroke.* Rockville, Md: Aspen Publishers Inc; 1987.

16 Tardieu G, Tardieu C. Muscle hypoextensibility in children with cerebral palsy, part I: clinical and experimental observations and part II: therapeutic implications. *Arch Phys Med Rehabil.* 1982;63:97–102, 103–107.

17 Gorden J. Anticipatory guidance from a motor control perspective. Program notes from *Anticipatory Motor Control: Sensory Processing, Motor Planning, and Functional Performance*; July 10–12, 1992.

Commentaries

Following are two commentaries on both "Clinical Use of Neuromuscular Stimulation for Children With Cerebral Palsy, Part 1: Lower Extremity" and "Clinical Use of Neuromuscular Electrical Stimulation for Children With Cerebral Palsy, Part 2: Upper Extremity."

I appreciate having the opportunity to compliment Ms Carmick for pursuing and reporting on her innovative use of neuromuscular electrical stimulation with children with cerebral palsy. We, as therapists, frequently rely on traditional neurological approaches, or integration of these approaches, to improve functional motor control of individuals with neurological dysfunction. These neurological approaches are labor and time intensive for the patient and the therapist. Results often evolve slowly and in small increments. In the past decade, therapists working with individuals with neurological problems have broadened their view of the patient's problems and have learned to incorporate principles of orthopedic physical therapy management (ie, assessment and treatment of joint and soft tissue mobility) into their overall treatment plan. Ms Carmick and others have taken us a step further in looking at another aspect of physical therapy management, neuromuscular electrical stimulation, which although not traditionally used with this patient population, appears to dramatically improve therapeutic effectiveness.

The therapeutic approach reported in this two-part case report provides an example of how to incorporate available technology into the comprehensive management of the patient with neurological dysfunction. As reported by Pape and Hirsh,[1] use of technology as an adjunct to treatment enables individuals with disabilities to pursue peak performance in a similar manner as that used by athletes. It also provides a mechanism for patients and their families to take an active role in their treatment program. By incorporating electrical stimulation into a home program, this apparently effective therapeutic modality can be utilized several times a week in a very cost-effective manner. Patients and their families also assume responsibility for their treatment program, improving their self-confidence and independence.

By reporting multiple case studies, Ms Carmick has shown use of neuromuscular electrical stimulation in conjunction with a dynamic, functionally based physical therapy program to be effective in children with hemiplegic cerebral palsy. The children represented very different age groups and levels of functional movement skill. The functional changes demonstrated by these children, in a relatively short time frame, are well described and supported by photographs. Use of functional, measurable outcomes such as the physiological cost index and measurement of gait parameters provides objective evidence of the changes made. These findings are certainly exciting and should encourage the author and other therapists to continue this avenue of study with larger, more varied samples of children with cerebral palsy.

Several interesting questions are raised by the findings reported. For instance, why was stimulation of the triceps surae muscle alone more effective in improving plantigrade gait than stimulation of tibialis anterior muscle. Our traditional approach of looking at the overactivity of the triceps surae muscle as contributing to toe walking would certainly lead us away from stimulating it any further. It would seem more logical to stimulate the antagonists of the spastic muscles, and this approach has been taken by others using electrical stimulation in their treatment of children with cerebral palsy.[2,3] Ms Carmick provides several intriguing hypotheses, including the concept of different muscle activation patterns in early walkers as compared with older children. Strengthening of active muscle contraction, alterations of the timing with which muscles are activated during functional activities, and producing fatigue in the spastic muscles may also be valid theories as to why the electrical stimulation is effective.

Other questions need to be explored if the most effective use of electrical stimulation technology is to be defined for working with children with cerebral palsy. What is the optimal intensity level? How often and for how long should the electrical stimulation be used? Exactly what does the electrical stimulation do to the muscles and how? What muscle groups should be stimulated and when?

Ms Carmick has provided clues to her clinical problem-solving model in her description of how electrical stimulation was used to decrease toe walking and to decrease unwanted rotation and asymmetry as one of the children learned to run. I hope that as she and other clinicians continue refining this approach to treatment, they try to document their problem solving with all of its trials and errors. This information, when synthesized, would be invaluable to other therapists as they try to incorporate neuromuscular electrical stimulation into their treatment programs.

Dr Pape and her colleagues at the Magee Clinic in Ontario, Canada, have also found electrical stimulation to be of benefit for children with neurological dysfunction. In the treatment model used in this clinic, the children use the electrical stimulation unit while they are sleeping and continue in their regular active therapy programs. A low-level stimulation is used that does not produce a fused contraction. They hypothesized that the stimulation promotes muscle and bone growth, as well as improves the balance between agonist and antagonist muscles. By utilizing the sleeping hours, the group feels that the stress of fitting therapy into the child's daytime schedule is lessened. It is also thought that the child's level of spasticity is often less while asleep and that the sleep cycle is a natural time for growth and repair functions to occur. Although this approach is different than that discussed by Ms Carmick, it has also been reported to be effective. Improvements in motor function have been reported for children with spastic diplegic cerebral palsy, spastic hemiplegic cerebral palsy, and spina bifida. Children with spina bifida have demonstrated improvement in bowel and bladder function as well as motor function.[1,2,4]

Again, I applaud Ms Carmick and other therapists who are exploring the effectiveness of using electrical stimulation as an adjunct to the active therapy programs of children with cerebral palsy and other neurological dysfunction. The dramatic results reported in this two-part case report have certainly intrigued me and leave me wanting to know more. Hopefully, many other pediatric physical therapists feel the same way and will continue from where Ms Carmick has left us. As further study of the use of electrical stimulation evolves, it will be important to continue to use objective outcome measures. These outcome measures should be directed at the main focus of our interventions as physical therapists: functional gains for our patients. It will not be enough to say that a child's range of motion or muscle strength has improved. Instead, functional changes must be reported. Ms Carmick has reported improved efficiency of movement and gait changes. How did these outcomes influence the children's overall functional performance? Perhaps in future studies standardized functional assessment instruments such as the Pediatric Evaluation of Disability Inventory[5] can also be included to help the therapist, the child, and the family put all of the reported improvements into perspective.

Donna J Cech, PT, PCS
Assistant Professor
Department of Physical Therapy
University of Health Science/Chicago Medical School
3333 Green Bay Rd
North Chicago, IL 60064

References

1 Pape KE, Hirsch SE. Priorities for treatment of children with spastic diplegia: technology-assisted self-care in the treatment of spastic diplegia. In: Sussman MD, ed. *The Diplegic Child: Evaluation and Management.* Rosemont, Ill: American Academy of Orthopedic Surgeons; 1992.

2 Pape KE, Hirsch SE, Bugaresti JM. New therapies in spastic cerebral palsy. *Contemporary Pediatrics.* May/June 1990:6–13.

3 Atwater SW, Tatarka ME, Kathrein JE, Shapiro S. Electromyography-triggered electrical muscle stimulation for children with cerebral palsy: a pilot study. *Pediatric Physical Therapy.* 1991;3:190–199.

4 Pape KE, Kirsh SE, McLorie G. Residual function uncovered: effects of therapeutic electrical stimulation (TES) on locomotor, bowel and bladder function in spina bifida patients. *Clinical and Investigative Medicine.* 1990; 13(4):B101.

5 Haley SM, Coster WJ, Ludlow LH, et al. *Pediatric Evaluation of Disability Inventory (PEDI).* Boston, Mass: New England Medical Center Hospitals; 1992.

I thank Ms Carmick for sharing her experiences using neuromuscular electrical stimulation (NMES) with children who have cerebral palsy. Not only do I appreciate learning about an intervention that could be helpful to other children, but I appreciate her effort in preparing the case study for publication. Many of us have had experiences that are worthy of sharing through case reports, but few of us have expended the effort necessary to publish them so that others can also benefit from our successes and failures.

As I think is common among pediatric physical therapists, until quite recently, I paid little attention to electrical stimulation and other interventions that seemed to conflict with a traditional neurodevelopmental approach to treatment of children with cerebral palsy. Contemporary models of motor development and motor control, however, have removed many of the former constraints, opening the way for NMES and other previously neglected interventions that may prove to be effective. Because my knowledge of the application of NMES to children with cerebral palsy is limited, I have chosen to focus my comments on other aspects of Ms Carmick's case reports and on the contribution that these and other case reports can make to physical therapy practice.

Case reports have long been recognized as a means by which information and experiences can be shared, contributing to the expansion of knowledge in a field. Much of the current common knowledge in clinical psychology, for example, was initially revealed through case reports.[1] Medicine, business, law, and social work are other fields that have benefited from extensive publication of case reports. Because our use of case reports in physical therapy has been more limited, the profession is probably yet to benefit fully from their potential contribution.

Case reports serve a number of purposes, several of which were nicely demonstrated by Ms Carmick's articles. A primary purpose is to share both successful and unsuccessful experiences with other clinicians.[2] Because little has been published about use of electrical stimulation with children who have cerebral palsy, Ms Carmick's two-part report is likely to prompt other pediatric physical therapists to try NMES with other children. To enhance the probability of similar success, therapists should, at least initially, attempt to replicate the intervention, as described in the case reports. This requires that the case report clearly and thoroughly describe the subjects, the interventions used, and the decision-making process that led to any modifications of the intervention. Clear and complete descriptions are also necessary to identify common subject and intervention characteristics across a series of reported case studies.

The subjects in these articles were, generally, well-described, and the descriptions could assist other physical therapists in identifying children with similar characteristics. The hand function of the child in case 2 was especially well-depicted and could serve as a model for other therapists attempting to describe movement characteristics. Because cognitive functioning can influence motor outcomes, it would have been helpful to have had information about the boys' cognitive functioning, and I was somewhat confused about the diagnosis of the child described in case 2. It would also have been helpful to know why the older boys, in particular, were referred for physical therapy and why the author selected these three children for NMES and for presentation in the case study. Use of NMES with at least five other children was touched on, but never discussed.

The specific intervention that was used was less well-defined than the subjects, and I think it would be difficult for most therapists to replicate. At various times, for example, the general therapeutic approach was described as "a task-oriented or systems-based model of physical therapy," "a task-oriented model of motor control," "a task-oriented model of motor learning," "a task-oriented motor model," and "a dynamic-systems or contemporary motor-learning physical therapy program." The author described minor features of the approach and gave a general reference, or two, but the overall physical therapy programs, including the home program of the boy in case 3, were unclear. Given the "preliminary evidence for the usefulness of NMES as an adjunct to the physical therapy program," it would have been helpful if the approach had been described in detail.

I was concerned by the author's statements that the 6.7- and 10-year-old boys were "beyond the age that physical therapy is expected to be beneficial." Dynamic systems theory supports my own experience and the limited research that suggests that when the focus of physical therapy is on functional outcomes, older children and children with severe disabilities can often make measurable and meaningful progress. It is when physical therapy focuses on reflex inhibition, fundamental patterns of movement, and developmental milestones that the benefits are doubtful. The intervention described in these case reports led to improvement in both basic movement patterns and functional skills, which is important. I think it is also important, though, to recognize that children with functional needs can benefit from physical therapy, even if their basic movement patterns do not improve.

Another important purpose for case reports, in addition to sharing information, is to provide a broad base of descriptive information that can be used to build theory and generate hypotheses for future research.[3] Case studies are often considered to be preliminary to research because, unlike well-designed qualitative or quantitative studies, their internal validity is weak and generalizability is limited.[4] They can usually provide more information than research studies, however, as demonstrated by the wealth of descriptive detail included in Ms Carmick's case reports. The finding that stimulation of the triceps surae muscle resulted in a more plantigrade foot position than stimulation of the tibialis anterior muscle is especially intriguing.

This is a time of exciting change in pediatric physical therapy. New knowledge in motor development and motor control is challenging many of the beliefs that have been fundamental to our practices with children who have neuromotor impairments, and increasing attention to principles of motor learning is prompting other questions about the manner in which we provide our services. Ms Carmick's articles are excellent examples of the way in which case studies can "assist in placing the 'meat' on the 'theoretical skeleton' "[5] of physical therapy practice. She has provided real-life descriptions of the successful application of contemporary theories of motor control and motor learning to intervention with children who have cerebral palsy. Our profession needs many more such practical examples that enhance or cast doubt upon these and other theories that are currently influencing our practices. I urge other physical therapy practitioners to follow Ms Carmick's lead by scrutinizing their own practices for good prospective or retrospective case studies and preparing them for submission to a journal. Clinicians often question their ability to write for publication, but the clinical experience is the important aspect of a clinical case study. The written expression can be aided, if necessary, by a colleague or an editor. I look forward to reading many more case studies in *Physical Therapy* in the months and years to come.

Irene R McEwen, PhD, PT, PCS
Associate Professor
Department of Physical Therapy
University of Oklahoma Health Sciences Center
PO Box 26901
Oklahoma City, OK 73190

References

1 Bolgar H. The case study method. In: Wolman BB, ed. *Handbook of Clinical Psychology.* New York, NY: McGraw-Hill Inc; 1965;28–39.

2 McEwen IR, Karlan GR. Case studies: why and how. *Augmentative and Alternative Communication.* 1990;6:69–75.

3 Barlow DH, Hersen M. *Single-Case Experimental Designs.* 2nd ed. New York, NY: Pergamon Press Inc; 1984.

4 Portney LG, Watkins MP. *Foundations of Clinical Research: Applications to Practice.* East Norwalk, Conn: Appleton & Lange; 1993;233–235.

5 Lazarus AA, Davison GC. Clinical innovation in research and practice. In: Bergen AE, Garfield SL, eds. *Handbook of Psychotherapy and Behavior Change: An Empirical Analysis.* New York, NY: John Wiley & Sons Inc; 1971:196–213.

Author Response

I thank Ms Cech and Dr McEwen for their encouraging and uplifting comments on my two case reports as well as for their thoughtful ideas and suggestions.

Ms Cech expressed interest in my finding that stimulating the triceps surae muscle alone was more effective in improving plantigrade gait than stimulation of the tibialis anterior muscle. Dr McEwen also found this to be intriguing. The finding is in contrast to the traditional idea that the triceps surae muscle is overactive and contributes to toe-walking. The traditional viewpoint would cause one to stimulate the tibialis anterior muscle rather than the triceps surae muscle. Ms Cech mentions fatigue and strengthening of active muscle contraction as possible valid theories for the effectiveness of neuromuscular electrical stimulation (NMES). I strongly agree that strengthening of the triceps surae muscle does help achieve a plantigrade gait, but I disagree with the suggestion about fatigue of the spastic muscles. The triceps surae muscle is already weak and ineffective. This muscle does not need to be fatigued; it needs to be strengthened.

I find it helpful to keep in mind that plantar flexors are normally responsible for two thirds of the total concentric work of gait.[1] Olney,[1] Dietz et al,[2] and Berger and colleagues,[3] among others, led me to this viewpoint on why NMES was so effective on the triceps surae muscle and not on the tibialis anterior muscle. It does not appear that the triceps surae muscle causes toe-walking in all children with cerebral palsy, as has been the traditional thinking. With stimulation to this muscle to increase the strength or control of the muscle contraction of the child in case 1, the child's foot became plantigrade. Over time, the triceps surae muscle gained strength and control in all three subjects in this case study, and no increased spasticity or loss of range of motion of the ankle was found.

With regard to Dr McEwen's questions concerning the children in cases 2 and 3, the child in case 2 had a stroke at birth from meconium aspiration. He attends a regular school, is considered above average in intelligence, and does have difficulties with writing and attention span. When he returned to my clinic to replace outgrown orthotic devices, it was decided to try NMES because of the progress of the child in case 1, who was felt to be similar in functional needs.

The entire home program of the child in case 3 was as described in part 1. He spent 15 minutes walking with NMES, triggered by the remote-control switch, also doing active dorsiflexion and plantar-flexion exercises in sitting and standing three times a week. There was nothing more. The child in case 3 was referred to physical therapy initially for a brace and physical therapy consultation. When he returned because of an outgrown brace, it was decided to try NMES.

The subjects were chosen because they were all of the same general diagnosis but of various ages. Also, the use of NMES on a child with only a one- or two-extremity involvement is simpler to describe than the application to children with more complicated problems (athetosis or diplegia). Comparing the children in cases 1 and 2 was felt to be of additional interest, considering that the child in case 1 received physical therapy with a contemporary or dynamic-systems model of motor control at the start with NMES added at the young age of 19 months, whereas the child in case 2 had received a neurodevelopmental therapy program of physical therapy and occupational therapy before changing to the program that the child in case 1 was given.

Dr McEwen expressed a desire for more references on motor control. There were six references on motor control listed at the end of part 1 (ie, references 6, 8, 10, 16, 17, and 18) and one (ie, reference 17) in part 2. Three are chapters from books in which the entire book discusses the subject. As I mentioned, most of the references concern adults, as there is very little written about motor control in pediatrics.

I certainly agree with Dr McEwen that when physical therapy is based on functional outcomes, older children and children with severe disabilities often make measurable and meaningful progress. Unfortunately, we do not have enough documentation in the literature to prove this. Published works by physicians[4–7] imply just the opposite—that children after 6 or 7 years of age do not progress. It has been my experience that local physicians and those working for California Childrens Services, a state agency serving children with disabilities through medical-therapy units in school settings, base their decisions for continuing physical therapy on the findings and guidelines of Bleck[4,6] and Molnar.[5,7]

In 1985, Molnar[5] stated

> Most children achieve maximal level of gross motor function including ambulatory potential, by 6–7 years. After this age physical therapy, regardless of its intensity, is unlikely to produce further functional gains.

In 1987, Bleck[4] reviewed several physicians' research on the effectiveness of physical therapy. All felt that there was a plateau by age 7 years and that motor improvement of children with spastic diplegia levels off. Bleck recommended that physical therapy be discontinued when the child is able to play outdoors with his or her peers, at 6 or 7 years of age. Bleck[6] published his Locomotor Prognosis Test in 1975. This test bases its score on the presence or absence of certain reflexes in the child who is at least 1 year of age. The prognosis was accurate in 94.5% of the 73 children studied. Bleck also stated that the "probability of a child walking after the age of seven is remote."

Bleck's test may be of further service to physical therapists besides the main function of prognostication. The underlying research was carried out over 20 years ago, and the results may reflect the skills of physical therapists at that time. Physical therapy has made many advances since then, and I feel the skills of the therapist are much improved. It may now be possible to show a greater percentage of children who can walk and make significant functional gains when they were not "expected" to do so. It is suggested that therapists working with young children routinely use a locomotor prognosis test during evaluation and then record pertinent data on the children who do or do not become functional ambulators.

We see, in our clinics, children who fail Bleck's test and then walk, children who walk after 8 years of age, children who walk but do not sit by 4 years of age, and children who otherwise make significant functional gains. We need to show that physical therapy has improved since the mid-1970s when Bleck and Molnar published their findings and that physical therapy can make significant functional changes where none are "expected." Physical therapists also need to demonstrate to physicians and health administrators that physical therapy is more than just obtaining a goal of ambulation by age 6 or 7 years without regard to movement quality and efficiency. I hope that documenting measurable significant changes on two children, who were not expected to progress according to Bleck and Molnar, will help to further these goals.

Judy Carmick, PT

References

1. Olney SJ. Work and power in hemiplegic cerebral palsy gait. *Phys Ther.* 1990;70:431–438.

2 Dietz V, Quintern J, Berger W. Electrophysiological studies of gait in spasticity and rigidity: evidence that altered mechanical properties of muscle contribute to hypertonia. *Brain.* 1981;104:431–439.

3 Berger W, Altenmueller E, Dietz V. Normal and impaired development of children's gait. *Human Neurobiology.* 1984;3:163–170.

4 Bleck E. *Orthopaedic Management in Cerebral Palsy.* Philadelphia, Pa: Mac Keith Press; 1987:168.

5 Molnar GE. Cerebral palsy. In: Molnar GE, ed. *Pediatric Rehabilitation.* Baltimore, Md: Williams & Wilkins; 1985:455.

6 Bleck E. Locomotor prognosis in cerebral palsy. *Dev Med Child Neurol.* 1975;17:18–25.

7 Molnar GE, Gordon SU. Cerebral palsy: predictive value of selective clinical signs for early prognostication of motor function. *Arch Phys Med Rehabil.* 1976;57:153–158.

Case Report

Effects of Prenatal Alcohol Exposure on Neuromotor and Cognitive Development During Early Childhood: A Series of Case Reports

The purpose of this article is to present a series of case reports of infants and young children who were exposed to alcohol prenatally. The five infants and two 5-year-old twins in this series all presented facial features characteristic of prenatal alcohol exposure, and all had medical histories of maternal alcohol abuse. The neuromotor and cognitive development of these seven children is described by presenting results of standardized tests administered longitudinally. In addition, clinical observations of growth, behavior, feeding, and musculoskeletal development are provided. Following a discussion of these assessment results, implications for physical therapy intervention and the need for clinical research are provided. Because children with fetal alcohol syndrome or alcohol-related birth defects present a spectrum of developmental differences that often include areas of concern to physical therapists, we need to increase our involvement in the assessment and treatment of these children as well as in research efforts to examine the efficacy of these interventions. [Harris SR, Osborn JA, Weinberg J, et al. Effects of prenatal alcohol exposure on neuromotor and cognitive development during early childhood: a series of case reports. Phys Ther. 1993;73:608–617.]

Key Words: *Cognitive development, Fetal alcohol syndrome, Neuromotor development.*

Susan R Harris
Jill A Osborn
Joanne Weinberg
Christine Loock
Kate Junaid

Despite the publication of "several thousand scientific communications" concerning the teratogenic effects of prenatal alcohol exposure[1] since fetal alcohol syndrome (FAS) was first recognized in 1973,[2] no reports could be located in the physical therapy literature describing the assessment or treatment of individuals with FAS. The purpose of this report, written as a companion article to the clinical perspective on FAS by Osborn and colleagues in this issue, is to present a series of case reports of infants and young children with either FAS or alcohol-related birth defects (ARBD) who have been assessed longitudinally by physical therapists and other health professionals. To be diagnosed with FAS, individuals must be characterized by abnormal signs in each of three areas: growth retardation; central nervous system (CNS) involvement; and characteristic facial features including short palpebral fissures, flat nasal bridge, flat philtrum, thin upper

SR Harris, PhD, PT, FAPTA, is Associate Professor, School of Rehabilitation Sciences, Faculty of Medicine, University of British Columbia, T325-2211 Wesbrook Mall, Vancouver, British Columbia, Canada V6T 2B5, and Faculty Clinical Associate, Sunny Hill Hospital for Children, 3644 Slocan St, Vancouver, British Columbia, Canada V5M 3E8. Address all correspondence to Dr Harris at the first address.

JA Osborn, PT, is a graduate student, Division of Neuroscience, Faculty of Medicine, University of British Columbia, 2177 Wesbrook Mall, Vancouver, British Columbia, Canada V6T 1Z3.

J Weinberg, PhD, is Professor, Department of Anatomy, Faculty of Medicine, University of British Columbia.

C Loock, MD, is Clinical Assistant Professor, Division of Developmental Medicine, Department of Paediatrics, Faculty of Medicine, University of British Columbia.

K Junaid, PT, is Section Head of Physiotherapy, Sunny Hill Hospital for Children.

This work was supported in part by a grant from the National Institute on Alcohol Abuse and Alcoholism (Dr Weinberg). Ms Osborn is supported by a Medical Research Council of Canada Studentship.

This article was submitted August 18, 1992, and was accepted April 23, 1993.

lip, and flattened maxilla.[1] The term *alcohol-related birth defects* was coined recently to describe "attribution of an observed anatomic or functional outcome to the impact of alcohol on the offspring" and has been recommended to replace the term *fetal alcohol effects.*[1(p598)]

The primary goal of the following case reports is to describe the neuromotor and cognitive development of these children and discuss behavioral characteristics that may differentiate them from typically developing children. A secondary goal is to suggest implications for treatment based on these assessment findings.

Although a number of published studies have described neonatal behavioral differences in infants with FAS[3–5] as well as developmental motor outcomes at a variety of different ages,[6–11] none of these reports have provided assessment data collected at repeated intervals (eg, every 4 to 6 months during infancy and early childhood). Following are case reports for five infants with histories of prenatal alcohol exposure who were assessed at least three times during the first 2 years of life. These case reports describing infant development are followed by case reports of a set of female monozygotic twins who were followed longitudinally from the age of 2 years 6 months to the age of 5 years 1 month by an interdisciplinary developmental assessment team. Emphasis will be placed on describing the two most recent developmental assessments of the twins.

In presenting these seven cases of children with FAS or ARBD, our goal is to highlight the neuromotor and cognitive findings resulting from the administration of standardized tests. Growth, behavioral, feeding, and musculoskeletal concerns will also be presented. Implications for physical therapy intervention and clinical research will follow the presentation of the case reports.

Case Reports of Infants With FAS or ARBD

All five infants were tested by the senior author (SRH) as part of a longitudinal development follow-up program for infants with diagnoses of neonatal addiction syndrome. All testing took place at Sunny Hill Hospital for Children in Vancouver, British Columbia, Canada, from 1990 to 1992. Tests administered included the Movement Assessment of Infants (MAI),[12] a 65-item neuromotor assessment tool that was administered at the first two visits (at approximately 4 and 8 months of age), and the Mental and Motor Scales of the Bayley Scales of Infant Development,[13] a standardized, norm-referenced assessment tool that has been used widely in longitudinal follow-up of high-risk infants. The Bayley Scales were administered at each of the follow-up visits. The MAI and the Bayley Scales were selected as appropriate tools for use in our follow-up clinic because infants exposed to drugs prenatally are at risk for neuromotor as well as cognitive deficits.[14,15] The purpose of the testing was to discriminate which infants were in need of early intervention services. The senior author has extensive clinical and research experience in administering these tests and also has provided numerous workshops on administration of each of these tools.

Based on a sample of 35 high-risk infants, the authors of the MAI manual have suggested the following ranges for total risk scores at 4 months of age: 0–7=within normal limits, 8–12=suspect, and ≥13=abnormal.[12] For the 8-month profile, a total risk score of >10 is considered cause for concern. Both the Mental Developmental Index (MDI) and the Psychomotor Developmental Index (PDI) of the Bayley Scales have a mean of 100 and a standard deviation of 16.[13] The standard errors of measurement (68% confidence intervals) for the MDI and PDI vary, depending on the infant's age at testing (Tab. 1).

The five infants tested in this series all showed facial features suggestive of prenatal alcohol exposure and were born to mothers with histories of prenatal alcohol abuse. Many of the mothers also smoked during pregnancy. Other drugs used during pregnancy included cocaine, heroin, diazepam (Valium®*), triazolam (Halcion®†), and lorazepam (Ativan®‡). As is typical of children with FAS/ARBD, all children described in the case reports were prenatally exposed to other drugs in addition to alcohol. Thus, it is virtually impossible to sort out the effects of the alcohol from the effects of the other drugs. For four of the five infants, the initial developmental assessment took place between 4 and 6 months of age; the infant described in the fourth case report was almost 9 months of age when first assessed. Subsequent follow-up visits were scheduled to occur at approximately 8, 12, and 18 months. Most of the infants were assessed within ±1 month of these scheduled visits (Tab. 1).

Infant 1

The first infant was a Native American boy who had been in foster care since early infancy. According to his hospital chart, his mother had a history of "drug and alcohol ingestion" during pregnancy. He was assessed initially at 5 months of age; his fourth and most recent assessment was conducted at 18 months. Because he presented abnormal characteristics in all three categories associated with prenatal alcohol exposure (growth retardation, CNS involvement, and characteristic facial features), a diagnosis of FAS was made. Although initially in the 25th percentile for height and weight and above the 10th percentile for head circumference, the infant's growth parameters fell off

*Roche Laboratories, Div of Hoffman-La Roche Inc, Nutley, NJ 07110.

†The Upjohn Company, Kalamazoo, MI 49001.

‡Wyeth-Ayerst Laboratories, Div of American Home Products Corp, PO Box 8299, Philadelphia, PA 19101.

Table 1. *Bayley Mental Development Index (MDI) and Psychomotor Developmental Index (PDI) and Movement Assessment of Infants (MAI) Test Scores at Each Follow-up Assessment*[a]

Infant and Assessment Tool	Age Range (mo)			
	4–6	7–9	11–13	18–20
Infant 1				
Bayley MDI	86	73[b]	60[b]	81[b]
Bayley PDI	80[b]	73[b]	75[b]	75[b]
MAI	6	15[b]	...	...
Infant 2				
Bayley MDI	89	77[b]	<50[b]	<50[b]
Bayley PDI	108	67[b]	55[b]	62[b]
MAI	14[b]	...	...	...
Infant 3				
Bayley MDI	104	83[b]	92	...
Bayley PDI	118	96	97	...
MAI	1	3	...	...
Infant 4				
Bayley MDI	...	<50[b]	50[b]	<50[b]
Bayley PDI	...	69[b]	59[b]	<50[b]
MAI	...	24[b]	...	...
Infant 5				
Bayley MDI	91	69[b]	84	100
Bayley PDI	85	80[b]	98	94
MAI	8[b]	10[b]	...	...

[a]Standard errors of measurement (68% confidence interval) for the Bayley MDI are ±4.6–5.7 at 4–6 months, ±6.9 at 7–9 months, ±6.7 at 11–13 months, and ±5.3 at 18–20 months; those for the Bayley PDI are ±5.4–7.0 at 4–6 months, ±6.6 at 7–9 months, ±5.8 at 11–13 months, and ±4.6–5.5 at 18–20 months.[13]

[b]Scores that are suspect or abnormal.

such that, at 18 months, he was below the 5th percentile for height, weight, and head circumference.

Craniofacial features characteristic of FAS included brachycephaly, short palpebral fissures, low-set ears, small nose, smooth philtrum, and thin upper lip. The infant demonstrated other characteristics associated with prenatal alcohol exposure such as abnormal palmar creases, small fifth fingers, and pectus excavatum. Although his 4-month MAI total risk score was within normal limits (Tab. 1), his 8-month risk score was 15, which is above the recommended cut-off score of 10 and thus suggests movement concerns. At both of these early visits, MAI concerns included generalized hypotonia, persistent primitive reflexes (asymmetrical tonic neck reflex, tonic labyrinthine reflex-supine, trunk incurvation reflex), delayed head-righting reactions, tremulousness, and delays in fine and gross motor milestones.

The infant's Bayley MDI had shown considerable variability. Although his initial assessment was in the low normal range, subsequent MDIs were from 1.0 to 2.5 standard deviations below the mean. His Bayley PDI was quite consistent across the four visits, ranging from about 1.0 to 1.5 standard deviations below the mean (Tab. 1).

As is typical of infants exposed to alcohol or other drugs prenatally, the infant had frequent episodes of profuse sweating (diaphoresis). He also has had a history of feeding and drinking difficulties, gagging on anything other than pureed food at age 12 months and eating only pureed or junior baby foods at age 18 months. He continued to drink from a bottle at age 18 months. During the first year postnatally, he also had a history of vomiting and constipation. He showed persistent and sustained attention during administration of the Bayley Scales at his most recent visit at 18 months. At each of the four testing sessions, he was noted to be very sociable and cooperative.

Infant 2

The infant described in the second case report was a boy of apparently mixed Native American and Caucasian heritage. He was born at 36 to 37 weeks' gestational age and had been in foster care since hospital discharge in early infancy. Prenatal maternal history included periodic drinking bouts (seven to eight beers) as well as use of heroin, intravenous cocaine, Valium®, Halcion®, and Ativan®. He was assessed initially at 4 months of age (corrected for prematurity), at which time a number of dysmorphic features were noted including short palpebral fissures, epicanthal folds, flat nasal bridge, flat philtrum, thin upper lip, bilateral hair whorls, and low-set ears. Because his growth had consistently fallen between the 60th and 90th percentiles, he would not qualify for a diagnosis of FAS but rather would be described as having ARBD, in spite of the fact that his developmental delays were much more significant than those of infant 1.

When assessed initially at 4 months, his Bayley scores were both within normal limits, although the MDI was in the low normal range. His MAI total risk score, however, was considered abnormal due to a predominance of risk items reflecting generalized hypotonia, persistent primitive reflexes (asymmetrical tonic neck reflex, palmar grasp, and tonic labyrinthine reflex-supine), delayed head-righting reactions, and failure to show any response (eg, eye widening, stilling) to the sound of the Bayley bell or rattle. He was noted also to have astasia (refusal to bear weight on his feet when placed in supported standing). Because of the MAI concerns, this infant was reassessed at approximately 6.5 months' corrected age, at which time his Bayley MDI had dropped to about 1.5 standard deviations below the mean and his PDI had decreased to 2.0 standard deviations below the mean. At his two most recent visits (approximately 12 and 19 months' corrected age), his MDI had dropped to >3.0 standard deviations below the mean and his PDI had decreased to about 2.5 standard deviations below the mean.

Musculoskeletal concerns noted in this infant at the first visit were bilateral talipes equinovarus and tibial bowing, for which he was treated with corrective shoes prescribed by a pediatric orthopedist. Because the infant could actively dorsiflex his ankle and evert his foot following tactile stimulation of the lateral border of the foot, the equinovarus appeared to be functional rather than structural. It had resolved by his last visit, although there was still some evidence of tibial bowing, which became particularly noticeable after he started walking. Another concern noted at the 4- and 6.5-month visits was lack of auditory responses to the Bayley bell and rattle. A subsequent audiology assessment at 10 months of age, however, indicated his hearing was normal.

The infant had consistently shown very unusual behaviors, including a flat affect, perseverant hand-waving, and staring at his left hand, at the initial 4-month visit. During his most recent visit, his mood fluctuated from extreme fussiness to smiling and laughing, with no apparent stimulus for either behavioral state. In addition, he demonstrated a number of "autistic-like" behaviors including intense stranger anxiety, unusual fears of inanimate objects, tactile and oral hypersensitivity, perseverant motor behaviors and vocalizations, rocking and other self-stimulatory behaviors, and obsessive interest in spinning the wheels on his stroller.

The infant had also had persistent feeding problems and, at the corrected age of 19 months, would eat only pureed foods and drink only from a bottle. He would not finger-feed nor had he ever brought food, toys, or any other objects to his mouth to either taste or explore them—behaviors that are universally characteristic of typically developing infants.

Infant 3

The third infant, also a Native American boy, had some characteristics to suggest ARBD. By physician's report, his mother consumed 4 to 6 beers per day during the first month of pregnancy. She also smoked cigarettes and took other drugs until about the fourth month of gestation. Although not growth-retarded, the most noticeable physical characteristic of this infant was microphthalmia (small eyes). Other characteristic features include a broad, flat nasal bridge and low-set ears. Although his growth continued to be within normal limits, his weight and head circumference had dropped at his most recent visit (approximately 13.5 months of age) from the 50th to the 25th percentile.

At his initial assessment at about 5.5 months of age, the infant had Bayley and MAI scores that were well within normal limits; his Bayley PDI was >1.0 standard deviation above the mean (Tab. 1). At his second visit, at age 9 months, his MDI had dropped to 83, which is just slightly greater than 1.0 standard deviation below the mean. Reportedly, his mother was continuing to drink and abuse drugs while this infant and his two older brothers were living with her. Just after his second follow-up visit, this infant and his brothers were taken from his mother to be cared for by their maternal grandparents.

By the child's third follow-up visit at about 13.5 months of age, he had been living with his grandparents for the past 3.5 months in an environment that was obviously much more stable and nurturing than his previous home situation. At that most recent visit, his MDI had increased 9 points such that it was again within normal limits, albeit on the low side of normal. His PDI remained solidly within normal limits. There are at least two possible explanations for the increase in his cognitive score. The standard error of the mean for the Bayley Mental Scale was approximately 6 to 7 points at these latter two assessment ages. His "true score," therefore, was ±6 to 7 points at each of the assessments, a factor that could easily have contributed to the 9-point improvement noted. Another, more tempting hypothesis is that the change in home environment may have positively influenced his performance.

Based on his overall performance, this infant was the least impaired of the five infants in this series. His growth was still within normal limits, and his most recent developmental testing demonstrated age-appropriate performance. He was very cooperative and compliant during all three evaluation sessions.

Infant 4

The fourth infant in this series, a girl, was assessed initially at almost 9 months of age. Of apparently mixed (Native American and Caucasian) heritage, this infant was born at 38 weeks' gestational age and weighed 2,400 g. She had been in foster care since 4 months of age. At birth, a "mildly sunken nasal bridge" as well as tremors, excessive crying, sneezing, diarrhea, and irritability were observed by the hospital pediatrician. Other dysmorphic characteristics were a small upturned nose, epicanthal folds, flat midface, thin upper lip, flat philtrum, and dysplastic toenails. Her mother had a long history of drug use, including cocaine, marijuana, and alcohol. This infant's growth had varied between the 10th and 50th percentiles, but her growth rate did not appear to be decelerating.

Table 2. *Characteristic Features of Prenatal Alcohol Exposure and Their Presence in the Five Infants Studied*[a]

Characteristic	Infant No. 1	2	3	4	5
Growth retardation (<10th percentile)	+	–	–	–	–
Characteristic facial features	+	+	+	+	+
Cognitive delay	+	+	–	+	±
Motor delay	+	+	±	+	±
Generalized hypotonia	+	+	–	+	±
Feeding/oral-motor concerns	+	+	–	–	–
Orthopedic abnormalities	+	+	–	–	–
Behavioral concerns	–	+	–	+	+

[a] + = characteristic was present, – = characteristic was not present, ± = variability in appearance of the characteristic across repeated assessments.

Developmentally, this infant demonstrated consistent and significant delays during all three testing sessions. At her initial assessment, both Bayley scores and the MAI score were abnormal (Tab. 1). The MAI total risk score of 24 reflected the following concerns: generalized hypotonia, tremulousness, delayed automatic reactions, inconsistent auditory and visual responses, and delayed gross motor and fine motor skills. Many of these concerns persisted into the second visit at approximately 13.5 months. Other behavioral concerns noted at the second visit included a flat affect and stranger anxiety.

By the third and final follow-up visit at almost 20 months of age, the infant's Bayley scores were >3.0 standard deviations below the mean. She had a very stiff quality of movement and persistent W-sitting posture. Other unusual behaviors noted were frequent dropping or throwing of test materials, abnormal fear of inanimate objects (eg, the small Bayley ball), and self-abusive face-slapping. Her foster mother reported twice-daily temper tantrums, tactile hypersensitivity of the scalp, and an abnormal fear of being placed in the bathtub. The infant's flat affect persisted, with the only changes in expression resulting from her unusual fears or her tantrums. Both developmentally and behaviorally, this infant exhibited severe disturbances that were somewhat similar to those of the infant in case report 2.

Infant 5

The fifth and final infant in this series was a Native American girl whose mother was reported to have consumed beer and other alcoholic beverages and to have smoked marijuana during pregnancy. Born full-term at 3,360 g, this infant showed signs of withdrawal including sneezing, irritability, diarrhea, and diaphoresis. Characteristic facial features included flat nasal bridge, short palpebral fissures, and ocular hypertelorism. This infant was also noted to have a high arched palate. Her growth continued at ≥50th percentile.

The infant was assessed initially at almost 5 months of age, at which time her Bayley scores were in the low normal range and her MAI total risk score was in the suspect range (Tab. 1). Risk behaviors noted on the MAI included increased tone in hip adductors, retention of tonic labyrinthine reflex-supine, upper-extremity tremulousness, astasia, and immaturity in development of automatic reactions.

During the infant's second visit at almost 9 months of age, her Bayley MDI had dropped to almost 2.0 standard deviations below the mean and her Bayley PDI had decreased only slightly to just greater than 1.0 standard deviation below the mean. The MAI total risk score was right at the cutoff for being concerning; muscle tone (as assessed by consistency, extensibility, and antigravity postures) and primitive reflexes were observed to be within normal limits, but automatic reactions were slightly immature. At 13 months of age, both Bayley scores improved considerably such that they were both within normal limits again. The child's foster mother reported a number of behavioral concerns, however, including screaming and "thrashing of arms" and throwing herself backward both when challenged or when unprovoked. Other concerns expressed included the child's lack of fear, lack of realization of dangers, pulling her hair out, hitting herself and others, and sudden outbursts of temper.

Summary of Infant Cases With Implications for Treatment and Research

As can be seen from these case reports, prenatal exposure to alcohol and other drugs results in a variety of neuromotor, cognitive, behavioral, and musculoskeletal abnormalities (Tab. 2). Only one of the five infants (infant 1) is currently growth retarded and, therefore, the only one with a diagnosis of full FAS. Interestingly, this infant has fared much better developmentally and behaviorally than two of the other infants (2 and 4) who would be classified as having ARBD, reinforcing the notion that prenatal alcohol exposure results in a diverse continuum of disabilities. Physical therapists should be aware that alcohol exposure can result in a wide spectrum of developmental delays and behavioral concerns in

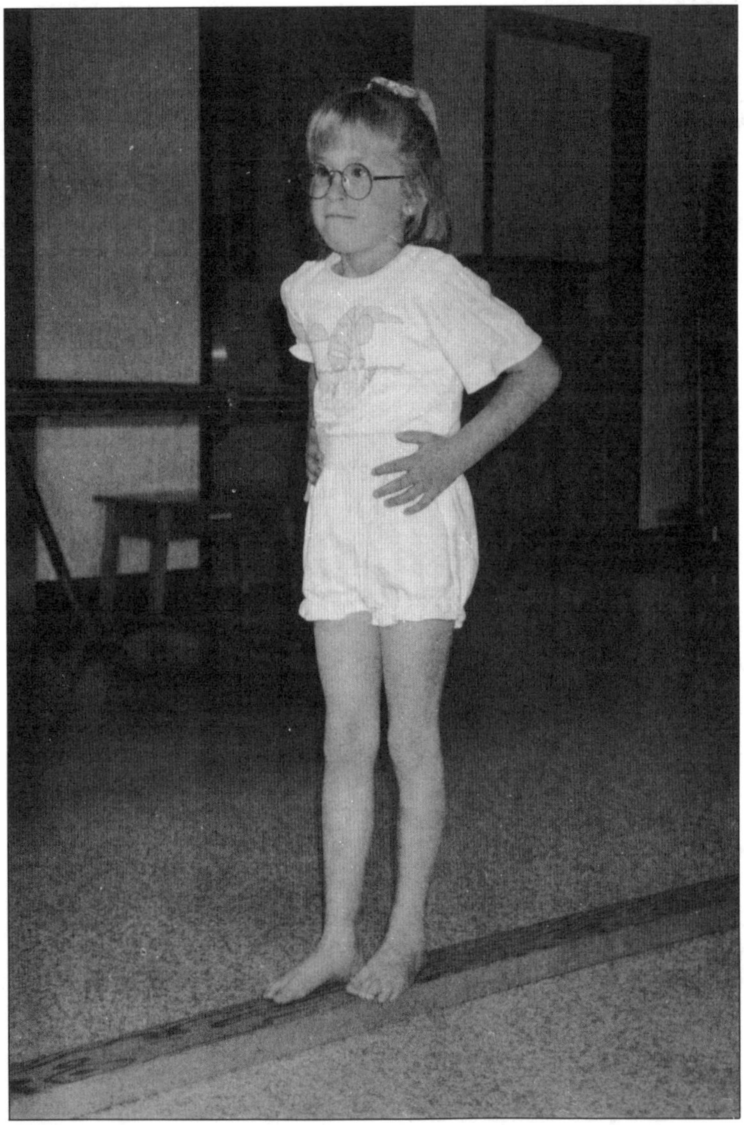

Figure 1. *Twin A walking forward on balance board, hands on hips (item 143 from Peabody Gross Motor Scale).*

both infants with diagnoses of FAS and infants with ARBD.

Each of these five infants is enrolled in a provincially funded Infant Development Program (IDP) that provides home-based early intervention and family consultation approximately twice a month. In addition, three of the infants (1, 2, and 4) receive physical therapy services through their IDP. During their first 12 to 15 months postnatally, the physical therapy was developmentally based direct service and included activities such as promoting hands-to-midline and hands-to-knees, encouraging active trunk rotation and movement into and out of sitting, facilitating quadrupedal and kneel-standing activities, and encouraging independent walking. Once these children attained independent ambulation, physical therapy intervention changed to a consultation or monitoring model with emphasis on balance activities (balance board, balance beam) and developmentally appropriate play activities. For example, the consultation program for infant 4 involved a series of gross motor and fine motor activities at various stations in a large room in the preschool where she was encouraged to move from station to station and engage in the various activities. Because the ability to play spontaneously is frequently lacking in these children, these are very appropriate and functionally oriented activities.

In the case of infant 2, the physical therapy focus changed from gross motor activities during the first postnatal year to consultation regarding his feeding and behavioral concerns. A recent visit by the senior author to this child's preschool classroom indicated that, at the age of 27 months, he was still refusing to eat any solid foods, such as crackers, cookies, or fruit. Attempts by the senior author at using tactile desensitization strategies in the oral area with this youngster resulted in his taking a small bite of a banana. It would be interesting to involve children similar to this child in single-subject research designs aimed at improving their eating abilities through either neurodevelopmental or behavioral intervention strategies.

There have been no published studies in which the effectiveness of early-intervention strategies has been assessed for children with FAS or ARBD. The use of treatment techniques to influence target behaviors, such as oral-motor therapy for feeding difficulties or balance activities to enhance balance or postural control, should be assessed. Physical therapists who are involved in the care and treatment of these children could contribute greatly to the examination of treatment efficacy for these children.

Case Reports: 5-Year-Old Identical Twins With FAS

The next two case reports describe a set of Caucasian monozygous female

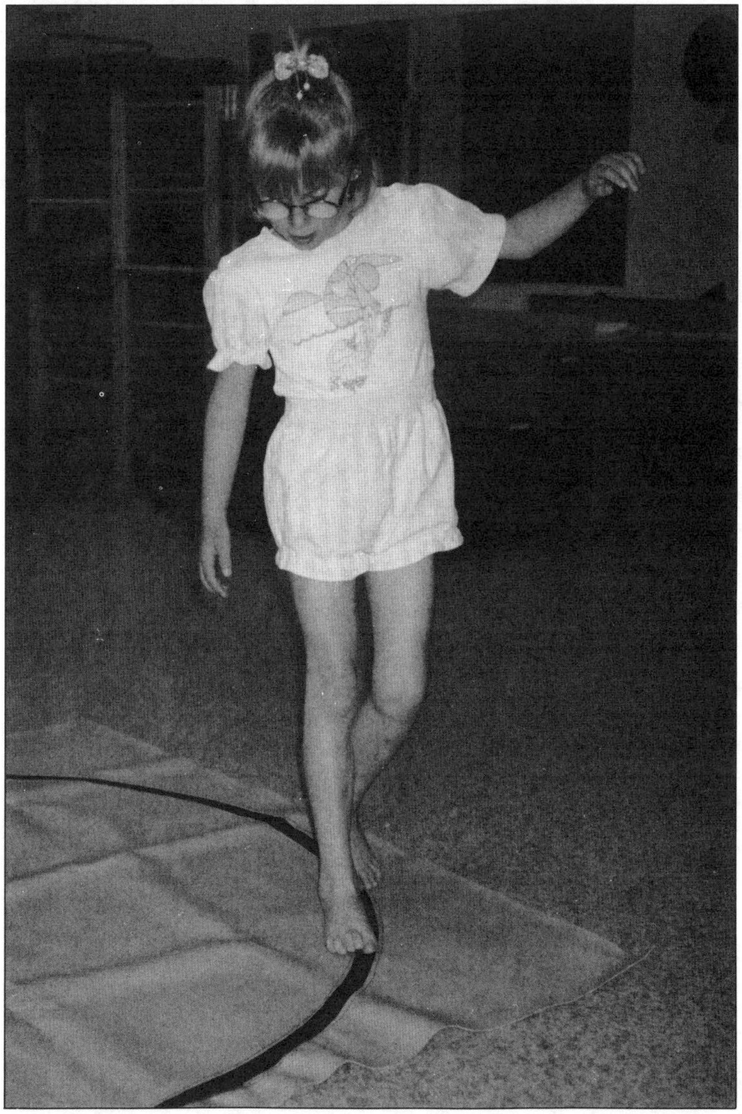

Figure 2. *Twin A walking forward on 1.2-m (4-ft) circle (item 100 from Peabody Gross Motor Scale).*

twins with FAS who were tested most recently at the age of 5 years 1 month. Born at term, twin A weighed 2,530 g and twin B weighed 1,820 g (a birth weight of <2,500 g at term is considered small for gestational age). Delivery was by emergency cesarean section due to fetal distress. The pregnancy was unplanned and was not confirmed until the fourth month of gestation. The birth mother was employed as a cocktail waitress and recalled drinking two or three Irish coffees each evening after work, five or six nights per week. Based on physician reports in her hospital chart, she had been a heavy smoker (approximately one pack per day) and may also have used marijuana. Private adoption was planned prior to delivery and took place when the twins were 3 weeks of age.

Early history was significant for sleep disturbances and difficulties with feeding. The twins were referred for pediatric and developmental assessments at 8 months of age because of hypotonia and delays in motor milestones; they had poor head control and were unable to sit independently. Chromosome assessment revealed normal karyotypes. Fetal alcohol syndrome was subsequently diagnosed at 25 months of age based on the overall developmental delays; growth retardation (height and weight at ≤10th percentile); and characteristic facial features including short palpebral fissures, flattened midface, long philtrum, and thin upper lip.

Twin A

Twin A was assessed initially at 33 weeks of age on the Gesell Developmental Schedules[16]; her gross motor level was found to be at 20 weeks or roughly 60% of her age level. At 22½ months on the Gesell measure, she was functioning at 13 to 15 months in gross motor skills. The Bayley Mental Scale was administered at 28 months, with a resultant MDI of 67; twin A's estimated level of gross motor development at 28 months was 16 to 18 months. She was assessed initially on the Gross Motor Scale of the Peabody Developmental Motor Scales (PDMS)[17] at 41 months of age, at which time her age equivalent was 18 to 23 months (about 50% of age level).

The most recent interdisciplinary assessments for both twins occurred at the age of 4 years 5 months (53 months). Psychological assessment for twin A showed a Stanford-Binet IQ of 71 (low average range), with relative strengths in auditory and language tasks and relative weaknesses in complex visual tasks, auditory memory, and spatial relations. Receptive and expressive vocabulary were at the 3-year–9-month (45-month) level, with visuomotor integration at the 38-month level. Physical therapy assessment reported low truncal tone, mildly lordotic posture, tight heelcords, and a tendency to run stiffly and on her toes; her gross motor age equivalent on the PDMS was 29 to 35

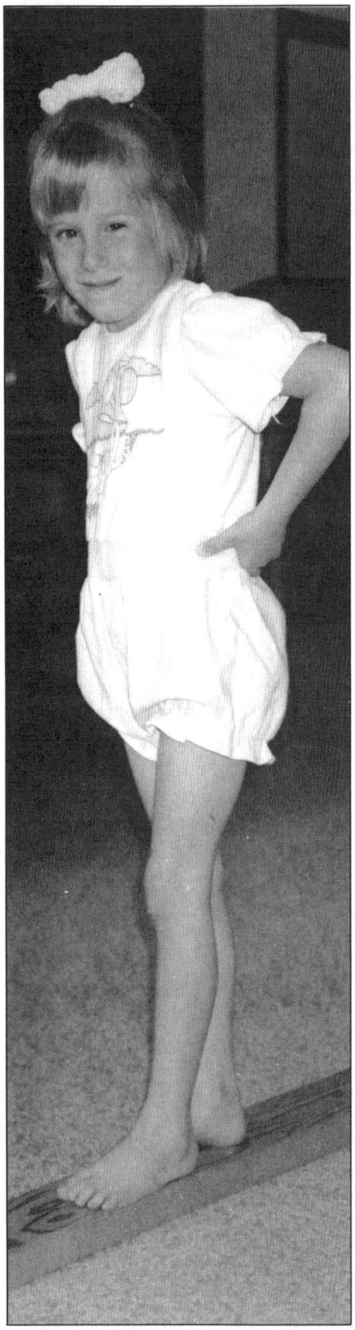

Figure 3. *Twin B walking forward on balance board, hands on hips (item 143 from Peabody Gross Motor Scale).*

months (about 60% of age level). Medical concerns noted at this visit included recurrent serous otitis media, a history of esotropia, and a history of tremulousness.

At 5 years 1 month (61 months), the Gross Motor Scale of the PDMS[15] was administered to twin A by a physical therapist (senior author). The PDMS was chosen because it is a standardized, norm-referenced test that has been used extensively for assessing motor development of children with a variety of different developmental delays. During and immediately following administration of the PDMS, clinical observations of muscle tone, range of motion, and automatic reactions were made. Apparent joint hyperextensibility was noted, as evidenced by slight elbow hyperextension and slight genu recurvatum (Fig. 1). Primitive reflexes had all been integrated. She had sufficient automatic reactions to maintain upright balance while running or walking on a balance beam. Twin A was noted to be able to run, hop on one foot, walk on the balance board, attempt to skip, and walk on a circle (Fig. 2). She had a basal age on the PDMS of 18 to 23 months and a ceiling age level of 54 to 59 months. Her gross motor age equivalent was 39 to 40 months, which was approximately 65% of age level. Percentile scores for the gross motor subtests and the total score were all at either the 1st or 2nd percentile, indicating that 98% to 99% of her agemates were performing at higher levels.

Twin A was noted to be cooperative during testing, although she became somewhat tired and frustrated toward the end of the 2-hour testing session.

Twin B

Like her sister, twin B was assessed initially on the Gesell instrument at 33 weeks of age; her gross motor level was 24 weeks or about 70% of age level. At 23 months, her gross motor skills were in the 12- to 15-month range on the Gesell measure (about 60% of age level). Her Bayley MDI at 28 months was 69, and her gross motor age level was estimated at 16 to 18 months (60% of age level). At the interdisciplinary assessment at 4 years 5 months (53 months), twin B received a Stanford-Binet IQ score of 72 (low average range), with relative strength in visual memory and relative weaknesses in spatial tasks and short-term auditory memory. Receptive and expressive vocabulary were at the 3-year–7-month level as was visuomotor integration. As with twin A, physical therapy assessment at this time reported truncal hypotonia and a mildly lordotic posture; her gross motor age equivalent on the PDMS was equivalent to that of her sister (29–35 months) at about 60% of age level. Medical concerns included recurrent serous otitis media and a history of tremulousness.

The Gross Motor Scale of the PDMS was readministered to twin B at 5 years 1 month (61 months) by a physical therapist (KJ). Clinical observations indicated that muscle tone and range of motion, although not assessed, appeared to be within normal limits. Automatic reactions included the ability to stand on the dominant foot (one-footed balance) for up to 6 seconds and on the nondominant foot for 3 seconds. Twin B, like her sister, was able to walk on a balance board with skills close to her age level (Fig. 3). Her ball skills (receipt and propulsion) were at about a 4-year level (Fig. 4).

Although they differed in performance on certain items, twin B's overall performance on the Peabody Gross Motor Scale was identical to that of her sister. She had a basal level at 18 to 23 months and a ceiling level at 54 to 59 months, with an overall age equivalent of 39 to 40 months (65% of age level); percentile scores were all at the 1st or 2nd percentile. Twin B was alert and cooperative throughout the PDMS testing.

Summary of Twins and Clinical Implications

Neither of these girls would appear to be developmentally different to the average observer. Because they are both small for their ages, their gross motor delays may not seem as signifi-

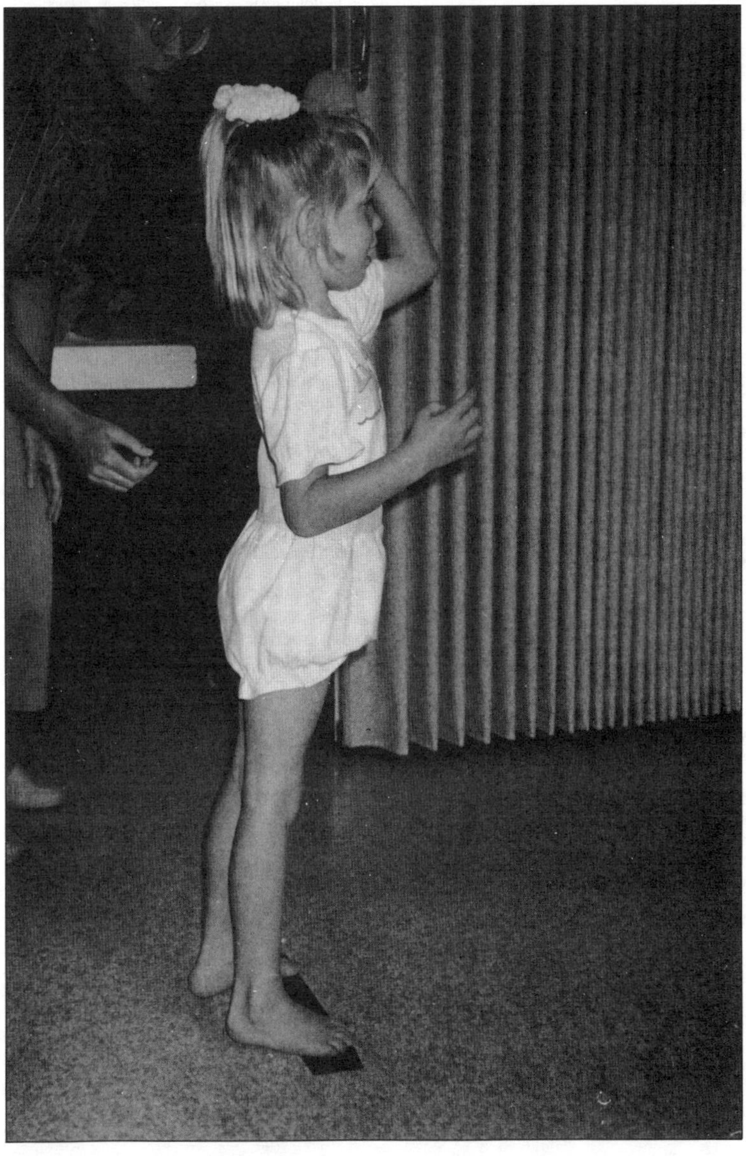

Figure 4. *Twin B throwing tennis ball at wall target (item 150 from Peabody Gross Motor Scale).*

cant as they actually are. As can be seen from the photographs, these children might appear, to the average layperson, to be typical preschoolers.

The twins are enrolled in a special needs preschool and receive speech and language therapy through that program as well as privately. They do not receive individualized physical therapy or occupational therapy but did partake in gymnastics classes between the ages of 3 and 4.5 years. Both children showed relative strengths in balance board activities, which may be a reflection of their involvement in gymnastics. Such community-based activities are probably more appropriate for children with these types of developmental delays than individualized, clinically based therapies. Children with FAS or ARBD who show more significant delays in both motor and cognitive areas, however, may be candidates for direct physical therapy.

Conclusions

As can be gleaned from these seven case reports, children with FAS or ARBD show great diversity in neuromotor and cognitive delays. Caution should be exercised, however, in interpreting results from the various standardized tests in that no Native American children were included in the normative samples for any of these tests and the normative data for the Bayley Scales of Infant Development have been criticized recently for being out-of-date.[18,19] Furthermore, the within-infant variability noted in the Bayley scores during the first postnatal year in the infant case reports is similar to findings reported by Coryell and colleagues[20] in their longitudinal assessments of full-term and preterm infants using the Bayley Motor Scale. As these authors noted,[20] clinical decisions regarding referral for intervention or discontinuation of follow-up should never be made based on an isolated test score. It is encouraging to note that the Bayley Scales are being revised and new normative data are currently being collected.[21]

Additional impairments such as feeding disorders and behavioral disturbances also vary widely. The children in this series who have diagnoses of full FAS are actually less severely involved and more functional than some of the children described here who lack the full syndrome.

Because the children in our series were born to mothers with prenatal histories of abusing other drugs, in addition to alcohol, it is impossible to sort out which of the developmental delays among our children are due solely to the alcohol exposure. Our clinical experience, however, as well as recent reports in the literature, suggest that "there does not appear to be developmental sequelae associated with prenatal narcotic exposure."[22(p597)]

The developmental motor delays, musculoskeletal abnormalities, and feeding difficulties (see clinical perspective by Osborn and colleagues in this issue) that can result from prenatal alcohol exposure are areas of concern to physical therapists. What remains to be examined, however, is what effect we might have in remediating these difficulties or in minimizing the emergence of functional impairments. Single-subject research designs provide an appropriate experimental model for clinically evaluating the effectiveness of physical therapy interventions. Such research is needed to further assess our role and usefulness in the management of infants and young children with FAS or ARBD.

Acknowledgments

We wish to thank the children and families who participated in the assessments that led to these case reports. We are also grateful to Dr Ann P Streissguth of the University of Washington for her support and encouragement in the development of this report and to Robert Stickney of Sunny Hill Hospital for Children for the photographs of the twins.

References

1 Sokol RJ, Clarren SK. Guidelines for use of terminology describing the impact of prenatal alcohol on the offspring. *Alcohol Clin Exp Res.* 1989;13:587–598.

2 Jones KL, Smith DW. Recognition of the fetal alcohol syndrome in early infancy. *Lancet.* 1973;2:999–1001.

3 Peirog S, Chandavasu O, Wexler I. Withdrawal symptoms in infants with fetal alcohol syndrome. *J Pediatr.* 1977;90:630–633.

4 Hill RM, Tennyson LM. An historical review and longitudinal study of an infant with fetal alcohol syndrome. In: Messiha FS, Tyner GS, eds. *Alcoholism: A Perspective.* Westbury, NY: Plenum Press; 1980:177–201.

5 Landesman-Dwyer SL, Keller L, Streissguth AP. Naturalistic observations of newborn: effects of maternal alcohol intake. *Alcohol Clin Exp Res.* 1978;2:171–177.

6 Streissguth AP, Sampson PD, Barr HM. Neurobehavioral dose response effects of prenatal alcohol exposure in humans from infancy to adulthood. *Ann NY Acad Sci.* 1989;562:145–158.

7 Golden NL, Sokol RJ, Kuhnert BR, Bottoms S. Maternal alcohol use and infant development. *Pediatrics.* 1982;70:931–934.

8 Streissguth AP, Clarren SK, Jones KL. Natural history of the fetal alcohol syndrome: a ten-year follow-up of eleven patients. *Lancet.* 1985;4:85–92.

9 Conry J. Neuropsychological deficits in fetal alcohol syndrome and fetal alcohol effects. *Alcohol Clin Exp Res.* 1990;14:650–655.

10 Kyllerman M, Aronson M, Sabel KG, et al. Children of alcoholic mothers: growth and motor performance compared to matched controls. *Acta Paediatr Scand.* 1985;74:20–26.

11 Barr HM, Streissguth AP, Darby DL, Sampson PD. Prenatal exposure to alcohol, tobacco, and aspirin: effects on fine and gross motor performance in 4-year-old children. *Dev Psychol.* 1990;26:339–348.

12 Chandler LS, Andrews MS, Swanson MW. *The Movement Assessment of Infants: A Manual.* Rollingbay, Wash: Chandler, Andrews, & Swanson; 1980:1–53.

13 Bayley N. *The Bayley Scales of Infant Development.* New York, NY: The Psychological Corporation; 1969.

14 Schneider JW, Chasnoff IJ. Motor assessment of cocaine/polydrug-exposed infants at age 4 months. *Neurotoxicol Teratol.* 1992;14:97–101.

15 Autti-Ramo I, Granstrom ML. The psychomotor development during the first year of life of infants exposed to intrauterine alcohol of various duration: fetal alcohol exposure and development. *Neuropediatrics.* 1991;22:59–64.

16 Knobloch H, Stevens F, Malone AF. *Manual of Developmental Diagnosis: The Administration and Interpretation of the Revised Gesell and Amatruda Developmental and Neurologic Examination.* Hagerstown, Md: Harper & Row, Publishers Inc; 1980.

17 Folio MR, Fewell RR. *Peabody Developmental Motor Scales and Activity Cards.* Allen, Tex: DLM Teaching Resources; 1983.

18 Campbell SK, Siegel E, Parr CA, Ramey CT. Evidence of the need to renorm the Bayley Scales of Infant Development based on the performance of a population-based sample of 12-month-old infants. *Topics in Early Childhood Special Education.* 1986;6(2):83–96.

19 Washington KA, Harris SR. Mental and motor performance of low-birthweight infants with normal developmental outcomes. *Pediatric Physical Therapy.* 1989;1:159–165.

20 Coryell J, Provost B, Wilhelm IJ, Campbell SK. Stability of Bayley Motor Scale scores in the first year of life. *Phys Ther.* 1989;69:834–841.

21 Aylward GP. Prediction of outcome for at-risk infants: application of the Bayley Infant Neurodevelopmental Screener to the Risk-route Model. *Dev Med Child Neurol Suppl.* 1992;66:33.

22 Kaltenbach KA, Finnegan LP. Prenatal narcotic exposure: perinatal and developmental effects. *Neurotoxicology.* 1989;10:597–604.

Letters to the Editor

Role of Ankle Plantar Flexors in Children With CP

To the Editor:

I am a physical therapist who works with children with cerebral palsy. I was most interested in Judy Carmick's article "Clinical Use of Neuromuscular Electrical Stimulation for Children With Cerebral Palsy, Part 1: Lower Extremity" in the August 1993 issue of *Physical Therapy.* As a clinician, I find the time spent in working on concentric and eccentric ankle plantar flexion invaluable. I was not surprised, therefore, to see that Ms Carmick found that stimulating the ankle plantar flexors (especially in case 1) changed the gait characteristics significantly, whereas stimulating the ankle dorsiflexors had an adverse effect. Several long-held beliefs about the ankle in gait in children with cerebral palsy are seriously questioned when the results Ms Carmick reports are studied. Although I have never used neuromuscular electrical stimulation with children with cerebral palsy, I have found the study and clinical application of gait analysis in children with cerebral palsy led me to look much harder at the role of the ankle plantar flexors.

The ankle plantar flexors play a far more important role in stance stability, energy conservation, and forward shift of the center of gravity in gait than do the dorsiflexors.[1-3] Yet, we as clinicians have always focused on the dorsiflexors in treatment, probably because we see the ankle usually assume a plantar-flexed position throughout the gait cycle in children with cerebral palsy. Electromyographic studies show us that in children with cerebral palsy, the ankle dorsiflexors are often active and of prolonged duration[4,5] in the gait cycle, that the plantar flexors are often silent during the swing phase when the ankle is in a plantar-flexed position,[5] that the ankle plantar flexors are weak,[2,6] and that the plantar flexors' stretch reflex is often delayed.[7] Additional information about muscle response to immobilization is yet another area we are only beginning to learn about. Immobile muscles may increase their stiffness and resist passive and active range of motion to oppose them.[1,8] Yet, the plantar flexors continue to be implicated as spastic, unwanted muscles that must be inhibited. So we stretch them, then immobilize them in a variety of orthotic devices, and surgically lengthen them if there are contractures. Then, we wonder why the 2-year-old toe walker becomes the 14-year-old crouch walker with such an energy costly gait that the person is in danger of losing ambulation altogether.

Although Bleck[1] states that there is a plateau in motor improvement in children with cerebral palsy, I see not only a plateau, but a decline in gait function in children whose gait has not been addressed with attention to the muscles that provide control and stability from heel-strike to mid-stance—specifically, the hip extensors, hip abductors, and ankle plantar flexors.[6] Children with cerebral palsy certainly walk after the age of 7 or 8 years, and so contradict Bleck's statement of motor plateau, but deterioration of gait is also quite common.

I do not know all the reasons why stimulating the ankle plantar flexors allowed a more plantigrade foot in the child in Ms Carmick's study. I believe that there could be several reasons. In assisting the plantar-flexor activity during the stance phase of gait, it is likely that the child was able to prolong the stance phase on that side and learn to shift weight over the lower extremity. This would give him the opportunity to develop other muscle groups needed for stance phase control. It would also be likely that the step length increased as the opposite leg had more time to complete deceleration in swing, with the possibility of bringing the center of mass forward over the stance foot. In repeating the stimulation with each cycle, the child would be more likely to assist eccentric soleus muscle activity as the muscle lengthens. It is during the mid-stance to heel-off phase of gait that the muscle would then more passively lengthen as the stance phase increased, thereby allowing more range of motion into dorsiflexion as a possibility. By actively lengthening the plantar flexors, the child may also be decreasing muscle stiffness. More range of motion into dorsiflexion could result. If the range of motion was available, and the plantar flexors not so stiff, active dorsiflexion during swing could result if prolonged co-contraction at the ankle is not too great.

I agree with Ms Carmick's response to the commentaries that the plantar flexors need to be strengthened in children with cerebral palsy in order to make gait as energy efficient as possible. The strengthening needs to take place throughout the muscle groups' entire range of motion, both concentrically and eccentrically. This work needs to be done in the context of a functional synergy for gait (ie, concen-

Letters to the Editor *should relate specifically to material published in the Journal or to research/clinical issues of relevance to the physical therapy profession.*

To be considered for publication, letters responding to articles must be received within 8 weeks of publication of the article. Letters must be submitted double-spaced, with two copies provided. Receipt of Letters to the Editor is not acknowledged; however, correspondents will be notified if the letter has been accepted for publication.

Authors of the article in question will be invited to respond to the letter. Accepted Letters to the Editor will be printed with the author response whenever possible. Letters and responses should be signed by all authors.

The Journal reserves the right to copyedit Letters to the Editor. Unless extensive editing is required, correspondents will not be sent a copy of the edited version to review.

tric and eccentric plantar flexion with hip and knee extension with the hip in slight lateral [external] rotation).

Marcia Hornbrook, PT
Owner, Marcia Hornbrook Stamer, PT, PC
817 Crawford Ave
Augusta, GA 30904

References

1 Bleck EE. *Orthopaedic Management in Cerebral Palsy.* New York, NY: Mac Keith Press; 1987.

2 Gage JR. *Gait Analysis in Cerebral Palsy.* New York, NY: Mac Keith Press; 1991:104.

3 Sutherland DH, Cooper L, Daniel D. The role of the ankle plantar flexors in normal walking. *J Bone Joint Surg [Am].* 1980;62:354–363.

4 Leonard CT, Hirschfeld H, Forssberg H. The development of independent walking in children with cerebral palsy. *Dev Med Child Neurol.* 1991;33:567–577.

5 Dietz V, Quintern J, Berger W. Electrophysiological studies of gait in spasticity and rigidity. *Brain.* 1981;104:431–449.

6 Sutherland DH, Cooper L. The pathomechanics of progressive crouch gait in spastic diplegia. *Orthop Clin North Am.* 1978;9:143–154.

7 Nashner LM, Shumway-Cook A, Marin O. Stance posture control in select groups of children with cerebral palsy: deficits in sensory organization and muscular coordination. *Exp Brain Res.* 1983;49:393–409.

8 Carey JR, Burghardt TP. Movement dysfunction following central nervous system lesions: a problem of neurologic or muscular impairment? *Phys Ther.* 1993;73:538–547.

Response:

I thank Marcia Hornbrook for her supportive and thoughtful comments on my case study. My experiences agree with hers—children do walk after age 7 years, and there is a decline, with age and growth, in gait function of children who do not gain strength in the antigravity muscles of gait. Bleck's research underlying his Locomotor Prognosis Test[1] may have reflected the efficacy of physical therapy at the time. Physicians[2] are still influenced by these findings when referring children for physical therapy and when deciding how long to follow children's progress during research projects.[3]

Ms Hornbrook references the importance of strength of the ankle plantar flexors and expresses concern that these muscles are not generally strengthened but ignored or weakened. I emphatically agree. Unfortunately, it is a generally accepted assumption that many children with cerebral palsy will have heel-cord lengthening in order to weaken the calf muscles.[4] Perhaps because equinus is the most common problem in children with spastic cerebral palsy[5] and heel-cord surgery is done on 20% to 25% of all children with cerebral palsy,[6] parents of children who are newly diagnosed as having cerebral palsy are often told that they do not need to worry, as the child can be helped in the future by doing heel-cord lengthening. It is a widespread medical assumption even when the child is only a babe-in-arms.

Classical teaching leads physical therapists and physicians to be concerned about strengthening the supposedly overactive spastic muscles.[7,8] The fear that I might have been increasing spasticity to the ankle plantar-flexor muscles, or the finger flexors of the hand, led me back to stimulating the tibialis anterior muscles in the leg and stopping stimulation of the finger flexors in the arm. It was only with time that I really became convinced that each time the tibialis anterior muscle was stimulated, the child in case 1 regressed. Each time I stopped stimulating the finger flexors before the child gained functional grasp and release, he would lose the ability to maintain grasp. I did not have to worry about increasing spasticity—it did not occur.

Ms Hornbrook discusses references on how important the plantar-flexor muscles are, and she expresses concern that we, as clinicians, focus on the dorsiflexor muscles. I strongly agree with her. Several authors have expressed concern that weakening needed muscles can be detrimental to the child.[9] Winters et al[10] categorized children and young adults with spastic hemiplegia into four groups based on patterns of gait. The average age of the groups increased from 9.5 years for group 1 through 12.5 years for group 4. The disability of each group was also progressive, beginning with a drop foot to additional problems in the foot, knee, and hip of the subjects in group 4. The authors found that surgery was contraindicated for group 1. Surgery and bracing were recommended in all the groups except group 1. To me, it appears that these groups are divided by biomechanical and not neurological changes. These biomechanical characteristics might be changed or prevented from progressing by active strengthening of the calf and gluteus maximus muscle groups.

It has been shown that the posterior calf muscles are extremely important, and when weakened are detrimental to the gait.[11,12] It has also been shown that when 40% of the body weight of adults with spastic hemiplegia is supported, the subjects' gait on a treadmill is much improved. Electromyographic studies showed decreased or normal activity, and the subjects walked straighter and faster with increased stride length and single-support time.[13] In the light of studies such as these, it would appear that there is a major relationship between body weight and needed body strength in order to maintain or increase independent function as the subject grows.

Physical therapists have been experimenting with strengthening spastic muscle without increasing spasticity or decreasing function.[14] Perhaps it would be helpful to study strengthening the triceps surae muscle in subjects who have been categorized according to the method of Winters and colleagues[10] to determine how strength does effect function and the need for surgery.

Judy Carmick, PT
3060 Miranda Ave
Alamo, CA 94507-1611

References

1 Bleck EE. Locomotor prognosis in cerebral palsy. *Dev Med Child Neurol.* 1975;17:18–25.

2 Rang M. Cerebral palsy. In: Lovell WW, Winter RB, eds. *Paediatric Orthopaedics, Volume 1.* Philadelphia Pa: JB Lippincott Co; 1986.

3 Watt JM, Robertson CMT, Grace MGA. Early prognosis for ambulation of neonatal intensive care survivors with cerebral palsy. *Dev Med Child Neurol.* 1989;31:766–773.

4 Strecker WB, Via MW, Oliver SR, Schoenecker PL. Heel cord advancement for the treatment of equinus deformity in cerebral palsy. *J Pediatr Orthop.* 1990;10:105–108.

5 Bennet GC, Rang M, Jones D. Varus and valgus deformities of the foot in cerebral palsy. *Dev Med Child Neurol.* 1982;24:499–503.

6 Etnyre B, Chambers CS, Scarborough NH, Cain TE. Preoperative and postoperative assessment of surgical intervention for equinus gait in children with cerebral palsy. *J Pediatr Orthop.* 1993;13:24–31.

7 Bobath B. *Adult Hemiplegia: Evaluation and Treatment.* London, England: William Heinemann Medical Books Ltd; 1970.

8 Alfieri V. Electrical treatment of spasticity. *Scand J Rehabil Med.* 1982;14:177–182.

9 Gage JR. Gait analysis: an essential tool in the treatment of cerebral palsy. *Clin Orthop.* 1993;288:127–134.

10 Winters TF, Gage JR, Hicks R. Gait patterns in spastic hemiplegia in children and young adults. *J Bone Joint Surg [Am].* 1987;69:437–441.

11 Simon SR, Mann RA, Hagy JL, Larsen LJ. Role of the posterior calf muscles in normal gait. *J Bone Joint Surg [Am].* 1978;60:465–471.

12 Sutherland DH, Cooper L, Daniel D. The role of ankle planar flexors in normal walking. *J Bone Joint Surg [Am]*. 1980;62:354–363.

13 Visintin M, Barbeau H. The effects of body weight support on the locomotor pattern of spastic paretic patients. *Can J Neurol Sci*. 1989; 16:315–325.

14 Bohannon RW. Relevance of muscle strength to gait performance in patients with neurologic disability. *J Neurol Rehabil*. 1989;3:97–100.

Part II: Orthotics and Devices

Reciprocal Action Skiis in the Treatment of Cerebral Palsy

Robertine St. James, R.P.T.T.

It is the purpose of this article to present a newly designed apparatus for the cerebral palsied child which is simple enough in construction to warrant a place in every department treating this type of case. The apparatus, to be referred to as "reciprocal action skiis," consists of a plurality of parts, assembled in such manner that the completed mechanism affords a means of rehabilitation, aimed toward assisting such patients to regain ambulatory function.

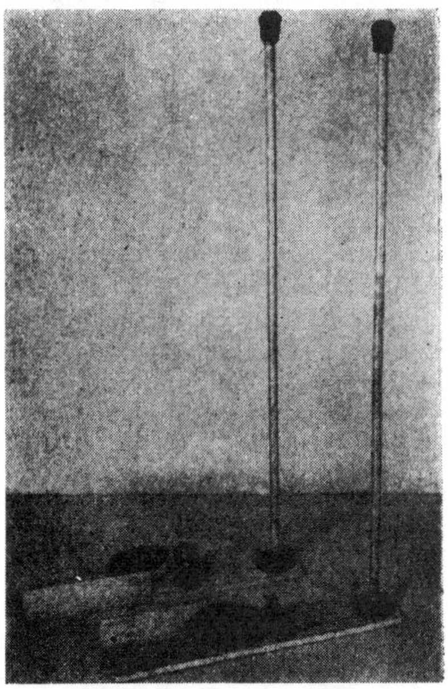

Figure 1. Ski poles.

Miss Mary Trainor, of the Children's Hospital, Boston, Massachusetts, has used ski-skates for several years to correct and improve the leg function of cerebral palsied children and the cord injured group of patients. They give a steadier base, and because the skate extends beyond the foot, heels are encouraged to approximate the floor. In stair walking, the skate blocks itself against the riser, causing trunk and hip action to be made easier by this stabilizing factor. They are especially helpful in correcting a scissors gait.

More recently Dr. Winthrop Phelps began to use larger skiis with poles attached in front (Fig. 1) for walking training at the Children's Rehabilitation Institute, Cockeysville, Maryland. These are indispensable for teaching balance, leg reciprocation, and for strengthening various muscle groups, but they offer little arm activity beyond a reach and grasp. The reciprocal action skiis, which are to be considered a progression from the ski-poles, and not a substitute for them, seem to suggest a solution to that problem.

Figure 2 demonstrates the essential difference between the ski-poles and the reciprocal action skiis. In the latter, canes at the sides replace the poles in front. This not only presents a better body alignment but allows normal arm and leg reciprocation. It also helps to develop lateral balance, while the ski-poles encourage antero-posterior balance. The canes are anchored just off center and are provided with a hand grip which should be extensible by about six inches in order that they can be adapted to several different children if necessary. They are supported and

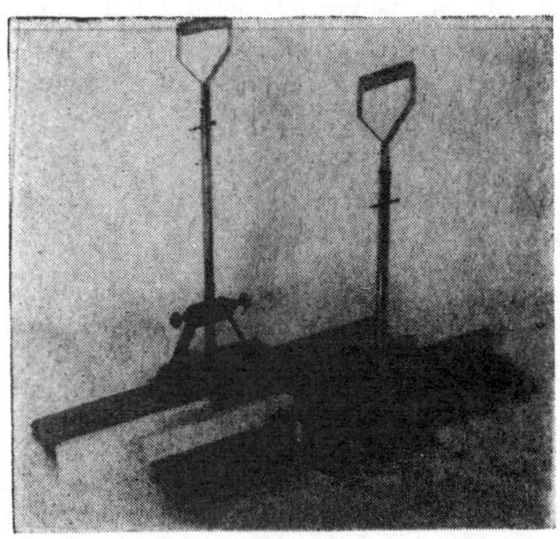

Figure 2. Reciprocal action skiis.

Cerebral Palsy Unit, State Hospital for Crippled Children, Elizabethtown, Pa.

This paper has been read and favorably commented upon by Dr. Winthrop Phelps, 3038 St. Paul St., Baltimore, Maryland; Miss Mary Trainor, The Children's Hospital, Boston, Massachusetts, and Dr. Tom Outland, Chief Surgeon, State Hospital for Crippled Children, Elizabethtown, Pa.

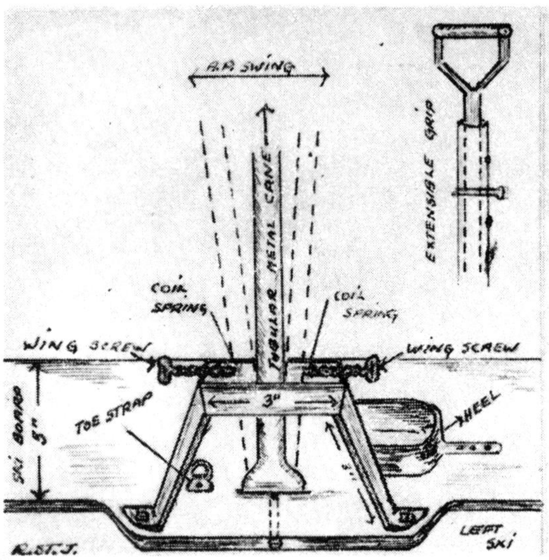

Figure 3. *Metal brace (left).*

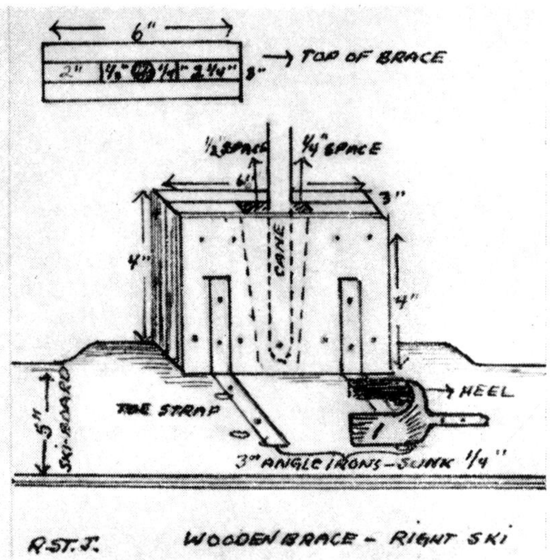

Figure 4. *Wooden brace (right).*

controlled by braces, whose composition may be metal, plastic or wood. The brace (Fig. 3) is arranged to give antero-posterior play. By means of wing screws with lock nuts, the range of swing is adjustable to the point of preference, or the cane may be made stationary for preliminary work and standing balance. Very light coil springs, inserted between the cane and brace, cause the cane to return to neutral and allow some resilience of action. In juxtaposition to the pivotal mounting are suitable foot attachments on the ski board.

For practical purposes a wooden brace acting on the same principle has been tried and found to be very satisfactory. This is shown in Figure 4. The measurements listed insure its stability, and a pair of three-inch angle irons give adequate reinforcement at the point of greatest strain. Minute adjustments in the degree of antero-posterior swing are not possible here, but with the cane blocked posteriorly at ¼" and anteriorly at ½", a twenty-inch cane would have a five-inch total swing. Wedges are used for fixation when it is desired. A metal cane (piping) with a tubular extension still is to be preferred for adjustability.

The ski itself is made approximately three times the length of the foot, with the foot piece placed on the middle third. This, however, is no set rule, for individual differences may necessitate readjustments. One child may find his center of balance directly in the middle, while another may find his slightly forward or more to the rear. A width of five inches has been used, with a projection at the site of the brace to allow for its attachment without interferring with the foot placement. The cane is attached about two and one-half inches ahead of the lateral malleolus.

Side boards may be added in front (inside) to eliminate internal rotation, or in back to eliminate external rotation. If more active dorsiflexion is desired the foot is placed more toward the front. In the case of a heel walker it is placed farther back.

The logical progression with the reciprocal action skiis would be standing balance, assisted walking and unassisted walking with the canes stationary. This is to be followed by arm reciprocation standing (passive, assisted and active), then to combine arm and leg reciprocation. A series of maneuvers such as turning, side-stepping, backing up, sitting down and getting up encourages independence within the child.

Bracing for Cerebral Palsy

Rebecca B. Hastings, B.S.

Some years ago when I first became interested in cerebral palsy, many of us had the attitude that bracing was contraindicated and was of no value to the cerebral palsied individual. This no doubt was true because of the construction, application and amount of bracing.

Many persons still have this impression and as I visit various units and see these children in clinics, it occurs to me that there is a need for more information, study and interest concerning brace procedures for this particular type of dysfunction. Articles have been written about the technics used in physical, occupational and speech therapy, but to my knowledge no article has been published giving personal impressions in regard to bracing for these children.

We know the reasons for bracing are to prevent deformities, to correct deformities and to aid in locomotion. In addition, we may add that in cerebral palsy there is better control of extraneous motions, there is an increase in stability for sitting and standing, and there is an improvement in leg posture which increases our ability to strengthen the proper muscles needed in locomotion.

Paramount reasons for applying braces to younger children is to prevent deformity if we discover they are developing, and in older youngsters braces are used because muscle weakness, spasticity, athetosis or rigidity has developed malpositions which need correction.

In the matter of aiding locomotion, the proper amount of bracing gives assistance to the control of extraneous athetoid motions of the legs and places them in a more functional position for reciprocal motion during walking. Steindler[1] states that "Skillful or perfect motion always involves the least expenditure of effort while unskillful motion requires much more." The athetoid control brace (Fig. 1) does assist in controling the unskillful motion and creates more stability for sitting, standing and walking.

It might be well to remember Steindler's phrase and strive to carry out this thought in all types of training for the cerebral palsied, whether it be during physical, occupational or speech therapy.

The spastic paraplegia, or other cerebral palsy types with paraplegia, is aided in locomotion by using the same type brace, and better leg posture assists the individual in learning to use the legs in a reciprocal manner.

During sitting, if the legs of the athetoid or spastic are not able to rest on the table or seat of the chair, sitting balance is practically impossible. However, with braces holding the thighs down, legs in abduction and by preventing rotation with a pelvic band, the leg position is greatly improved. Thus many times children who have been unable to sit without using their hands for support suddenly are able to maintain sitting balance, leaving their arms free to learn hand activities.

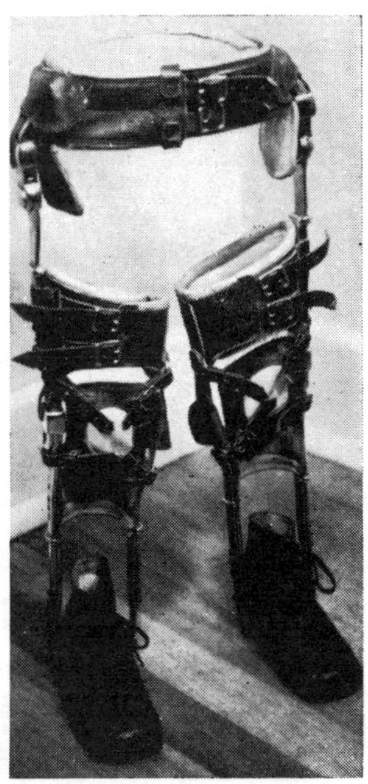

Figure 1. Athetoid control brace.

In the spastic who presents the typical paraplegia, it is difficult for the therapist to work for muscle strengthening when the position we desire to correct returns immediately after the exercise period. Bracing by long leg brace with pelvic band assists in maintaining good leg posture after exercise and also assists in strengthening the proper muscles during locomotion because they are now in a position of function. A good example of this is shown when a child constantly stands in a knee flexed position. The therapist is endeavoring to strengthen the knee extensors but during the remaining hours

1107 North Front St., Harrisburg, Pa.

of the day, the knee is in flexion. If long leg braces are used with a knee lock, extension can be obtained, and when the child walks, he still maintains knee extension. When standing in a standing table or practicing standing balance, it is very interesting to observe how well and how many contractions the quadriceps groups are able to accomplish. Naturally, this helps in increasing strength.

Before considering surgery to correct a deformity it is well to see if the desired position can be obtained by applying external fixation. This correction may be gained by bracing, thus eliminating the need for surgery. If a new deformity is caused by the use of external bracing, we can then adjust the brace to correct the condition. If surgery has caused this factor it is more difficult to correct.

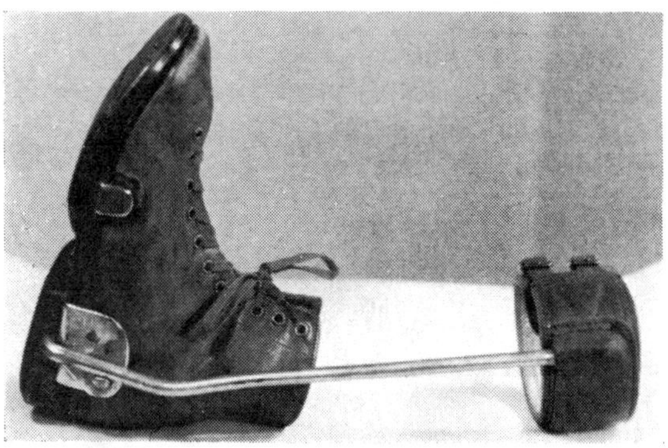

Figure 2. Short single bar caliper night brace.

For example, let us consider the typical equinus position of the foot. The conservative procedure would be to apply a short caliper double brace with the foot stop at 90 degrees for day wear, and a short single bar caliper night brace (Fig. 2) to correct the position at night. When using a night brace it is well to apply the caliper box and brace to an old shoe as this will help eliminate pressure caused by stiffness of a new shoe. An old shoe will fit snugly around the ankle and hold the heel in place. If the shoe is too large the foot will move around and this will cause much discomfort and rubbing. When the shoe is too short, the box or toe of the shoe can be removed allowing the toes more freedom. It is also well to add a long metal plate either on the outside or inside of the shoe depending upon the size, so that the plantar flexor power does not allow a forefoot drop, which will eliminate some of the stretching ability of the brace.

For a night brace, we must decide whether to apply the single bar on the lateral or medial aspect of the shoe. If the foot is in a position of supination or inversion, it is best to apply an inside bar so that the foot can be pronated to a neutral position. An outside T strap will be added to assist in correcting the varus position. If the foot is in pronation or valgus the bar should be applied on the outside as it will be possible to bend the bar to cause supination or varus.

One thing that is important to remember when stretching a heel cord is to watch the position of the foot. When a heel cord is short and being stretched, often times the foot is forced into pronation and there is an apparent lengthening of the tendon; however, if you force that foot into dorsiflexion and inversion it can be seen that the Achilles tendon is not elongating. We then can bend the night caliper bar into supination and begin dorsiflexing the foot by bending the bar upward. The heel cord then can be stretched without as much damage to the arch.

The best way to determine the amount of dorsiflexion a foot is able to tolerate is to (1) apply the shoe to the foot being sure that the heel is well down and laced to the third hole from the top of the high shoe, (2) place the caliper bar in the caliper box, (3) the bar is in front of the stop which is placed on the flange at about 90 degrees, (4) the therapist then extends the knee and holds the sole of the foot, (5) add pressure *gently* until the foot will not allow further dorsiflexion, (6) while the brace is on, the brace man then bends the bar back *to* the stop and the brace is adjusted. If one follows this procedure it is certain that the stop is not set too high so that pressure sores will result, nor is it set too low so that stretching is not effective. After the foot has been held in this position for several weeks, the same test can be given and if the bar leaves the stop we know it is again time to bend the bar back to the stop. When using a night caliper it also may be necessary to apply double bar short leg caliper day brace so that the patient is able to keep the foot on the floor and walk with a heel toe sequence. When applying this brace, it is well to place the desired corrections on the shoe before applying the caliper box. It also is well to be sure that the caliper pins are straight across the heel. If the inner portion of the caliper pin is toward the front of the heel and the outer caliper is further back, this will necessarily turn the foot out which sometimes causes difficulty if the foot is pronated.

The double bar brace will cause more stability than the single bar brace as a single bar day brace sometimes causes lateral deviation of the knee joint. If there is an extreme amount of pronation it is well to add an inside wedge just below the sole and then place the caliper box on the shoe. By placing the raise between the sole of the shoe and the caliper box, it is possible to gain more correction than by placing it on the bottom of the heel. We must align the brace bars perpendicular to the floor so that the knee is not forced out of line.

It has been advocated by a well known authority that often a single bar day brace is more effective than the double bar brace, as it is possible to adjust the foot position by simply bending the caliper bar to create the desired foot position. Another difficulty with the pronated foot can be noticed when the scaphoid bone is prominent and a red area develops. This can be alleviated by applying a longitudinal sponge rubber arch pad covered by leather. The foot then will not rest so heavily against the counter.

When using a bilateral short leg brace, or long leg brace for that matter, we must adjust the stops on the shoe with exceptional accuracy. The flange of the caliper box will hold the drill rod pin which is used as a stop. When trying to determine where the stop should be placed, we must consider the amount of tension or lack of tension in the heel cord. In considering the first point, it may appear that the foot will not relax to 90 degrees; however, if you hold the knee in flexion or extension and slowly but gently push the foot into dorsiflexion and wait for the release of tension, you may discover that the foot will come up to neutral position. This indicates that it is not necessary to raise the heel of the shoe to accommodate for equinus. We are then able to apply the drill rod stop on the inner and outer flange of both shoes so that the caliper bars are perpendicular to the floor, or at 90 degrees. All drill rod pins must be placed so that each bar is perpendicular to the floor; if this is not done it will be noticed that twisting will occur in the foot because of the marked plantar thrust and standing balance will be disturbed.

After the brace has been constructed and before the stop is applied, it is well to let the patient use the brace for several weeks. During this time standing balance is practiced and the therapist watches closely to see where the center of balance is found. When the child falls backward, there may be some spot where he can catch his balance, then we can mark the flange on the outer and inner side of both shoes and the drill rod stop is placed at this spot. If the child loses balance forward, we watch to see where he catches his balance and mark those spots for the placement of the drill rod.

When practicing standing balance after stops have been applied, and the child constantly loses balance either forward or backward, we can place a piece of metal between the stop and the brace bar. An ordinary key or several keys can be used. If balance is secured with this additional thickness the stop can be moved to take up the slack. Often it is customary to bend the bar back to the stop to create this additional degree of change; however, by doing this the entire brace is now out of alignment and further difficulty will result in other areas. After the correction of equinus we can then determine the muscle power of the foot. Perhaps the tendo achilles had been stretched, allowing passive dorsiflexion beyond 90 degrees, but what is the power of the dorsiflexors? It may be that the position of the foot has now assumed a calcaneous deformity because of spastic dorsiflexors if we have not been able to watch the case frequently. We then can retrain the gastrocnemius and lower the night brace to 90 degrees, thus correcting the new foot position which is undesirable. It may be that no power returns to the dorsiflexors, and if we can keep the heel cord stretched out until full growth is reached, we can at least expect to obtain a gait without equinus. It may be that when the tension of equinus is released and the cord stretched out that there will be power in the dorsiflexors and a heel toe sequence will be possible. If surgery had first been done on this type of foot the results would have been very gratifying and successful. When the patient is able to walk with a heel-toe sequence, we can then remove the day brace.

If the gastrocnemius is weak and unable to function, the foot will assume a calcaneous position and balance will be lost forward. This can be corrected by adding a forward stop. In some cases the foot shows poor function in both dorsiflexion and planter flexion. It has been found advantageous in these cases to use a double stop.

At the knee joint, the problem is to decide how a brace must be used; i.e., whether the child should walk with the knee locked or unlocked and to determine what type of knee cap will best function for this particular knee. If it is necessary to have long leg braces with pelvic band to aid in abduction or to keep the hips from internally rotating, and if the knee has full range of motion actively, we then can use a free joint without a drop lock.

To determine whether or not a drop lock is necessary we must test the position of the knees on weight bearing. If there is a degree of flexion which cannot be overcome by the child while standing or walking a drop lock should be added to the brace. The knee must remain locked until the child can maintain extension both standing and walking without using the lock. When he is able to maintain knee extension standing and walking, we then keep the knee joint unlocked.

Should the knee present a flexion contracture it will be found that by keeping the braces locked for most of the 24 hours and by tightening or loosening the knee cap, a great deal of correction will occur over a short period of time if the tightness is due to muscle pull or tension.

In the morning the braces are removed for bathing and this is an excellent time to look at the legs for red marks or pressure areas which will warn us that the brace or shoe is not fitting properly. It might be well to mention here that socks with holes or seams may cause rubbing just as much as socks that are too large.

During weight bearing, we may find a knee that shows evidence of hyperextension. This may be caused by two factors, weakness of hamstrings or tightness of the heel cord. If it is due to weakness of the hamstrings the knee joint will prevent hyperextension; however, if it is due to tension in the heel cord, a 90 degree stop or forcing the foot to just a little above a right angle will help flex the knee.

For a knock knee position, the type of knee cap that pulls the knee to the outer bar rather than the usual knock knee pad that is placed on the inner bar above the knee joint is preferable. If there is bowing of the leg, the knee cap can be so constructed that pressure will come from the outside of the knee to the inside bar.

In dealing with the hips and when trying to determine whether or not a pelvic band is indicated, we must be aware of the amount of active motion, strength of motion, and here again we must consider weight bearing as an important factor. If it is impossible for the child to maintain abduction, external rotation while standing and walking, the application of a pelvic band will greatly aid in walking and help to maintain these positions for the training period. If a pelvic band is used, it must be strong enough so the child cannot draw the legs together or roll the legs inward. I have seen pelvic bands applied, and yet if the therapist puts these braces on the treatment table, she is able to abduct and adduct the leg portion of the brace with ease. Imagine how a child, with marked tension in the adductors, could draw the leg portion of the brace together so that the knee joints lock when he is trying to take a step forward. The pelvic band is then of little value if the patient has no abductor power. Occasionally, we see a strong pelvic band but weak thigh bars; the same will happen under this circumstance. When the child is able to maintain abduction and does not internally rotate, the pelvic band can be removed. One advantage of the caliper box brace is that shoes can remain on the child while the brace can be removed to see what picture the gait is showing, and the child is also able to practice walking under supervision without braces. When his legs have gained a good walking pattern, the braces can be removed for short periods of time until he has complete control. If there is recurrence of the difficulty because of growth, the braces can be reapplied.

For the trunk position we must again decide according to the child's functional ability whether or not the application of a back brace is necessary and what type would benefit the child. During sitting and standing if good trunk posture can be controlled it will not be necessary to add support. If, however, the child cannot sit erect and the trunk is always in a flexed position, upright bars can be added to the pelvic band. Here again we must be sure they are strong enough to accomplish the purpose for which they were applied.

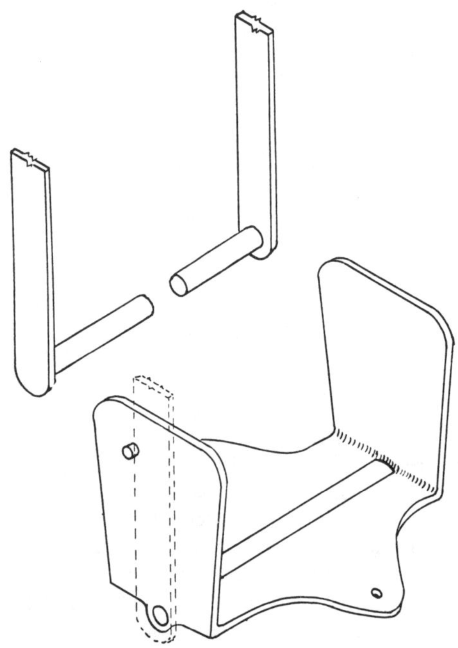

Figure 3. Caliper box.

During standing we study the posture of the hip as well as the trunk. When the child stands with trunk erect but constantly flexes at the hip, we know that hip locks added to the pelvic band will greatly assist in teaching standing balance. If the hips are held firmly so that flexion is not possible, and the trunk still falls forward, a back brace should be added.

It might be well to mention here that braces for the cerebral palsied child must necessarily be constructed differently than those for the infantile paralysis patient.

The cerebral palsied child usually presents a great amount of muscle strength and braces must be constructed so that they are stronger than the muscle power which the brace is attempting to block. In the infantile paralysis case, lightness is the best quality for construction because of muscle weakness, and the support is given to eliminate strain placed on stronger muscles which do not present an increased amount of strength.

BRACE CONSTRUCTION

Throughout the country, braces are constructed on similar patterns and many different materials are used. If one is familiar with the appearance of a brace it often is possible to tell at a glance what brace house constructed the appliance.

From my own limited personal experience, I should like to outline how braces are constructed at the State Hospital for Crippled Children in Elizabethtown, Pa., because I feel that those braces have offered a great deal in the training program for cerebral palsied individuals.

Mr. Alfonz Glaubitz, superintendent of the shop, has spent many years with the problems confronting us and has worked out quite a successful method for the construction of braces for the cerebral palsied group.

At Elizabethtown the braces are hand-forged and nickel plated. Hand-forged bars have a decided advantage as they can be held heavy at joints and other sections when necessary and tapered down where the stress is not so great.

The caliper box (Fig. 3) usually is made of 14 guage soft, cold rolled steel and the tubing is brazed to the caliper plate that holds the pins for the ankle stops. Whenever such stops are used, a metal plate inside the shoe is indispensable and should extend

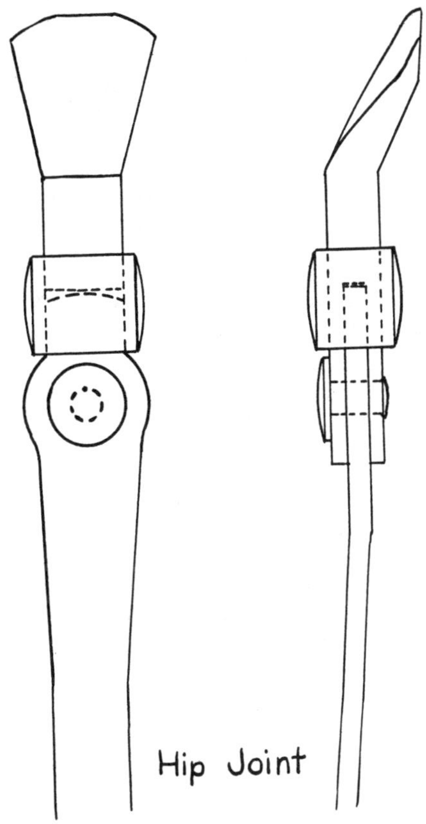

Figure 5.

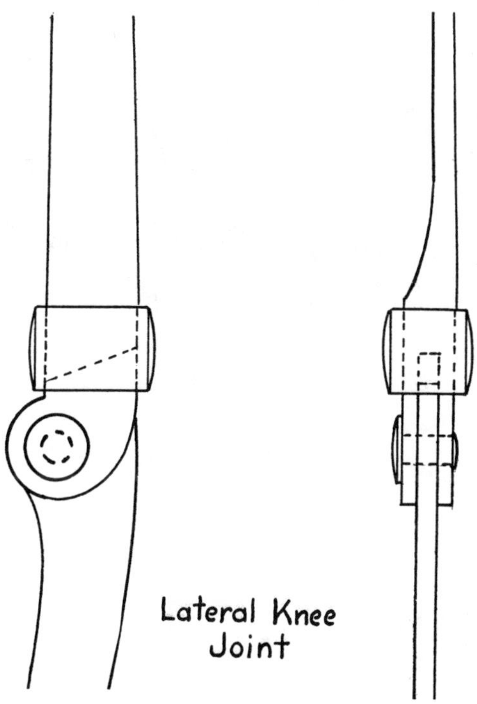

Figure 4.

to the first metatarsal and sometimes beyond. Without this metal plate the foot position in relation to the leg cannot be maintained for any length of time. The shoe will break down at the arch and the desired 90 degrees of limited plantar flexion motion would be lost. Because the patient has to depend on these stops for balance, a heavy inner footplate is to be selected. The stops are made of $\frac{3}{16}''$ drill rod.

The knee joint (Fig. 4) is constructed with the box type joint as greater stability is gained, and better motion is obtained under strain. The lock is held up by the use of a flat spring which is made of blue spring steel. It is riveted to the bar above the joint and when holding the lock up, flexion is possible or when the lock is down, knee extension is maintained. Care must be taken so that the lock does not slip up in walking; this can be done by being sure that the drop lock fits well around the joint. The box hip joint (Fig. 5) need not have motion limited in hip extension unless necessary. When the muscle pull constantly holds the hip in hyperextension then the joint is constructed to eliminate this. It is well to realize that if the thigh bar which fits into the box hip joint is a little smaller than the box joint the tension of the adductors will cause the hip joint to bind and motions of flexion and extension will be difficult. Special attention should be given to the pelvic band. As mentioned before, it controls the legs in establishing a walking pattern. The complete pelvic band and hip joint must be strong enough to hold the legs in the desired position. A ¼″ metal band is a daily routine and pelvic metal bands of heavier metal will be necessary for larger patients. A longer than normal trochanter bar will be advantageous. The pelvic extension bars play an important role in holding the legs abducted and they should, therefore, be strong between the hip joint and the loop of the thigh bar. This can be accomplished without difficulty if one uses hand forged bars. If a single leg brace is used with a pelvic band, a whole band is desirable.

When a patient is using a pelvic band and long leg braces, it is well for the patient to be able to sit with the knees locked and not have the pelvic band touch the back. This also is necessary in sitting with knees flexed. As a matter of fact, it is not necessary for the brace bars or thigh and calf bands to fit the legs too snugly. If any brace fits too snugly and causes pressure in any area, the child will fight the brace and more tension, overflow and inability to do activities will be the result. Calf bands are made of surgical steel and should be strongly constructed and cut or hammered to shape. The upper thigh cuff should be approximately 1″ in width at the peritoneum and should widen toward the lateral side to twice the width. This band should never be less than $\frac{1}{16}$″ in thickness but heavier if the case requires it.

Single night brace bars are made of $\frac{3}{16}$″ round surgical steel for patients whose length from knee to floor does not extend over 8″. If the length is between 8″ and 12″, round bars of surgical steel of ¼″ is used, and for all lengths above 12″, $\frac{5}{16}$″ round steel is used. The calf band of ¾″ by $\frac{1}{16}$″ should embrace the calf of the leg. The caliper pin should extend the width of the heel. The foot plate should extend the full length of the shoe and be constructed of heavy metal. Bars for night braces are made of "Rezistal" type of stainless steel and can be bought as stock material.

Knee caps are best held in position by "D" rings. The straps are stitched on the knee cap at a 30 degree angle, with the exception of the lower lateral strap which has no "D" ring. It is stitched to the knee cap at a 45 degree angle, and the strap goes around the lateral bar. This arrangement will allow the knee cap to slip up a little in a sitting position. Knee caps should have a hole cut over the patella, and padded with cotton or lambs wool covered with fine horsehide.

Buckles of about ½″ are used throughout the braces. Children will manage their dressing problems with greater ease if buckles are used on the pelvic strap thigh cuff and knee caps. Lacings or buckles are dispensed with on the calf band and it is open in front. Leather used in braces should be of the best quality. Elk, calf and Russett leather is used for coverings and straps; cream and pearl horse for linings.

Whenever braces are in need of repair, it is of importance that the shoes of the patient also be sent to the bracemaker, as without them he cannot balance the braces. Oiling braces once a week will save hours of work and help keep the braces in good function.

References

1. Steindler, Arthur: The Mechanics of Normal and Pathological Locomotion in Man. Charles Thomas, Baltimore, Maryland, 1935, p. 13.
2. Murphy, Eugene F.: Persons and Organizations Interested in Research on Braces. Mimeographed, Washington 25, D. C., May 20, 1947.
3. Jordan, Henry H.: Orthopedic Appliances. Oxford University Press, New York City, 1939.
4. Braces Today. News Letter of The Pope Foundation, Inc., 197 South West Avenue, Kankakee, Illinois.

The Physical Therapy Review

(Formerly The Physiotherapy Review)

Official Publication of The American Physical Therapy Association

Volume 29 **January 1949** **Number 1**

Toys, Games and Apparatus

For Children with Cerebral Palsy

Gladys Gage Rogers and Leah Thomas

(Editor's Note: There have been so many requests for this article that the authors were asked to revise it for republication. It originally appeared in the January-February 1935 issue of THE PHYSICAL THERAPY REVIEW.*)*

During recent years the medical profession and the public have become increasingly aware of the large number of children with cerebral palsy. This group has been a challenge to the medical profession, and today, from coast to coast, there are special clinics for their care. They urgently need an opportunity for education and now many of them are in schools throughout the country. Many of us who are watching this impetus know that new state institutions are just around the corner. "Institution" is not the correct word; "school" is not the correct word either. We must find a new word suggesting a combination of home, school and hospital. These new centers must provide facilities for medical care and education in many specialized fields which at present are available only in widely separated cities and towns.

From the many already well-established clinics the physicians are selecting the children who have the mental capacity and physical ability to compete with normal children. These children are the lucky few. They have an opportunity to gain a normal education, each making progress at his own rate of speed. Some of these children will be self-supporting.

The larger group is made up of children with normal mentality but with physical disabilities which prevent them from competing with normal children. This is the group for whom the new state centers must be planned. Physicians, physical therapists, nurses and the public should plan now to prevent lowering the standards of the group with normal mentality by not permitting the inclusion in these centers of those children with subnormal mentality.

The centers will not be hospitals or schools alone. These centers will be homes first of all. Improved physical skills and education will be the goal of every child there. For children with cerebral palsy, skills and education are gained only by an uphill road over which they fight with courage and determination. Most of these children will live in these centers for many, many years. We must all work with imagination to give them an opportunity to find "the joy of living."

The following suggestions are a small part of the type and kind of material which physical therapists should be gathering in order to have ready a new creative program for this particular group. The search for toys, games and apparatus is nationwide. However, it seems impossible to make these lists without first mentioning two far more important factors than the toys themselves. One factor is the setting or environment in which the toys are used, the other factor is the psychology of their use. These factors are of paramount importance because the principles underlying the therapeutic value of using toys must be applied, not for a few years, but for fifteen or twenty years.

The child must discover the way open to him through his own efforts, an effort that calls into

Ascutney, Vermont.

play all the capacity for activity that he has. We must see that a child has within his reach, if he will make an effort, toys that stimulate him to continued activity. This activity must bring satisfaction and a sense of accomplishment.

A specific example is the peg board which is well known to all. No child with normal mentality can be expected to enjoy placing pegs in this board for two or five years not to mention the possible need of this exercise for ten years. A step of imagination will lead us to realize that there is an equal amount of therapeutic value in placing faggots on a fire in an Indian village. The anticipation of lighting the fire in evening when the hunters return with their deer is stimulation enough to lay a large fire of which the child may well be proud. This means that the exercise has been repeated willingly many more times than would be possible with a monotonous peg board.

The demand for persistence and exertion which does not bring satisfaction to the child produces instead discouragement and an unwillingness to exert himself again. Ordinarily the little child has a strong desire to roll, creep and later to walk. He will make vigorous effort to reach for and manipulate objects. Too often the handicapped child finds that his efforts have been futile; there is nothing in his environment that he can successfully control except his parent. If his own activity gives him no satisfaction, he will demand entertainment provided by others, or passively accept defeat. There should never be discouragement or impatience; never let the child think you are disappointed, and always make him think he has done better than you expected him to do. Remember that the tone of the voice means as much to the little child or perhaps more than do the words. Some teachers advocate a daily chart for exercise to let the child watch the improvement curve. It seems wiser not to start the chart until you are sure that the daily improvement will be large enough to encourage him. To set a goal, "when you can walk," if far beyond the child's present ability, may be a discouragement rather than a stimulus. There should never be competition or a time element unless it is all made a happy joke. Daily exercises, under the direction of a person trained in this work, must keep the muscles in condition to function, prevent contractures, demonstrate new motions, but the actual control of the muscles depends upon the purposeful effort expended by the child.

Each toy should be selected for its therapeutic value. The first principle is to make certain he will not be discouraged by finding it too difficult to manipulate. If the child is eager to play with a certain thing, complete frustration is apt to make him tense and nervous. A phlegmatic child will simply cease to try. Always have a suitable toy within reach which he can pick up and hold in his hand if he cares to. If it is something he enjoys, he does not think of it as an exercise, but as a game.

Education, play and exercise should be of therapeutic value. These should go on continuously throughout the day without the child being conscious that most of his activities have been planned to this end. In this way far greater progress will be made than the usual half hour of intensive muscle training and little or no occupation for the remainder of the waking hours.

Suggestions for Finger, Hand, and Arm Exercises Sitting at a Table

1. A musical dinner gong, such as is used in dining cars affords great joy.
2. Cover the entire table with a large sheet of paper tacked down with thumb tacks. Use large jumbo crayons which can be grasped easily.
3. Put paper clips on letters and words. Use magnet to draw out letters and form words—in same way draw out words to form sentences. (Milton Bradley school material.)
4. Magnetic toys demand less skill of motion than the above suggestion. (5 and 10 cent stores.)
5. Fishing with a magnet on the end of a string. Have fish in a basket and catch them by dropping magnet into basket. On each fish have a problem or letter or word. ($2 + 3 = 5$, or A, B, C, or ran —horse, etc.)
6. Dusting with a cloth always seems to give pleasure, and helps with big arm movements. A paper napkin in each hand to wipe the table is enjoyed a few times.
7. A large dishpan of water in which to push around floating toys.
8. A table with a two inch rim on three sides and one-half inch on front side will prevent toys from constantly dropping to the floor. Bore holes in opposite rims and tie strings in these holes so that the strings run lengthwise across the table. Fasten spools, buttons, beads, blocks on the strings. Use toys which may serve a constructive purpose. Count spools or buttons, learn colors with beads, name the animals, have letters or words on the blocks. If the child is not old enough for this suggestion, tie on soft stuffed animals or dolls to play with. Stretch colored elastic bands across the table in the same way the string is fastened. Pull these bands forward, then let them snap back to place, knocking down wooden men or small toy nine pins. Count the pins and add the score each time.
9. A large plate of flour, make finger patterns.
10. Jack stones are too difficult to play the cor-

rect game, but children enjoy moving them about.

11. Printing pad: animal stamps as well as letters and words can be found for this purpose.

12. Printing set or printaprimer.

13. Anagrams.

14. Make tracks like animals—use water color on end of fingers or make tracks in plasticene.

15. Small sand box on the table.

16. Bread dough—the children like the feeling of bread dough and will mold this long before they show interest in plasticene.

17. Clothes pins—these can be fastened together to make queer designs. This has an advantage of using both hands. A few colors or faces on the pins will make them more interesting. Push clothes pins or different shaped pegs into clay.

18. Roll balls across table—try to hit object. Rubber balls covered with worsted netting are desirable in certain cases.

19. Roly-poly toys are excellent. One child made her first successful attempts with hand exercises playing with these.

20. Piling up large square bean bags is not so discouraging a task as blocks.

21. Tinker toys—these demand more degree of skill than most other suggestions.

22. Bead numerical frames—different colored beads are pushed back and forth on wires. Colors may be learned. Addition and subtraction in arithmetic may be made interesting.

23. A large peg board—put large different colored pegs in holes in board—then put a corresponding wooden colored cap on each peg. (Milton Bradley.)

24. Hammer and nail set. (Milton Bradley.)

25. Clay molds.

26. Spatter work.

27. Soap bubbles.

28. Cut art stencils to crayon.

29. Large wooden beads—round and square—one half inch to one inch size.

30. Bell—similar to those on teachers' desks.

31. A, B, C weaving looms.

32. Circular or straight knitting frames.

33. Finger painting. This has been very successful when done to flowing music. Two of our children used their bare feet with great enjoyment and made very interesting pictures.

Suggestions for Children Lying on a Mat on the Floor

If the child can lie prone this is the best position—he will then use his back and neck muscles to great advantage.

34. Small furry animals or rag doll to pick up.

35. Small bean bags—the shape of a half moon will fit the hand. Small turtles and a Chinaman that can be held by his queue are interesting.

36. Small bells to shake.

37. Rubber toys of all descriptions—when squeezed they make a noise or squirt water.

38. Blowing feathers.

39. Blowing or hitting balloons.

40. Jumping toys—bunnies, ducks and frogs which hop along by squeezing bulb.

41. Push around floating toys in low pan of water.

42. If outdoors—put mattress where child can pick grass, clover and wild flowers.

43. Change beans or wooden beads from one bowl to another.

44. Rattles disguised with more grown up ornaments.

Suggestions of Toys Which May Be Used Sitting or Standing Without a Table

45. Leather string with soft toy on end to whirl around in big arm circles.

46. Toy clothes pins and line for doll clothes. (a) wash tub; (b) wringer; (c) iron.

47. Wooden dishes.

48. Toy brushes with dust pan. Feather duster.

49. Dish mops with faces.

50. Building blocks of every description.

51. Pretty boxes or toy eggs to open and close. Smaller ones inside of larger ones.

52. String to pull and ring a bell or a row of bells.

53. String to pull on and turn off electric light.

54. Watering pot—used in bath tub with great glee as well as out of doors.

55. Ball on elastic—this can be thrown at a distance and will come back to child.

56. Accordion.

57. Tambourine.

58. Drum.

59. Wrist bells.

60. Xylophone.

61. Harmonica.

62. Toy piano.

63. Other rhythm band instruments.

64. Blowing out paper toys—these are long narrow strips of paper with a feather on the end.

65. Sandbox—have a long narrow sandbox where the children may stand beside each other rather than opposite. This will prevent the accidental throwing of sand in other's faces. Children who cannot stand alone may be strapped to the box if given support around the hips and low back. Others can stand between a wall in back of them and the sandbox in front. Many of them stand in their walkers which may be pushed close to the sand.

66. Wooden sand toys.
67. Wheelbarrow—to fit particular child—this toy necessitates using both hands. This will be a great aid in maintaining balance, if instead of one wheel, two wheels are used across the front. These wheels are on an axle the same as two wheels from a doll carriage. Fasten the box part of the wheelbarrow on to this axle.
68. Doll carriage. Weight with stones or sand bags.
69. Toys on ropes to be pulled.
70. Small buckets to wind up on string or chain. These can hold water or sand and be drawn from over a wall.
71. Light punching bag—burlap stuffed with rags will answer the purpose.
72. Ring toss. Use rubber rings.
73. Ball board—balls roll on an incline and drop with a click into holes. Each hole is numbered and scores may be kept.
74. Waterproof dolls—these can be tubbed like real children.
75. Telephone with dial.
76. Raffia or yarn—if braiding is difficult strands of different colors may be wound around each other.
77. Toy money.
78. Cash register.
79. Inexpensive typewriter with letters on a dial.
80. Sewing cards.
81. Enlarged art crayons — wax, hexagonal in shape four and one-half inches long and one-half inch thick.
82. Large pencil—Eagle brand, 75-12 automatic, eight inches long, three-quarters inch in diameter.
83. Magnetized letters for a blackboard—they cling to the board or may be pushed about.
84. A bar or pulley handles.
85. Balloons.
86. Set of flags—twenty-three nations. (Educational Playthings, Inc.)
87. Telegraph set—a child may learn to tap by the Morse Code.
88. Winding mechanical toys or victrola.
89. Marbles.
90. Twister toys.

We suggest that mothers and physical therapists send for catalogues from

Milton Bradley Company,
Springfield, Mass.

Educational Playthings, Inc.
20 East 69th Street,
New York City.

The Ideal Line—Distributed by
J. L. Hammett Co.,
Cambridge, Mass.

J. L. Hammett Co.,
Kendall Square,
Cambridge, Mass.

Childhood, Inc.
32 East 65th Street,
New York City.

Montessori Material,
J. L. Hammett Co.
Kendall Square
Cambridge, Mass.

GAMES

Group games afford the happiest moments of the day. Almost every game must be adapted in some way for these children. Many of them are changed beyond recognition, but this in no way decreases the joy and good spirit of the games. Almost every child in our group has experienced from three to eight years of a lonely, inactive life. Each child has been the center of his own world. His life goes on at a tempo which he sets. His activities are governed by his physical limitations. His interests and education depend entirely upon those of his parents, many times one parent.

We believe for these children suitable group games will have educational value. This type of child tends to react slowly to external stimuli. They are slow to think, to hear, to observe, to see and to do. At first many of them appear to be almost oblivious to what goes on around them. In proportion to the improvement possible with these children, we are certain they react to group games as favorably as a group of normal children.

Sense perceptions are quickened; each child grasps more quickly that it is his turn, that the balloon is coming his way, that he is in danger of losing by a wrong guess. He hears footsteps behind him. He soon knows what to do when his name or number is called. Will-power develops and inhibitions vanish through games. A social sense which leads to social cooperation and good will is, for these children, one of the most valuable assets to be learned through games. During the game hour they are in a world of many people. Since these children are alone so many hours of every day, the game time should be carefully planned to give them every advantage of group play.

Tests of skill or strength, methods of capture, running, competition and all the usual excitement which accompanies games are barred to us. Such activities are not necessary because we must find games that have their value in a "carry-over" which can be applied in an inactive world.

Singing games are, no doubt, the best beginning for play with these particular children. They are simple in content, the pianist can set a slow rhythm and the activity naturally cannot extend beyond what the piano is telling us to do.

To the surprise of the instructors "Ten Little Indians" served a bigger purpose than ever before in the history of its being sung. During Indian week we come to assembly dressed as Indians. There are one, two or three feathers in our hair. Some of us carry newspaper tomahawks, while others carry tom-toms made of oatmeal boxes. The pianist surprised us all by arriving with a papoose strapped to her back. The day before we made a teepee and laid the fire mentioned elsewhere in this chapter. We have had real Indian dishes at meals and we have read Indian stories. So, this morning at assembly we are not playing Indians, but we are actually living Indians, and for the first time we are living the Indian stories we have heard.

In such a setting we are not going to have time to regret that we cannot hide in ambush and spring upon the enemy or that we cannot perform the authentic war dance. It is enough for us to be content with less. We are all sitting in a circle. One child is named as the first Indian. As we sing "One Little Indian" he stands before his chair—"Two Little Indians," the next child is helped to his feet and then he proudly stands alone to the end of the verse. "Three Little Indians," the next child is helped to stand and is assisted in standing throughout the verse. When ten little Indians are standing the first verse is ended. Beginning with the tenth Indian we sit down, one by one, as we sing through the second verse. The children loved this song and frequently asked for it. The action is so simple that we can readily assume that each child felt a satisfaction in doing his full share in the group activity. There is no reason for apologizing for this simplicity in action because at four, five or six years of age, many times standing up and sitting down are envied performances which these children have seen accomplished by other children, whom they secretly know are still babies. It is a valuable exercise for these children to stand up and sit down to music. They are so distracted by the fun of doing it this way that most of them do not seem like the same children attempting to stand at the direct command of an adult.

We have a prayer to the Indian Sun God. The children refuse to be left out of this worship. A councilor with perhaps less spiritual enthusiasm for this particular form of worship, kneels beside a child who needs assistance, holds him in balance and raises his head, arms and hands in benediction. In circle formation we are kneeling on the floor. The body is bent forward with the head touching the floor and arms extended forward overhead. As we sing, "Wa-Kon-da-dhe-dhu. Wa-pa-dhin-a-ton-he," we raise our heads from the floor and extend the arms upward to the sky. During the second verse we return slowly to the starting position. The difficulty in balancing is somewhat forgotten by the aid of the soft flowing music. Before Indian week is over most of us have learned to do this exercise in a more relaxed degree than we did at our first attempts.

Indian music and Indian dances give us many avenues leading directly to beneficial muscle training. Of equal importance is our endeavor to create so vivid a story of Indian life that our week of Indian games may be the foundation of a real and lasting interest in Indian history. We aim to make the high points of each week so broad and far reaching that these interests will grow, and leave less time for regrets that our physical prowess is not greater.

"How do you like to go up in a swing" a song with words by Robert Louis Stevenson, music by Reginald de Koven is another favorite. We stand in a circle, partners facing each other and holding hands. Last summer we had three "walkers" in the circle. Through the verses and chorus the arms swing from side to side in slow rhythm. During the chorus "Swinging, swinging, swinging, etc.", one child runs under the swinging arms and continues around the circle until the music stops. When the song has been learned thoroughly and the first enthusiasm is lessened by repetition, select a child in one of the walkers to go around the circle as the others have done in turn. There is a hushed outstanding joy surrounding the group as each set of couples silently moves to adjust the formation of the circle to allow adequate space for the walker. At the suggestion of the children this game never ceased until, with awkwardness and patience the other two children in walkers had been pushed around with the gaiety and spirit of fairy dancers. We had all danced a solo part from start to finish. The mother of one of our oldest children told us that her daughter had been practicing standing alone during the winter, because she enjoyed the dance so much she wished to show us her improvement in executing it the following summer. She did accomplish this end.

The action of the words in "Hansel and Gretel Dance" can well be carried out sitting in a circle. Instead of turning in place standing as we sing "Round and round and back again" we make big arm circles.

Another game is that of rolling a big ball across a circle trying to make it go out between persons in the circle. It is called Circle Stride Ball on playgrounds. We sit in a circle and allow the children to kick with the feet or hit with the hands. This is an excellent game because there is no waiting for the slower children. The ball is always in play. Within a short time there is marked improvement in skill.

It is impossible to give further details of games but a short list of those we have used successfully follows:

Singing Games

Oats, Peas, Beans and Barley Grow	The Steeple Bells
Shifty Shadow	Snail
Did You Ever See a Lassie?	Row, Row, Row Your Boat
Farmer in the Dell	Little Bo Peep
Looby Loo	Sing a Song of Sixpence
Muffin Man	My Old Dan
Mulberry Bush	Round and Round the Village
Nuts in May	

Games Without Music

Balloon games	Hide the Thimble

Guessing Games

One variation we make is to whisper to one child some action which he can do while the others guess —such as an airplane or shoveling coal on the fire, going upstairs.

Simon Says.

Pass two bean bags around circle.

Nine Pins.

Games which children may play in smaller groups according to physical limitations

Croquet.

Dart game—we hesitate to mention this but the children ask for it daily. It is a special favorite for rainy days.

Simple ball games with enough councilors to keep the ball in play.

Tether Ball. (Miniature pole braced on table.)

Bean Bag.

Peggoty.

Throwing dice for many games where men are moved about on a board.

Spinning for numbers to move men in such games as mentioned above.

Dominoes.

Tit tat toe.

Apparatus

1. A rather heavy table similar to the old fashioned kitchen table is very useful. Cut a round hole in the top eight inches in diameter. Put wooden rims, two inches high on all four edges of the table. This will prevent play toys from dropping to the ground. The child can stand inside this table and have excellent support. Casters on the legs for indoors or larger wheels for out-of-doors will allow the child to move about and make the play time more interesting.

2. A small table with the legs cut short the correct height for the child when kneeling is excellent for children who cannot stand, but can kneel. If they fall because the knees slip forward under the table, place a board in front of the legs at one end. This gives the child a chance to brace his knees. With this support at the knees and the top of the table giving support at the height of the chest, children can crayon, look at books, or play games on the table. Children will remain in this position for a long time without fatigue. It is an important step toward strengthening the back muscles.

3. Jungle gym—during the summer we live in medieval England, so, the jungle gym is not a jungle gym, but a beautiful castle which stands near Sherwood Forest. There are several long lanes of pipes leading to it. These are not pipes to which we must cling and pull along to reach the framework and there attempt to do certain exercises we have tried to do for days or weeks past. These pipes are avenues leading to the castle to which we have been invited to make a visit. We frequently refurnish the castle and then we explore from top to bottom and tell what we find as we travel from room to room. Knights in armour on white chargers are sometimes at the door and we go racing off with them after the castle inspection is over. Beside the jungle gym are sand tables by which the children in walkers are playing. They can hear the conversation during the castle adventure and frequently the piles of sand tell the same story of the beautiful castle and its white chargers.

4. A ladder will be found more useful if it is fastened to the side of the wall. This will give support to the toes and prevent the feet slipping forward as the foot is placed on the rung. This ladder may well serve as the bar on which the child may pull himself from a sitting to a standing position.

5. A see-saw is enjoyed. At each end, in front of the sitting space, have an upright with handles to which the child may cling or be tied with straps.

6. Heavy book racks similar to music stands may be placed by the tables in which the children stand. There is no possibility of the child hitting this with his hands and he may read or ask another child to turn the pages as they look at pictures together.

7. Tricycle—fasten a board six inches wide, vertical to the rear axle. It should extend from this axle to a height of the child's shoulders. Fasten it at the axle and back of seat. Strap the child to this board with one strap under his arms and another around his hips. Tie the feet on to the pedals with two-inch straps made of inner tire tubes. These

are strong and will cling to the foot, the ankles and the pedals the same as a bias piece of cloth. Tie the hands securely with bandages, over and over the handle bars and around the wrists. Fastened this way, a child of tetraplegia type felt so secure that she would relax and ride up and down the corridors and in the ward of a hospital. Within a few weeks she could travel about alone. When sitting at a table she could not control her arm movements. Her fingers were in constant motion and she could not pick up anything from the table. With her hands tied around the handle bars and feet tied to the pedals she gained muscle strength and coordination in learning to steer and pedal.

8. A velocipede is better for some children than a tricycle.

9. A blackboard serves many purposes. Lines and circles drawn to music are helpful. If the child cannot hold an eraser, a dust cloth will serve as well. Chalk can be purchased one inch in diameter. Tie this to a string fastened to the top of the frame to prevent the chalk from falling to the floor. Magnetized letters will cling and can be pushed around on the board. We have found that sticking an end of the chalk in a soft ball or inside of a ball of cotton is an aid in helping the child hold it.

10. Ramps used instead of steps by the porches are as valuable as any apparatus we have found.

Our book, "New Pathways for Children with Cerebral Palsy," contains more practical material for group instruction than we have been able to locate in any other publication and no doubt would be of value to anyone wanting toys, games and apparatus for children with cerebral palsy. This book was published by Macmillan in 1935 and is now out of print. It could be found in medical libraries only.

Reciprocal Motion Skiis*

for Cerebral Palsied Children

Joan C. Kuhnen

A newly designed pair of Reciprocal Motion Skiis for the treatment of cerebral palsied children have been developed at Lenox Hill Cerebral Palsy Center where Dr. George G. Deaver is the Medical Director. They have proved to be of great value in teaching a reciprocal pattern of walking, strengthening various muscle groups, and teaching balance while in motion. They teach the child the proper distribution of body weight; that is, to balance the upper right quadrant over the lower left quadrant; the upper left quadrant over the lower right quadrant. They also allow the child to practice walking backwards.

Previous work has been done with skiis of different types, notably by Dr. Winthrop M. Phelps of Children's Rehabilitation Institute, Cockeysville, Maryland, who pioneered the use of skiis with poles for cerebral palsied children; ski-skates devised by Miss Mary Trainor of Children's Hospital, Boston, Massachusetts, and reciprocal action skiis designed by Miss Robertine St. James of Children's Rehabilitation Institute, Cockeysville, Maryland.[1]

The basic concept of the Reciprocal Motion Skiis is the establishment of a reciprocal pattern of walking. The importance of teaching this reciprocal pattern is well known. Dr. Temple Fay of Philadelphia, Pennsylvania, has for several years studied the importance of the simultaneous movement of the opposite arm and leg. He refers to this reciprocal action as a "crossed pattern" movement.[2]

In teaching a reciprocal pattern of walking, the physical therapist begins with table or mat exercise in a supine or prone position and progresses to reciprocal crawling and then to reciprocal walking in parallel bars. Finally, before the child learns to walk unassisted he is taught to walk in skiis. The skiis provide the necessary balance, they strengthen the leg muscles and teach leg reciprocation. They are an essential part of every training program for cerebral palsied children.

Reciprocal Motion Skiis are a natural development of older types of skiis. They have stable poles which are crossed near the base so that the right hand grasps the pole attached to the left ski, and the left hand grasps the pole attached to the right ski. Because the poles are stable and attached in this manner the child can walk in the skiis only with a true reciprocal pattern. When the left leg moves forward the right arm will likewise advance. In other words with each step the opposite arm and leg move simultaneously following the natural reciprocal pattern of walking.

These skiis teach the child to distribute his body weight properly and to balance while in motion. That is, to balance the upper right quadrant over the lower left quadrant of the opposite side; the upper left quadrant over the lower right quadrant of the opposite side. The motion of the opposite arm and leg occurring automatically with each step promotes proper distribution of body weight when walking.

The Reciprocal Motion Skiis have vertical guides running from front to back along the inner edges. These prevent internal and external rotation of the hips and prohibit a scissor gait. There are U-shaped locks which prevent the child from crossing the skiis but which allow them to move parallel to each other. By preventing crossing of the skiis either in front or in back, the physical therapist can teach the child to walk backwards also. This will help to strengthen the extensors of the hips and give him confidence.

For the child who is making progress in independent walking but who needs strengthening of leg muscles, the physical therapist places sandbags

Coordinator, Lenox Hill Cerebral Palsy Center, Lenox Hill Hospital, New York, N. Y.

*Purchased through Reciprocal Motion Skiis, 513 West 54th Street, New York, N. Y. Patent Pending.

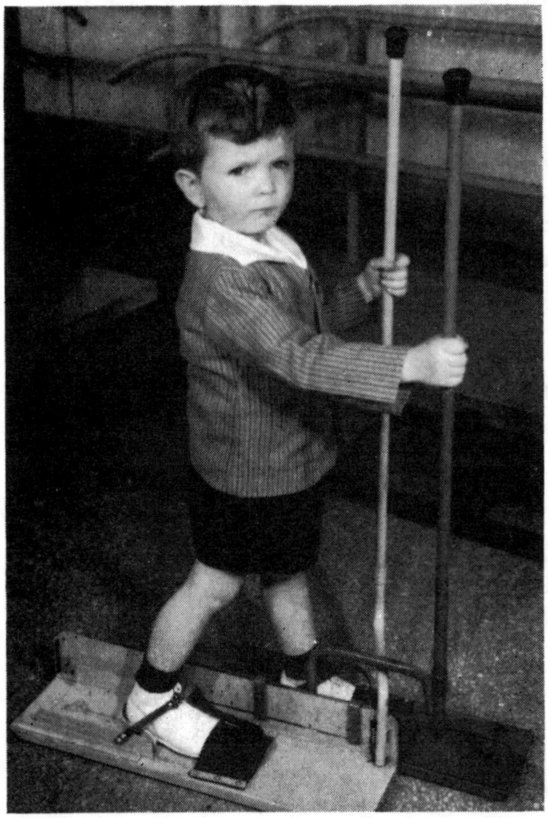

Child in position to use Reciprocal Motion Skiis

in the back of each ski. The weight of the sandbags gives resistance to walking and strengthens the muscles. In either forward or backward walking, strengthening of various muscle groups occurs, i.e., quadriceps, hamstrings, extensors of the hips, flexors of the hips, and so forth.

These skiis are built purposely on a very broad base to prevent the child from tipping over. At a treatment center the child can practice without the guidance of the physical therapist and still be perfectly safe. In other words, after the child has finished his treatment the physical therapist can put him in the skiis knowing that he is practicing a true reciprocal pattern of walking, strengthening various muscle groups, learning balancing and the proper distribution of body weight, and yet he is perfectly safe even though he is unattended. This leaves her free to treat another child while the one in the skiis learns independence.

Another feature of the skiis is their use of color. These skiis are finished in red and yellow. The opposite arm and leg to be moved simultaneously in the reciprocal pattern are attached to a ski and pole which are the same color. Thus the child associates the movement of the right arm and left leg with red, and the movement of the left arm and right leg with yellow. This use of color permits visual learning as well as kinesthetic learning.

The use of two colors has been worked into a series of activities designed to establish a pattern of reciprocal motion. A red ribbon is placed on the right wrist and left shoe; a yellow ribbon on the left wrist and right shoe. The child walks in parallel bars and is instructed to move the two red ribbons (right arm and left leg); then the two yellow (left arm and right leg). He is walking with reciprocal motion of the arms and legs.

From parallel bars he progresses to Reciprocal Motion Skiis where the same two colors are used. The right hand holds the red pole which is attached to the left ski which is also red. The left hand holds the yellow pole which is attached to the right ski and which is also yellow. The child is instructed to move the two red, then the two yellow. With each step the child has reciprocal motion of the arms and legs. By making possible reciprocal walking in the ski-stage of the cerebral palsy training program, Reciprocal Motion Skiis provide a continuity of treatment heretofore unattainable. They are a natural and essential bridge from parallel bars to walking unassisted.

From Reciprocal Motion Skiis the child progresses to crutch walking if it is indicated. When using crutches a red ribbon is attached to the right crutch and the left shoe, and a yellow ribbon to the left crutch and the right shoe. This time the child is instructed to move the red crutch, yellow shoe, yellow crutch, red shoe. This produces a four-point gait. For a two-point gait the child is instructed to move the two yellow, then the two red.

When he learns to walk without the aid of crutches, ribbons are placed on his shoes and index fingers. He is instructed to move the two red, then the two yellow. This produces a reciprocal pattern of walking which in time will become his natural gait.

REFERENCES

1. St. James, Robertine: Reciprocal Action Skiis in the Treatment of Cerebral Palsy. Physical Therapy Review, September 1943.
2. Fay, Temple: The Neurophysical Aspect of Therapy in Cerebral Palsy. Archives of Physical Medicine, June 1948.
   Fay, Temple: Problems of Rehabilitation in Patients with Cerebral Palsy. Delaware State Medical Journal, March 1946.
   Fay, Temple: Observations on the Rehabilitation of Movements in Cerebral Palsy Problems. West Virginia Medical Journal, April 1946.

The Physical Therapy Review

(Formerly The Physiotherapy Review)

Official Publication of The American Physical Therapy Association

Volume 29 December 1949 Number 12

The Importance of Bracing in the Treatment of Cerebral Palsy

Herbert E. Hipps, M.D., F.A.C.S., and Genevieve Waters

The judicious use of braces is an extremely valuable adjunct in the training program of the cerebral palsied. Much surgery can be eliminated and the development of desired purposive muscle actions can be accelerated by their use.

General Indications

The multiple, wayward muscle actions of the athetoid that hinder purposive action can be restrained in an extremity by a brace, thus permitting the patient to concentrate his attention on one joint movement at a time, and thus, by simplifying the purposive action pattern, make it more easy to learn.

Many weakened muscles, weak and ineffective from overstretching by a more powerful spastic antagonist, often can regain sufficient strength to become effective, if supported by a brace during the early part of the training period.

The development of purposive muscle action can be accelerated by supporting a joint of an extremity in the desired position of optimum function, or by supporting the joint in any position that makes it easier for the patient to use the involved muscles.

Many deformities, such as an equinus foot or a palmar flexed wrist, frequently can be corrected permanently by the wearing of a spring action brace.

Beginning deformities, due to improper muscle action, can be prevented.

Illustrative Cases

K. M.—Spastic hemiplegia, age 12. His left arm was held in rigid extension at the elbow and was carried uselessly behind him when he stood or walked. His wrist was rigidly dorsiflexed, and the fingers remained tightly flexed into the palm of his hand. He could not voluntarily extend the fingers, nor flex the elbow, and he could not bring the arm forward to the front of his body. This patient never had made any attempt to use his hand and fingers, principally because he could not get the hand to the front of the body in a position where it could be used.

He had been treated by the usual physical therapy methods many times before and had never shown any improvement.

A brace was applied holding the elbow in 90 degrees flexion and the wrist in a neutral position (Fig. 1).

He was given one exercise and only one to perform. This was to flex his shoulder, bringing the arm forward to the front of his body. He

1604 Columbus, Waco, Texas, and Crippled Children's Hospital, 1501 North Eighteenth, Waco, Texas.

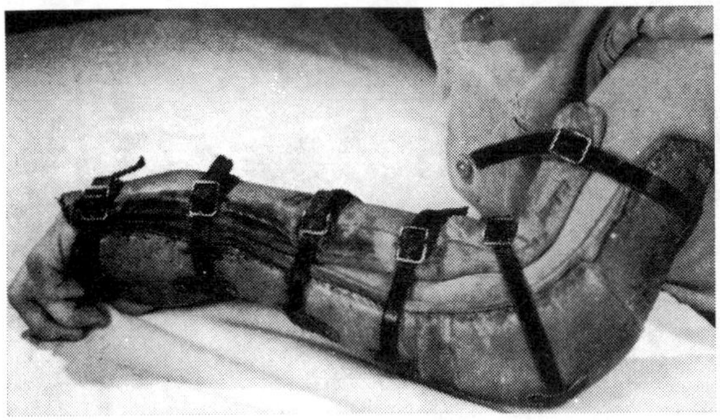

Figure 1.

did this many times a day. He practiced continually under our rather strict and constant supervision, and he learned how to do this one thing fairly well in approximately thirty days.

Now the brace was removed part of the time each day and he was given exercises in flexing and extending the elbow. He wore it all the rest of the time, day and night.

At the end of three months the brace was cut off to just below the elbow joint. The upper part of the brace was no longer needed. He held the arm down by the side of his body, he could bring it forward, and he could flex and extend the elbow slowly but with good control.

The brace, now supporting the wrist only, was still worn night and day. He was started on finger exercises. His other arm was tied down against his body so that he had to use his left arm and fingers for everything.

He worked with his left hand constantly. We saw to it that he did.

Within three more months this remaining part of the brace was removed. He could use his hand and fingers creditably and he had formed the habit of using his hand in most of his activities.

He has been seen at intervals since then and is showing a constant improvement.

M. P.—Spastic monoplegia, age 6. He walked with his left knee bent and on the toes of his left foot. The heel cord was tight. It could not be stretched enough to permit the foot to come to a right angle.

A drop ankle brace, with springs in it to stretch the heel cord, was applied. He wore this night and day for four months. Then it was left off during the daytime and he wore it at night. All during this time he was given exercises in extension of the foot.

In three more months he no longer needed the brace. He walked well. He got his heel down on the floor with every step.

He is being rechecked at intervals. His brace has not been used at any time during the last six months, but if any heel cord tightness should recur, then again he would be advised to wear the brace each night until it was again corrected.

D. T.—Athetoid, age 14. She had fair use of both arms and hands, but she could not stand or walk. Uncontrolled, wayward movements of the legs occurred when she attempted to take a step.

Long thigh-length braces were applied to both legs. This permitted her to concentrate attention on hip motions only, as the knees and feet were held relatively immobile in the braces. She learned to stand alone and to walk between rails fairly well within six months time and is now walking for short distances with crutches.

Within another eight or ten months one brace probably will be cut off just below the knee; still later the other one will be done likewise, and perhaps still much later the feet may be liberated.

H. Z.—Spastic hemiplegia, age 16. He had never used his right hand, which was small and palmar-flexed acutely at the wrist. He could flex and extend the fingers slightly. The fingers remained, most of the time, in extension. The wrist could be extended passively but he could not hold it this way.

Obviously this patient could never learn to use his hand and fingers properly as long as the wrist remained in this deformed position. His overstretched extensors were too weak to make much progress against the stronger flexors. Hence, a plastic brace was applied holding the wrist in dorsiflexion but permitting free finger motion. He wore this night and day for four months (Fig. 2).

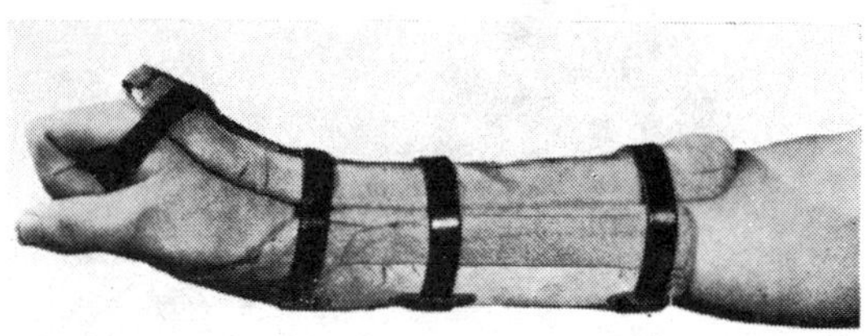

Figure 2.

He was given things to do with his hand. He was kept busy all day long. He was not allowed to rest.

At the end of four months he could flex the fingers completely and he could extend them almost to completion. He had good control over them. Then the brace was removed for short intervals each day while finger and hand work continued. Later it was removed all day, but he continued to wear it at night.

He is still wearing it every night and is using

his hand without the brace all day. He has good use of this formerly useless hand.

P. F.—Mild athetoid, age 8. She walked awkwardly, popping the right knee backward with each step. The knee had thus developed a mild degree of genu recurvatum that was constantly getting worse.

Because of an apparent tightness in the heel cord, a short leg drop ankle brace was applied. Springs in the brace stretched her heel cord.

This did not help her in controlling the back-knee tendency.

Then two curved bars were added to the brace, holding the knee in about 20 degrees flexion (Fig. 3). She wore this for six months. After this, little by little, the brace was left off, and she was given exercises in trying to stand and walk without popping the knee backward. She gradually learned this and is now walking without a brace, but we have applied a one-inch elevation on the right heel. Only when she becomes excited or tries to run does she ever let it return into the genu recurvatum deformity.

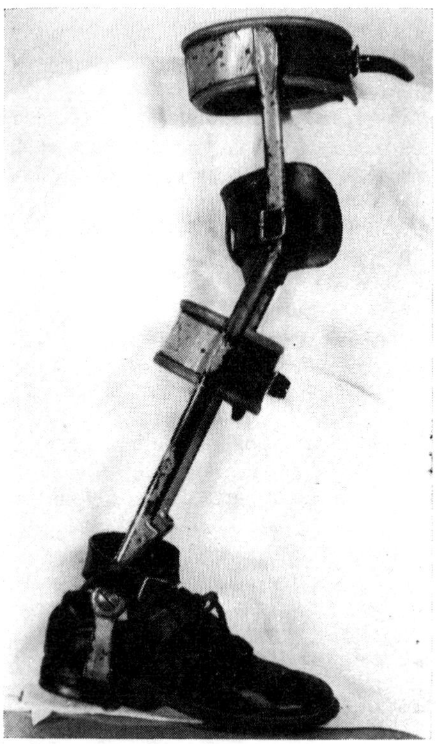

Figure 3.

J. V.—Spastic monoplegia, age 7. He had one wrist that was acutely and rigidly palmar-flexed. He could not extend it and it was impossible to extend it passively. Because of this awkward position, he could not use his fingers.

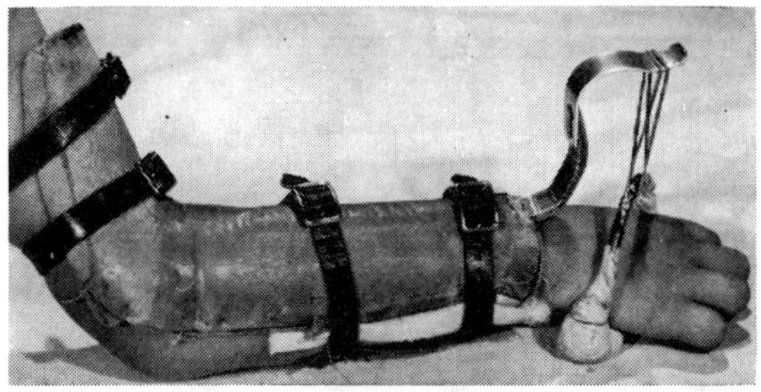

Figure 4.

A brace was applied with a rubber band traction device on it that pulled upward constantly on the hand, gradually pulling the wrist into extension (Fig. 4). He wore this splint night and day for six months, during which time the splint was adjusted at the necessary intervals, to keep a constant, mild upward pull on the hand.

By this time the wrist had been brought into full dorsiflexion but he was not able to hold it there. Accordingly, a smaller, rigid, cock-up splint was applied to hold the correction that had been obtained and he was started on active finger exercises.

K. J.—Spastic hemiplegia, had good use of her involved left leg and of all the joints of the left upper extremity. However, when she flexed the fingers to grasp objects, the thumb pulled in under the flexing fingers and got in the way. She could not abduct the thumb. She could not keep it out of the way of the flexing fingers.

Long and persistent training at home and by competent physical therapists had failed to correct this.

A short wrist splint with an extension to hold the thumb in full abduction was applied (Fig. 5). She wore this night and day for five months. During this time she continully used her hand.

Then the splint was removed for short intervals

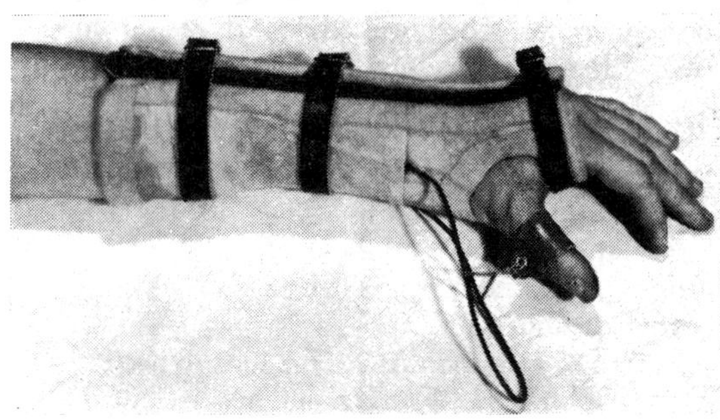

Figure 5.

each day and she was taught thumb abduction and opposition. The intervals were increased as she gained in ability to control the thumb.

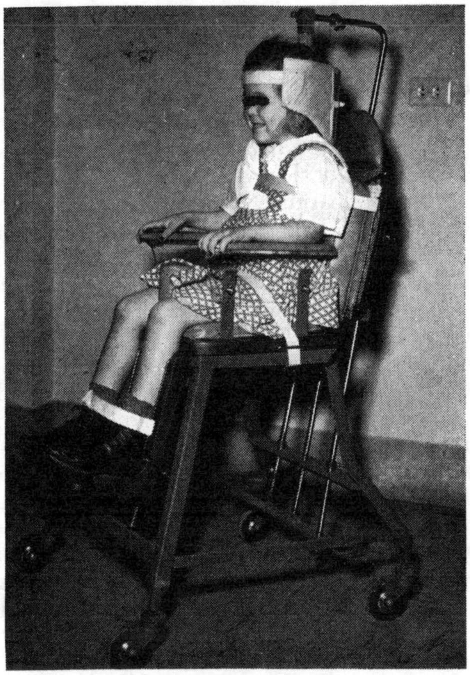

Figure 6.

Now she wears the splint only at night. She can abduct and oppose the thumb slowly but fairly well and it no longer pulls down in the way of the flexing fingers.

M. F.—Spastic, age 3. She could not stand, walk, sit alone, or hold up her head. She had no voluntary control of her hands and arms. She had been considered as a "hopeless case."

A chair-brace was built for her (Fig. 6). She was held in this chair by straps across the legs, lap, pelvis and chest. A movable head piece supported the head, while permitting rotary movements of the head.

She was kept in this chair-brace practically all day long every day. As she moved her head from side to side, to see things of interest, she gained control of the neck muscles. Gradually the head support was left off as she learned to balance the head. Then little by little the back piece of the chair-brace and the chest strap was lowered. She then became able to sit alone without any back support, but with the side arm supports. Now these too were lowered and were moved away from her body slowly a little at a time, until she finally was able to sit alone on the chair seat unsupported in any way. During all this time she also was learning to use her hands and arms.

She is now ready for the application of long leg braces so that she may learn to walk.

* * * * * *

These cases clearly indicate the following specific benefits that can be gained from the use of braces in cerebral palsy:

(1) Learning muscle control is accelerated.

(2) Many surgical procedures are eliminated.

(3) Some deformities can be corrected.

(4) Beginning deformities can be prevented.

There are many instances where the use of braces is an absolute necessity for the recovery of function in an extremity.

A Support for Teaching Head Control in Cerebral Palsy

S. Malvern Dorinson, M.D., Mary Markus
Patricia McLaughlin

One of the problems frequently encountered in the treatment of the athetoid type of cerebral palsy is the lack of head balance. In the early years of life this is due mainly to the weakness of the neck extensors, which fail to maintain the head in the erect position, (there is also poor coordination between neck flexors and extensors). Later, as the muscles become stronger the athetosis becomes more severe causing increased difficulty in head control.

Poor head control interferes with many functional activities. It slows the attainment of sitting and standing balance and handicaps walking in two ways. First, the child cannot focus on one object long enough to measure distance before the movement of his head has pulled his eyes away. Second, the moving of his head upsets his balance and causes exaggerated movements of other parts of his body to compensate, all of which make for an unsafe and ungainly pattern of walking.

Even in sitting activities of which feeding, reading, and speech are of major importance, poor head control is a handicap to successful training. It does little good to teach hand to mouth coordination if the mouth is constantly moving away from the hand.

Most efforts at feeding training stress upper extremity control without giving due consideration to control of the head, jaw, and neck.

Similarly in attempting to read, these children scan the line of words by turning their head from side to side instead of moving their eyes from left to right. Some of these children do have an internal strabismus and a primary weakness of the external rectus muscle, but even those children with a normal forward gaze have poor ability to move the eyes laterally. This can easily be seen when the head is held still by the examiner and the child is asked to look to one side. The child struggles to release his head to turn to that side rather than turn his eyes. The fluency of reading will be delayed until some eye control can be established.

Again, in learning to speak the child must have the head balanced without tension in the neck and throat. He must be able to focus his eyes on one object whether it be his image in a mirror or a set of letters and pictures. Most of the previous training has been to teach a type of conscious relaxation. This is only partially successful and when head balance is really needed for efforts requiring concentration, the relaxation is seldom maintained.

Another method of dealing with the problem is to provide a posterior head support and have the head fixed by a lateral support so that it cannot be turned from side to side. This type of apparatus is exceedingly frustrating to the child and consequently its practical value is greatly diminished.

In an effort to combat this, a type of headsling similar to that used in Sayre neck traction was devised. Normally the Sayre headsling is of a 2-point suspension and secures its leverage under the chin and the occiput. This basic principle was modified to provide suspension of the head by 4-points in order to control the anterior and posterior motion as well as the lateral motion. The head straps were made to fit around the forehead as well as the chin and occiput in order to gain a better purchase on the head. These straps were easily and simply made from ¾ inch webbing with proper buckles attached and then hooked to a portable-type stand which could be adjusted for the height of the chair and the size of the child. Our stand was made of metal with its own broad base rather than attached to the back of the chair so that the headsling could be brought to the child rather than the child to the apparatus.

The children were placed in these slings for short periods of time in the beginning to accustom them to the limitation of motion. Since there was no rigid fixation there was less tendency for the child to fight the apparatus. Nevertheless, it took several weeks for a child to learn to relax enough in the sling to do some additional

S. M. Dorinson, M.D., Director, Department of Physical Medicine and Rehabilitation, Maimonides Health Center and Garden Hospitals, San Francisco.
Miss Markus, Physical Therapist; Miss McLaughlin, Occupational Therapist; Conyer School, Visalia, Calif.

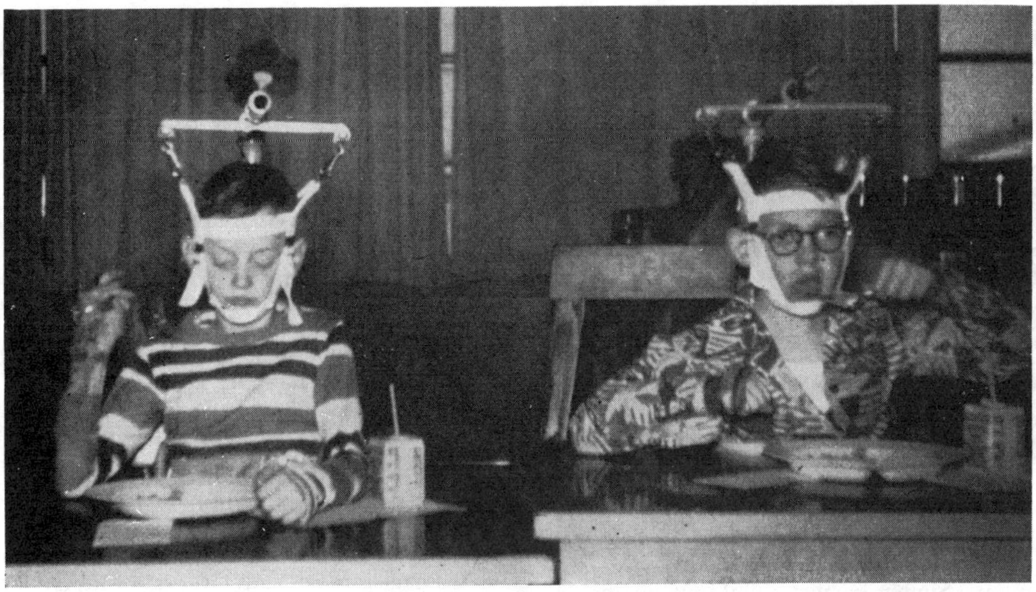

Figure 1. Two athetoid children in their head slings eating lunch. Note normal position of head in relation to plate.

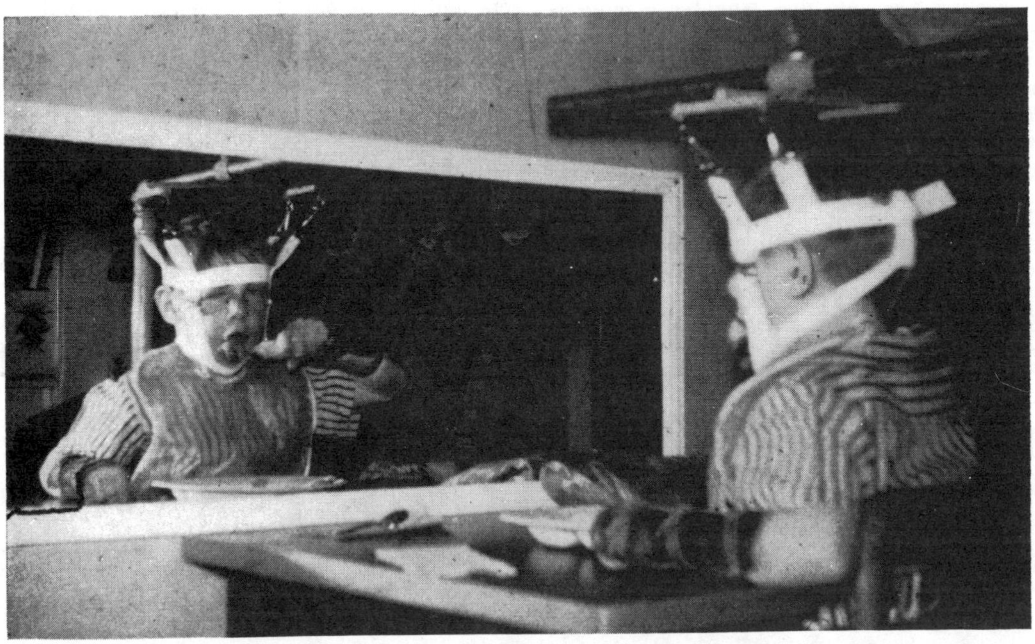

Figure 2. Feeding training in front of mirror. Note posterior arrangement of sling.

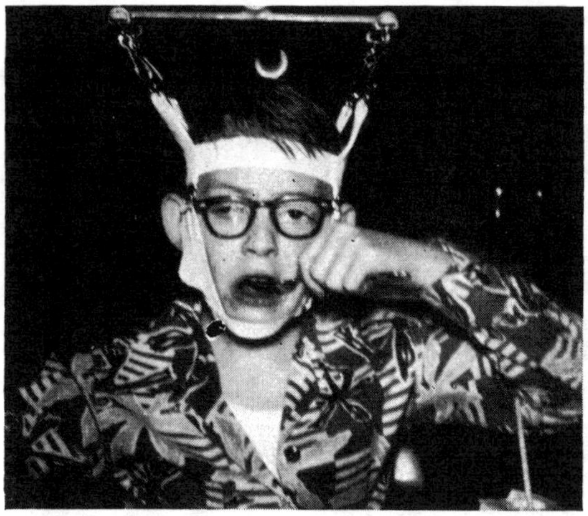

Figure 3. Close-up of head sling. Note strap across the forehead gives greater stability yet does not interfere with jaw action.

activities. Simply having a child sit in this apparatus has brought about the greatest improvement in conscious relaxation that we have been able to obtain with these children, and this relaxation persisted for some time after the child's head was removed from the sling. Later, while in the sling the child was taught eye motions, particularly in a lateral and upward direction while maintaining the head motionless. This was done by the physical therapist and was considered to be not only a treatment procedure for physical therapy but actually a prereading exercise to be carried over into the schoolroom. The occupational therapist began some feeding training also with the head held in the sling. At a later date the child was placed in this apparatus during some of the school activities such as reading so as to maintain the head in a position for optimal control of head and allow the eyes to scan the reading material in front of him.

Figures 1 to 3 show several of the children eating their lunch while in these slings. It is evident from the pictures that there is no rigid fixation, that the child is fully capable of moving enough to carry on his activities and yet the head is held in the best position for feeding training. The child's head is not down on the table almost on the level of the plate with his hand shoveling in the food as is usually seen; instead, the head is up in the usual position and the hand is bringing the food up to the mouth in a normal manner.

This apparatus was first designed for use in a cerebral palsy treatment center and in conjunction with classroom activities. However, it has proved so safe and effective that parents are instructed in its use, and often small children, ages 2 and 3, are able to use such apparatus at home.

Our experience with the sling has been extremely encouraging. The therapists, the teachers and the parents have been able to note improvement in many aspects of the child's functional activities following institution of its use in therapy, classroom and dining room. In conclusion, we feel the use of a headsling will greatly accelerate the process of gaining head control and thus improve walking, speech, feeding, and other hand skills.

Vol. 39, No. 5 THE PHYSICAL THERAPY REVIEW 319

Suggestions from the Field

A Stand-Up Chair for Cerebral Palsied Children

Laura V. Bosworth, B.A.

The "Stand-Up Chair" offers child-initiated reaching, sitting, and standing experience repetitively and in a protected situation. It consists essentially of a seat and a series of horizontal bars placed before it. The entire structure is mounted on a platform with free-rolling casters. In using it the child is induced to reach forward, thus getting his upper trunk weight properly located over his feet, and to pull himself to the upright posture without assistance. He thus learns to utilize his hands and arms for an assistive purpose and to coordinate pull of hands with push of feet in a properly coordinated manner. (Most normal children gain this experience in a playpen. Cerebral palsied children rarely need a playpen and so miss this opportunity.)

The construction of the stand-up chair can be varied in many ways. It is desirable to have an adjustable seat. It is also desirable to have a detachable bar at one side so that the child can, with assistance, step in and out instead of being lifted. The upper two horizontal bars in front should be removable so that as the child gains in ability, the height of security can be decreased. An adjustable toe-board is essential, to be placed so that the reach will exceed the distance of the toes from the front of the chair when the child is standing. A few children tend to pull their feet back and under them. For these children the board is placed behind the heels and toe straps used to keep the feet straight. In some situations the added feature of a drop-leaf tray is good. It is located in front and usually at the level of the second horizontal bar. It is positioned for use when the child is standing and is useful when a table of proper height is not available. At other times the tray is in the lowered position.

This chair has been particularly applicable to the child having athetosis. His uncontrolled motions require that he be tied in any other chair so that most normal experiences of helping himself are thwarted. It has also been useful for the slowly-developing or mentally retarded child. These children go through a long period of

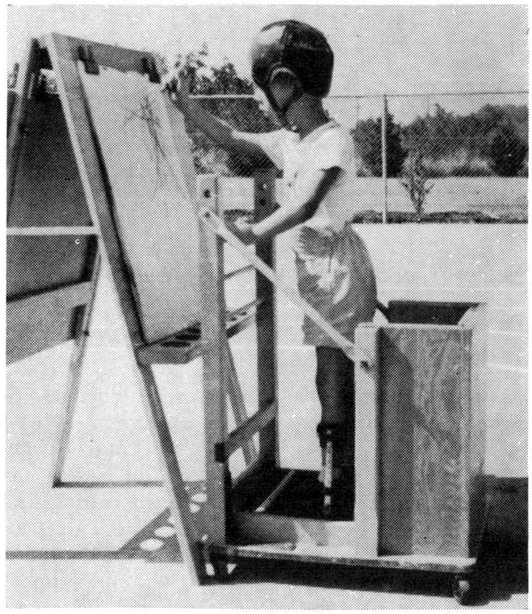

Figure 1. The Stand-Up Chair at the easel.

"floor-sitting," rigidly fearful because they do not know what to do with their hands or feet, or some go through a long period of the "pulling to standing" phase without achieving standing balance because they have no sense of correct foot placement. The feet can be strapped in position and the child will enjoy a secure standing balance. Also, tendencies toward pronation of the feet and hyperextension of the knees, often prevalent in these children, can be avoided. The spastic child too gains in ability and mobility through repetitive use of such a chair.

The stand-up chair was designed for use in the kindergarten or primary school rooms, but in selected situations it has been used satisfactorily in the home. It can be easily moved from classroom to playground. The standing balance practiced during movement, using his own hands for guidance, is a pleasurable and worthwhile experience for the child. In the classroom he can stand at the easel for painting or near book or project shelves. One of the finest possibilities is during speech activities where children spontaneously stand to express themselves. On the playground the child can stand and play ball or stand at the sand box. Whatever the situation, the child is free to sit or stand, impelled by his own desires.

Physical Therapist, Shadelands School, Concord, California.

Diagram and dimensions are available upon request of the author.

Suggestions from the Field

Design and Measurement of Training Chairs for the Cerebral Palsied Child

Gordon G. Robertson, M.A.

Introduction

An understanding of the basic sequences of growth is a prime requisite for any therapist who is responsible for a training program of encephalopalsied children. Dr. Arnold Gesell has described certain behavior patterns which are characteristic of normal growth. Basically, an infant can be expected to lift his head and hold it erect momentarily at 6 weeks, sit without support from 6 to 8 months, crawl by 7 months, stand without support by 1 year, and walk at the age of 12 to 15 months. Cerebral palsied children cannot be expected to maintain this schedule, and various artificial devices must be provided to enable them to accomplish these developmental norms.

One of these devices is the special training, or relaxation, chair that is designed to meet the individual difficulties of the child. To satisfy the needs of a general therapy program, the chair must be comfortable, as no child can be expected to tolerate a position which constantly irritates and antagonizes him; and it should be durable since this equipment, with minor adjustments, may serve the patient for several years. Frequently two, and in rare cases, even three chairs are needed as the child grows. Ease of handling, which makes it possible to transport the chair in and out of doors, adds to its usefulness.

We have excellent facilities for the construction and maintenance of these training chairs at our Institute. A modern, well-equipped, wood shop is located adjacent to the physical therapy department, and a carpenter is available to build, repair, and modify the chairs and other equipment.

Physical Therapist, Cerebral Palsy Institute, Norman, Oklahoma.

Types of Relaxation Chairs

We use two types of relaxation chairs, *bucket* and *standard.*

The *bucket* model is designed primarily for patients with an opisthotonos or a tonic neck reflex and/or those who have extreme difficulty with head and sitting control. Its construction permits the seat-back-footrest portion to be pivoted as far as 45 degrees from the perpendicular by means of a dowel rod. This type of chair is usually indicated for children diagnosed as tension athetoids, rigidities, and the most severe custodial cases.

The *standard* model has no moving parts, but is constructed so that the seat-back-footrest portion of the chair is tilted 5 degrees from the perpendicular. Its design is identical to that of the bucket chair except the dowel rod is eliminated. It is recommended for ataxics, most spastics, and for the moderately involved patient who has good head balance.

Description of Materials

After years of experimentation we have selected ¾ inch plywood for the seat, sides, back, arms, and footrest portions of the chairs. Formerly redwood and white pine were used, but these materials were too unstable; however, maple, oak, birch, and other hardwoods can be ideally substituted. The base structure is composed of two, 1 inch by 4 inch planks and four, 2 inch by 4 inch boards. A ¾ inch wood dowel is used for the bucket models. Three inch casters are used on both types of chairs.

Measurements

In order to insure a perfect fit an order form sheet is filled out and sent to the wood shop. (Fig. 1) This sheet contains all information pertinent to the completion of the chair. Miscellaneous information such as foot control positions and placement of trunk supports is included under *Remarks* or on the reverse side of the paper. It is suggested that periodic checks be made with the carpenter and therapy staff while the chair is under construction.

The type of chair to be used is prescribed by the orthopedic consultant. His prescription may

CEREBRAL PALSY INSTITUTE

Order Form for Special Equipment

SPECIAL CHAIR

TYPE OF CHAIR__________ NECK REST__________ PADDING__________

Height of Back__________ Width of Seat__________

Depth of Seat__________ Height of Tray__________

Angle of Back with Seat__________ Degree of Tilt__________

Seat to Footboard__________ Angle of Footboard Tilt__________

TRAY:

Width__________ Length__________ Depth of Cutout__________

Width of Cutout__________

DATE PROMISED__________

REMARKS__________

NAME OF CHILD__________

PARENTS' NAME__________

ADDRESS__________

Figure 1.

include such accessories as headrests, trunk supports, and degrees of tilt.

As a preliminary to the actual measurement, the patient while using his braces is placed in either a regular straight back chair, a stool set against the wall, or an available training chair. The latter is preferred by our department though any of the above would be acceptable. The parents or a therapy aide steadies the patient during the fitting. The following formulas are used to determine the various measurements:

1. *Height of back* is measured from the seat to the first thoracic vertebra.
2. *Depth of seat* dimensions may be determined by measuring the distance from the back of the trial chair or the wall to the knee joint, less 1 inch.
3. *Seat to footboard* is obtained by measuring from the knee joint to the tuberosity of the calcaneus, minus 1½ inches.
4. *Width of seat* varies according to the diagnosis. Patients with tremor and athetoids are fitted snugly, allowing as little as ½ inch clearance on each side, whereas the measurement of a spastic child allows from 1 to 2 inches on each side, according to the individual requirements for training.
5. *Height of tray* is determined by measuring from the xiphoid process to the seat. We have used many other methods in the past for this dimension but now believe this to be the most accurate. At times, however, the tray may be raised an inch for occupational therapy activities.
6. *Angle of back with seat* should be 90 degrees, unless a severe extension thrust would dictate an 85, 80, or even 75 degree angle.
7. *Angle of footboard tilt* should measure 90 degrees, unless an angle of 85 degrees would permit better foot placement.
8. *Degrees of tilt:* All *standard* chairs are usually tilted 5 degrees from the perpendicular. *Bucket* chairs are made to tilt from 30 degrees to 45 degrees.
9. *Tray:* An 18 inch width and 22 inch length is used for small children. The length is often increased to encourage reach, grasp, and release ac-

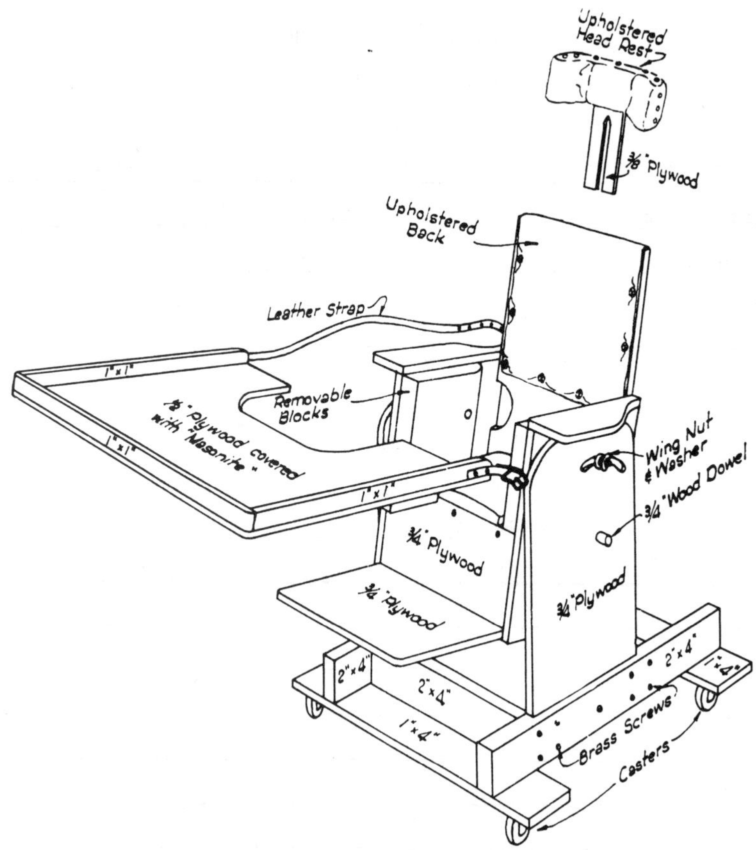

Figure 2.

tivities, but the width is rarely changed. A U-shaped cutout fits snugly around the thorax; this prevents the hands and arms from slipping under the tray, aids in teaching sitting balance, and promotes better feeding technics.

ACCESSORIES

1. *Headrests*

The head supports are constructed from blocks 4 inches by 4 inches that are cut into a concave shape to give support to the occiput as well as to the sides of the head. Recently, we have been experimenting with a V-shaped block and have found it to be quite satisfactory. A 3/8 inch by 3 inch plywood board is used to attach the headrest to the chair back (See fig. 2). A 3/8 inch slot is cut in the center of the plywood and the headrest is anchored at the desired height with a wing nut that extends through the back of the chair. (Height adjustment is thus easily made by a simple twist of the wing nut.) One inch by 1 inch blocks about 5 inches long are placed on either side of the slotted board to give added support and prevent excessive lateral movement.

2. *Trays*

The surface of the tray or desk is made of Masonite glued to ½ inch plyboard. Borders of birch 1 inch high are placed across the front and sides of the tray. Two small L-shaped boards cut from 2 inch by 2 inch blocks are installed on the under side of the tray in such a manner as to permit the tray to slide into position over the armrests and still give firm lateral support. The tray is held in position by a ¾ inch leather strap that buckles behind the chair.

3. *Trunk supports*

Occasionally a pair of thoracic supports are needed to aid in the training of head and sitting balance. These supports may be easily attached to the back of the chair so that they extend under the axilla. Cut to the desired length, 2 inch by

2 inch pieces are usually sufficient when padded with foam rubber or rubber axillary pads from a set of crutches.

4. *Foot control boards*

When stabilization of the feet is indicated a tracing of the child's shoes is made and an identical pattern is cut with a jigsaw in an inch board. The board, with its shoe-windows, is then placed on the footrest and straps are attached in order to prevent the feet from slipping out of the wells. This design insures more accurate and secure placement of the feet.

5. *False sides*

Minor adjustments, such as lowering the footrests and raising the tray or back, may be made by simply adding a board cut to the required dimensions; however, a revision in the width of the seat requires a maximum repair effort. This problem may be solved by adding a block in the sides of the seat. (Fig. 2) The block may be removed or decreased in width when added space is required.

6. *Posture straps*

Possibly the most useful accessory on the chairs is the posture tie. This strap enables the patient to maintain a more correct posture and also serves as a valuable safety belt.

Each chair is constructed with two small half-moon shaped openings in the back about 1 inch above the seat. From the front of the chair, a piece of orthopedic stockinette is inserted in one of these openings, pulled behind the chair, and back through the other slot. A single overhand knot is tied so that the knot fits firmly against the back of the chair and the two ends are draped down the middle of the seat and over the footrest. The child is then placed in the chair. The loose ends are brought up between the legs, crossed over each thigh and reinserted through the slots. A firm bowknot completes the procedure after the stockinette is drawn tightly enough to force the buttocks against the back of the chair.

PADDING

A seat and back of $\frac{1}{2}$ inch firm slab sponge rubber are placed in all chairs to insure the maximum of comfort. Plastic leatherette with re-inforced backing is used to cover the sponge rubber and is held in place by ball-topped upholstery tacks. Felt, orthopedic stockinette, sheet wadding, and gauze may be used, in addition to the sponge rubber, to prevent irritation to various parts of the body.

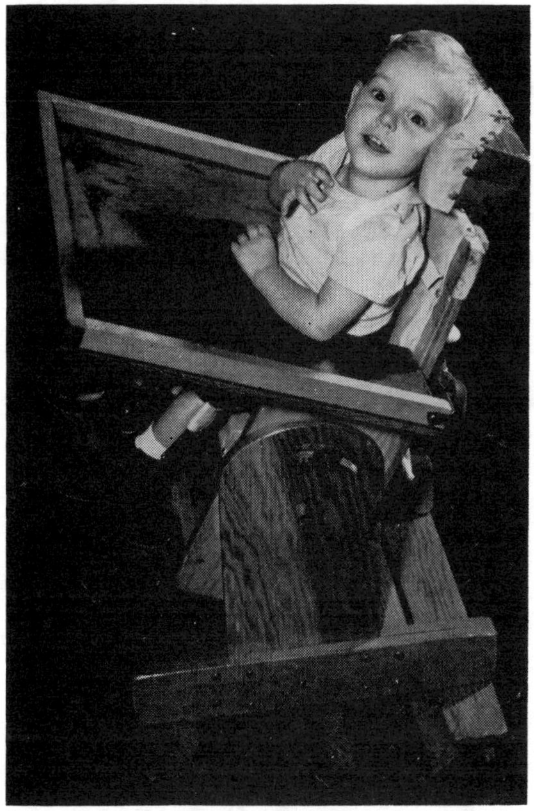

Figure 3.

CARE AND CLEANING

It is recommended that all chairs and trays be cleaned daily with a soap detergent and hot water. A monthly lubrication of the wheels is desirable to prevent rust and malfunction. We have found a liquid rubber lubricant or three-in-one oil to be the most satisfactory. Additional coats of shellac and varnish may be applied to eliminate chipping or splintering.

REVIEW WITH PARENTS

When the chair is finished it is moved to the physical therapy department where the upholstery is tacked into place. The parents are present when the chair is fitted and if any corrections or additions are necessary they are completed while the parents wait.

The parents receive a detailed explanation of the chair's use. This includes: (1) why the chair is being provided, (2) how to place the child in the chair properly, (3) recommended time in the chair, (4) a brief explanation of the parts and working order, and (5) instructions regarding care and cleaning.

After instructions have been completed and questions answered, the parents are asked to review verbally the entire procedure before leaving. When the child is recommended for in-patient training, this chair accompanies him and serves as an excellent transportation device in addition to its primary function of balance training.

REFERENCES

1. Egel, Paula F.: Technique of Treatment for the Cerebral Palsy Child, St. Louis, The C. V. Mosby Company, 1948.
2. Cruickshank, William M. and Raus, George M.: Cerebral Palsy, Its Individual and Community Problems, Syracuse University Press, 1955.
3. Cerebral Palsy Issue, Phys. Ther. Rev., 28:3 (May-June) 1948.
4. Spencer, Helen: Balance training in cerebral palsy: Principles and procedures, Phys. Ther. Rev. 37:8 (Aug.) 1957.

Suggestions from the Field

Head Support for Gait Training of Patients with Cerebral Palsy

Helen J. Mayes*

This head support was devised primarily as a temporary supplemental aid in posture and gait training. It can be utilized most effectively by patients with cerebral palsy whose head is not held erect because of lack of control rather than weakness.

Basically, this device consists of a chin support with lateral bars resting on two vertical uprights. Variations may be necessary for individuals, but the following measurements were used on this basic device: (1) A chin support upon which the head rests is a metal piece 3½ inches by 4 inches across, padded and curved to fit the chin. (2) The two vertical uprights support the chin rest, provide attachment for the lateral bars, and have slots for height adjustment. They are made of sturdy metal that is flexible to permit bending. They are 11 inches long with a 7 inch piece across the top where the chin support rests and the lateral bars attach. (3) There are two lateral bars 4 inches long and set 5 inches apart that control sideward motion of the head. They have holes for adjustment and a wooden block at the top of each 1½ inches by 1¾ inches padded with sponge rubber for comfort.

This head support may be attached to a walker. (Fig. 1.) This is done by means of two clamps that vary according to the walker size and may be padded with sponge rubber to prevent play. (Fig. 2.)

A third vertical bar is added for attaching to a tricycle. This attaches at the upper end of the basic device by means of horizontal bar. (Fig. 3.) At the lower end, it attaches to the tricycle by means of a C-clamp. (Fig. 4.) The third vertical bar is slightly curved, 12½ inches in length and has a slot one half its length for height adjustment. The horizontal bar is 7 inches wide and the third rounded clamp varies with the size of the tricycle.

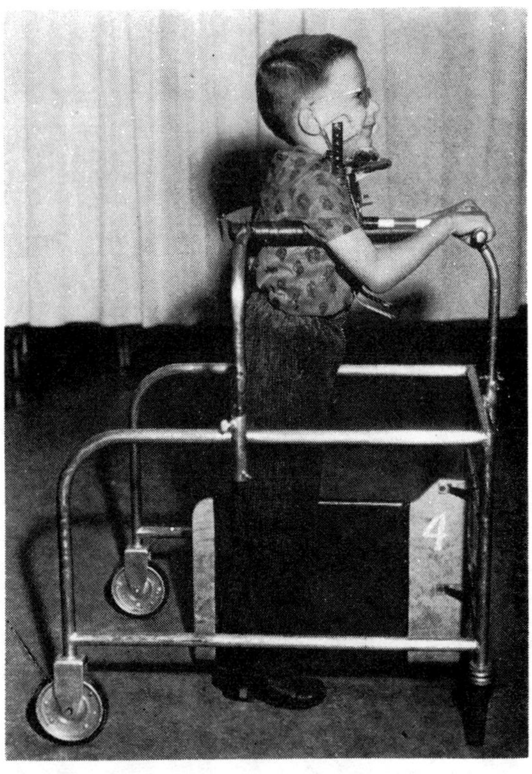

Fig. 1. Device in use on a walker.

In using this head support the following suggestions may be helpful: (1) This entire device whether fitted to the walker or tricycle may be tilted and adjusted as necessary to keep the child erect. (2) In many cases a back rest and un-

* Physical Therapist, Jane A. Neil School for Handicapped Children, Chicago, Illinois.

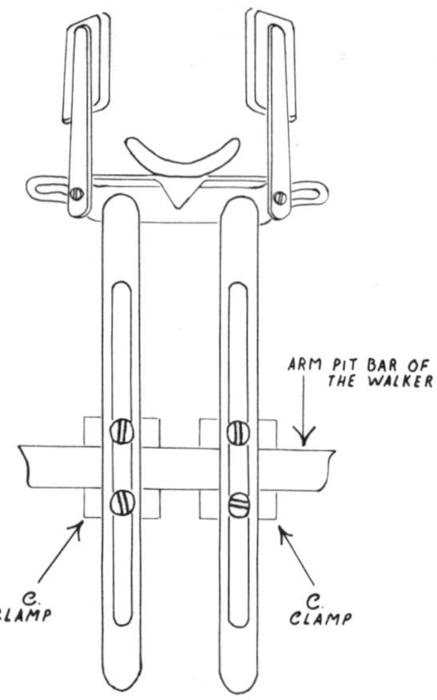

FIG. 2. Method of attaching the device to the walker. Bar is semi-circular and passes under the arms. It is adjustable to keep the body erect, and is completed in the rear by a strap that fastens for safety.

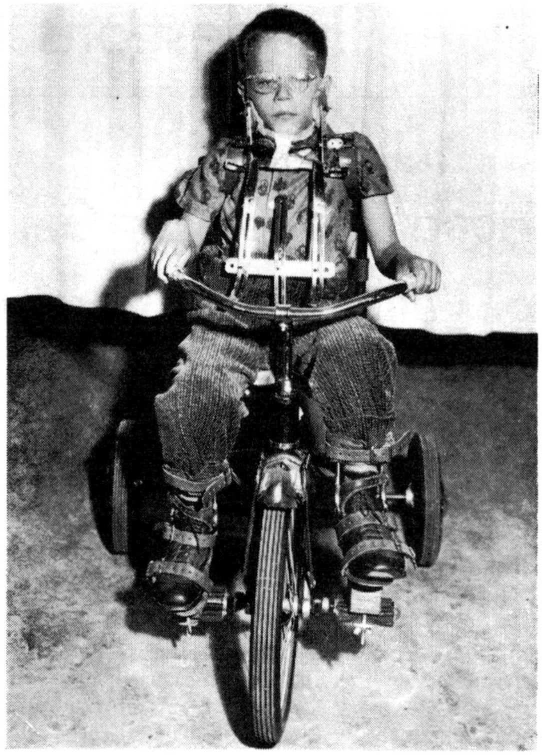

FIG. 4. Method of attaching to a tricycle.

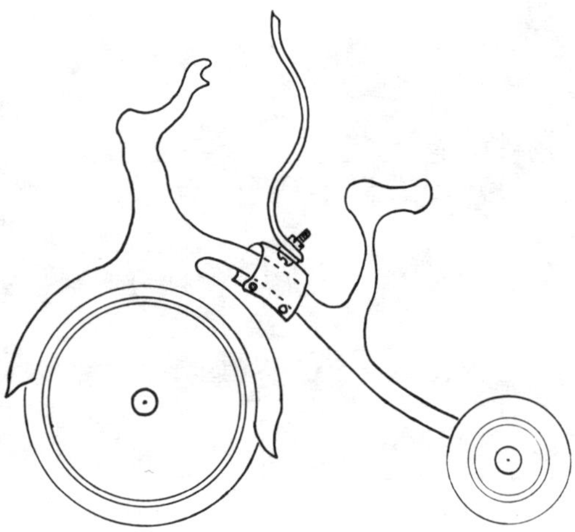

FIG. 3. Device in use on a tricycle.

derarm straps are desirable on the tricycle for safety and posturing. (3) To allow for leg clearance on the tricycle the two vertical uprights may be bent to preserve their length for anticipated future use. (4) An ordinary leather strap may be slipped through the slots of the chin rest and brought behind the head if the child tends to slip out of the head support posteriorly. (5) Metal screws proved superior to wood screws.

Acknowledgment: I wish to thank the staff for their enthusiastic co-operation. Gratitude is also expressed to Hughey Dixon of the Rehabilitation Institute of Chicago for the diagrams and to the parents who contributed materials for the device.

NEW CONCEPTS IN BRACING FOR CEREBRAL PALSY

ALICE L. GARRETT, M.D., MARILYN LISTER, B.S., and JERELYN BRESNAN, B.S.

THERE ARE MANY INDICATIONS that the treatment of cerebral palsy is undergoing a revolution. This is similar, in many ways, to the radical changes that occurred in the treatment of poliomyelitis shortly after World War II. Large quantities of information have been gathered by a number of different specialties, including the behavioral sciences and the basic researchers. We are all struggling to make sense of this confusing maze of facts and theory and from it draw an organized plan of action that will benefit our particular patients.

Physical therapists as a group have led in the challenge of older methods of treatment. But in developing more effective methods of treatment, let us beware of the overzealous following of a narrow pathway of theory, and try to keep an open mind for the new developments in all fields, not only that of physical therapy.

From the Rancho Los Amigos Hospital, Downey, California.

Adapted from a paper presented at the Symposium on The Child with Central Nervous System Deficit: Physical Therapy Aspects, September 13–17, 1965, Stanford University, Palo Alto, California.

THREE POINTS OF VIEW

Orthotics as a specialty has contributed much in the past and today, particularly, is rapidly developing into a mature scientific discipline. One should give full regard to these developments in the search for new methods. Before discussing specific bracing, we need to consider three concepts involving basic points of view.

Unencumbered Re-education

The first concept may be introduced with an analogy. Before Sister Kenny, poliomyelitis was treated with prolonged rest and immobilization. She introduced the revolutionary concept of muscle re-education, movement, and the discarding of braces. With time, the pendulum swung back and a combination of re-education, exercise, bracing, and surgery is now generally accepted. Controversy is limited to only the finer points.

The treatment of cerebral palsy has swung far in the direction of unencumbered re-education. Bracing and surgery are condemned by some as interfering with the natural development of normal function. The newer methods of treatment have given rise to many questions about the heavy rigid bracing often used to enable standing at any cost. However, it is also well to consider that spasticity may be controlled by other methods besides the laying on of the physical therapist's hands; a brace that could control spasticity would have an added advantage of being applied for a longer time than the physical therapist's hands are available. The elimination of a spastic pattern for the full twenty-four hour day would be a most desirable goal.

Bracing at present is often considered as the last resort. This belief is not to be discounted—it is based on the experience of many qualified professionals who believe the problems it engenders are greater than the benefits. However, instead of dismissing the whole concept, perhaps revisions of design could be developed to preserve the benefits but lessen the problems.

Make a Reasonable Prognosis

The second concept for consideration concerns prognosis. One of the greatest deficits in the treatment of cerebral palsy is our inability to provide an early prognosis. We are reticent to acknowledge permanent disability in the individual patient until very late. It is misleading to start every preschool child on a program aimed at future normal function. When the patient reaches the teen years, the obvious permanent dysfunction cannot be denied. The family cannot accept this sudden change in our attitude. We need to prepare families for a limited prognosis rather than develop their attitude of co-operating diligently with the physical therapist toward the goal of normalcy.

Years ago the same problem was faced in the treatment of poliomyelitis. At one time reeducation of paralyzed muscles was continued far too long. Today we can admit there is a limit to the return of function that will occur, and substitution patterns of motion, braces, and surgery are used to gain maximal function within the limits set by the residual paralysis. Parents of a Mongoloid child have fared much better because diagnosis, with its prognosis, is made at birth, and false hopes are not fostered.

Admittedly an early prognosis is more difficult in cerebral palsy, but it is not impossible. In fact, many patients and many parents unconsciously reach this point before the physical therapist does. Usually, interested parents will carry out a home program with great enthusiasm as long as progress is being made; but they lose interest when a plateau is reached. This is especially evident in treatment programs connected with a day school. When school is recessed in the summer, the number of patients falls off drastically, because neither parents nor children will make the added effort to attend a therapy session unless changes in function are evident. When fall comes and the children are again bussed to school, therapy is again demanded by parents who feel guilty that they may have interrupted this march toward normalcy.

When progress is very slow and the disability great, might it not be better to accept permanent disability, substitute early for some of the dysfunction, and concentrate efforts on the more likely or vital abilities? Let the drive toward normalcy be limited to those with at least a ghost of a chance of getting there.

Undertake a Reasonable Patient Load

The third concept is allied to the second. There is a great discrepancy between the number of brain-injured children and the number of physical therapists available to treat them. Too often the problem is solved by giving inadequate treatment, too few times, to too many children. As a result little progress is made but everyone is loath to discharge the patient, and treatment drags on.

If, instead, physical therapists worked with the child in a concentrated manner daily and adequately evaluated progress, when a plateau is reached the level of activity could be maintained at home and in school. Bracing and other forms of positioning could be used to maintain the activity while the child becomes more proficient at tasks already learned. Then, after a period of time when he is ready to take another progressive step, another concentrated course of therapy could be started. In this manner interest in treatment would not die out, maximal benefit would be obtained and more patients would be adequately treated. Premium professional therapy hours would be fully utilized and more physical therapists would maintain a vital interest in this field of work.

BASIC FUNCTIONS

The field of orthotics has an unrealized contribution to make to the treatment of cerebral palsy. Bracing can be used concomitantly with the other methods of treatment to accomplish

BRACING IN CEREBRAL PALSY

two different basic functions—one is to block unwanted motion and the other is to provide stability.

Block Unwanted Motion

If the goal for the patient is the path toward more normal function, it would be helpful to block an undesirable overpowering spastic pattern so the patient can use his active voluntary control. Abduction splints are frequently used to control subluxing hips in cerebral palsy patients. It was noted that young children who wore this splint a few months showed markedly decreased adductor spasticity and extensor thrust; and voluntary control of both legs was much more advanced.

As a result of this observation a brace was devised that blocked hip adductor spasticity but allowed free motion under the patient's

FIG 1. (Top) Brace to limit undesirable motion of adduction but allow abduction. (Bottom) Hip joints of brace can allow free flexion and extension or can be blocked to limit range of motion at any point.

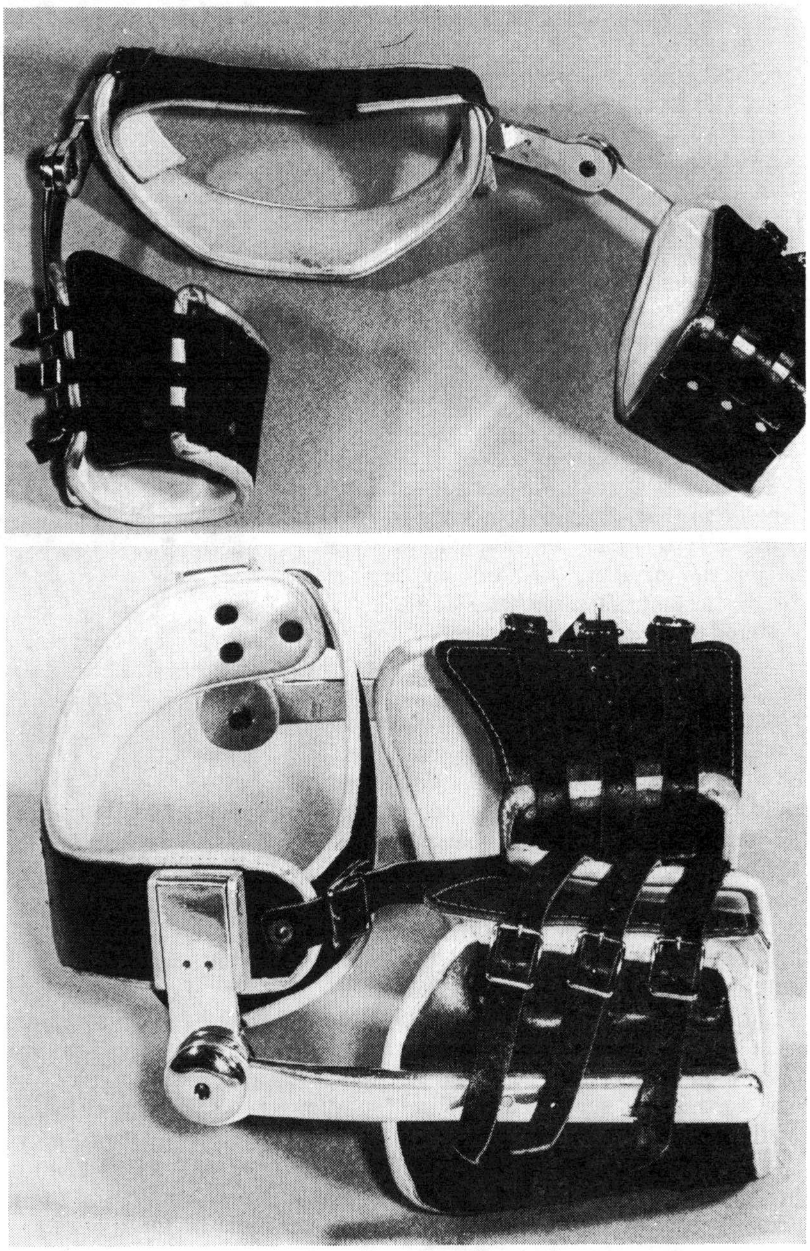

control. It could be applied to a child who can assume the kneeling or crawling position but cannot maintain the position unless the physical therapist manually blocks the unwanted adductor spasticity. The brace would have the added advantage of being with the patient for a prolonged period of time.

An even greater application of this principle may be observed in a child who can walk, but walks with the typical scissors pattern. If he can maintain stance without eliciting the extensor pattern, then this brace should block the spastic scissoring and allow a more normal gait.

In this way ambulation could be permitted earlier, with the obvious advantages of free locomotion in accomplishing other activities of childhood.

The brace which has been devised to limit undesirable motion while permitting controlled motion is in need of further improvement, but is a step in the right direction. This brace consists of a pelvic band fitted below the anterior-superior spines, hip joints, and two thigh cuffs. The hip joints allow free abduction but prevent adduction. Flexion and extension can be free or they can be blocked to give a limited range of motion at any point (Fig. 1).

Provide Stability

The second function of bracing is to provide stability so that the patient has fewer joints to control. If the patient's disability is so great that he cannot approach normalcy he may be able to accomplish some tasks if he has only a limited number of motions to control. If a patient lacks, eye, head, and trunk control, and has not made significant progress in acquiring this control after an adequate concentrated program, such bracing should be considered. If the head and trunk were stabilized, the patient could concentrate on developing control of the eye musculature, and thus enhance visual perception. A head support attached to a body jacket can provide this stability. Often the patient will have good control of rotation of the head but be unable to hold the head upright.

Limited use is made of the neck muscles when upright because the head remains flexed forward or to the side. It would be desirable then for the head support to stabilize but allow rotation.

A head support has been designed to meet these criteria. It is fitted to the head like a helmet. A pivot point at the top of the head allows rotation but all other motion is blocked (*see* Fig. 2). With this support the patient has been able to function with the head and trunk in the upright position throughout the day.

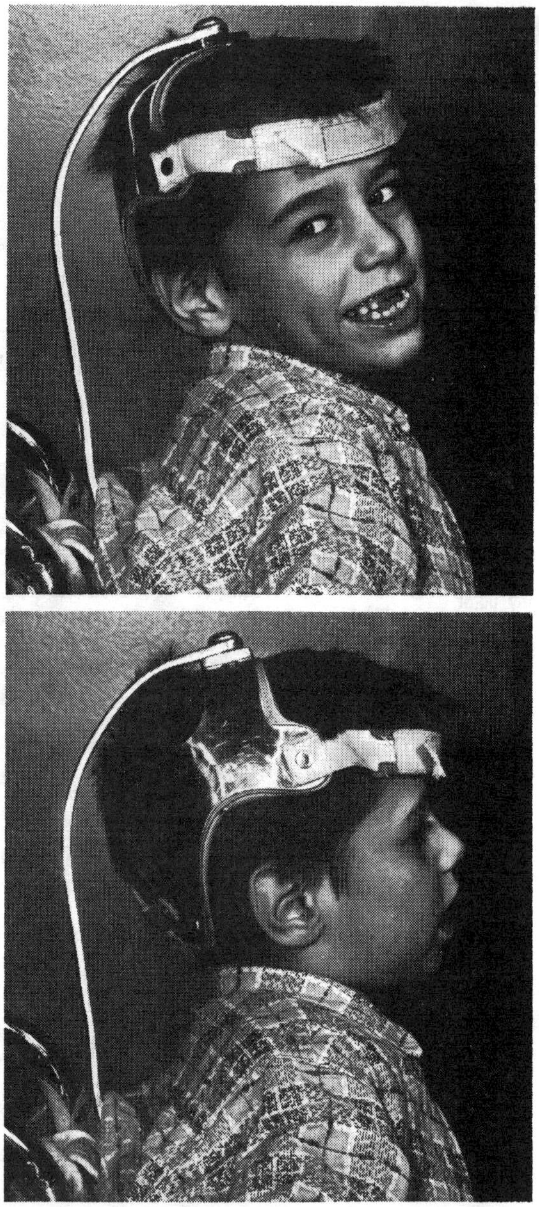

FIG. 2. (Top, bottom) Head support with pivot point at top to allow rotation of head. All other motions are blocked.

It has been surprising to see the gain in the patient's ability to hold the head upright, as well as to control the eyes, after wearing this support for several months. Probably the reason for the gain is that the child is using

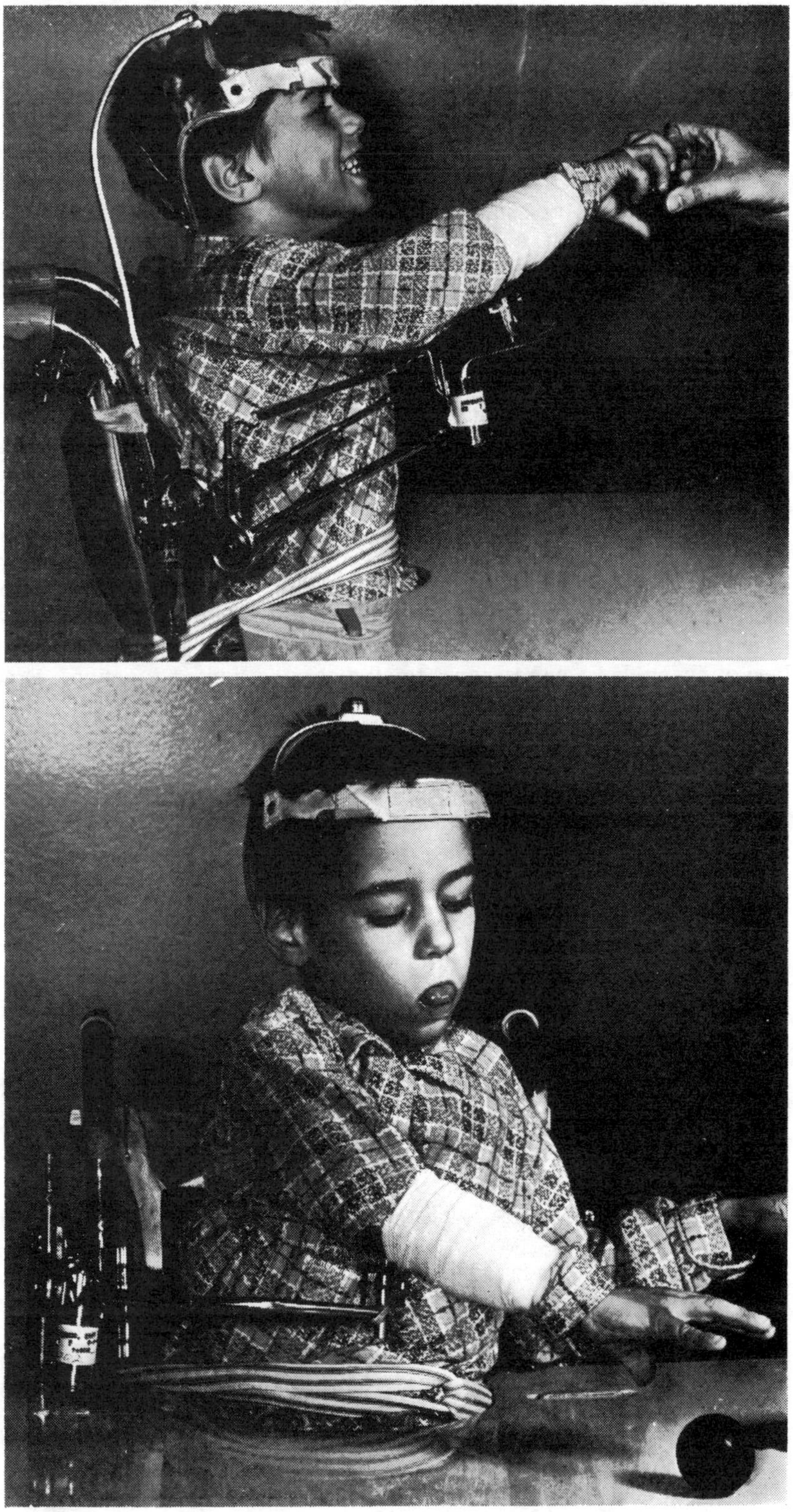

FIG. 3. (Top, bottom) Elevating proximal arm added to friction mobile arm support to allow free elevation while the friction joints continue to control horizontal shoulder motions. External rotation is also blocked.

neck and eye muscles for a greater total time during the day through spontaneous functional activity.

The next step for this brace will be to add another joint to give a limited range of flexion and extension and yet provide enough stability to prevent the head from falling into the typical resting position of full forward or lateral flexion.

Severely involved hypotonic athetoids without intelligible speech and without arm control have no means of communication. These children appear to have a degree of intelligence that cannot be tapped and yet they appear to respond to their surroundings to a greater degree than expected. Education has little to offer them because of this lack of communication.

If these children could gain sufficient eye and hand control to use an electric typewriter, communication could be established. Besides the trunk and head support, there is also a need to block the involuntary abduction–external rotation of the shoulder in order to gain the necessary control. Friction mobile arm supports have been tried in the past to give arm control but they have the disadvantage of giving the same resistance to all motion. Elevating proximal arms can be added to the mobile arm support which will allow free elevation while friction joints control horizontal shoulder motions and a block can be added to prevent external rotation. These additions seem to be a change for the better but are far from the final answer (Fig. 3).

A different type of joint is needed to replace the friction joint. It would be desirable to stop quick uncontrolled motion but still permit free motion when it is under voluntary control. One possibility which is in the process of development at the present time is a hydraulic joint similar in principle to that used in the prosthetic knee. When motion is sudden, the resistance to the motion is marked, but with slow motion there is minimal resistance.

SUMMARY

The braces illustrated demonstrate that bracing is not inconsistent with the newer concepts of physical therapy, but can be used as a training device to supplement a treatment program. If such bracing can increase function without interfering with development of control, then it provides a valuable tool which hastens motion learning. In patients with severe disability and total dependence, bracing may offer the hope of providing some practical though limited function. Bracing along these lines is in its infancy. Its potential will be realized when it is incorporated in the total treatment program.

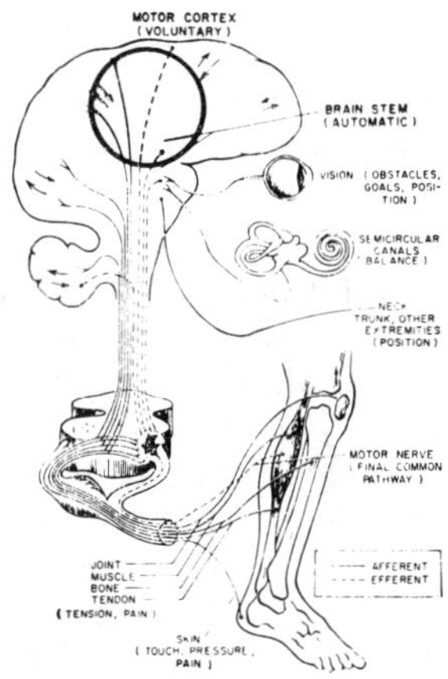

CONTROL DYSFUNCTION

I. Pathomechanics

JACQUELIN PERRY, M.D.

THE INABILITY to walk because cervical or thoracic spinal cord injuries have disrupted the motor and sensory message tracts is a relatively simple type of control dysfunction. Intellect, sensation and motor function are normal above the level of lesion. The separation between normal and disabled is not as obvious when the lesion is in the brain and intellect may also be impaired. This has been one of the areas of confusion in evaluating patients with cerebral palsy, strokes or brain trauma.

A second point of confusion is the fact that there are two levels of motor control within the brain (Fig. 1). Simple reflex synergies for

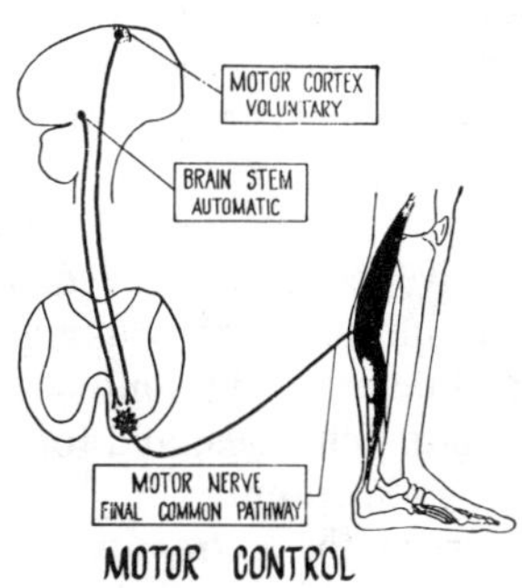

FIG. 1. Motor instructions are sent to the anterior horn cells from two areas within the brain: The cortex for selective motion and the brain stem for primitive patterns.

CONTROL DYSFUNCTION

mass patterns of action reside within the residual primitive centers of the brain as representatives of simpler forms of life; selective and precise motor function originates in the cortical structures which are unique to man.[1]

The third aspect of the complexity of control dysfunction rests with the significance of sensation which is so readily overlooked. Persons learn to know exactly where their hand or foot is by the senses of stretch, pain and pressure within the joint structures, muscles, and skin (Fig. 2). These are related to the person's mental image of his body. When either the proprioceptive clues or the body image are distorted, subsequent motor performance which depended on this information is abnormal.

Another problem of motor function is a dependence on the mild, or normal, stretch reflex to provide protection when the extreme ranges of motion are approached. The sensitivity of the muscle to stretch encourages it to contract before the joint capsule or ligaments are stretched, and hence these tissues are protected from a damaging strain by prompt muscular action. The subtlety of response to stretch is lost when the selective motor control centers are damaged. As a result, there is an excessive response called spasticity. The final motor performance in the brain damaged patient is a composite of impaired–to–absent selective control, reflex pattern activity and spasticity.

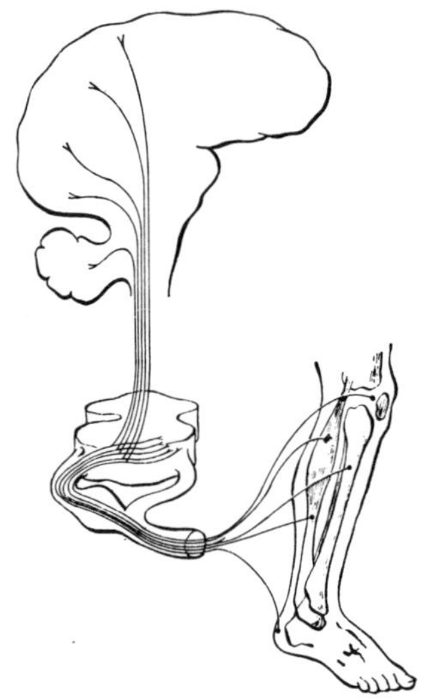

FIG. 2. Sensations of joint position, muscle tension, pain, and pressure, etc., are relayed to the cord and appropriate centers within the brain for assimilation and interpretation in order to guide the motor control centers as to proper motor instructions.

THE WALKING CYCLE AND CONTROL DYSFUNCTION

The relative values of selective versus patterned motion can be appreciated by a brief review of the walking cycle. For stereotyped movement the basic synergies of simultaneous hip, knee and ankle flexion or extension are utilized, as at the onset of the stance or swing phase. Selective control is needed, however, for further refinements of walking to accommodate for differences in limb length as the extremity position changes, and for the efficient utilization of momentum.

Stabilization of the extremity in the weight accepting phase of stance consists of simultaneous hip, knee and ankle extension (Fig. 3). This corresponds to the primitive extensor reflex pattern. The pick-up phase of swing is also a reflex pattern, as there is simultaneous flexion of the hip, knee and ankle (Fig. 4). Thus, a patient with only primitive patterns remaining, can walk by alternately using the mass flexor and extensor responses appropriately. On the other hand, normal walking requires maintenance of hip and ankle flexion as the knee is extended when the person reaches for the next step (Fig. 5). Gradual lessening of ankle extension, with continuous effort by the hip and knee extensors, is required as the trunk glides forward over the flat foot (Fig. 6). A marked increase in ankle plantar flexion is needed to push the person forward (Fig. 7). During the balance assist phase the ankle extensor muscles must be active at the same time the hip and knee flexors are contracting (Fig. 8).

In each of these phases of a normal gait cycle there is a mixture of flexion and extension patterns, or a variation in their strength. This requires selective coordination which is beyond the capability of the person with brain damage. As a result, these patients can be trained or equipped for safe and effective walking, but a normal pattern is not attainable unless there is complete neurological recovery.

REFERENCE

1. Krieg, Wendell J. S., Functional Neuroanatomy. First Edition. Blakiston Company, New York, 1945.

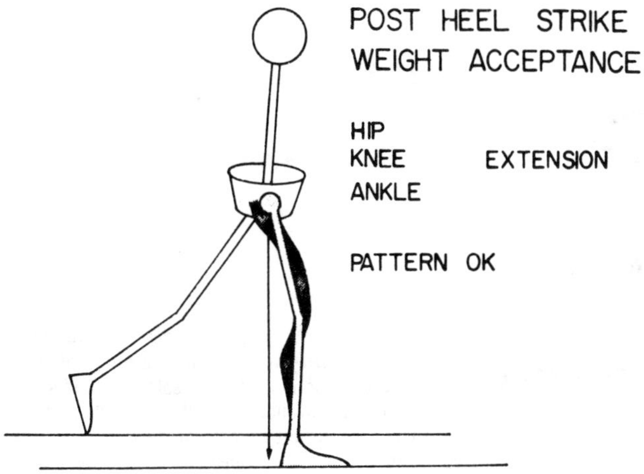

FIG. 3. A person can successfully support his weight with only the primitive extensor pattern since it corresponds to the normal simultaneous activity of the hip, knee, and ankle extensors as they stabilize the extremity for weight acceptance.

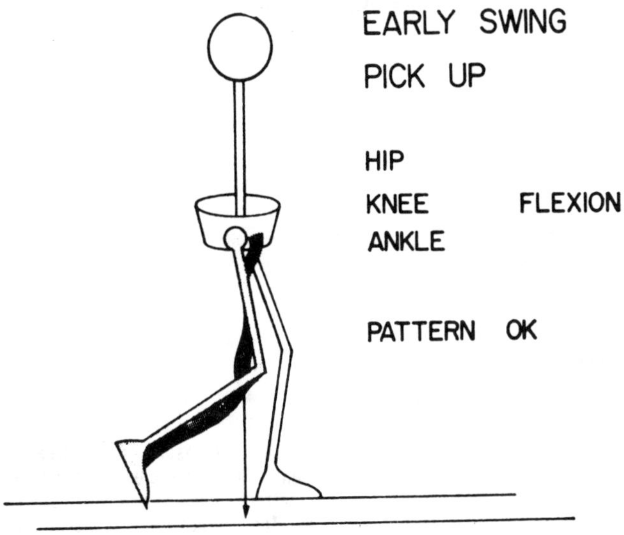

FIG. 4. The patient who depends entirely on primitive patterns can take a step because this action corresponds to the normal simultaneous hip, knee, and ankle flexion of the pick-up task in early swing.

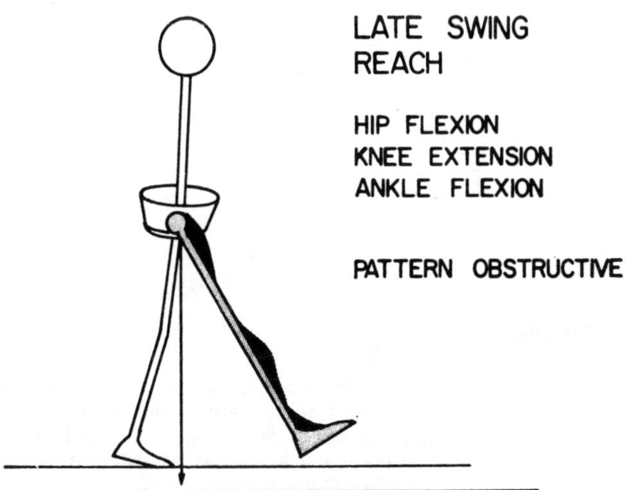

FIG. 5. The patient dependent on primitive synergies for movement cannot take a step of normal length unless he falls forward as he is unable to extend his knee while keeping the hip and ankle flexed.

CONTROL DYSFUNCTION

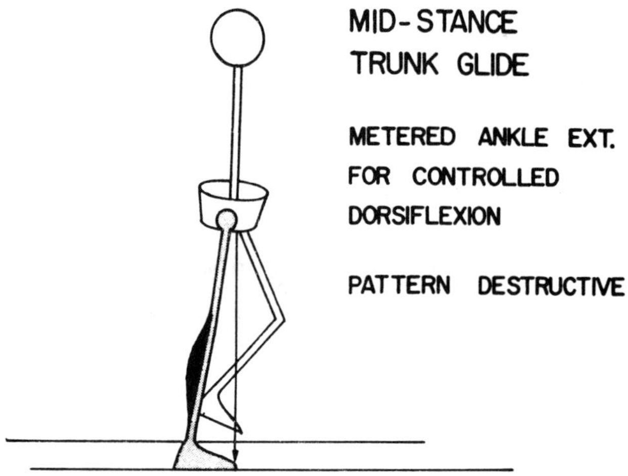

FIG. 6. The trunk normally glides forward over the flat foot by the gradual lessening of the plantar-flexion action of the soleus. Graduated control is not available to the patient who is dependent on primitive control patterns. To accomodate to the fixed ankle equinus which prevents his trunk balance over the foot, he quickly shifts his weight to the other foot. This results in shortening of the length of step taken by the normal leg in the hemiplegic patient.

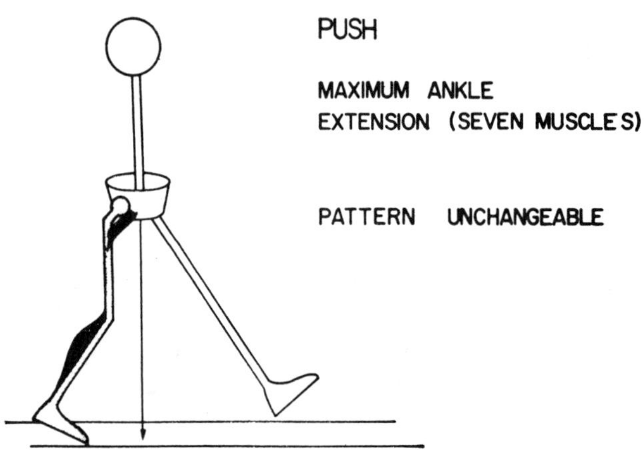

FIG. 7. Normal push force results from increased action of the plantar flexor muscles. The patient using primitive patterns cannot vary the activity of his muscles. The suggestion of push force that some patients evidence is due to the elasticity of the tense muscles or any contracture present.

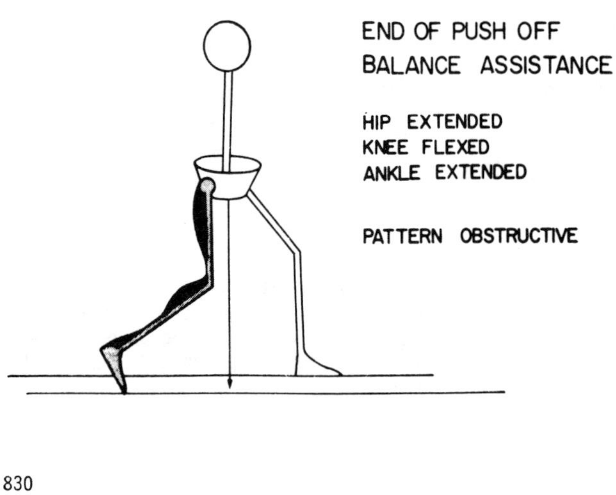

FIG. 8. The limb depending on primitive patterns cannot let the knee relax in flexion while there is active plantar flexion. Thus there will be no assistance with balance as he shifts his weight onto the other foot.

II. Control of Lower Extremity Movement in Cerebral Palsy

Selective Control Bracing

VIRGINIA SCARAMUZZA, B.S.

THE PRINCIPAL LIMITING factors in the control of lower extremity movement in cerebral palsy are defective voluntary muscular control and perceptual dysfunction. The manner in which the child receives and interprets sensory stimuli affects his motor performance. Children with cerebral palsy perform activities in gross patterns of movement. These patterns of movement can either be useful or they can interfere with function depending on the balance of their components.

Miss Scaramuzza is Physical Therapy Supervisor, Arthritis and Childrens' Services, Rancho Los Amigos Hospital, Downey, California.

The major components of the lower extremity extension pattern are hip extension, knee extension, and ankle plantar flexion. The flexion pattern consists primarily of hip flexion, knee flexion, and ankle dorsiflexion. Children with cerebral palsy often have mixed patterns of movement as demonstrated in the typical extensor thrust which combines extension with adduction. Treatment goals are based on blocking the interfering, and developing the useful patterns of motion. The goals are attained through an integrated program of physical therapy, bracing, and surgery.

The traditional type of bracing for children

BRACING IN CEREBRAL PALSY

with cerebral palsy is the bilateral, double-upright, long leg brace with a pelvic band constructed with the intent of restricting movement (Fig. 1). These braces are heavy, cumbersome and definitely achieve their purpose of restricting motion. Such bracing provides a stable standing position but does not permit the amount of motion necessary for walking.

A more appropriate choice of brace design is that which restricts the interfering abnormal motor patterns and yet still permits the child freedom of movement. These braces are used only until the child has developed control of his useful patterns of movement and are considered to be an adjunct to physical therapy.

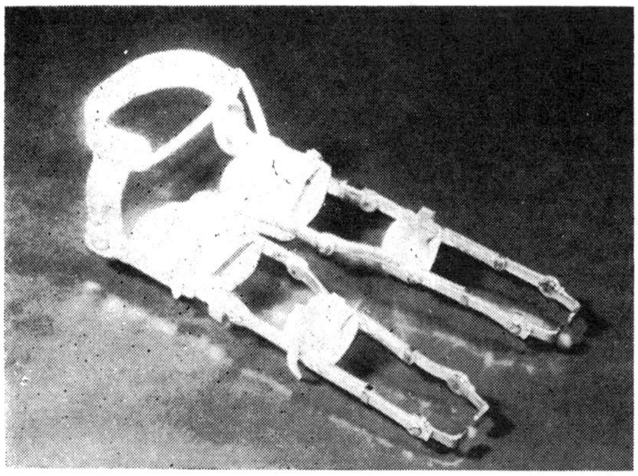

FIG. 1. Traditional bracing for patients with cerebral palsy consists of bilateral, double upright long-leg braces with a pelvic band.

PHYSICAL THERAPY

The first responsibility of the physical therapist is to observe and analyze the child's movements. The chronological sequence of motor development as observed in normal children has been universally used to assess the development of children with cerebral palsy. The child is observed while performing activities in the supine and prone positions, and when crawling, kneeling, standing, and walking. Of greatest importance is the level of development at which the child can perform with ease and also the level at which he has the most difficulty. It is at this next level—when the child is attempting to perform an activity with which he has difficulty—that an astute analysis of the movement is essential. The specific limiting factors that hinder the accomplishment of the activity must be determined.

The chronological sequence of development cannot be followed rigidly. Many normal children do not crawl before they walk. Furthermore, other factors such as neurological function and the presence of abnormal reflex patterns influence chronological development in children with cerebral palsy. As an example, a child with hemiplegia who is unable to crawl reciprocally may be able to walk in a reciprocal pattern (Fig. 2). He should not be detained from advancing to the next level which he is capable of performing. The child's ability to advance through this sequence depends on the maturation of the central nervous system, with resultant improvement in voluntary muscle control.

In analyzing the movement of children with cerebral palsy, the common terms used to describe problems in other diseases often are inappropriate. Terms such as "muscular weakness" or "lack of strength" may be meaningless in describing a child with defective voluntary muscular control. What is actually noted clinically is an overactivity of abnormal patterns of movement which limit useful activity. These patterns often result in deformity which further limits functional ability.

Because of the severe lack of voluntary muscular control, many children with cerebral palsy will not be able to walk. For these children, a treatment program, planned to develop control of the head, trunk, and upper extremity, is most practical. To walk, the child needs: (1) adequate head and trunk control to allow independent sitting balance (Fig. 3); and (2) adequate lower extremity reciprocal motion with voluntary control of flexion and extension.

Following the analysis of movement, a coordinated program is planned to develop useful patterns of movement. While head and trunk control are necessary for walking, the most useful pattern of movement in the lower extremities is control of flexion and extension. Various techniques can be used to influence muscular activity. Once the abnormal patterns of movement have been identified, methods of blocking those patterns such as the use of reflex-inhibiting postures or prolonged application of ice may be used. Useful patterns of movement can be encouraged through

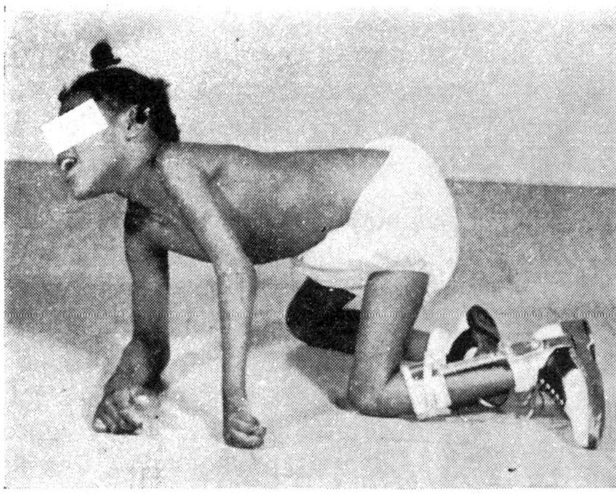

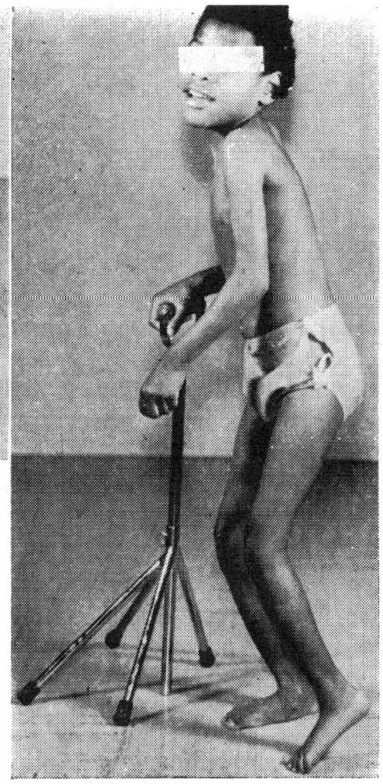

FIG. 2. Inability of this child to bear weight on her left arm (above) prevents her from crawling in a reciprocal pattern. The same child is able to walk with the support of one cane (right).

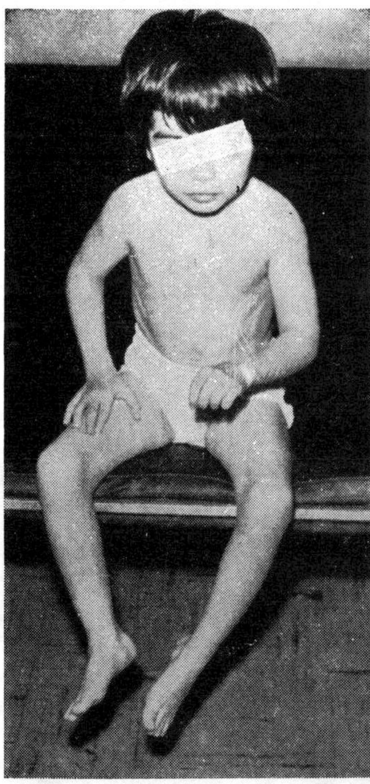

FIG. 3. Prerequisites for walking are independent sitting balance (left) and voluntary control of lower extremity flexion and extension (below).

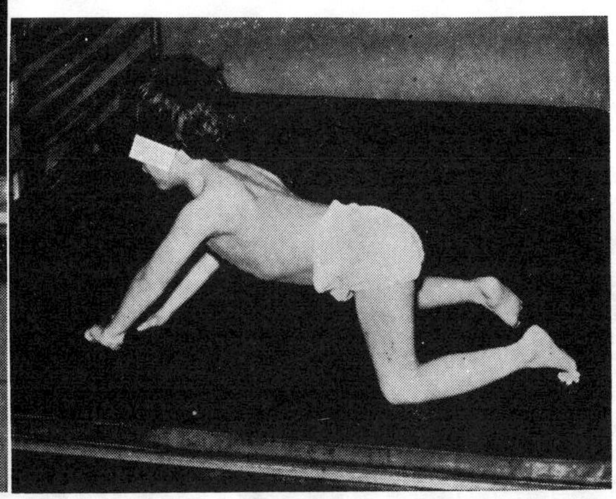

various facilitation techniques such as cutaneous stimulation or passively imposed patterns of movement. These methods are included in the standard treatment of children with cerebral palsy. However, these procedures are time-consuming and often are effective only during treatment.

Bracing with freedom of movement, except for selective control of unwanted movement, can increase the efficiency of treatment by prolonging the time the child's desired activity can be maintained. By the appropriate choice of brace design, unwanted movement can be limited while the child is permitted to move in useful patterns. This type of temporary selective control brace enables the child to practice desirable activity more hours in the day. Thus, he gains proficiency through prolonged repetition.

SELECTIVE CONTROL BRACES

After a careful analysis of the patient's performance in which the major obstacles to effective walking or crawling have been identified, a brace is selected which will restrict this undesired motion with little or no limitation of other motions within the walking pattern. The hip, or the knee, or the ankle is braced individually as needed. Care is taken not to allow the brace to obstruct any useful motion.

Hip

One of the prerequisites for ambulation is lower extremity reciprocation. Reciprocal motion in the child usually, but not always, begins in the crawling position. Spastic hip adductor muscles and an extensor thrust will interfere with the development of reciprocal crawling. (Fig. 4, left)

Abduction Splint for Crawling. In order to block the unwanted adductor pattern of motion, an Ilfeld splint can be used.[1] (Fig. 4, center) This is an abduction splint often prescribed by the physician to control dislocated or potentially dislocating hips. The splint consists of an adjustable spreader bar and two thigh cuffs. It prevents adduction, but allows some hip flexion and extension. Clinically, it has been observed that the splint is effective in blocking the spastic adductor muscles and allows the child to develop increased reciprocal motion. (Fig. 4, right) Not only are the adductors blocked, but the abductor muscles of the hip are allowed to develop once the overpull of the adductors is decreased. In these splints, the child can crawl for several hours daily, practicing reciprocal crawling and exploring his environment.

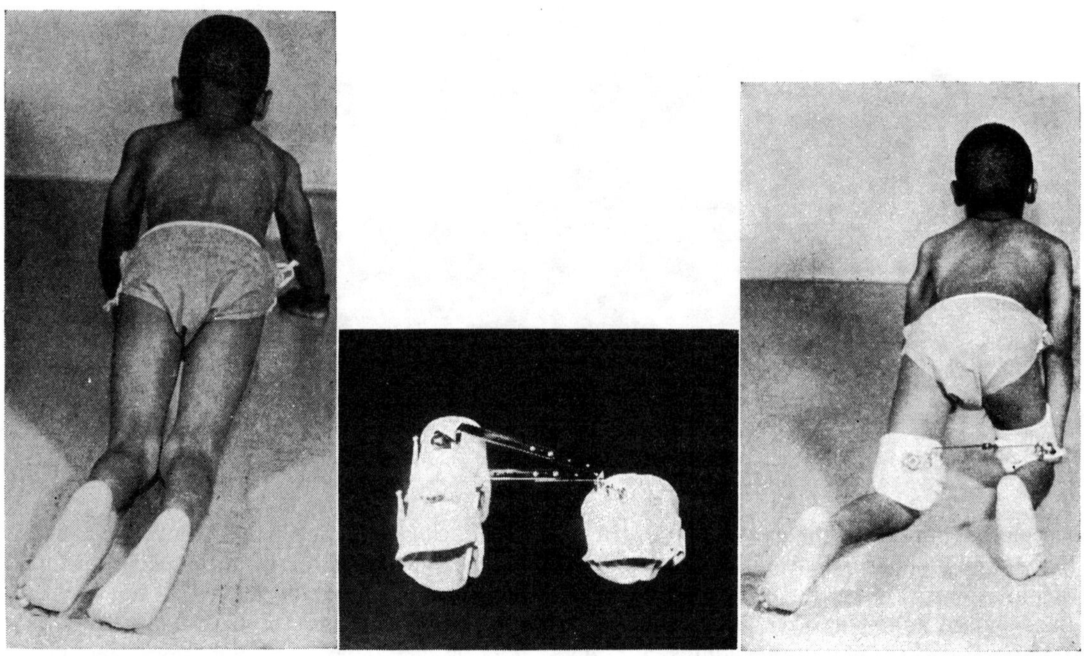

FIG. 4. Spastic hip adductor muscles (left) interfere with reciprocal movement. An Ilfeld abduction splint (center) with adjustable spreader bar and two thigh cuffs prevents hip adduction but allows flexion (right).

Hip Control Brace for Walking. As the child moves on to higher developmental activities (such as the complex mechanics of walking in contrast to crawling), more freedom of motion in flexion, extension, and abduction is needed. To control the spastic adductors and retain the other freedom, a hip control brace is used.[2] It consists of two leather thigh cuffs with hip joints attached to a pelvic band fitted below the anterior superior spines. The hip joints are constructed to permit free abduction and to prevent adduction. (Fig. 5) Just as the previously discussed abduction splint allowed the child to develop voluntary control of flexion and extension in the crawling position, this brace allows similar control to occur in the kneeling and standing positions. By eliminating the spreader bar, the hip control brace has the additional feature of permitting free flexion and extension of the hip which is necessary for reciprocal motion during walking. This brace decreases the unwanted adductor activity, and at the same time provides stability at the hips. The design of the brace provides stability by widening the base of support in the kneeling and standing positions. (Fig. 5)

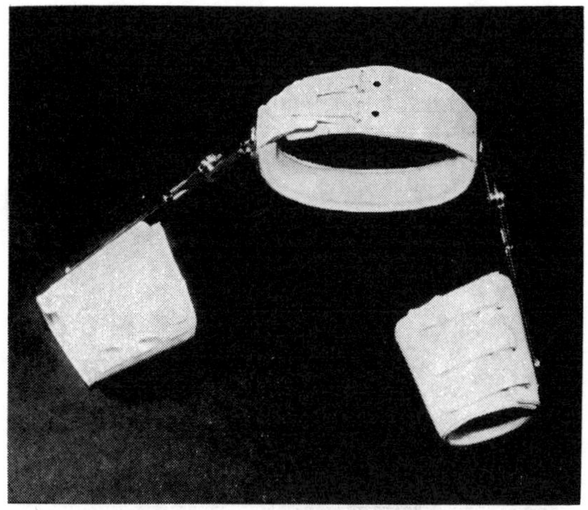

FIG. 5. The hip control brace (above) limits hip adduction and permits free abduction range of motion. It also permits an increased base of support (below).

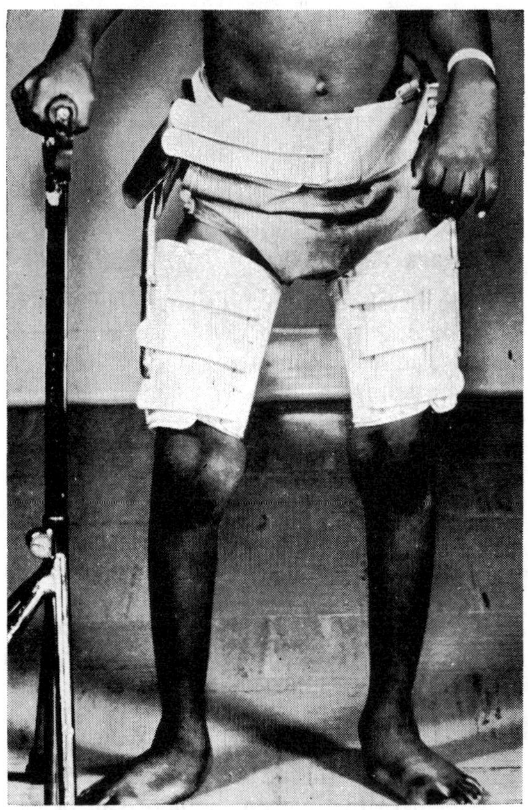

Either the extension or flexion pattern may dominate lower extremity movements in children with cerebral palsy; most commonly the flexion pattern is the stronger. Clinically, we have noted that when the hip control brace is first worn, the flexion pattern increases. That is, increased flexion occurs at the hips and the knees. This can be accounted for by the fact that muscles in the adductor group are also hip and knee flexors. Thus, when motion in one direction is restrained, tension of the muscles is concentrated in the other ranges. However, this increased flexion is a temporary situation as blocking of the adduction component of the flexion pattern permits the weaker extension pattern to be strengthened through increased weight bearing.

Twisters. Overactivity of the hip internal or external rotator muscles rarely is a problem in itself. Usually the rotation component is only part of a more complex pattern of movement. Twisters, which allow free flexion and extension, can be used to control either internal or external rotation when it exists as a single problem. It is often necessary to determine whether control of the rotation component alone will affect the total pattern. The twisters consist of four layers of steel helical weave encased in rubber tubing. (Fig. 6) The cables are attached to a pelvic band and to a caliper in the shoe or to the lateral upright of a brace.

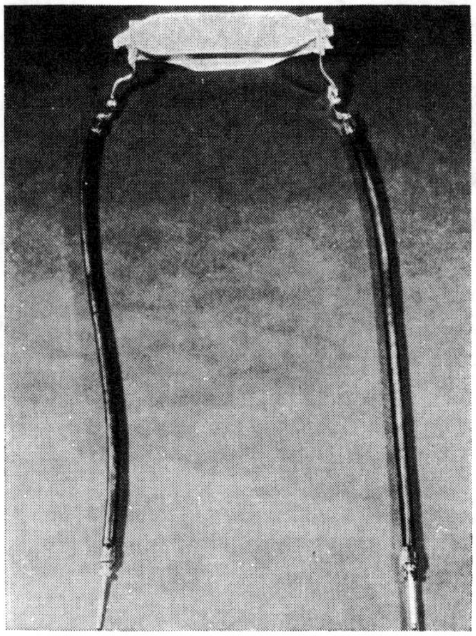

FIG. 6. Twisters may be used to control hip rotation.

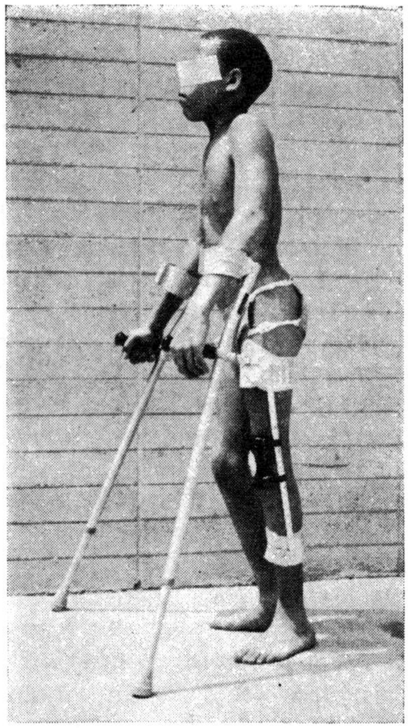

FIG. 7. A knee cage with an anterior knee control is used as a training aid to encourage the extensor pattern of motion.

Knee Cage for Extensor Pattern Assistance

Some cerebral palsied children are unable to walk despite having reciprocal control of flexion and extension because they have inadequate strength of the extensor pattern. Clinically it has been noted that joint compression augments the extension pattern and can be facilitated through prolonged standing in a standing box or on a standing table.

A knee cage may be used as an additional training aid to develop an adequate extension pattern while walking. (Fig. 7) The purpose of restricting knee flexion is not to provide knee stability, per se, but to support the child in extension so that he can develop his extensor pattern at the hip. Also, knee stability in itself is not usually the major problem in cerebral palsy. If hip control and a secure placement of the foot on the floor can be obtained, the knee is stable. Once again, this temporary brace will permit the child to start walking sooner and to develop extension power as he performs the activity. If the flexion pattern continues to be an overpowering force affecting the hip and knee, surgical release of the hip flexor muscles may be necessary to permit greater activity of the extension pattern.

Short Leg Brace for Ankle-Foot Stability

An analysis of the pattern of motion is essential if the factors that interfere with function are to be determined. In a child with hemiplegia, as an example, the common deterring factor to weight bearing is overactivity of the extension pattern. Two problems that result from excessive plantar flexion are marked equinus and inversion of the foot (either one or both place the foot in an unstable position) and extreme hyperextension of the knee on weight bearing. If the foot is not flat on the floor, but is held in equinus, the knee is forced into hyperextension as weight is taken on the extremity.

If the gastrocnemius-soleus spasticity is mild, a short leg brace blocked at 90 degrees can be used to hold the ankle in a stable weight bearing position. This brace not only puts the foot in a stable position, but also reduces the force that pulls the knee into hyperextension on weight bearing.

If, on the other hand, the problem is overactivity of the flexion pattern, then the problem will be excessive flexion of the hip, knee, and ankle. A short leg brace with the ankle set in slight plantar flexion may reduce the flexion pattern by preventing dorsiflexion of the ankle.

RELATIONSHIP WITH SURGERY

The treatment program described consists of physical therapy, bracing, and surgery. Bracing not only serves as a valuable adjunct to physical therapy, but can also be used to predict the effectiveness of surgery. If bracing has adequately fulfilled its function of limiting unwanted motion and providing stability, then a surgical procedure may be considered to permanently decrease the force of the unwanted motion or to provide the needed stability. For example, a hip control brace can be used to ascertain whether the child's function is improved by blocking adduction at the hip. If the brace is advantageous, then a surgical procedure to transfer the adductor muscles posteriorly may be indicated to decrease the force of this pattern permanently. In this procedure, the adductor muscles that attach anteriorly are moved to the ischial tuberosity to decrease adductor power and supplement the extension pattern. With the decrease in adductor power, the hip abductor muscles usually improve in strength.

SUMMARY

Children with cerebral palsy usually have the longest treatment records and the shortest list of functional achievement. Perhaps it is time that physical therapists investigate new approaches to treating these children—methods that are practical and oriented to function. As therapists, we must be able to recognize when, and then be willing to admit that the child has reached a plateau in improvement. At this point, the child needs the equipment that is best suited to permit freedom of motion while reducing the interfering patterns of movement. Selective control bracing will permit him to be active at home and school until he is ready to advance to another developmental level. With routine follow-up care, the physical therapist can continually reassess his status. The use of this orthotic equipment makes efficient use of professional time and allows the child the freedom of movement needed for further development.

The equipment proposed for such use was: the abduction splint, the hip control brace, the knee cage, twisters, and the short leg brace. They reflect the type of bracing that permits free movement and yet limits the overpowering spastic patterns. With these added dimensions of bracing that allow freedom of motion, the child can progress to more advanced patterns of movement. When the child learns to control these useful patterns without a brace, bracing should be discontinued.

REFERENCES

1. Ilfeld, F. W., The Management of Congenital Dislocation and Dysplasia of the Hip by Means of a Special Splint. J. Bone Jt. Surg., 39-A:99–109, 1957.
2. Garrett, A., M. Lister, and G. Bresnan, New Concepts in Bracing for Cerebral Palsy. J. Amer. Phys. Ther. Ass., 46:728–733, July 1966.

SUGGESTED READING

Holt, Kenneth S., Assessment of Cerebral Palsy. Lloyd-Luke Ltd., London, 1965.

SUGGESTIONS FROM THE FIELD

Weighted Shoulder Harness for Children with Cerebral Palsy

JACQUELINE FIKE DOHERTY, B.S.

A description of a suspender-like harness used for the attachment of shoulder weights on the child with athetoid cerebral palsy is presented. The harness is used primarily to stimulate postural reflexes, promoting trunk stability in both the ambulatory and the nonambulatory child without creating any restriction of movement in the upper extremities.

THE CHILD with cerebral palsy of the athetoid type has difficulty controlling his head and extremities due to instability in the trunk. In view of recently proposed theories of treatment, the traditional weighting method of cuffs and shoes is no longer adequate. A method of weighting has been developed to give resistance to and stimulate the basic postural reflexes, and to meet the objectives of comfort, compactness, and cleanliness; ease of application; interchangeable weight; nonrestriction of normal joint action; and usability by both ambulatory and nonambulatory patients.

The basic suspender-like harness is fitted first. Both the waistband and the extension piece which goes midway up the back are made of two-inch-wide elastic (A in Fig. 1). The waistband (B in Fig. 2) has hook-and-eye closure in front. A "D" ring (C in Fig. 1) is sewn to the elastic in back at a height approximating the tips of the scapulae. One-and-one-quarter-inch-wide elastic is sewn to the waistband at left front, extended up and over the

Mrs. Doherty is Chief of Therapy and Program Coordinator, Home of the Merciful Saviour for Crippled Children, Philadelphia, Pennsylvania.

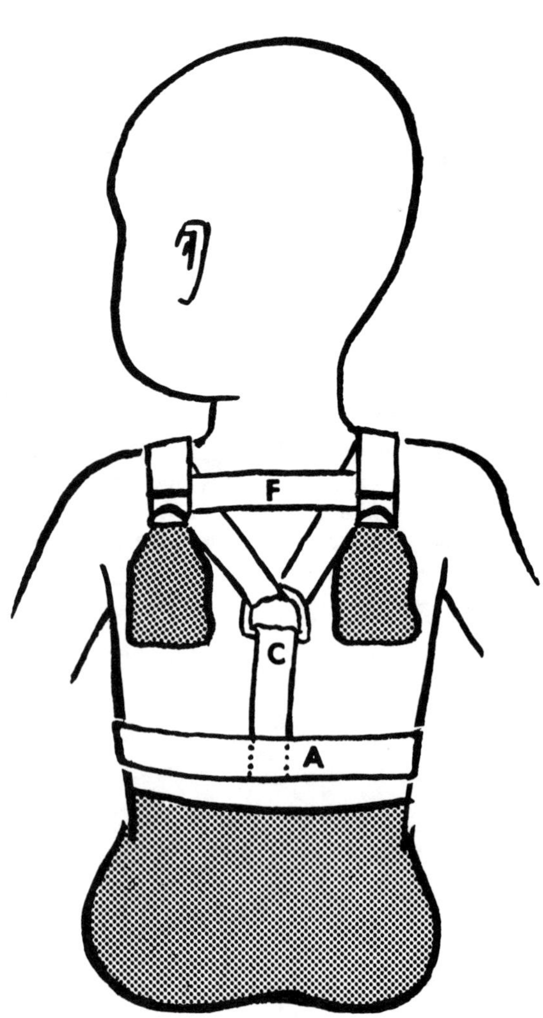

Fig. 1.

shoulder through the back ring, and then brought forward over the right shoulder and sewn to the right front of the waistband. To keep the shoulder straps from sliding off, a narrow piece of elastic, also with hook-and-eye fastening, is used across the chest (D in Fig 2). This completes the suspender harness.

The second step consists of cutting two pieces of cotton webbing, each measuring one and one-half inches wide and six to nine inches long. A wide metal-hook clip is attached to all four ends of these pieces, which are then laid over the shoulders and sewn on the basic suspender at midshoulder (E in Fig. 2). A piece of elastic (F in Fig. 1) connects the webbing strips to keep them from flipping to the side. No other attachment to the basic harness is necessary.

The weights are made of number 4 lead shot in a flat canvas bag which measures three and one-quarter inches square. Each bag has a permanently attached rectangular ring used to attach the bags to, and remove them from, the clips. In order to permit some free movement of the shot, which creates better adherence to body contour, the bags are not filled to capacity. They may be filled with lead shot weighing from one-half to one and three-quarter pounds each. Scotch Gard® is used for ease in cleaning.

This type of weighting has been found useful in the schoolroom as well as in various therapy programs. Because the child sits in his regular chair with more trunk stability, his arms are freed for specific skills. The therapist is then able to work on other areas of facilitation while pressure on the shoulders continues.

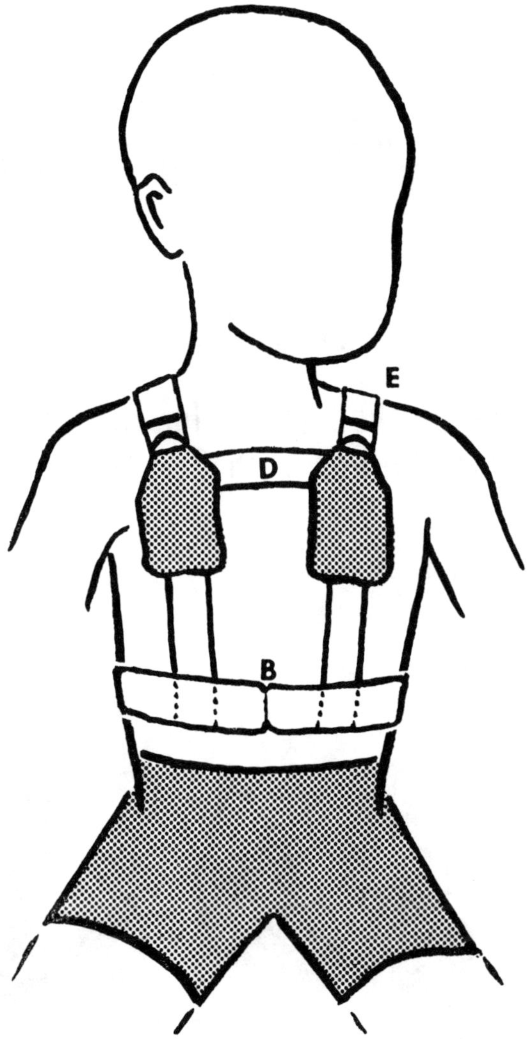

Fig. 2.

suggestions from the field

Wheelchair Insert for Hip and Trunk Support for Children with Cerebral Palsy

CAROL GILBERT, B.S.

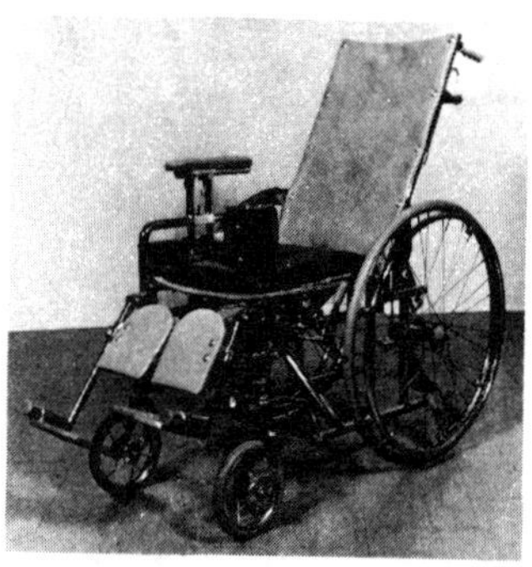

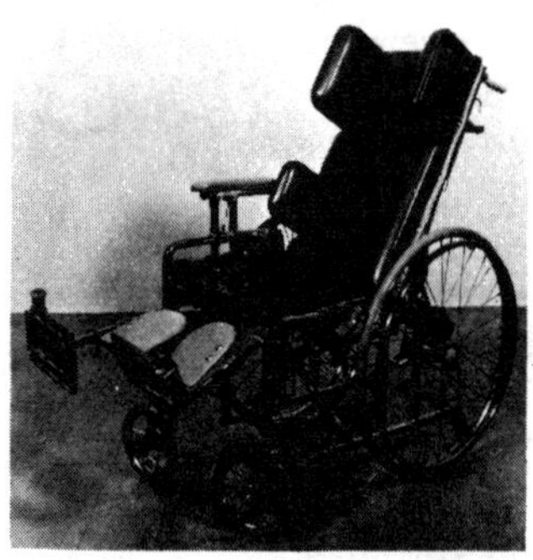

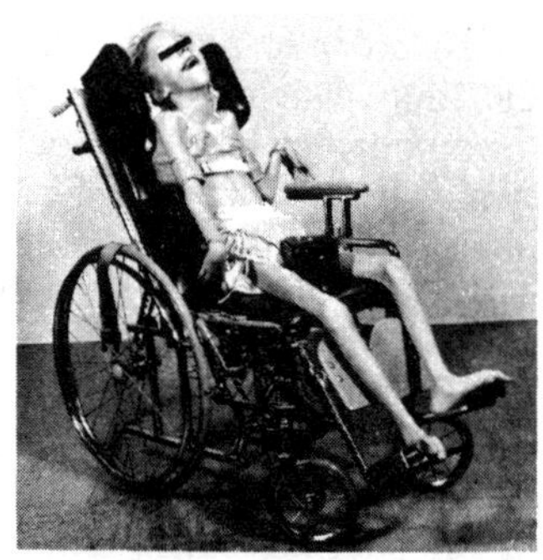

(Left to Right) Fig. 1. Seat insert with centered leg-spreader, which may be offset for patient with severe pelvic obliquity or abnormal leg posture. Fig. 2. Combined seat and back inserts with a single trunk support. Fig. 3. This patient with cerebral palsy has a dislocated left hip with limited flexion range and resultant leg length discrepancy.

In working with severely involved cerebral-palsied children, wheelchair positioning frequently becomes a problem of paramount importance, especially when spasticity, hip dislocation, scoliosis, and lack of head and trunk control are complicating factors. Our institution has developed a wheelchair insert which has proved to be helpful in meeting these problems and in maintaining the patient in a functional sitting position.

The insert consists of two parts: each may be used separately or may be attached with hinges as one unit (Figs. 1 and 2). Materials are relatively inexpensive: approximate cost for both pieces is $8.50 to $10.00. A 2-centimeter plywood base, measured to fit the patient's wheelchair, is covered with 2.5-centimeter styrene foam and then a naugahyde cover. Head wings and trunk supports (optional) are constructed in the same way and attached with shelf brackets. The seat insert (Fig. 1) has a triangular-shaped leg spreader, with each side

Mrs. Gilbert was staff physical therapist, Physical Therapy Department, Rancho Los Amigos Hospital, Downey, CA 90242, at the time this article was written.

Information may be requested from Mrs. Virginia Guess, Physical Therapy Department, Rancho Los Amigos Hospital, Downey, CA 90242.

13 x 13 centimeters, which is padded with foam and covered with naugahyde for comfort and which serves to appreciably decrease extensor and adductor tone by positioning the hips in an abducted position.

If active thrusting into extension is a major problem in maintaining a good sitting position, thicker padding may be added at the front of the seat insert to bring the hips into more flexion. This position will help reduce the total extensor tone and prevent the patient from thrusting out of position.

With this wheelchair insert, a seat belt or pelvic strap is usually sufficient to ensure patient safety, and numerous restraining straps are unnecessary (Fig. 3).

Electronic Sensory Aids as Treatment for Cerebral-Palsied Children

Inapproprioception: Part II

FREDRIC A. HARRIS, Ph.D.,
FRANCIS A. SPELMAN, M.S.E.E.,
and JOHN W. HYMER, B.S.E.E.

A new approach to treatment of children with athetoid cerebral palsy has been developed using electronic sensory aids to improve kinesthetic monitoring of the head and limbs. In this article, the theory underlying this approach is related to the concept of inapproprioception. *The electronic sensory aids and accessory devices used in the treatment program are described, as are the therapeutic activities which the children undertake while wearing the sensory aids. Exteroceptive systems (auditory and visual) are used as information carriers substituting for the proprioceptive system. The artificial sense organs built for this purpose convert movements of the head and limbs to proportionately varying electrical signals and thence to corresponding auditory and visual signals. The children are automatically reinforced for using these signals to establish control during postural and movement activities. Improvements in postural stability and in control of voluntary movements are observed within a few weeks of treatment, as illustrated in sample strip-chart recordings of movements made by the children. Cumulative improvements over weekly and then monthly periods of treatment are documented objectively in duration histograms summarizing such data.*

In an earlier article, Harris introduced the concept of *inapproprioception*—faulty kinesthetic monitoring resulting from defective proprioceptive feedback—in an effort to account for the production of athetoid movements.[1] He pointed out that the description of athetoid movements as "random and purposeless" (i.e., involuntary) is inaccurate and that the grossly incoordinated movements typical of the athetoid cerebral-palsied individual might reflect faulty limb and head position determination while voluntary movements are being attempted. In principle, such problems could be caused by desensitization of muscle stretch receptors, which would derange the position control system that makes postural stability and smooth transitional movements possible in the normal individual.[2] Based upon this concept, the suggestion was made that treatment should consist of improving the quality of kinesthetic sensory inflow from a given body part (head, elbow, wrist) and exercising that part separately with the rest of the body stabilized. The goals of such therapy would be postural stability of the head and limbs alternating with smooth, controlled movements.

Dr. Harris is Research Assistant Professor, Department of Physiology and Biophysics, University of Washington Medical School, Seattle, WA 98105.

Mr. Spelman is Senior Engineer, Regional Primate Research Center, University of Washington, Seattle, WA 98105.

Mr. Hymer is a Computer Systems Engineer for the Consolidated Electronics Corporation, Seattle, WA 98101.

Adapted from a paper presented at the fiftieth annual conference of the American Physical Therapy Association, Houston, TX, June 24-29, 1973.

This program was supported by a grant from the Bureau for Education of the Handicapped, under the Title VIb funding provision of PL 91-230.

Since that time, this concept and the related suggestions for therapy have been evaluated through initiation of a rehabilitation program involving the development and use of electronic artificial sense organs.[3] By means of these sensory aids, cerebral-palsied children are provided with accurate information about limb and head position over auditory and visual pathways, substituting for proprioception, as they work toward specific goals related to postural stability and quality of movement. The present article is a progress report on this program which involves design and production of the artificial sense organs, incorporation of these sense organs into substitute feedback systems, and use of the resulting sensory aids in therapeutic exercise for cerebral-palsied children.

The substitute feedback systems providing information for head and limb position control use sensors modeled after receptors in the vestibular system, joints, and muscles. The movement monitored by these sensors, which are mounted on the head or limbs, is converted into proportionately varying electrical signals and thence to auditory or visual signals. The patient attempts to control his head and limbs on the basis of these exteroceptive signals in a variety of situations. Provision is made for automatically rewarding the child for success in his efforts at position control using information obtained from each sensory aid. The approach is success oriented, since the child is presented with tasks of minimal difficulty at first and he proceeds from there at his own pace. Each task is meant to be challenging, but not overwhelming, in its demands on him.

Strip-chart recordings are made directly from the outputs of the movement sensors to provide for exact, quantitative comparisons of baseline performance and performance sampled at various times during long-term treatment. Sample strip-chart records and summary graphs derived from them are shown in the "Results" section to document the gains made by children participating in the program.

METHODS

Description of Devices

Head Control Device (HCD). This device, used to teach control and thereby stabilization of the head, employs two mechanoelectrical transducers (sensors which convert mechanical events into corresponding electrical signals) to monitor movements of the head. The transducers are mounted in an enclosure on top of a helmet worn by the child and consist of potentiometers with rotating shafts having pendulums attached to them. The two transducers are mounted at right angles to each other, so that one responds to front-to-back and the other to left-to-right movements of the head. (The pendulums are attached in gimbals fashion, so that tilt can also be registered in planes intermediate between the two vertical planes.)

The transduction is based on the fact that, as the head tilts away from the gravitationally neutral position, the weights attached to the pendulums tend to remain in the neutral position. Because of this, the potentiometer shafts are rotated by an amount corresponding to the angle through which the head has tilted. This rotation causes the electrical resistance of the potentiometers to change, and the voltage drop across them also changes by an amount proportional to the angle of tilt. This change in voltage is finally converted into a series of electrical pulses by a voltage-controlled oscillator circuit. (The frequency of the pulses is proportional to the change in voltage and thus to the amount of tilt of the head.) The oscillator, in turn, energizes a piezoelectric element (unimorph) which is mechanically deformed by each electrical pulse it receives, thus emitting a click sound for each pulse. Four unimorphs are mounted within the helmet worn by the child, each representing a particular direction of tilt (front, back, right, and left). The overall effect achieved electronically is that, as the head deviates from the neutral position, the subject hears clicks emanating from the unimorph on the side toward which the head is tilting. The greater the tilt, the faster is the rate of clicking. Thus, the child hears his head position in terms of the pattern of sound within the helmet, and steers toward a neutral head position indicated by near or total absence of sound in both front-back and left-right channels (Fig. 1).

Secondary visual feedback is provided by four light-emitting diodes (electrical elements which glow when current passes through them), each one representing the direction of tilt to

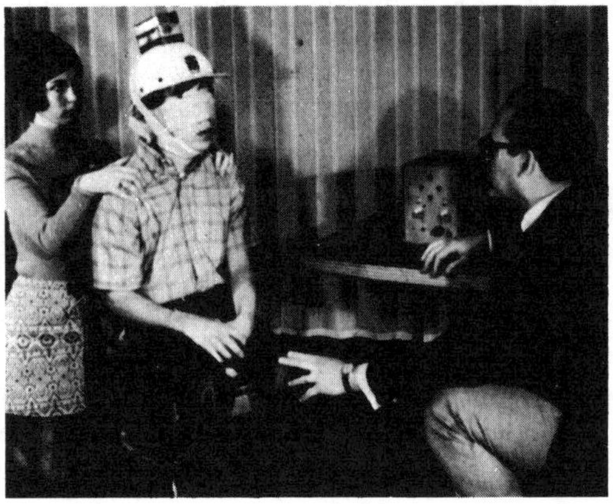

Fig. 1. Head control device. The helmet houses the gravity sensitive transducers and the auditory stimulators. The processing unit, near the author's right hand, regulates auditory feedback according to movement sensed by the transducers. (Use of the blindfold to preclude visual orientation, as shown here, is not routine procedure.)

which its illumination corresponds by its position on the control box panel. For example, as the child's head tilts forward, he sees a light glow representing the forward direction of tilt in addition to hearing clicks from the front of the helmet. The visual feedback, while not proportional, helps the child discover quickly the direction of deviation of his head. Those children who can use both auditory and visual cues simultaneously generally perform well.

An automatic positive reinforcement mechanism incorporated into the head control system is especially valuable for working with children who have difficulty understanding instructions or who otherwise lack motivation for using alternate sensory systems for monitoring head position. A control unit, receiving its input from the sensors, actuates a movie projector which runs as long as the head is held within set limits of tilt (Fig. 2). Films shown include both cartoons and educational material; each child makes his own selection. Again, to ensure partial success, the tilt limits are adjustable to suit the child's level of proficiency. The film drive and sound are stopped each time the head tilts too far, and reactuated when the head is brought back within the desired limits. A selector switch enables the therapist to determine whether the actuator will be governed by either channel of tilt separately or by both simultaneously.

Both 110-volt powered and portable, battery-powered versions of the head control system have been developed and tested. The latter unit provides only auditory feedback, but allows the child complete freedom of movement about the treatment area and home classroom. When the counter with which it is equipped is connected to a readout unit at the end of a trial session, the readout displays the number of pulses accumulated while the head was tilted away from the neutral position. The lower the count, the better the head control during the period of observation.

Limb Position Monitor (LPM). The limb position monitor also uses potentiometer-based transducers, which, in this case, measure the angle of rotation about the axis of individual joints. To date, sensors have been developed for the elbow and wrist joints. For each joint, the potentiometer is mounted on a goniometer positioned at the joint axis. The amount of potentiometer shaft rotation during movement corresponds to the angle between the goniometer arms which move with the body parts proximal and distal to the joint. As in the HCD,

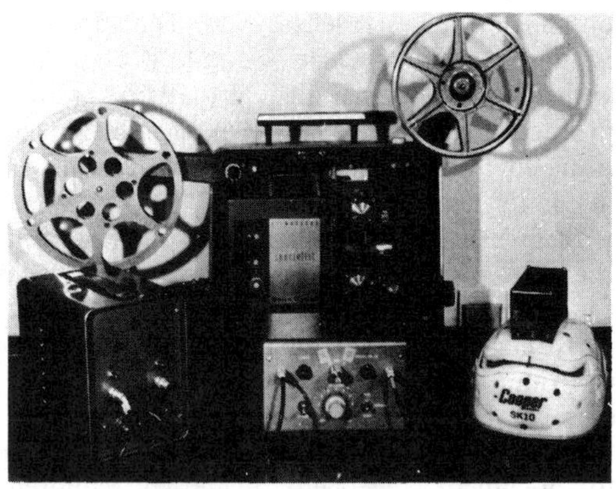

Fig. 2. Accessories used for automatic reinforcement. The helmet and processing unit bracket the actuator and projector used to reward the child automatically for his attempts to control his head on the basis of auditory feedback. The tilt tolerance on the actuator is adjustable to suit the stage of training. Whenever the preset limits are exceeded, the projector is shut off.

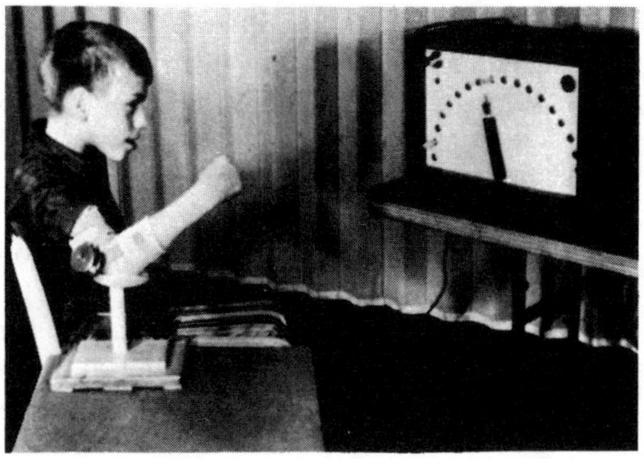

Fig. 3. Limb position monitor. An athetoid child intently watches the "dummy arm" of the limb position monitor, operated by a servomotor, duplicate his movements. The joint-angle transducer is mounted on a goniometer, which in turn is fastened to an elastic sleeve over the elbow (an improved mounting frame, fastened to the arm with Velcro straps, is currently in use). The cupped elbow support is used in early stages to prevent movement at the shoulder; the intent is to restrict movement to the joint which the child is attempting to control.

when the potentiometer shaft is rotated, the electrical resistance of the potentiometer varies and the voltage drop across the resistor changes in direct proportion to the amount of rotation. The voltage change, in turn, becomes the input signal for a servomotor which moves a small dummy arm through exactly the same angle. The child monitors the position of his own arm by watching the corresponding movements of the dummy arm. A display panel behind the dummy arm, in the form of a protractor with the pivot point of the joint represented in the middle of the baseline, indicates 180 degrees of possible rotation. Light sockets are provided at 10-degree intervals along the arc of the protractor; light-emitting diodes are plugged into these sockets to indicate positions at which the arm is to be held or to delimit the extremes of the desired range of motion to be attempted (Fig. 3). With two selector switches, the therapist can set the upper and lower thresholds for a sonalert (sound-emitting device) which is activated if the child's movement exceeds the desired limits. (The sonalert has been modified to produce a sound with gentle increase and decrease in volume in order to avoid evoking startle responses.) The occurrence of the sound when the arm movement exceeds the preset limits in effect tells the child he is "twisting the arm too far." The sound serves as a mild negative reinforcer because of its somewhat unpleasant quality, and the children try to avoid its production by keeping their movements within the limits set by the therapist.

Description of Therapeutic Activities

Activities Using the HCD. In daily prescribed activities, the child uses proportional auditory feedback to systematically exercise the neck muscles which stabilize his head. The activities include 1) experiencing passive motion to delineate the extremes of click frequency corresponding to the range of movement and the neutral position of each plane of tilt, 2) actively bringing the head to the neutral position from any starting point and holding it there, 3) returning to the neutral point and holding there after the therapist deliberately offsets the head a particular amount, and 4) slowly moving the head through the extremes of the range of movement in either direction for several repetitions and then stopping and holding at the neutral point.

Within the success-oriented frame of reference, the child practices with each feedback channel turned on separately before he attempts simultaneous control of both axes of tilt. Additionally, a sensitivity control on the oscillator circuit allows the therapist to diminish progressively the amount of tilt represented by a particular click rate as the child learns better control. (Initially, the child can make head swings of high amplitude without being bombarded with excessively high feedback click rates. As he begins to learn head control, the sensitivity then can be increased so that the child is immediately informed of successively smaller deviations.) The procedure is similar to *shaping* a desired behavior, as the term is used by experimental psychologists. Initially, the child succeeds at his task with behavior that is not much more refined than his presenting condition. Progressively better control of head position is demanded of him in the course of continuing treatment. The sensitivity control is set realistically so that the child is successful at least 50 percent of the time. This provides for the child's building a positive self-image on the basis of his achievements.

Activities Using the LPM. Initially, the child is asked to move his elbow or wrist joint over whatever range of motion and with whatever quality is permitted by his innate muscle tone and coordination. Then he is encouraged to move the part smoothly and to stop at the same upper and lower limits each time. Next, the child is instructed to move his arm or hand in such a fashion that the dummy arm swings smoothly back and forth between the extremes of a range of motion which the therapist indicates by positioning the marker lights as described earlier. If necessary, the sonalert system is used to remind the child not to exceed the limits of motion desired. As control is gained, the range of allowable motion is gradually diminished by moving the marker lights closer together. Finally, only one light is left on and the child is instructed to keep the finger of the dummy hand pointed at that light as long as he can by holding his own arm still. The child gains experience both in moving his arm and in holding the arm still at various positions with accurate visual feedback. The fascination of seeing the "action at a distance" of the dummy arm, caused by his own movements, ensures that the child watches the movements of the dummy arm even if he tends not to observe his own arm directly. This heightened attention is the reason an external indicator provides better visual feedback than the child's own body parts.

Data Collection

To date, eighteen athetoid cerebral-palsied children, ranging from seven to eighteen years old, have participated in the program. Eight are using, or have used, the LPM; nine are using the HCD. The most advanced child is using both devices simultaneously. All of the children have been given thirty minutes of therapy using the devices, some daily and others three times weekly, over total periods varying from two to twelve months during the 1971-1972 and 1972-1973 school years combined.

During the first year of the program, baseline sessions were filmed to document each child's presenting condition, and then the children's activities were filmed again at regular intervals during treatment. Daily progress notes were kept including objective data (instrument sensitivity settings, projector controller tilt thresholds, hand-timed duration of holding postures) and subjective comments pertaining to smoothness of movement, quality of muscle tone, occurrence of associated movements, and drooling.

During the second year, records of the transducer outputs were made using a three-channel strip-chart recorder. Since the transducer outputs corresponded directly to the movements of body parts, movements could be permanently recorded and the quality of movements and duration of holding fixed postures could be measured objectively and quantitatively. With three recording channels, the HCD and LPM could be monitored alone or simultaneously. In the latter situation, the effects of moving the arm on stability of the head, and vice versa, could be studied.

RESULTS

The various forms of data collected all showed that athetoid cerebral-palsied children could be assisted by using mechanoelectrical "artificial sense organs" to gain postural stability and improve control over voluntary movements.

All of the children using the HCD improved in head stability. Duration of holding a fixed posture with the head increased from a few seconds to more than five minutes in some cases, with concomitant normalization of tone in the neck muscles. Comparison of strip-chart records made at intervals during treatment demonstrates this (Fig. 4). For this particular child, the baseline record (4A) showed incessant, high amplitude (90°), and rapid (4 cycles/sec.) movements of the head, both front-to-back (FB) and left-to-right (LR). Control was slightly better in the FB plane than in the LR, the longest period of simultaneous stability in both channels being one second. After one month of treatment, the child showed striking improvement. Extended stretches of stability were evident in the individual channels, and two periods of simultaneous stability in both channels were approximately 10 seconds long. In a fifty-five-second period of time, the head made large-scale

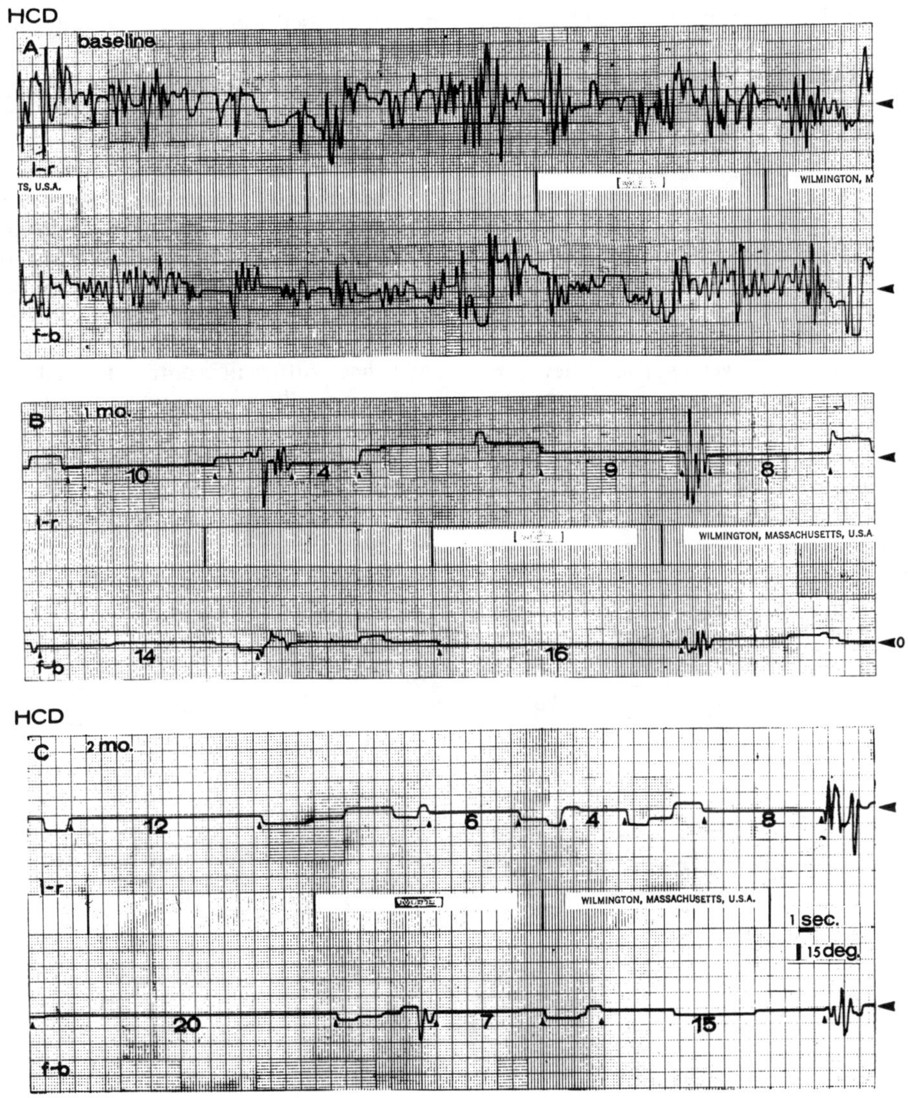

Fig. 4. Strip-chart records from head control device. Head position is indicated along the vertical dimension and time along the horizontal. Tilt from left to right is represented on the top tracing; from front to back, on the bottom. Tracings are all from the same child, taken at different times during treatment. The large arrowheads denote the neutral position for each plane of tilt; tilt to the left and tilt to the front are both represented as upward deflections. The small arrowheads denote the beginning and end of periods of stability, with the number at the center of the interval indicating the time in seconds during which stability was maintained. The calibration scale is one second per horizontal division and 15 degrees per vertical division.

movements only twice (4B). After a second month of treatment, the child was able to hold his head within five degrees to either side of the neutral position in both channels for the entire period shown, with the exception of a few seconds. The twenty-second stretch of perfect stability at the neutral position in the FB channel was particularly striking (4C). (Since this time, several of the children have attained neutral-point stability for periods exceeding five minutes at a stretch.)

All children using the LPM showed a

decrease or elimination of tremor and improvement in smoothness and accuracy of movements of their arms. Range of motion at the elbow joint also increased. Progress using the LPM is illustrated through the comparison of sequential strip-chart records for one of the children (Fig. 5). After one month of training, large scale oscillations (amplitude 50°, frequency 2/sec.) were present as the child moved his arm from one position to another, with an overshoot before the arm settled down to the new position. The child could hold his arm reasonably steady, however, at each new position. Note that as treatment continued within even a single session, the tremor was reduced in amplitude, and stability was improved (5A). Another stretch of recording made the same day revealed another kind of problem. Holding of fixed positions was good, with a shorter period of oscillation (having mainly high frequency components) during the transition from one position to another, but attempts at repetitive movements between 70 and 110 degrees of flexion revealed irregularity. Tremor increased during these movements (5B). After five additional treatments, the tremor was almost gone, holding was good, and repetitive movements had a more uniform, smoother profile. The child could make fine movements (10° at a time) without tremor or overshoot (5C). At the end of two months' treatment, the child had sufficient control to make either large- or small-scale movements with a minimum of tremor, could hold any position assumed, and could make repetitive movements of almost identical amplitude and time course (5D). At this time, the child was ready to progress to a tracking task, using a dynamic

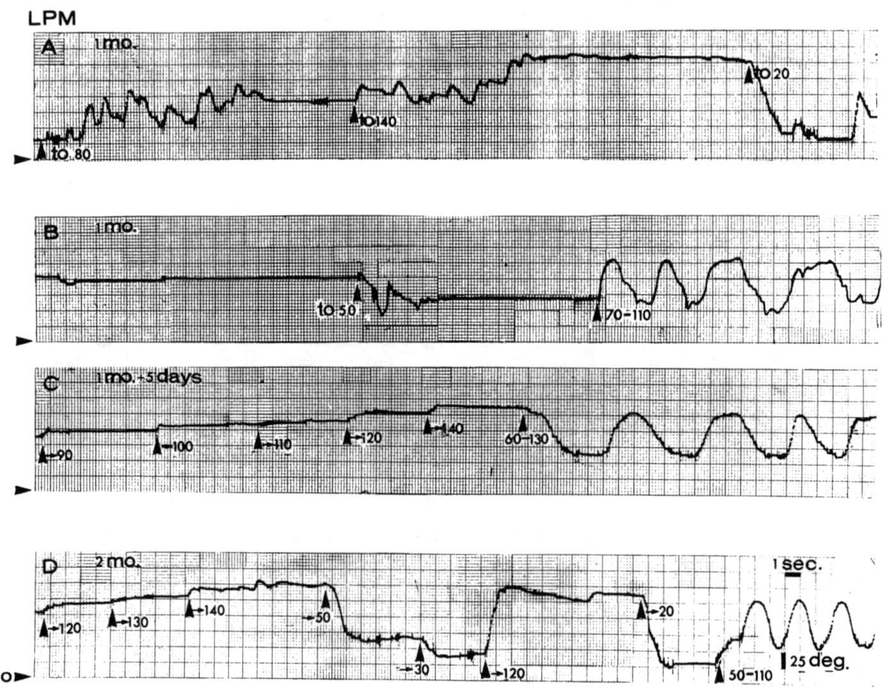

Fig. 5. Strip-chart records from limb position monitor. Elbow position in terms of degrees flexion is represented along the vertical dimension and time along the horizontal. Records A-D are all from the same child and taken at different times during treatment. The large arrowhead at the lower left corner of each record denotes full extension at the elbow. Each large arrowhead pointing upward denotes the beginning of a movement to a new position, and the adjacent numbers indicate the elbow joint position which the child is asked to attain in terms of degrees flexion. For repetitive movement between two points, the limits of the movement are expressed as a pair of numbers (e.g., 70-110). The calibration scale is one second per horizontal division and 25 degrees per vertical division.

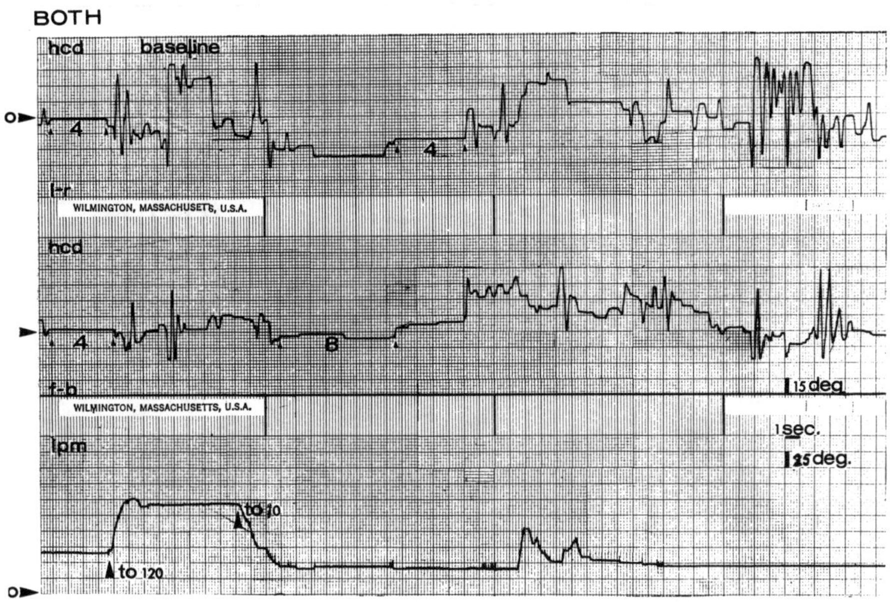

Fig. 6. Strip-chart records from HCD and LPM used simultaneously. The two head tilt channels are represented above and the single elbow flexion channel is represented below in the record, with the tracings automatically synchronized by the recorder. These particular tracings were taken the first time the child tried combining head and arm control and represent a baseline to which subsequent records will be compared. The time scale is the same for all three tracings; the position calibration is 15 degrees per vertical division for the HCD tracings and 25 degrees for the LPM tracing.

version of the LPM, where the requirement would be to move the arm continually to keep up with the position of a moving target, rather than slowly shifting the arm from one static position to another.

The study of both differentiation and coordination of head and arm movements has just begun, and only one child has progressed to the point of being able to do a fair job of controlling his head and arm at the same time. His first attempt at using the HCD and LPM simultaneously revealed that when an arm movement was made, the movement interfered with stability of the head. Moreover, a subsequent head movement in turn brought about a movement in the arm, showing that the association of movements could go in either direction (Fig. 6). This child's treatment is continuing with the goal of establishing independence of movements of the head and arms.

Duration histograms were used to present a complete, quantitative summary of each child's performance at various stages of training. Each graph shows the number of times the child held his head stable for periods of various lengths during a single therapy session or during a longer period of training (week, month, or longer). By comparing graphs for successive training sessions or for different times during the total treatment program, cumulative improvement in function can be evaluated objectively.

As one would expect, during the early treatment sessions short intervals of stability were most prevalent. Data from fifteen minutes of recording (five minutes at the end of each of three treatment sessions) during the first week are shown in Fig. 7A. During a comparable fifteen minutes of recording in the second week of treatment, longer intervals began to show up in the strip-chart records and secondary peaks emerged toward the right side of the graph (7B). In the third week, based again on fifteen minutes of recording, long periods of stability were increasingly prevalent (7C). (At the time of this writing, several children were able to

Fig. 7. Duration histograms for cumulative performance analysis. Graphs A to C follow one child through the first, second, and third weeks of his treatment using the HCD. Duration of intervals of stability is indicated on the horizontal axis and the number of times the child was able to stabilize his head for particular durations on the vertical axis. For example, in A the head was held stable with respect to L-R tilt twice for 10, once for 20, and once for 40 seconds. The left-right and front-back channels are plotted separately here, for at this stage the child may be able to stabilize better in one plane of tilt than in the other. (L-R tilt, dotted lines; F-B, solid.)

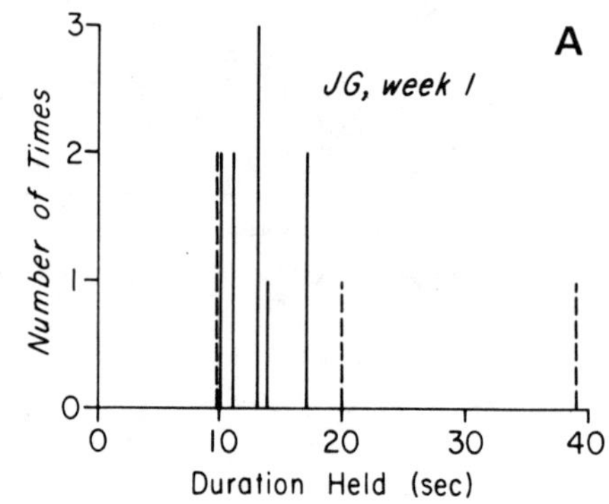

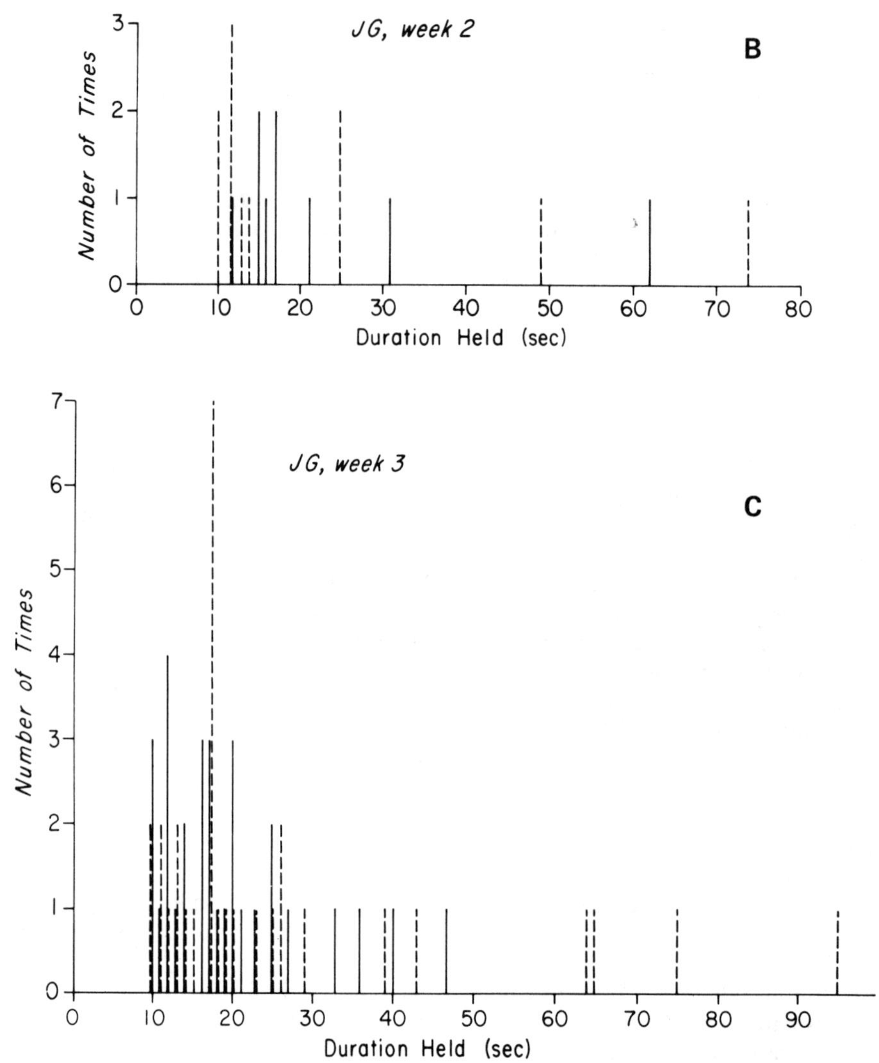

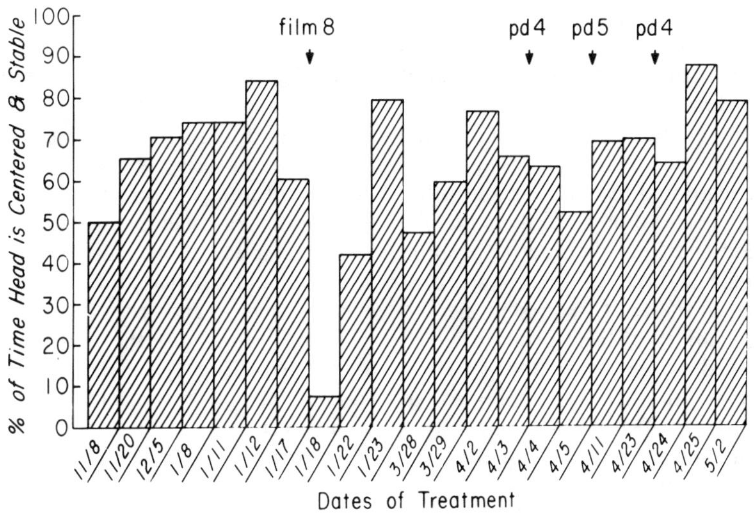

Fig. 8. Percentage stability time histograms. This graph shows the percentage of time for each day of treatment during which another child held his head within particular tilt tolerances. From 11/8 until 1/17, measurements were made of intervals during which the head was held within 20 degrees of the neutral position in both channels simultaneously on the basis of auditory feedback alone. Use of the movie projector for reinforcement was begun on 1/18; holding the head within a tilt tolerance of 25 degrees from neutral was necessary to keep the projector running (maximum setting of 8 on the controller). Subsequently, the tilt tolerance was adjusted three times; once to 15 degrees (setting 4), then to 17.5 degrees (setting 5) and then back to 15 degrees. At the end of the treatment period shown, the child was able to keep her head within 15 degrees of neutral in both planes of tilt approximately 80 percent of the time.

hold their head steady for periods exceeding those characteristic of a normal person's posture when he is not consciously trying to hold absolutely still.)

Another form of performance summary graph showed the percentage of the recording time for each day of treatment during which the child's head was held sufficiently steady to keep the movie projector running for reward (Fig. 8). The child's ability to hold his head within 20 degrees of the neutral point improved quite steadily without specific reward until the point at which reinforcement via the movie projector was introduced with the widest tilt tolerance setting; here the disruptive effect on performance of anything new in the procedure is illustrated. Performance dropped to a low level with the change in the task, but then climbed steadily as the child habituated to the sounds made by the projector and responded to the reinforcement it provided. Subsequently, the tolerance limits narrowed, in this case prematurely and too much, and performance fell again. The tilt tolerance was then widened by one step and performance improved again. After additional practice, the tilt tolerance was again diminished, and, despite this, the child could keep the projector running approximately 80 percent of the time. Thus, the child progressed in terms of two variables; the head was kept within progressively closer approximations to the neutral position for a progressively greater proportion of the time as treatment proceeded.

An important incidental observation in all cases was that while the child using one of these devices concentrated on controlling an individual limb or his head, extraneous, associated movements throughout the rest of his body seemed to lessen. The lessening of these movements may have reflected an increase in sensitivity of stretch receptors resulting from elevated gamma efferent outflow, thus permitting better control during the period of concentration.[4] In particular, movements of the mouth were minimized and drooling was less. This effect often persisted after the end of the therapy sessions.

Instances of functional carry-over of the beneficial effects of treatment using these devices have been noted by teachers and other staff members outside of physical therapy. One child could find and hold the neutral position for the first time without the use of a mirror when her speech therapist requested her to reproduce the stability of head position which she had achieved while using the HCD in physical therapy. Another was observed to make fewer errors than usual in typing with a head wand during the half-hour periods immediately following treatment using the HCD. Still another could hold a cane steady enough to touch my nose with it repeatedly after training with the LPM. And, most important, two children have made impressive gains toward independent ambulation as a consequence of improved head control. One of these children has progressed from use of crutches to independent walking, while the other has moved from dependence upon a rolling walker to the point where he slides a chair along in front of him for minimal support. The latter child is beginning training in the use of crutches.

DISCUSSION

The sample records and graphs are objective evidence that the approach advocated (i.e., improving sensory feedback) is effective for treatment of cerebral palsy. Postural stability and quality of movements can be improved by using electronic exteroceptive substitutes to supplant defective proprioceptive monitoring of body parts. The use of these substitutes, of course, raises the question of whether the child taught to control his movements using electronic sensory aids can maintain his improved function *without them* subsequently. The answer is probably "Yes, but you've got to explicitly provide for the transition in the training program." That is, the child must be slowly weaned from dependence on the devices after he has learned to function well using them. In order to accomplish this, he must be taught to correlate whatever residual intrinsic sources of body position information he has with the information he gets from the substitute feedback systems and to shift his attention gradually from the artificial feedback back to his natural sensory systems. He will have greater success in doing so if, as a result of therapy, his natural monitoring systems are *tuned* to a higher degree of sensitivity. We have seen indications of such a phenomenon occurring. For example, as the children watch the LPM monitor and try to control movement at the elbow, tremor and associated movements are lessened throughout the body. Resensitization of the stretch receptors via the gamma efferent system may be responsible for this phenomenon. Also, the child may be helped to cross-correlate artificial and natural systems by switching back and forth between them. For example, the unimorphs can be switched off in the portable version of the HCD so that the child can practice controlling his head without the auditory feedback for short periods of time. The degree of his success can be determined by the accumulation of pulse counts (which can still be made in the absence of any audible click production). Using the portable HCD in the classroom, in particular, will enable us to objectively measure carry-over of head position control learned during therapy sessions.

As mentioned in the "Results" section, we have *already* seen functional improvement implying carry-over of motor control learned during therapy, even without deliberate attempts to gradually wean the children from the devices. Perhaps the children in whom these improvements were noted have sufficient proprioceptive sensation intact to enable a cross-correlation with the information from the devices, and they had been doing this unconsciously. Others will require special training in order to accomplish this. Constant reminders to the children to *use* new skills may also be necessary. Two of the youngsters could respond immediately to a request to straighten up and hold their heads erect, with appropriate shifts in weight bearing and excellent final postures, but they did not *remember* to carry themselves this way all of the time. Perhaps with frequent reminders this posture will become more automatic. Still others may never succeed with the transfer and may have to wear miniaturized versions of the devices on a chronic basis in order to maintain proper postures. We hope that all our children, or at least the majority, can eventually be weaned from dependence on the devices; this may prove the most challenging part of the rehabilitation problem. We have come a long way, however, in demonstrating that electronic sensory aids can improve motor function, even on a short-term basis, while the child is using such assistive devices in therapy and in the classroom.

Future Projections

Additional artificial sense organs and substitute sensory systems have been devised to enable children to monitor, and therapists to record and modify, the position of other body parts critical for standing balance and ambulation. One of these systems is for establishing correct alignment of the foot and ensuring contact of both heel and toe with the floor. Another will teach the child to bring several body parts into the correct relative positions simultaneously and to train for self-feeding and other coordinated activities needed for independence. These devices will be evaluated through 1974. Our hope is that their success also will indicate the value of applying technology to rehabilitation and education of physically handicapped children.

Acknowledgment. Special recognition for her role in ensuring this project's success is due to Mrs. Barbara Harris, Supervisor of the Program for the Physically Handicapped, Department of Special Education, Seattle Public Schools. Her commitment to aiding the handicapped and foresight regarding technological applications in Special Education were invaluable in dealing with the complexities of incorporating an innovative program such as this into a public school setting.

REFERENCES

1. Harris FA: Inapproprioception: A possible sensory basis for athetoid movements. Phys Ther 51:761-770, 1971
2. Asanuma H: Cerebral cortical control of movement. Physiologist 15:3:143-166, 1973
3. Harris FA, Spelman FA, Hymer JW: Therapy for Cerebral Palsy Employing Artificial Sense Organs for Alternatives to Proprioceptive Feedback. Proceedings, 1972 Carnahan Conference on Electronic Prosthetics, 1-4, ORES Publications, College of Engineering, University of Kentucky, Dec. 1972
4. Harris FA: Control of gamma efferents through the reticular activating system. Am J Occup Ther 23:397-409, 1969

THE AUTHORS

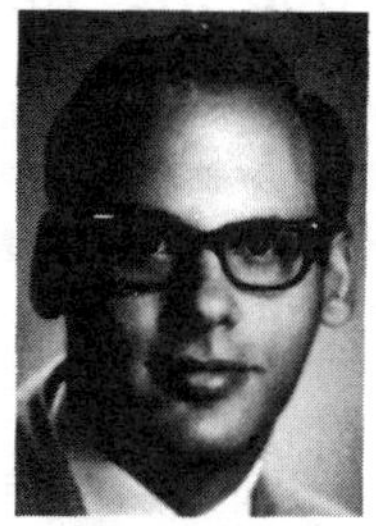

Fredric A. Harris received his Ph.D. degree in neurophysiology from the University of Washington in Seattle. Dr. Harris, investigator in charge of the program described in this paper and inventor of the HCD and LPM devices, carries out basic studies on the function of the nervous system in laboratory animals as well as working with physically handicapped children. He has been active in continuing education and basic curriculum instruction for both occupational and physical therapists and has given lectures and demonstrations of his cerebral palsy rehabilitation program throughout the United States during the past two years.

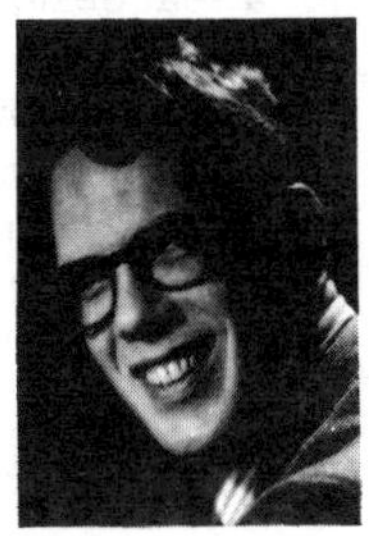

Francis A. Spelman, design engineer for the devices used in the program, received a baccalaureate degree in electrical engineering from Stanford University in 1959, a M.S.E.E. from the University of Washington in 1968, and is currently working on his doctoral dissertation at that university. Mr. Spelman has been senior engineer at the Regional Primate Research Center at the University of Washington since 1961.

John W. Hymer, electronics specialist responsible for construction and assembly of the devices used in the program, handled electronics maintenance on the DEW Line in Alaska from 1967 to 1968. He received his B.S.E.E. degree from the University of Washington in 1973 and is continuing work on his master's degree. He was involved in construction of electronic devices for research at the University's Primate Center from 1970 to 1972, and is currently a computer systems engineer for the Consolidated Electronics Corporation, Seattle, Washington.

clinical reports

Seating for Cerebral Palsied Children—The Sleek Seat

RUTH H. DUNKEL, BS,
and ELAINE TREFLER, BOT

Some children with cerebral palsy of the spastic or athetoid type, or both, exhibit excessive extensor tone manifested by a strong extensor thrust reflex or by pronounced extensor hypertonicity. Most commercially available seating is inadequate for these severely involved children. The obvious need is for a seat designed to hold the child comfortably in flexion with his shoulder girdle protracted, thereby decreasing the occurrence of the abnormal extensor reaction. The seat needs to be portable, aesthetic, durable, and adaptable to several bases, whether wheeled or otherwise.

DESIGN

One of the original designs for flexion seats comes from Dr. Winthrop Phelps who designed a "jack-knife" chair around 1957. Later, Mrs. Francis Corley at Les Passees Rehabilitation Center designed "the box-seat" for very young cerebral palsied children. This type of flexion seating is believed to be of functional and therapeutic value for children with excessive extensor tone.[1,2]

The Sleek Seat has been developed to meet functional and therapeutic criteria by the Rehabilitation Engineering Program in Memphis in cooperation with pediatric therapists in the Memphis area (Figure). The seat is constructed from "sleek" tubing which is used on construction sites as a mold for concrete columns. After the tube is cut with a jigsaw to form the shape needed, a sling of denim or strong sail cloth is attached to the tube with Velcro®*. The sling forms a hammock system which holds the child suspended in a flexed position. The side supports on the sling push the shoulder girdle into protraction and a lap belt across the angle of hip flexion holds the hips flexed and prevents a strong extensor thrust from pushing the child up out of the seat. Foam padding lines the entire edge of the tube to make contact with the edges comfortable for the child. The final step requires contact paper or paint for an attractive, washable exterior. The Sleek Seat is available in four sizes to accommodate children from 6 months to about 14 years of age.

RATIONALE

The therapeutic rationale for the design is based on the theory that if the athetoid child is correctly positioned in flexion most of the day from an early age the primitive extensor

Mrs. Dunkel is the physical therapist for the University of Tennessee Center for the Health Sciences, Rehabilitation Engineering Program, 1248 La Paloma Street, Memphis, TN 38114, and Instructor in the Department of Physical Therapy, University of Tennessee Center for the Health Sciences, College of Community and Allied Health Professions, Memphis, TN 38163.

Miss Trefler is the occupational therapist and senior research therapist for the University of Tennessee Center for the Health Sciences, Rehabilitation Engineering Program, and Assistant Professor, School of Occupational Therapy, University of Tennessee Center for the Health Sciences, College of Community and Allied Health Professions, Memphis, TN.

* Smalley & Bates, Inc, 88 Park Ave, Nutley, NJ 07110.

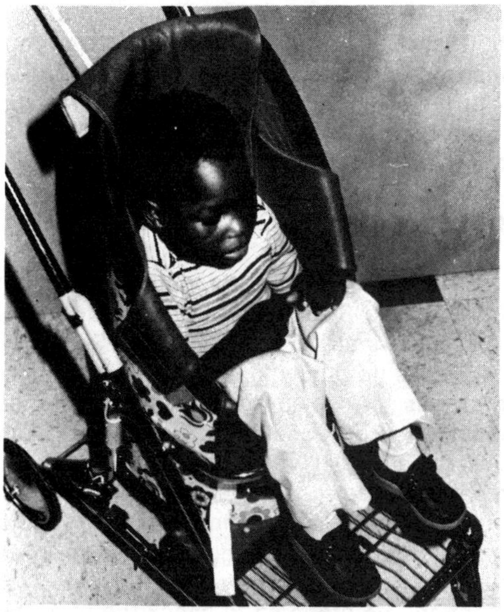

Figure. Sleek Seat with stroller base.

thrust pattern will not be reinforced and strengthened; for the spastic child, a flexed and relaxed position prevents constant contraction and strengthening of hypertonic extensor muscles. For both types of children, the maintained stretch on the trunk and hip extensors helps decrease the extensor tone and allows a more normal balance between the abdominal and back extensor muscles to develop.

Normal development is impossible for a child who spends most of his day in a total extension pattern with the shoulder girdle retracted and arms in the coronal plane. Even the development of a child's self image relies heavily on sensory input through exploration with his hands. A second advantage of the flexed position in the Sleek Seat is that the child is held erect with the shoulder girdle protracted and the arms forward. This position normalizes the tone of the shoulder girdle retractors and allows the child to bring his hands together in the midline for observation and exploration. Finally, the sling effect with side support assists the child in achieving midline orientation. Not only are his hands together and visible, but his head and trunk are stabilized in the midline position. The visual orientation that he now receives is of vertical things being vertical. A decrease of the asymmetrical tonic neck reflex is sometimes seen in children who have been placed in the midline position.

CASE HISTORY

D. W. is a $2^1/_2$ year old cerebral palsied child with severe spastic quadriplegia secondary to anoxia at birth. He demonstrates extreme extensor hypertonicity throughout the neck and trunk with strong shoulder retraction, fisted hands, and scissoring of the lower extremities. He was referred to the Rehabilitation Engineering Center for therapeutic seating to decrease excessive extensor tone. After evaluation by the clinic team, he was fitted with a Sleek Seat. When in the Sleek Seat, his general body tone was relaxed, his hands were together, his shoulders forward, and his lower extremities relaxed, flexed, and abducted. When the child was seen in review clinic six weeks after receiving the seat, both the attending therapist and physician noted improvement in head control and relaxation of extensor hypertonicity.

DISCUSSION

The severe extensor hypertonicity seen in D.W. is a frequent symptom of brain damage when lower brain structures function without higher central nervous system inhibition. Abnormal postural reflex mechanisms are "released" from central nervous system control, and become imprinted in the child's nervous system as "normal" because they are the only motor activities he has experienced.[3] The pediatric therapist must first prepare the way for gross motor control by inhibiting such abnormal reflexes and hypertonicity when inhibition of the child's central nervous system is insufficient or lacking. By inhibiting abnormal motor activity the therapist can attempt to facilitate more appropriate movement patterns.

Many therapists have experienced frustration in treating a child in a scheduled therapy session knowing that the child will not be properly positioned and handled the remainder of his day, thus negating much of the benefit of his therapy. The Sleek Seat provides an adjunct to therapy by providing a relaxed posture for home and school. The benefits of therapy as well as the benefits of a more normal quality of postural tone can be derived throughout the child's day.

In addition to therapeutic considerations, the Sleek Seat is designed to be light weight, attractive, and adaptable to the child's environment. Parents and teachers have reported its usefulness as a car seat, classroom seat, transport stroller, family-TV room chair, and feeding seat. The relaxed posture makes feeding easier for the child and the parent.

ADVANTAGE – DISADVANTAGE – PRECAUTIONS

The main advantage of the Sleek Seat is that when properly seated, the child is maintained in a relaxed posture. Some of the children when first in the seat either slump forward with their head on their knees or fight the feeling of flexion which is a new and unfamiliar posture. Most children, however, adjust quickly, exhibit relaxation of extensor hypertonicity, and actually enjoy the benefits of an upright sitting posture. When the child is out of the seat, spasticity is still present, but it is less severe and often relaxes with time. In the meantime, the child has been positioned correctly and has had the experience of being out of his extensor pattern.

The most effective use of the Sleek Seat is with very young children who are diagnosed early and can be treated before strong extensor patterns develop. As the young child grows, a combination of neurodevelopmental therapy techniques and relaxed postures assists him to develop more normal patterns of movement. The flexion seating can be discontinued when the child is in a stage such as creeping or no longer appears to be dominated by extensor hypertonicity.

As a precautionary note, any therapist would be remiss in failing to instruct the family in range-of-motion exercises and positioning to avoid contractures and to allow for developmental activities when the child is not in the Sleek Seat. It is usually important, for example, for both maintaining range of motion and encouraging sequential development that the child be involved in activities in a prone position. The child should not spend more than one or two consecutive hours in the Sleek Seat.

CONCLUSION

Proper evaluation of the child and correct fitting of the Sleek Seat are most important. The authors stress that the Sleek Seat concept does not apply to every child with cerebral palsy. An inappropriate selection of a child for a Sleek Seat or an improper fit of an appropriate child would be detrimental at the most and useless at the least. The person recommending and fitting a child should have a working knowledge of the neurophysiological concepts of cerebral palsy management and be prepared to check the fit of the seats on a regular basis.

An instruction manual on evaluation criteria, fitting, and fabrication techniques of Sleek Seats is being developed by the therapy department of the Rehabilitation Engineering Center in Memphis. Anyone interested in further information may contact the Center at the following address:

The University of Tennessee
Rehabilitation Engineering Program
Therapy Department
1248 La Paloma Street
Memphis, Tennessee 38114

Acknowledgment. Appreciation is expressed to the Les Passees Rehabilitation Center, Children's Division, and to Mrs. Francis Corley, RPT, who pioneered the concept of the flexion seat in Memphis.

REFERENCES

1. Christopher RP: Recent advances in mechanical aids in the management of children with brain damage. South Med J 67:400, 1974
2. Finnie NR: Handling the Young Cerebral Palsied Child at Home, ed 2. London, William Heinmann Medical Books LTD, 1974, pp 164–165
3. Pearson PH, Williams CE: Physical Therapy Services in the Developmental Disabilities. Springfield, Charles C Thomas, Publisher, 1975, pp 116–118

suggestions from the field

Dynamic Trunk Stabilizer for Children with Cerebral Palsy

PATRICIA MONTGOMERY, MA, and JAN GAUGER, BS

Children with cerebral palsy often have difficulty stabilizing their trunks to maintain good sitting posture. Static chest supports, which pull the patient back into the wheelchair, place a maintained stretch on tight musculature, particularly trunk flexors, and facilitate increased trunk flexion. This is probably due to the effect of stretch on the neuromuscular spindles.

A method of dynamic positioning for patients who lack trunk stability was described by Farber.[1] She used rubber tourniquet hose across the chest and over the patient's shoulders. The hose was anchored to the back of the chair to provide a downward and inward force to the trunk for vertical compression of vertebral joints. Joint compression of more than body weight has been demonstrated to be facilitory to the muscles around the joint. This compression, coupled with quick and maintained stretch provided by the hosing as the patient sits or moves, theoretically facilitates trunk cocontraction and well aligned posture of the trunk.

When this support was tested with a group of children with cerebral palsy two difficulties were encountered: 1) the tourniquet hose provided too much resistance for young children, and 2) the hosing would not stay in place when the children moved.

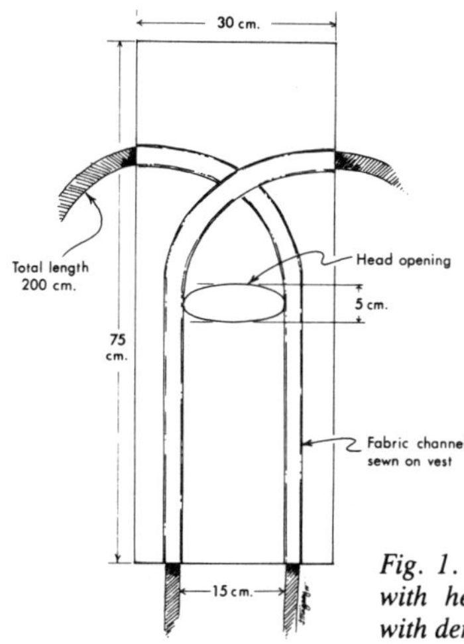

Fig. 1. Inside view of vest with hem facing threaded with dental dam.

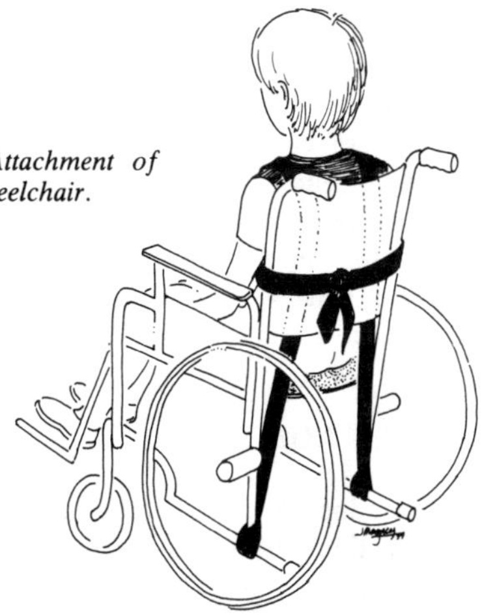

Fig. 2. Attachment of vest to wheelchair.

A cloth vest (75 cm x 30 cm with a hole 15 cm x 5 cm cut for the head) was devised (Fig. 1). Hem facing $4\frac{1}{2}$ cm wide and 70 cm long was sewn on the wrong side and threaded with dental dam, a soft elastic material available through dental supply firms. The dental dam was folded to a width of 4 cm and cut in lengths of 200 cm. The straps cross the chest of the patient and are tied in the back of the wheelchair. The other end of the straps pass over the shoulders and are secured beneath the wheelchair (Fig. 2).

Dental dam is easily removed when the vest is laundered. The vest prevents the elastic straps from slipping and has been used successfully with a number of children.

Mrs. Montgomery and Mrs. Gauger are Staff Physical Therapists at Bridge-View School, St. Paul Public Schools, 360 Colborne St, St. Paul, MN 55102.

REFERENCE

1. Farber SD, Huss AJ: Sensorimotor Evaluation and Treatment Procedures for Allied Health Personnel. Indianapolis, The Indiana University Foundation Press, 1974

suggestions from the field

Wheelchair Insert for Severely Handicapped Children

LAIRD D. WISELY, BS,
RAYMOND L. COSS, MD,
and EARL KNIFFEN

Numerous articles have been published in PHYSICAL THERAPY regarding orthopedic carts and special modifications for severly handicapped persons. We, too, at Good Samaritan Hospital, have had experience with patients having chronic conditions and deal with positioning of persons with severe cogenital and acquired deformities. Our past experience has been mainly with inpatients and contacts with their parents during our cerebral palsy and brace clinics. The parents expressed to us the inadequacy of "off the shelf" adapted wheelchairs to improve sitting stability effectively and to control the severe physical deformities of their children. Other deficiencies associated with these wheelchairs were inactivity while the child was in the wheelchair, low-level tolerance to sitting, and decreased mobility in his environment which ultimately led to alienation from the family circle and limited social interaction.

We, too, directed our efforts toward finding an "off the shelf" solution to these problems. With our efforts being fruitless, we designed and constructed the wheelchair insert.

DESCRIPTION

This adaptive device can be inserted into a standard reclining-back wheelchair with removable, or wide set, arm rests (Fig. 1), or, in particular cases, may be adapted to a collapsible, stroller-wheel unit. Modifications may include bilateral head and shoulder supports, a shoulder harness, lateral trunk stabilizers, and abductor U-bars. The insert is entirely lined with 5 cm (2 in) leather-covered foam padding which is affixed in interchangeable sections with Velco®* backing for incontinence considerations.

Mr. Wisely is Chief Physical Therapist, Good Samaritan Hospital, 605 N 12th St, Mt. Vernon, IL 62864.

Dr. Coss is Medical Director, Good Samaritan Hospital.

Mr. Kniffen is Chief Carpenter, Maintenance Section, Good Samaritan Hospital.

This article was submitted September 12, 1977, and accepted October 26, 1977.

* Smalley & Bates, Inc, 88 Park Ave, Nutley, NJ 07710.

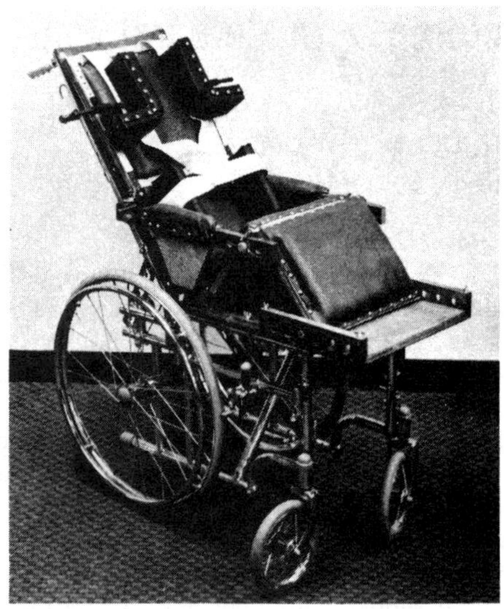

Fig. 1. The wheelchair insert in a reclining wheelchair with the armrests removed.

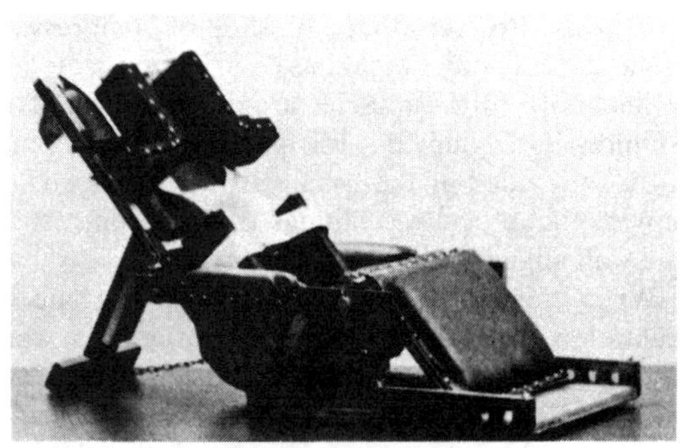

Fig. 2. The insert with a stabilizing T-bar.

The insert is adjustable at the knees, hips, and back and is removable from the wheelchair. The upper back support may be gatched down for possible use in providing bronchial drainage. The insert can be placed on flat surfaces such as the lawn or a table by the use of the posterior stabilizing T-bar with chain attachment (Fig. 2). Also optional is a multiposition patient lap tray that may be used with the insert in or out of the wheelchair. The insert is completely collapsible for ease of transportation.

The major objective for most patients using the insert is to improve sitting capability, tolerance to sitting, and mobility in his environment. Other objectives can be established and achieved through the use of different modifications. For instance, the physical variables such as adductor tightness, knee flexion contractures, hip flexion contractures, scoliotic type deformities, respiratory involvement, and poor sitting stability can be reduced by adjusting available modifications.

We believe that by providing for changes in the patient's physical setting, a definite positive effect will be experienced in visual stimulation and social interaction. We believe that the burden will be lessened for the parents and that greater participation and acceptance will be experienced.

We have been measuring patients for their inserts at our clinics by placing the patient into a form insert. This allows us to fit the insert to the patient's individual dimensions and to take into account individual needs caused by physical deformities.

We are continually trying to improve on this insert to meet all the patient needs and currently are trying to determine whether this type of insert can be constructed at home by the family for a reasonable cost. We have had an excellent response from various community groups in constructing the insert and purchasing materials for individual patients. In these ways, as little expense as possible is incurred by the family and third party payers.

Mobility Module Counteracting the Tonic Labyrinthine Reflex in a Cerebral Palsied Child

LINDA WAT, BS

Wheelchairs, walkers, canes, and crutches are the conventional devices used to provide physically limited persons with mobility. In a child with cerebral palsy, lack of control or strength in the trunk, arms, or legs, and poor coordination or balance may prevent the use of these methods. Muscular activity is often also dominated by primitive reflex patterns of movement and the child cannot control his limbs. An example is the tonic labyrinthine reflex (TLR) which is a major deterrent to independent mobility by a cerebral palsied child. Strong flexion of the extremities and neck when the child is placed in a prone position blocks the voluntary extension needed for crawling. Strong extension when the child is supine "pins" him to the floor.

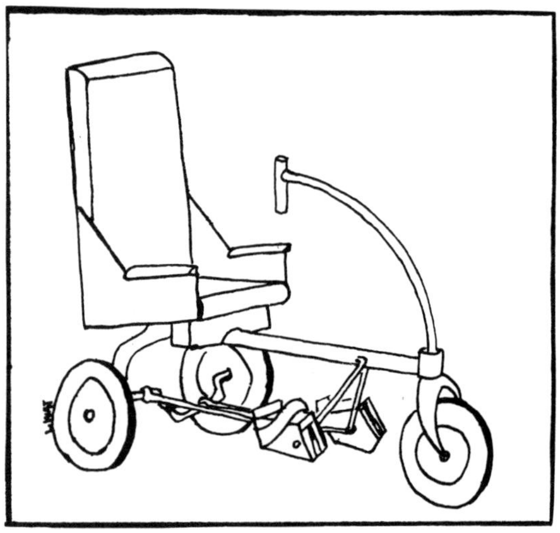

Fig. 1. (above) Toy tractor with camshaft-drive mechanism and modifications.

Case Study

P.S. is a 6-year-old boy with athetoid cerebral palsy. Confined to a wheelchair, he has inadequate trunk muscle control, lacks good sitting balance, and wears bilateral knee-ankle-foot orthoses with a trunk extension for support. He is unable to propel his wheelchair bcause of insufficient arm-hand control and is unable to crawl because of the TLR. His independent mobility is limited to rolling on the floor. P.S. has voluntary reciprocal flexion-extension of his legs. He has some control of grasp and arm motion in his left arm, but the right arm is more severely involved. An attempt to provide this child with a means of independent mobility initiated the following project.

Guidelines for the project were based on: 1) using reciprocal flexion-extension leg motion, 2) positioning the body to minimize the TLR effects, 3) providing maximal trunk stability with minimal motion restriction, 4) using the left arm for steering

Ms. Wat is a physical therapist for the Loma Linda University Medical Center Home Health Agency. Her address is PO Box 546, Loma Linda, CA 92354.

This article was submitted July 28, 1977, and accepted October 25, 1977.

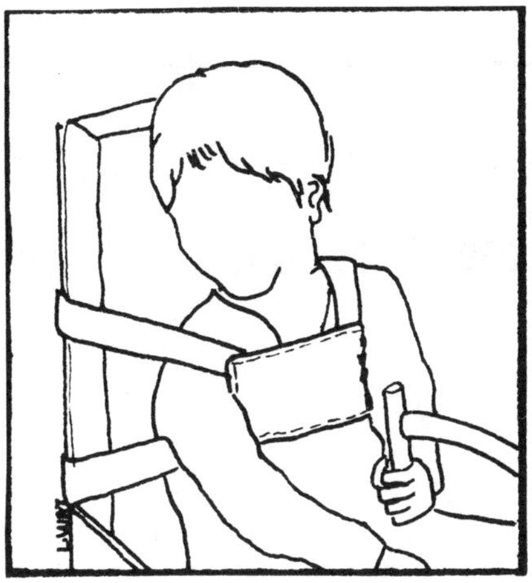

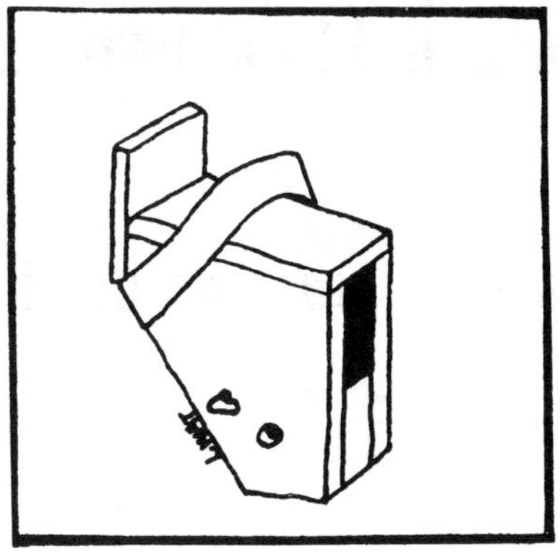

(LtoR) Fig. 2. Bib-style harness used to support child against back rest. Fig. 3. Close-up of built-up foot pedal.

control, and 5) harnessing the energies of a youthful desire to "Go!"

A toy tractor with a camshaft drive mechanism (Fig. 1) was used for the module base. This type of drive mechanism utilized available reciprocal leg motions and was easier to operate than the rotary motion of a conventional tricycle. Fastened to this base was a seating unit composed of a 26 in × 12 in × 1/2 in back joined at 90 degrees to a 12 in × 14 in × 3/4 in base. To provide the patient security while sitting and to minimize the TLR influence, the entire seat unit was then reclined 15 degrees from the horizontal. The sloping side panels and narrow width of the seat provided lateral trunk stabilization. The seat was cushioned with 2-inch foam rubber covered by denim. These cushions were fastened to the seat by 1 and 1/2 inch Velcro ®* strips and could be removed for washing.

The child was secured in the seat by a bib-style harness (Fig. 2) made from denim. Fastened behind the seat, the harness kept the upper trunk erect, yet seemed comfortable. The orthoses were not worn. The steering handle was aligned vertically to keep the forearm in a neutral position midway between pronation and supination. This positioning enabled steering without a downward pull which would stimulate an arm flexion pattern as a horizontal handle would have done. The steering shaft was improvised from a ski pole.

Built-up foot pedals (Fig. 3) were designed to keep the hip extensor muscles on a slight stretch for better "push power." Screw stops on the pedals limited plantarflexion to from 15 to 20 degrees thus directing motion forward, not downward.

* Smalley & Bates, Inc, 88 Park Ave, Nutley, NJ 07110.

After six 30 to 45-minute training sessions, P.S. was able to power the module adequately by himself and steer with minimal guidance. A 5-year-old spastic cerebral palsied boy with similar handicaps was also trained on the module and "soloed" after four training sessions. The module has provided a mobile alternative to two wheelchair-bound boys.

Materials

The module was specifically built for a child measuring about 40 inches and weighing 40 pounds, but it can be varied for children of different sizes. The approximate cost of the module was $40.00. The basic construction materials are below:

Camshaft toy tractor for the base. This might be obtained gratis from such groups as service clubs, firemen's associations, and Armed Forces Reserve Units. 12 in × 24 in × 3/4 in plywood for the seat base; 24 in × 36 in × 1/2 in plywood for the remaining parts; 1 1/2 in × 1 1/2 in × 12 in wood block for seat angulation; 1 in × 6 in dowel and 3 ft lightweight aluminum tubing for steering assembly; 24 in × 36 in × 2 in foam rubber for cushions; 2 yards denim for cushion covers, bib harness, and straps; 1 1/2 in Velcro and canvas webbing for foot straps, etc; 1 pint oil-base enamel paint, 2 oz contrast trim paint; assortment of nuts, screws, bolts, nails, and sandpaper.

Acknowledgment. The project was submitted as a senior requirement for the School of Allied Health Professions, Department of Physical Therapy, Loma Linda University. Advice and assistance were given by the Therapy Department of J.C. Carmack School-O.H., San Bernardino, California; Bo Ying Wat, MD; and Sharon Jantz.

suggestions from the field

Prone Standing Board for Use in the Classroom

EILEEN COHEN, BS

This device was fabricated as an alternative for certain wheelchair-bound students to spending all day in a wheelchair.

Commercially made prone boards tend to be expensive, whereas this device was made from easily accessible scrap material. The total cost for wood, foam rubber, hardware, and paint was about $5. The tricycle frame, training wheels, and naugehyde had been donated to the school. The versatility of the device allows a child to be moved from one area to another and gives a child the opportunity to participate in classroom activities while head stability and extensor tone are being promoted and encouraged.

The prone board was mounted on an old tricycle frame to which training wheels were added to promote greater stability (Fig. 1). The training wheels were attached by bolts and braces to the front fork. The board was made from 1.9 cm (3/4 in) pressboard covered with 5 cm (2 in) foam and water-resistant naugehyde. The measurements for the board were determined by measuring from axilla to instep, and from shoulder to shoulder at the broadest part. The board was then secured to the tricycle frame at the area where the seat would be and on the rear metal footplates. The footboard was attached by metal "L" bars that were drilled so as to make the footboard height adjustable. The footboard was made from 1.9 cm (3/4 in) pressboard with the front panel raised to allow the toes to fit through. Two wooden supports were inserted and nailed to the bottom of the board for proper alignment of the foot and leg when the child was in the semiupright position. To some extent, the prone board can be adjusted toward a more upright position by placing blocks of wood between the board and the area of the handlebars and the seat attachment.

The time spent by the child in the prone stander started with 10 minutes twice a day and has since increased to 30 minutes twice a day. The child and classroom teacher have both found the stander beneficial for certain classroom activities (ie, table top activities), and from the physical therapist's point of view, the stander has promoted extension of the child's head and trunk (Fig. 2).

Acknowledgment: Special thanks to Dennis Stephen, Head Custodian at the SPEED Developmental Center, for his time and skill in fabricating this board.

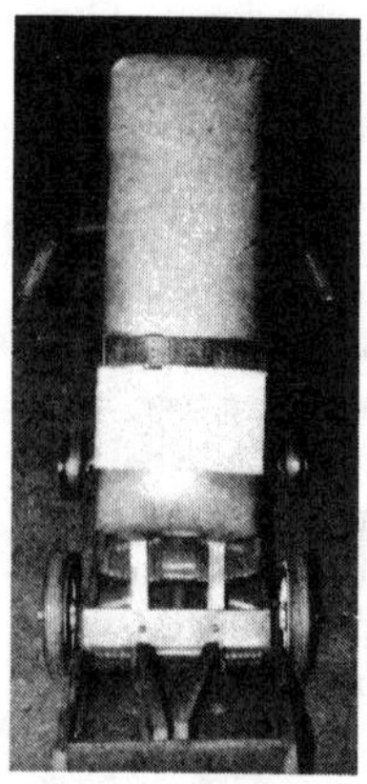

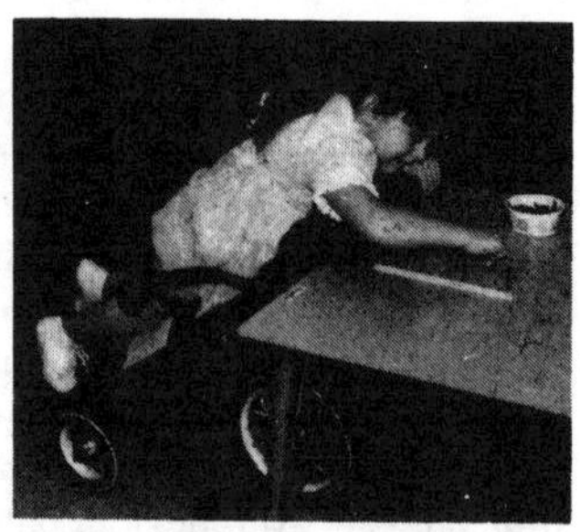

(L to R) Fig. 1. Improvised prone standing board on a tricycle base. Fig. 2. Student using prone standing board.

Ms. Cohen is a Staff Physical Therapist with SPEED Developmental Center, 1125 Division St, Chicago Heights, IL 60411.

This article was submitted December 20, 1977, and accepted February 23, 1978.

Nutritive Sucking in High-Risk Neonates After Perioral Stimulation

ELIZABETH LIPMAN LEONARD, MS,
LONNI E. TRYKOWSKI, MS,
and BARRY V. KIRKPATRICK, MD

Five high-risk neonates were selected from the population of newborns in the Neonatal Intensive Care Unit of the Medical College of Virginia Hospitals to investigate the effect of perioral stimulation on nutritive sucking ability. A polygraph and pressure transducer were used to record sucking activity over a four-minute interval for three successive feedings. During the first and third feedings, the infants received no stimulation. During the second feeding, infants received perioral stimulation whenever they stopped sucking for a two-second period. An analysis of variance showed a statistically significant effect from the stimulation sequence as well as a trend of decreasing sucking activity during the four-minute interval. The study indicated that perioral stimulation may be an effective method for increasing nutritive sucking ability of infants who are poor feeders.

Key Words: *Infant, newborn; Physical stimulation; Physical therapy; Sucking behavior.*

Recent advances in neonatal medicine have increased the number of viable high-risk newborns who require extended hospitalization and special care. This increase in high-risk newborns is important to physical therapists because of the growing tendency of pediatricians to refer infants to physical therapy departments for management of some common neonatal problems, particularly of impaired feeding and oral function.

That high-risk infants have a high incidence of feeding problems during the neonatal period is well documented.[1,2] Factors such as anesthesia of the mother during labor and delivery, hypoxia of the baby during delivery, and metabolic disorders are all well known to influence the baby's feeding ability. The resulting feeding disorders can be critical during the newborn period, when sufficient nutrients are essential to support life and sustain rapid growth.

Infants who cannot adequately suck and swallow must have their nutritional needs met through gavage and intravenous feedings. Although these procedures are well established, they may cause serious complications. For instance, gavage feedings may give rise to aspiration of food, esophageal perforation, and vagal stimulation that may lead to bradycardia and apnea. Intravenous hyperalimentation may result in electrolyte imbalance, thrombophlebitis, and septicemia. Thus, eliminating or reducing the need for gavage or intravenous feeding would be advantageous.

The purpose of this study was to determine whether perioral stimulation facilitates nutritive sucking ability in high-risk newborns. We anticipated that perioral stimulation would activate reflex behaviors such as rooting, sucking, and swallowing. We hoped that providing such stimulation before feeding would facilitate nutritive sucking ability and reduce or eliminate the need for gavage or intravenous feedings.

Ms. Leonard was Consultant, Pediatric Physical Therapy, Medical College of Virginia Hospitals, Richmond, VA 23298, when this study was done. She is now Consultant, in private practice, 505 N River Rd, Manchester, NH 03104.

Ms. Trykowski was Staff Physical Therapist, Physical Therapy Department, Medical College of Virginia Hospitals, when this study was done. She is now Field Physical Therapist, Petersburg Health Department, 35 W Fillmore St, PO Box 2081, Petersburg, VA 23803.

Dr. Kirkpatrick is Director, Neonatal Intensive Care Unit, Medical College of Virginia Hospitals.

An abstract of this paper was presented as a clinical investigative study at the Fifty-third Annual Conference of the American Physical Therapy Association, St. Louis, June 1977.

This article was submitted December 11, 1978, and accepted October 5, 1979.

LITERATURE REVIEW

Feeding behavior of newborns has only recently been investigated by physiological monitoring.[3-9] Such monitoring shows that the sucking pattern of the human newborn is organized in a temporal sequence linking sucking, swallowing, and respiration.[10] Infants can suck in either of two modes. In each mode there are characteristic differences in the temporal organization of the sucking pattern. In the nutritive sucking mode, the sucks are characteristically of long duration and consist of uninterrupted bursts of between 50 and 200 sucks. In the nonnutritive mode, sucking consists of a sucking period of short duration followed by a rest period and then the resumption of sucking. The respiration-to-suck ratio is 1:1 in nutritive sucking[9,10] and 2:1 in nonnutritive sucking.[11]

Wolff studied the serial organization of the sucking patterns in 40 healthy newborns following an uncomplicated pregnancy and gestational period and an uneventful vaginal delivery.[10] He noted little variation in the sucking patterns of normal babies after the fourth day of life. In examining premature infants aged 29 to 30 weeks, however, he found that they tended to suck in a disorganized pattern during the first week of life but that the pattern stabilized by two to three weeks of age.

Other researchers have investigated the relationship between mouthing activities and proprioceptive and exteroceptive cues that occur during sucking, swallowing, and respiration.[3,12,13] Mueller and Rood use tactile and proprioceptive stimulation to the face and oral cavity of children with CNS dysfunction in an effort to stimulate better sucking and swallowing patterns.[14-16] To stimulate sucking, they apply cutaneous stimulation to the face. To control oral-pharyngeal incoordination, they apply proprioceptive stimulation, such as stretching the skin overlying the masseter and buccinator muscles and applying pressure at the base of the tongue.

METHOD

Subjects

As they became available, five subjects were selected from the infants in the Newborn Intensive Care Unit of the Medical College of Virginia Hospitals. Only infants who were at least four days old were selected. This period allowed time for any CNS-depressing maternal medication in their bloodstreams to disappear. All infants were between 27 and 40 weeks of gestational age, determined by methods described by Dubowitz and co-workers[17] and Amiel-Tison.[18] Also, all had sustained a neurological insult of sufficient magnitude to be placed in a high-risk category for subsequent developmental delay. They had no evidence of respiratory distress syndrome but had a history of difficulty with feeding. Vital statistics are summarized in Table 1.

Research Design

A single-subject research design using repeated measures on a single variable was chosen. Each infant served as his own control, inasmuch as it was not feasible to assign infants to equivalent groups where they could be matched on identical variables.

Apparatus

An ordinary plastic nursing bottle was attached to a pressure transducer. A 5-mm (0,2-in.) hole was made on the side of the bottle 6 cm (2.4 in.) from the neck of the bottle. Inside the hole a 1.5-cm (0.6-in.) piece of plastic tubing was attached with a small plastic bolt. A piece of Y tubing was plugged into this piece of plastic, serving as a conduit. The transducer was attached to one side of the Y tube by means of a Leur lock. The transducer was attached to a polygraph with a low-level, direct-current preamplifier. On the other side of the Y tube was a plastic line

TABLE 1
Vital Statistics

Baby	Sex	Chronological Age (days)	Gestational Age (wks)	Birth weight (gm)	Apgar Scores	Problems
1	M	19	31	1,680	1, 3, 5	Asphyxia
2	M	22	33	1,680	1, ...,[a] ...[a]	Placenta previa, asphyxia
3	F	94	27	1,320	4, 5, 7	Seizures
4	M	13	40	1,740	9, 9, 9	Small for gestation
5	F	98	28	880	...,[a] ...,[a] ...[a]	Hydrocephalus

[a] Test not completed.

TABLE 2

Number of Sucks Per Minute

Subject	Minutes											
	Morning Feed				Afternoon Feed				Evening Feed			
	1	2	3	4	1	2	3	4	1	2	3	4
1	38	30	14	0	60	33	31	25	39	5	13	22
2	40	37	38	29	66	43	40	37	38	14	57	37
3	49	28	40	22	75	44	41	29	31	29	14	24
4	23	43	20	18	43	44	35	29	34	47	43	44
5	26	9	38	17	39	20	21	33	28	15	7	8
TOTAL	176	147	150	86	283	184	168	153	170	110	134	135
$\bar{X}$	35.2	29.4	30.0	17.2	56.6	36.8	33.6	30.6	34.0	22.0	26.8	27.0

attached to a water manometer. The manometer was fitted with a three-way stopcock so that the pressure generated at the tip of the nipple could be calibrated. This line was clamped off during the recording.

Infants were placed in an infant seat inclined 30 degrees from the horizontal to align the head and neck in the optimal anatomical position for swallowing. The infant's head was held in midline to avoid facilitating the rooting or tonic neck reflexes. The sucking apparatus was strapped to an overhead bar in order to prevent recording the infant's extraneous movements. Infants were fed a standard solution of five percent glucose in water that was at room temperature from a bottle fitted with a sterile premature nipple unit.

Procedure

Sucking measurements were made over a 9- to 12-hour period, depending on whether the infant was on a 3- or 4-hour feeding schedule. This procedure was intended to eliminate any carry-over or practice effects that may have occurred from trials administered on consecutive days. Changes in sucking activity that may have resulted from maturation were controlled by taking three measurements in one day. Three successive recordings were made on each infant and included a morning feed, an afternoon feed, and an evening feed. Recordings were made one-half hour before the usual feeding time. This was done to assure that the infants would be motivated to suck, inasmuch as the strength of the sucking reflex is in part determined by whether the infant is hungry.

The first recording (morning feed) was taken to establish a base-line sucking pattern for each infant. The nipple was placed in the infant's mouth and the sucking-pattern was recorded. All recordings were taken in four consecutive minute intervals so that sucking-activity changes could be monitored and evaluated as a function of time. Subsequently, each recording was divided into one-minute intervals and analyzed for the number of sucks per minute. The paper speed for each recording was 6 mm (2.4 in.) per second.

During the second recording (afternoon feed), a similar procedure was followed. However, when the infant stopped sucking for two seconds, the skin overlying the masseter and buccinator muscles was stimulated by manually applying a quick touch-pressure stimulus that lasted approximately one second. This was done in the area of the buccal fat pad by simultaneously squeezing both cheeks. The pressure applied was approximately 200 gm/cm^2.

The third tracing (evening feed) was identical to the tracing taken in the morning and was made to see if the initial base-line could be reobtained after the stimulation sequence.

RESULTS

A mean score indicating the number of sucks per minute was calculated for each of the three trials for each infant. For the group of five subjects, the means were 28.0, 39.4, and 27.5 sucks/second for the morning, afternoon, and evening trials, respectively. The means for each minute interval for all 12 trials are shown in Table 2.

An analysis of variance for the stimulation conditions indicated a significant effect from the stimulation trials ($F = 6.06$; $df = 2, 8$; $p < .05$). The analysis of variance also indicated that the stimulation had a significant effect for the number of sucks per minute that occurred over the four-minute intervals ($F = 5.20$; $df = 3,12$; $p<.05$). No significant interaction between the time intervals and the stimulation conditions was observed.

A Tukey Multiple Comparisons Test was administered to determine between which stimulus conditions significance occurred. The trial with the perioral stimulation (afternoon feed) was found to be statistically significant (hsd = 10.40; df = 3,57; p<.05). A Tukey Multiple Comparisons Test also showed a significant difference between the mean scores for the number of sucks per minute that occurred during the first and fourth minutes of the trials (hsd = 7.30; df = 4,56; p<.01).

DISCUSSION

Our results support the experimental hypothesis that perioral stimulation will facilitate nutritive sucking in high-risk neonates. A decreasing trend in the amount of sucking activity was also observed during the four-minute interval. This trend may have been caused by satiation and fatigue, because feeding is very energy consuming for extremely small infants.

CONCLUSIONS

A therapeutically applied feeding program using perioral stimulation is beneficial in managing newborns with feeding dysfunction.

A feeding program for high-risk infants could be effective in improving decreased or absent feeding abilities. This type of program can also provide an opportunity for developing maternal contact and caretaking. This therapeutic feeding procedure can be easily taught to parents. When feasible, parents could be allowed to feed their infants while the infants are in intensive care and thereby help to provide for both their nutritional and emotional needs through feeding and handling.

Acknowledgment. The authors would like to thank Dr. Edwin C. Myer for the loan of his equipment.

REFERENCES

1. Lubehenco LO, Delivoria-Papadopoulos M, Butterfield LJ, et al: Long-term follow-up studies of prematurely born infants: 1. Relationship of handicaps to nursery routines. J Pediatr 80:501–508, 1972
2. Drillien CM: Abnormal neurologic signs in the first year of life in low-birthweight infants: Possible prognostic significance. Dev Med Child Neurol 14:575–584, 1972
3. Thach BT, Weiffenbach JM: The lateral tongue reflex in low-birthweight infants. In Bosma JF (ed): Oral Sensation and Perception: Development in the Fetus and Infant. Fogarty International Center Proceedings Number 21. Springfield, IL, Charles C Thomas, Publisher, 1973, pp 370–382
4. Bosma JF: Form and function in the infant's mouth and pharynx. In Bosma JF (ed): Oral Sensation and Perception: The Mouth of the Infant. Fogarty International Center Proceedings Number 17. Springfield, IL, Charles C Thomas, Publisher, 1972, pp 3–27
5. Kron RE: Instrumental conditioning of nutritive sucking behavior in the newborn. Recent Advances in Biological Psychiatry 9:295–300, 1966
6. Kron RE: The effect of arousal and learning upon sucking behavior in the newborn. Recent Advances in Biological Psychiatry 10:302–313, 1968
7. Kron RE, Litt M: Fluid mechanics of nutritive sucking behavior: The infant's oral apparatus analyzed as a hydraulic pump. Medical and Biological Engineering 9:45–60, 1971
8. Kron RE, Stein M, Goddard KE, et al: Effect of nutrient sucking behavior of newborn infants. Psychosom Med 29: 24–32, 1967
9. Peiper A: Cerebral function in infancy and childhood. New York, Consultant Bureau, 1963, pp 396–485
10. Wolff PH: The serial organization of sucking in the young infant. Pediatrics 42:943–956, 1968
11. Wolff PH: The interaction of state and nonnutritive sucking. In Bosma JF (ed): Oral Sensation and Perception: The Mouth of the Infant. Fogarty International Center Proceedings Number 17. Springfield, IL, Charles C Thomas, Publisher, 1972, pp 293–312
12. Soentgen ML, Pierce L, Brenman HS: Mouthing activities in the human neonatal sucking act. Arch Oral Biol 14:1159–1167, 1969
13. Sameroff A: Reflexive and operant aspects of sucking behavior in early infancy. In Bosma JF (ed): Oral Sensation and Perception: Development in the Fetus and Infant. Fogarty International Center Proceedings Number 21. Springfield, IL, Charles C Thomas, Publisher, 1973, pp 135–151
14. Mueller HA: Feeding. In Finnie N (ed): Handling the Young Cerebral Palsied Child at Home. New York, E. P. Dutton & Co, Inc, 1975, pp 113–140
15. Mueller HA: Facilitating feeding and prespeech. In Pearsons PH, Williams CS (eds): Physical Therapy Services in the Developmental Disabilities. Springfield, IL, Charles C Thomas, Publisher, 1972, pp 283–310
16. Rood MS: A neurophysiological approach to the remediation of central nervous system dysfunction. Read at the meeting of the Committee for Continuing Education in Sensory Integration, Madison, WI, 1974
17. Dubowitz LMS, Dubowitz V, Goldberg C: Clinical assessment of gestational age in the newborn infant. J Pediatr 77:1–10, 1970
18. Amiel-Tison C: Neurological evaluation of maturity of newborn infants. Arch Dis Child 43:98–93, 1968

suggestions from the field

Rollermobile for Children with Cerebral Palsy

ANN IVEY, BS,
and DONALD D. ROBLYER, MS

Children with severe neurological deficits m. work for years in therapy to gain basic head contr(and pelvic and shoulder girdle stability. Functional play activities that allow them to use these slowly gained abilities are limited. We adapted, from Nancy Finnie's book, a wheeled roller seat for use by severely involved, elementary-school-aged children with cerebral palsy (Fig. 1).[1] On the roller seat, the children may use whatever control they have gained in therapy to move themselves around. They can be stabilized in a fairly therapeutic position. They adore their "car," which is an excellent motivator for progress during therapy sessions.

CONSTRUCTION

The rollermobile is made from half a sheet of ¾-in* plywood, 72 in of ¾-in hardwood (we used ash), 36 square in of ⅛-in pliable plastic, a 1-in dowel, 5-in platform casters, 36 square in of ½-in rug padding, 36 square in of vinyl, 3 automobile seat belts, 2 yd of Velcro, nails, clevis pins, wood screws, hinges, staples, carriage bolts, and wing nuts. The materials can be purchased for just under $100.

The body is constructed of two solid plywood ends, 9 in wide at the base, 12 in high, and 4½ in in radius. Five plywood ribs, 7½ in by 30 in, are nailed into notches on the ends. The plastic is stretched over the ribs and fastened with a staple gun on all four sides. Each caster is attached to the end of a hardwood board 3 in by 12 in. Each board is screwed underneath the body of the "car" at a 15-degree angle.

*1 in = 2.54 cm.

Ms. Ivey is Consulting Physical Therapist, Arlington Independent School District, Arlington, TX 76012 (USA).

Mr. Roblyer is a special education teacher, Life and Work Awareness Program, Veda Knox School, Arlington, TX 76012.

This article was submitted February 21, 1980, and accepted March 7, 1980.

The hood and trunk are plywood boxes 4 in by 12 in by 12 in, fastened to a slightly wider base. The top of each box is hinged to open as a door, so that adjustment knobs for the dashboard and seat back can be reached. The hood and trunk are screwed to the tops of the caster boards, not to the body.

A triangular seat with rounded corners is made of plywood. It is then covered with padding and vinyl and screwed through the plastic to the ribs.

For the dashboard, 12-in by 12-in plywood vertical sides are slatted. Holes are placed so that the dowel handpiece can be adjusted when in position. A 12-in by 16-in board is screwed horizontally into the slots in the vertical pieces. A vertical piece 12 in by 24 in, with two vertical slots at the base, is cut and screwed between the two other vertical pieces to make the front of the dashboard. Carriage bolts and wing nuts are placed in the slots and are attached to the front of the body, so that the base is adjustable in height (Fig. 2). The dowel is held in place with clevis pins.

The back is made with a 30-in by 12-in piece of wood, vertically slotted at the base. Side wings (16 in x 6 in) are screwed to each side. Notches are cut at hip level for seat-belt attachment. The inside is padded and covered with vinyl. The back is attached to the posterior end of the base with carriage bolts and wing nuts.

Seat belts secure the child's pelvis. Each thigh is secured in hip flexion and abduction. Velcro is attached to the top posterior portion of each back wing so that the child's arms may be secured in hyperextension and external rotation. The rollermobile is painted with pictures of a radiator grill, speedometer, radio, fuel tank, and license plate.

USE

We let children use the rollermobile on days when regular therapy sessions are not scheduled. Arm positions vary, depending on the abilities of the children:

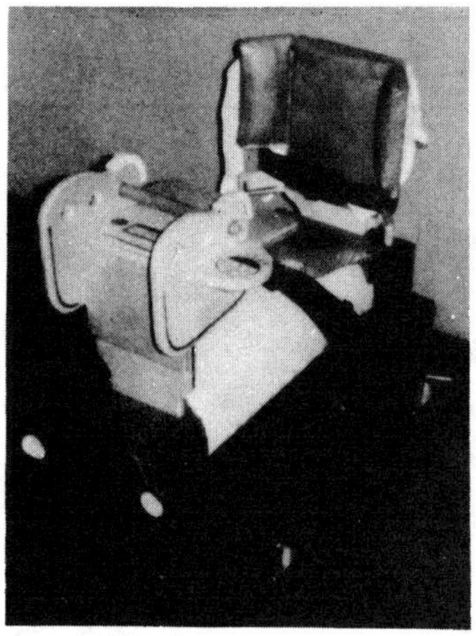

Fig. 1. Rollermobile for children with cerebral palsy.

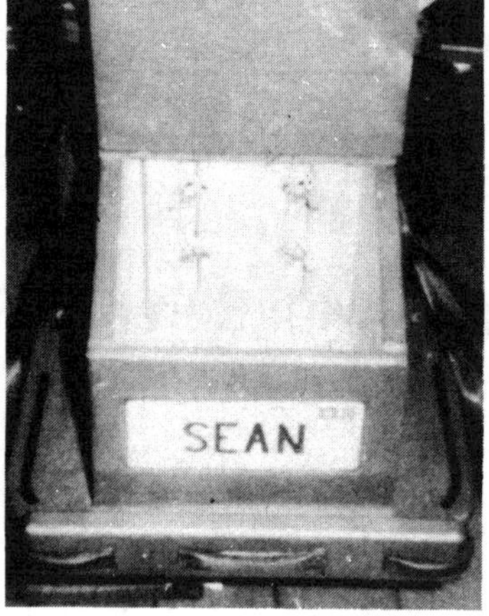

Fig. 2. Height-adjustment mechanism for back and dashboard.

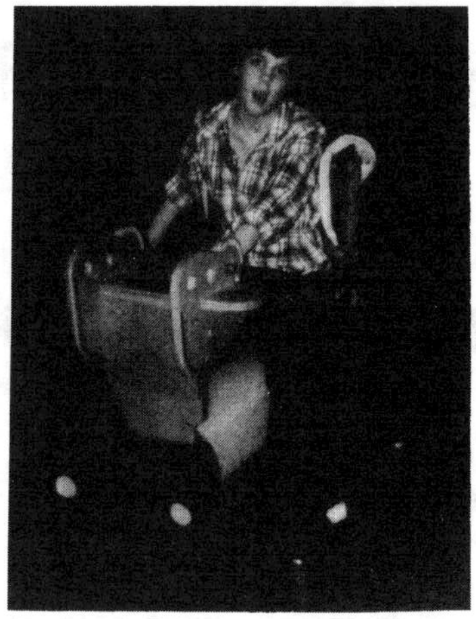

Fig. 3. Child with limited upper extremity function grasping dowel, pelvis stabilized.

their arms may be secured at the back, or they may grasp the dowel on the dashboard (Fig. 3) with one or both hands. They are belted in at the hip and thigh and allowed to move freely about the school. The disadvantage of its use is an initial increase in abnormal tone because of the child's excitement and the excessive effort required in moving. Advantages are proximal trunk stabilization in a reflex-inhibiting position and functional use of the body in movement.

We have noticed improvement in head control, trunk stability, sitting balance, and arm and hand control with use of the rollermobile. Motivation in therapy is much improved, because therapy activities are explained in terms of the child's ability to "drive the car" more successfully. We are pleased to be able to combine treatment principles with a recreational activity for the children. We recommend its use at home and school for severely involved children with cerebral palsy.

REFERENCE

1. Finnie N: Handling the Young Cerebral Palsied Child at Home. New York, E.P. Dutton & Co, Inc, 1975

Evaluating the Adult with Cerebral Palsy for Specialized Adaptive Seating

LYNDA HOLLETT HUNDERTMARK

Physical therapists may not expect to have a pronounced effect on the neurodevelopmental function of the cerebral palsied adult because the neuroplasticity of the child is no longer present in the adult. Adapting the environment to such an adult, therefore, becomes of utmost importance. The wheelchair may be the most important structure of the environment for cerebral palsied adults. I present methods for assessing the severely involved adult client and evaluating adaptations of the wheelchair for therapeutic seating. The anterior and posterior tilt of the pelvis and the vertical angle of the backrest are emphasized in achieving therapeutic seating for the severely multiply handicapped adult.

Key Words: *Adult, Cerebral palsy, Wheelchair.*

Adaptive seating for severely disabled cerebral palsied children has been a subject of increasing concern in recent years. The literature, however, has rarely addressed the needs of adults with cerebral palsy. As physical therapists, we have often focused our attention on mobile and changing children with cerebral palsy. Many severely multiply handicapped adults, however, also require the knowledge and skills of physical therapists to adapt the environment to individual needs. Adaptive seating may be the most important device available for any client who cannot be comfortably, safely, and functionally seated in a commercially available wheelchair.

The adaptive wheelchair should be "therapeutically" designed to improve the overall function of the client. Goals may include providing increased mobility for the client or improving the client's posture, muscle tone, or ability to eat, digest, and breathe properly. Interaction with the environment from the upright position may also enhance psychosocial and cognitive development of the client.

In my experience, most adult clients requiring highly specialized seating have severe extensor spasticity. Nearly all these clients have severe scoliosis with vertebral rotation, and many retain early developmental reflexes (tonic labyrinthine reflex and tonic neck reflexes) that impair or prevent normal functioning. With rare exceptions, adult clients have moderate or severe contractures that are often permanently fixed. These problems often preclude seating in commercial wheelchairs without extensive adaptations.

The therapeutic success of the adapted seat depends on the accuracy and comprehensiveness of the initial seating assessment. Sitting posture, tone, reflex patterns, and musculoskeletal limitations must be accurately assessed in the upright position. The appearance of symmetrical posture is often deceptive when the trunk, pelvis, hip, and knees are not carefully observed with clothing removed. The purpose of this article is to suggest a method for assessing severely multiply handicapped adults for adaptive seating. I discuss observations of changes of tone, reflexes, and normal reactions as seating positions are altered. I explain the "fitting chair" and assessment of the orientation of the client in relation to gravity in the chair. Finally, I present problems inherent in wedging the wheelchair seat and reclining the seat insert to overcome extensor spasticity.

ASSESSMENT

The therapist working with children may assess changes of postural tone and reflexes as they are carried, moved in the lap of the therapist, and placed in different positions. Children may often be hypotonic rather than spastic, are also more mobile, and will almost certainly change during the growing process.[1] Adults, on the other hand, are frequently more fixed in their movement patterns. They may have learned to use abnormal reflexes functionally or to "fix" with spasticity against a backrest or calf panel for stability. Only a careful and precise assessment of the client can determine how the client may gain or lose function with various adaptations.

The client should be evaluated in the sitting position over the side of a mat table. Beginning at the pelvis,[2–4] particular attention must be paid to anterior and posterior tilt and to lateral symmetry because restriction in any direction will cause changes throughout the body. For the very involved client, the therapist may assume a position behind the client, knees astride the client, and hands on the pelvic crests. An assistant may stabilize the client's feet and knees at or as near 90 degrees as possible with the thighs evenly supported on the mat. With this high degree of support and control at the pelvis, the therapist slowly shifts the client's weight laterally, forward, and backward. The therapist may need to use her own body to shift the client's entire trunk forward from the pelvis, sometimes rotating the client's trunk to encourage relaxation. The therapist must accurately assess the position of the superior iliac spines as the trunk is moved to assure that apparent movement of the pelvis is not in fact occurring in the back. The therapist should note if reflexes or abnormal

Ms. Hundertmark was Program Coordinator for Physical Therapy, Wassaic Developmental Center, Wassaic, NY, at the time this article was written. She is now a consultant and educator in the field of adaptive equipment and developmental disabilities in private practice, R.D. 2, Clove Valley Rd, LaGrangeville, NY 12540 (USA).

This article was submitted March 16, 1984; was with the author for revision 14 weeks; and was accepted August 16, 1984.

movement patterns increase or decrease as the pelvis and trunk are moved in all planes.

Lateral mobility of the pelvis must be assessed with attention to uneven distribution of the weight-bearing surface. Lateral movement may be severely restricted in the scoliotic client, and frequently one pelvic crest and the lowest rib are very near each other. Because the goal is to distribute the client's weight as evenly as possible, changes in posture must be observed as the weight is shifted more evenly over both ischia.

The therapist should observe the impact of righting reactions on sitting posture. As the pelvis is tilted anteriorly, righting and equilibrium reactions may result in head and trunk extension and hip and knee flexion. If the pelvis is tilted posteriorly in the presence of righting reactions, the client will often bear weight on the sacrum and flex forward. With the neck in flexion, the head may right into extension or may remain in flexion, leaving the client looking down. Equally important, a posterior tilt in sitting may permit, and even encourage, extension of the hips, which widens the 90-degree hip angle and may then trigger the full extensor pattern.[5] Although clinicians widely recognize that the hips must maintain an angle of 90 degrees or less to prevent extensor spasticity,[2,3,6] the posterior pelvic tilt is often overlooked as a starting point of hip extension in the sitting position.

Righting reactions will also influence posture if the client's back is reclined, regardless of the angle of the hips.[7] At only 5 degrees of a reclined position, the client may tend to flex the head slightly forward as we do in the seat of a car. If reclined more than 15 degrees, a client with righting responses may begin to curl the trunk into flexion.

Changes in the lower extremities must be observed as the pelvis is moved. Because the hamstrings are two-joint muscles, stabilizing below the knee with a heel or leg support of any sort in the presence of hamstring spasticity may result in undesirable hip extension and posterior pelvic tilt. The client then may "sit on the sacrum, always slipping forward out of the wheelchair."[5(p280)]

Positions of the pelvis and trunk also significantly affect head position and control. As noted above, flexion of the head sometimes occurs when a seat is reclined. More often, however, contact of the back of the head with an extended backrest in a reclined or tilted position may trigger extensor spasticity. A therapist may, therefore, find it beneficial to avoid use of an extended backrest or head support and bring the client fully upright. The head may then extend freely without contributing to the full extensor pattern.

Finally, the therapist must observe the position and function of the upper extremities as the head, trunk, and pelvis are changed. As extensor tone of the trunk is reduced through positional changes, the arms may be needed to maintain stability. A tray may provide some support, but the client who must lean on the elbows to keep from slumping forward may be free to do little else with the upper extremities. The arms may also demonstrate increase or decrease of the symmetric or asymmetric tonic neck reflexes with postural changes. The overall effect of the tonic reflexes on function should determine whether posture responses should be stimulated or inhibited by the adaptive unit.

The position of the body in relation to gravity must also be assessed. Nwaobi et al, in a recent EMG study of low back extensor activity of spastic cerebral palsied children, suggested that "orientation of the body with respect to gravitational force" may be as important a factor in hyperactivity of extensors as the angle of the hip.[7(p180)] Because we cannot readily assess the effect of body orientation with the hips at predetermined angles (usually 90°) while the client sits over the side of a mat, a "fitting chair" must be used for this assessment.

THE FITTING CHAIR

Only during a trial phase in a wheelchair can we see the *in situ* effects of each adjustment. Then, the goals resulting from the previous seating assessment can be applied in a "fitting chair." Whether a specially made fitting chair, or simply an available wheelchair is used, adjustability is the key. We must adjust width; depth; height of the footboard, armrests, and backrest; and the angle of the seat to the client's measurements and medical and therapeutic needs. If the client is using a wheelchair, a simple seat insert of tri-wall* (triple-density cardboard) may be angled by placing "spacers" of wood, tri-wall, or other material along the front edge of the seat. The angle of the backrest may be altered in the same manner. Pieces of foam or blocks may provide all the adjustability needed in width and depth of the seat.

The optimal position for seating a client is 90 degrees horizontal for the seat and 90 degrees vertical for the backrest.[2] The client should be placed in the fitting chair as close to this ideal position as possible. Accommodations for a scoliosis, such as a back contour of foam or other material, should be included. The pelvis should be positioned in neutral in the following three planes: with slight anterior tilt, equal weight bearing on the ischia, and iliac crests equally against the backrest to straighten pelvis and trunk rotation if "windblown" posture is present. The therapist may find it necessary to place the client to one side of the seat and allow the knees to drift to the opposite side to assure that the pelvis and trunk are not rotated. The corrected position may then be maintained by the use of a wedge-shaped cushion along the abducted femur. Any other contractures and deformities must also be accommodated in the fitting chair.

As the angles of the seat and backrest are altered, the therapist can observe changes in the client. The seat angle may be altered by use of spacers, and a block moved behind the backrest from bottom to top will vary the trunk angles. The tilt of the entire unit may be changed by placing a wedge beneath the front casters and moving it slowly until the best angle is noted by the client's posture (Fig. 1).

Remember, it is the tilt of the pelvis that influences posture and tone throughout the body. The optimal position of the pelvis in sitting is slight anterior tilt. Various methods may be used during the assessment to achieve this position. Bergen and Colangelo suggested cutting out the area of the backrest that the buttocks contact so that the lower part of the pelvis extends further back in the chair than the trunk.[2] Wedging the top of a back insert forward may also tilt the pelvis and trunk anteriorly and in my clinical experience, excellent results have been attained using this method with some very spastic clients. A soft ethafoam lumbar roll, usually 2 in† thick, may work well to prevent a persistent posterior tilt in a

* Tri-wall Containers, Inc, Wassaic, NY 12592.
† 1 in = 2.54 cm.

limited number of clients, who often have low muscle tone rather than high muscle tone.

Therapists should assess the foot-support system in the fitting chair. Because many clients for adaptive seating have hamstring spasticity or knee flexion contractures beyond 75 degrees, footrests extended in front of the casters in the usual position are not appropriate. To prevent the hamstrings from functioning as hip extensors, a foot box or lengthened foot support may be used to allow 90 degrees or more of flexion at the knees (Fig. 2). The foot box should extend forward beyond the reach of the heels and back under the seat as needed. Calf panels or pads should not be used with this type of foot box to avoid hamstring facilitation.

When the client is seated fully upright, a tray may be suitable for support much the way we use a table or desk top. Plans for the tray should usually be determined during the assessment process. The fit, height, and tilt of the tray are important in achieving the best posture and muscle tone. A tilted tray may help to maintain hands in midline and in contact with each other. A tray may also be essential for clients whose muscle tone decreases excessively when the hips and trunk are at a 90-degree angle. The tray may be provided with a high inner rim for trunk support, or it may provide support only through the arms as the elbows rest on the tray.

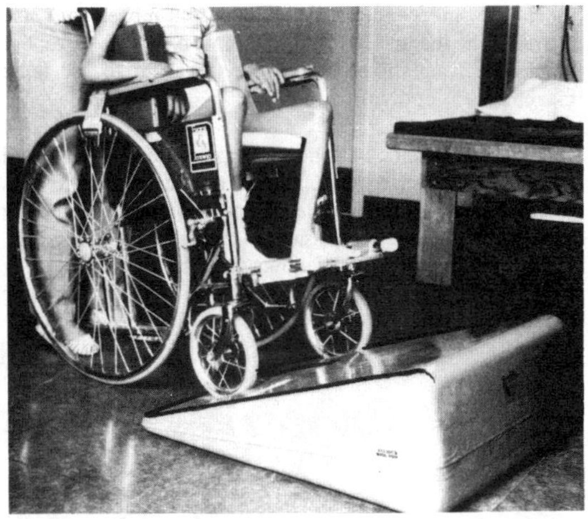

Fig. 1. Optimal angle of the seating unit can be determined by placing a wedge beneath front casters to observe varying angles of tilt.

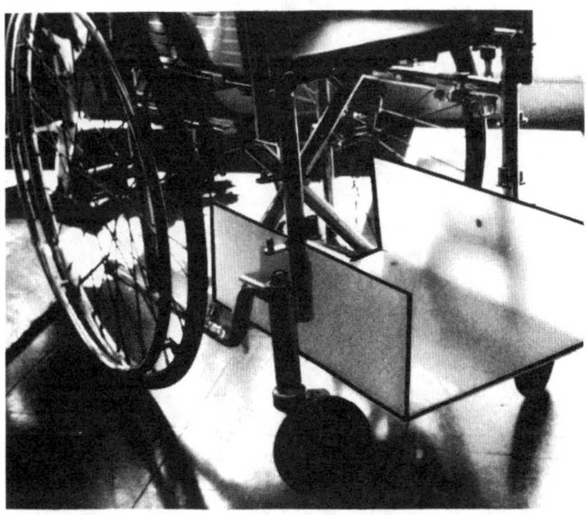

Fig. 2. A foot box extended back behind the uprights and under the seat prevents the hamstrings from extending the hips.

DISCUSSION

Bergen and Colangelo noted that "a majority of clients with disorders of tone show a posterior pelvic tilt when sitting" because of "overactivity of hip extensors."[2(p 5)] They also noted that the posterior tilt leads to the full extension pattern. The pelvis must, therefore, approximate as nearly as possible the normal anterior tilt position in sitting. Wedging the seat invariably increases the posterior tilt in clients who lack full hip mobility. This loss of the anterior tilt is the reason that wedging of the seat has often been unsuccessful in correcting the problem of extensor spasticity in sitting.

Underlying the practice of wedging is the firm belief that reducing the angle of the hips to 90 degrees or less inhibits extensor spasticity. That premise is not in question here. If the pelvis is tilted posteriorly, however, the hip angle may only appear to be 90 degrees. The true angle of the hip will often be significantly greater than 90 degrees. The true angle determines whether spasticity will be inhibited.

The reclining position, often used with a wedged seat for severely spastic clients, is successful only in a passive sense. As spasticity subsides and the client relaxes, he may sink back into the seat rather than extending out of the wheelchair. Moreover, extensor activity is not reduced by reclining and may actually increase. In the aforementioned EMG study by Nwaobi et al, reclining the back as little as 15 degrees with the hips maintained at 90 degrees flexion produced more low back extensor myoelectric activity than when the back was straight upright.[7] At 30 degrees of a reclined position, with the hips maintained at 90 degrees, extensor tone was still higher. The results of this study suggest that reclining a client either elicits the supine tonic labyrinthine reflex, or contact of the back or the head with a headrest initiates the extensor response. Nwaobi et al do not speculate on either of these reactions as possible contributing factors.[7] In either event, we must be aware of the results of this study and carefully assess the effects of reclining the backrest or tilting the insert when positioning our severely involved cerebral palsied clients.

CONCLUSION

Not all clients can be positioned or assessed as I have described, and so these procedures have exceptions. Some clients may require surgical correction before they can be brought to an upright position. Those with severe hydrocephalus or very low tone may be unable to bear the full weight of the head and trunk vertically. The fitting chair will reveal instances where clients have used postural reflexes or hypertonicity for function. Unfortunately, it may not be possible to provide a substitute that will allow the client as much function or independence as the abnormal movements may provide. The therapist has little alternative, in such cases, but to provide adaptations that enable the client to use these movements as optimally as possible.

Acknowledgments. I extend my appreciation to Mary Ann Delaney, whose neurodevelopmental training and discussions greatly broadened my knowledge and awareness of handling and evaluating cerebral palsied clients; and to Ed Mohler, MD, whose questions and willingness to listen led to learning and discovery. I give special thanks to Gil Recchia, Adaptive Equipment Specialist, who accepts the impossible as a challenge to his own creativity.

REFERENCES

1. Bobath KA: A Neurophysical Basis for the Treatment of Cerebral Palsy. Philadelphia, PA, JB Lippincott Co, 1980
2. Bergen AF, Colangelo C: Positioning the Client with Central Nervous System Deficits: The Wheelchair and Other Adapted Equipment. Valhalla, NY, Valhalla Rehabilitation Publications, 1982
3. Trefler E, Hanks S, Huggins P, et al: A modular seating system for cerebral palsied children. Dev Med Child Neurol 20:199–204, 1978
4. Finnie NR: Handling the Young Cerebral Palsied Child at Home, rev ed. New York, NY, EP Dutton Inc, 1970
5. Rang M, Douglas G, Bennet G, et al: Seating for children with cerebral palsy. J Pediatr Orthop 1:279–287, 1981
6. Carrington E: A seating position for a cerebral palsied child. Journal of Occupational Therapy 32:179–181, 1978
7. Nwaobi O, Brubaker C, Cusick B, et al: Electromyographic investigation of extensor activity in cerebral palsied children in different seating positions. Dev Med Child Neurol 25:175–183, 1983

Splints and Casts

Managing Foot Deformity in Children with Neuromotor Disorders

BEVERLY D. CUSICK

This article presents methods by which physical therapists can use splints and casts to intervene directly in pediatric foot deformity management, preprescription evaluation, rehabilitation, and new splint designs for children with neuromotor disorders. Recent advances in biomechanics, engineering, and orthotics have introduced new methods of preventing or reducing foot deformity while facilitating optimal function. Several splint styles are described with current indications and contraindications for their use. The use of casts in serial applications to reduce soft tissue contracture rather than to reduce muscle tone is discussed.

Key Words: *Biomechanics; Foot deformities; Orthotics/splints/casts, lower extremity; Pediatrics.*

Lower extremity alignment, structural integrity, and mobility differ markedly in infants and toddlers with normal (unimpaired) neuromotor function compared with older children and adults with normal neuromotor function.[1-10] The child's foot is malleable and is affected by chronic deviations in postural alignment, laxity in the supporting ligaments, or disturbances in motor function in the trunk and lower extremity.[2,11-18] The child with a neuromotor disorder, therefore, is a predictable candidate for structural abnormality and dysfunction in the lower extremities, particularly the feet, as a result of creep. *Creep* is the slow development of deformity related to soft tissue adaptation to the chronic application of abnormal stresses.[1,19]

The pediatric team that manages problems of foot deformity ideally consists of physical therapists and occupational therapists, a pediatric orthopedist, an orthotist, and, in some facilities, a physiatrist, a podiatrist, and an orthopedic technician. The team's resources include an increasingly sophisticated knowledge of age-specific biomechanics related to the lower extremity and such principles as floor-reaction forces and the closed kinetic chain.[1,2,6,7,20-25]

Management of motor disorders that involve abnormalities in muscle tone regulation and unique functional compensations is a complicated process. Despite recent developments in biomechanics and orthotic intervention, the potential effectiveness of an orthosis can be anticipated but not predicted at the time of prescription. Its functional impact can only be ascertained after supervised implementation.[26] The expense incurred in this process, both in time and financial resources, becomes prohibitive when the orthosis fails to meet the team's goals and the patient's needs for comfort, deformity prevention, and adequate support for optimal function.

Clinicians, therefore, have turned to plaster and low-cost splinting materials for several reasons. The purpose of this article is to present some methods by which physical therapists can use splints and casts to intervene directly in deformity management, preprescription evaluation, rehabilitation, and design of new devices for children with congenital and acquired neuromotor disorders. Four aspects of current trends and rationale for the implementation of splints and plaster casts are discussed: 1) recent events that helped establish principles of orthotic intervention and the application of those principles to the design of splints for the foot and ankle, 2) new findings in developmental biomechanics, 3) clinical research and experience related to the use of casts, and 4) availability of improved splinting materials.

GOALS OF PEDIATRIC ORTHOTIC INTERVENTION

The following goals of pediatric orthotic intervention were drawn from the literature, although the authors varied in their emphases.

1. Prevention of deformity. This is the most common orthotic application in pediatrics. The main target is the deforming influence of creep. Because the process of ossification is incomplete in the young child, abnormal forces of weight-bearing and muscle tension will result in deformity of bone structure.[1,2,21,26-29]
2. Correction of soft tissue deformity. By using casts, splints, and orthoses to reduce deformity in the soft tissue structures in the foot of the growing child, creep is implemented in reverse in the prolonged application of corrective (rather than deforming) forces. Body weight, size, and skin tolerance are limiting factors in this application.[1,26,30]
3. Control of undesirable motions of the affected supporting segments while permitting motion where it occurs normally.[31]
4. Protection of weak stabilizing muscles, either following surgery[11,17,29,32] or secondary to hypotonia.[33]
5. Control of deviations associated with tonus abnormality (N. Hylton and R. P. Jordan; personal communication; March 18, 1988).[13,23,29,33]
6. Enhancement of experience. The child who is otherwise unable to stand or walk can experience upright posture with biomechanical support devices while gaining the physiologic benefits of the standing position.[14,34]

HISTORICAL PERSPECTIVE

Well-documented, diverse events in recent decades contributed to our current management of foot deformity in children with nonparalytic neuromotor disorders. Changes occurred simultaneously in the design and use of casts and

B. Cusick, MS-CCT, PT, is a physical therapy consultant, Cardinal Hill Hospital, 2050 Versailles Rd, Lexington, KY 40504; and a part-time staff member and consultant, Lexington Physical Therapy, Inc, Lexington, KY. Address correspondence to 332 Lafayette Ave, PO Box 11426, Lexington, KY 40502 (USA).

orthoses. The developmental process continues with the recent emergence of lower extremity functional splints as an alternative intervention.

Beginning in the 1950s, the high-top shoe with double-upright, short leg brace was commonly used and has since been recognized for its shortcomings in securing the spastic foot and ankle in neutral alignment and a plantigrade position. The leather shoe quickly conforms to the shape dictated by the deforming forces that cross the ankle and foot.[11,23,33] In the 1950s, however, the Helfet heel seat—a small, U-shaped insert—was developed to treat flexible flatfoot (pes planus) in children and helped usher in a new concept in minimum stabilization of the calcaneus.[35]

In the late 1960s, high-temperature plastics such as polypropylene appeared as an orthotic medium and sparked the development of lightweight, total-contact devices and the need for a systematic, biomechanical approach to design and implementation of orthotic systems.[22,23,31,32,36,37] With total-contact devices came an abundance of clinical problems related to functional impact and skin tolerance, particularly in individuals with neuromotor impairment. A shift occurred in the concept of bracing as a shoring up of falling structures to a more dynamic definition of promoting improved functional efficiency.[31,38]

The University of California Biomechanics Laboratory (UCBL) shoe insert was developed in the 1960s to treat flexible pes planus. The UCBL shoe insert applied principles of floor-reaction forces to the goal of using minimum stabilization to reduce foot deformity.[39] By 1977, research showed that both the Helfet heel seat and the UCBL shoe insert effectively reduced flexible flatfoot deformity with a plantar-flexed talus in healthy children under the age of 9 years.[30] Other researchers later advocated the use of properly fabricated UCBL shoe inserts for certain children with cerebral palsy.[23,40]

By 1975, research showed that a fixed-ankle, below-knee orthosis with the ankle set at 5 degrees of dorsiflexion effectively reduced the genu recurvatum (knee hyperextension) that occurs in combination with equinus deformity in children with cerebral palsy.[41] Floor-reaction principles were effectively applied to the problem of minimizing external apparatus to control knee alignment and function.

Early in the 1980s, the floor-reaction principles at work in Saltiel's patellar tendon-bearing, knee-locking ankle-foot orthosis for paralytic disability[42] were applied to the problem of crouch deformity in children with cerebral palsy. The anterior floor-reaction orthosis (AFRO) was created as a result.[43] The solid crouch-control ankle-foot splint (AFS) was developed concurrently with the AFRO, although without the benefit of influence.

CHANGING CONCEPTS IN CASTING

The rationale and techniques related to the use of casts in the management of neuromotor disorder has varied over time and among different regions of the world. In the 1950s, physicians in California and South Africa used plaster casts to conservatively manage both structural (soft tissue) and functional limitations imposed by lower extremity spasticity.[44,45] Westin and Dye reported on 27 years of success in using long leg casts to manage contractures in patients with cerebral palsy.[44] In 1960, the identification of the tonic reflexes of the foot led to the design of a contoured footboard, which was incorporated into the "inhibitive cast," known also as the Seattle cast.[46,47] The footboard is designed to reduce the pressure stimuli that elicit the tonic foot reflexes. By 1970, long leg casts were an integral part of cerebral palsy management in Australia.[48]

During the late 1970s, below-knee "plasters" (K. Bobath and B. Bobath, unpublished article, November 1966), also known as inhibitory casts, were introduced in the eastern United States in conjunction with training in neurodevelopmental treatment.[49] Built with a toe support and posted to flatten the sole for optimal efficiency in weight-bearing, plasters offered a primitive means by which to apply the principles of floor-reaction forces to promote stability. Plasters were used as an extra pair of hands to enhance therapeutic exercise aimed at promoting equilibrium and control against gravity in the proximal joints and trunk (J. D. Mohr, personal consultation, March 1977).

In 1977, therapists at the Children's Rehabilitation Center (CRC) in Charlottesville, Va, initiated the use of plasters in the treatment of children with functional rather than fixed equinus deformity and related postural disturbances.[50] In 1979, the CRC began to use bivalved casts and footboards[48] (L. Yates, personal consultation, April 1979) and relied on polypropylene orthoses for follow-up.[51] Although the casts were bivalved, their cumbersome features and functional limitations highlighted the need for techniques that would offer minimum stabilization and optimal biomechanical alignment and function.

In recent years, several authors have described their experience using inhibitive casts and orthoses[47,50,52–54] and neurophysiological and tone-reducing ankle-foot orthoses (TRAFOs).[55,56] These devices incorporate design features that inhibit hypertonus resulting from four potential problems: 1) spasticity, 2) tonic reflexes in the foot, 3) the positive-support reflex, and 4) abnormal toe grasp. The TRAFO also purportedly uses biomechanical alignment of the foot structure to facilitate improved function.[55] Researchers, however, have yet to quantify or substantiate the effects of TRAFOs,[57–59] despite an abundance of clinical and empirical evidence of improved joint mobility and function.*

Given the improved alternative management options, since 1984 I have joined numerous authors in advocating the use of casts in only serial applications to conservatively reduce fixed contracture related to chronic hypertonus (see article by Selby in this issue).[2,17,26,44,62–64] The main tissues involved in serial casting for children with neuromotor impairment are the knee flexors, ankle plantar flexors, and neighboring connective tissues. Serial plaster casts are used to increase joint mobility. If serial cast treatment fails, surgery is considered, and a postsurgical splint or orthosis is used as necessary for maintenance and protection of weakened tissues or to enhance stability in upright positions.

Selection criteria among the alternative cast and orthotic interventions have changed as increasingly sophisticated research supports and discards their efficacy. Current trends reflect new technologies, making improved materials available to the innovator. Splints have emerged in this process.

SPLINTS—A NEW ALTERNATIVE

At CRC in 1981, we learned that Aquaplast® splinting material† had been revised to eliminate stickiness and was being used in foot-deformity manage-

* 44, 45, 47–52, 54, 55, 57–62.

† WFR/Aquaplast Corp, PO Box 635, Wykoff, NJ 07481.

ment for children with myelodysplasia at Children's Hospital in New Orleans, La. We began to use Aquaplast® for children with cerebral palsy after, and eventually instead of, bivalved below-knee casts. By 1985, nearly all bivalved-cast use had ceased at CRC.

The orthosis has become an established and valuable tool in the effective management of children with a neuromotor disorder. The use of orthoses is not likely to diminish as new materials and design concepts improve their effectiveness. The introduction of functional splints for the lower extremity offers a management option that supplements orthoses and casts as interventions for selected children. A distinction, therefore, has developed between orthoses and splints according to three factors: 1) materials, 2) durability, and 3) the provider.

Orthoses are usually fabricated from high-temperature plastics, acrylics, leather, or metal, individually or in combination, and are intended for long-term use. They are made by certified orthotists and some podiatrists. Lower extremity splints, although often modeled after orthoses, are made of low-temperature thermoplastics and are limited in durability. Splints are made by trained therapists, orthopedic technicians, and some podiatrists and orthotists. Training in splint- and cast-fabrication methods usually requires one day of supervised practicum after a thorough review of normal and abnormal developmental and closed-chain biomechanics, and a discussion of selection criteria and other management concerns (see article by Lockard in this issue).

Six primary uses for splints have been identified in the management of children with neuromotor disorders:

1. An alternative to high-temperature orthoses for small, active children. Splints provide months of support for most ambulatory children who weigh less than 50 lb‡ and can easily be revised or replaced to accommodate changes in functional ability or growth.
2. Night splints. Lightweight and easily fabricated and revised.
3. Immediate postoperative immobilization of the distal lower extremity. Muscle lengthenings at the knee and ankle usually require a brief period of immobilization in plaster. Partial hip adductor tenotomy, iliopsoas muscle release, or selective dorsal rhizotomy, however, do not warrant plaster casts on the distal lower extremities, although a measure of distal stability provided by a splint might be helpful during the postoperative rehabilitation process (R. P. Jordan; personal communication; November 11, 1987).[65] Because the desired period of postoperative protection for weakened muscles is often less than six months, an orthosis made to last for years exceeds the needs for short-term, immediate distal stability. One or two splints can be expected to suffice for the desired duration and can be discontinued gradually at the surgeon's request. Periodic monitoring is advised.
4. Evaluation before prescribing specific designs in high-temperature orthoses. A splint replicating the proposed orthosis can be tested to determine the potential functional impact of the suggested orthosis.
5. Training aids in a rehabilitation setting or program. Splints can be implemented promptly, and any changes that occur with the patient's recovery (eg, those observed in rehabilitation after head injury) can be accommodated expediently by modifying the splint design.
6. Interim support. If a time lag is expected between molding and providing a high-temperature orthosis, a splint can be used during the waiting period. Necessary support is provided without compromising consistency of care.

At CRC, we discovered that the use of Aquaplast-T®† to make splints offered several advantages:

1. Low cost. Splints often cost only 20% to 25% of the price of orthoses of comparable design. Reduced costs for replacement required by growth eliminate substantial health care expenses.
2. Speed and simplicity of fabrication. After the practitioner (ie, the physical therapist, orthotist, orthopedic technician, or physical therapist assistant) is trained, most devices can be fabricated within 20 to 60 minutes. In most cases, two trained individuals, one of them a therapist, collaborate to take the mold, which sets within 5 minutes. The remaining time is spent trimming and finishing the device.
3. Flexibility of the splint material. Because the foot is an intricately adaptive segment, a small measure of resilience is often desirable, particularly for infants and older children.
4. Design creativity. Team members can experiment with logical design adaptations to meet individual needs for support or function. The cost effectiveness of the creative process promotes the development of new design concepts. The fit and functional impact of the design is readily apparent at fitting, and failures can be discarded while their lessons are retained.

The disadvantages of using Aquaplast-T® in its current formula include 1) bulkiness, 2) limited durability with increased loading forces, 3) slight shrinkage (up to 2%), and 4) the capacity for the finished splint to melt in a sunny window or near a strong heat source. An alternative material, Orfit®,§ resembles Aquaplast® in handling properties, does not shrink, softens at a lower temperature, and must be applied directly to the skin during molding. Orfit® devices also melt near a strong heat source.

PROBLEM-SPECIFIC MANAGEMENT WITH SPLINTS

Most problems of deformity and function in the lower extremities of children with nonparalytic neuromotor disorders occur in the presence of one of two conditions: 1) hypertonus, including spasticity and compensatory muscle overactivity of the stabilizing type, or 2) weakness, either as a feature of hypotonia or as a consequence of surgical lengthening of the supporting musculature.[2,7,11,19] Primary or secondary laxity of the supporting ligaments can occur with either abnormality.[2,11] Management approaches differ for each type of problem.

Hypertonicity

Limitation of full ankle dorsiflexion mobility, diagnosed as equinus, is the most common problem of foot and ankle alignment and function in children with hypertonic neuromotor disorders.[11] Lack of full ankle mobility results in severe biomechanical consequences at the foot, knee, and hip in standing and gait.[6,7,11,13,23,41,66]

The beginning walker normally reveals excessive coactivation of the knee

‡ 1 lb = 0.4536 kg.

§ Available through Se Pro Healthcare, Inc, 140 Domorah Dr, Montgomeryville, PA 18936.

and ankle muscles on electromyographic analysis, contacting the floor with the whole foot and demonstrating a gradual increase in reciprocal and timely activation of the extensor and flexor muscles in the swing and stance phases of gait.[67,68] This initial coactivation period is replicated when a solid AFO is worn by a child with neuromotor impairment who cannot actively provide such distal stability.

The normal gait pattern at the knee and ankle is mature at the age of 3 years when the knee extends before heel-strike during the swing phase.[67,68] As stance progresses before heel-off, the ankle dorsiflexes up to 10 to 15 degrees past neutral as the tibia rotates forward over the stable plantigrade foot.[6,68–70] By contrast, equinus gait lacks both normal heel-strike with knee extension and midstance motion of the tibia over the plantigrade foot. The tibia remains posterior to the ankle, resulting in one of two compensations: 1) The knee hyperextends as the child attempts to lower the heel to the ground, or 2) toe-standing persists with knee flexion to allow forward progression.[2,6,66,69] The result is a shortened stride length and a reduction in walking velocity.[66,68,70] Equinus deformity commonly occurs in combination with other deformities (ie, knee flexion contracture, knee hyperextension, equinovalgus, or equinovarus).

Knee flexion contracture. Knee flexion contracture is caused by overactivity in the gastrocnemius or hamstring muscles, or both.[2,11,13,44] Any device applied at the ankle to reduce equinus must be accompanied by intervention to regain knee extension mobility. One or more of the following methods are commonly used: 1) reciprocal innervation via activation of the quadriceps femoris musculature[49]; 2) mobilization at the posterior hip joint capsule[71]; 3) night splinting[15]; 4) long leg serial casting[2,26,43,44,63]; 5) positioning in long sitting, maintaining the pelvis in a vertical position[15,49]; or 6) surgical lengthening.[11]

Knee hyperextension. The child stands with limited range of ankle dorsiflexion and attempts to lower the heel of the plantar-flexed foot to the ground by hyperextending the knee joint (Fig. 1).[2,6,23,26,41,66] Knee hyperextension of less than 10 to 15 degrees is often managed successfully by maintaining the ankle in 5 degrees of dorsiflexion (Fig. 2).[41] Floor-reaction forces impose flexion at the knee by applying pressure to the posterior aspect of the proximal tibia on weight-bearing.[23,26,41]

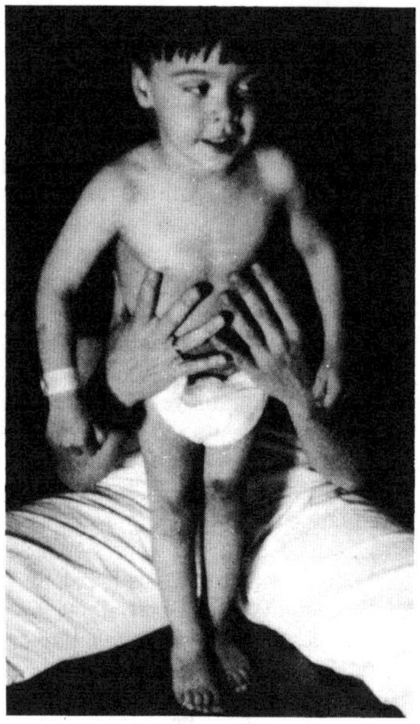

Fig. 1. Child exhibiting knee hyperextension associated with functional equinus.

Equinovalgus (equinus with pronation of the foot). Over half of the children with bilateral hypertonus have equinovalgus.[11] Structurally, the hypertonic muscles within the triceps surae muscle group elevate the posterior calcaneus, causing it to plantar flex within the foot (equinus). Simultaneously, the elements of pronation of the subtalar and midtarsal joints are expressed, usually imposed by excessive weight-bearing on the medial (internal) aspect of the forefoot. The plantar-flexed calcaneus everts at the subtalar joint; the talus plantar flexes and migrates medially and forward; the forefoot abducts and everts, uncovering most of the medial surface of the head of the talus; the rays rotate inwardly; and the toes claw with a lateral (external) deviation.[6,7,11,70] The tibia and fibula follow the talar motions by way of the ankle mortice.[6,7] Shortening develops in the peroneal muscles and lateral ligaments at the subtalar and ankle joints.

Persistence of femoral antetorsion often contributes to pronation in children with spastic diplegia. The abnormal medial twist of the femoral shaft imposes medial weight-bearing forces on the foot and vice versa.[2,6,7,11]

The causative mechanism of equinovalgus deformity is currently being debated, questioning whether the primary problem is tightness in the triceps surae muscle or spasticity in the peroneal muscles.[7,11] Both viewpoints offer potentially valid explanations that may apply to individual cases.

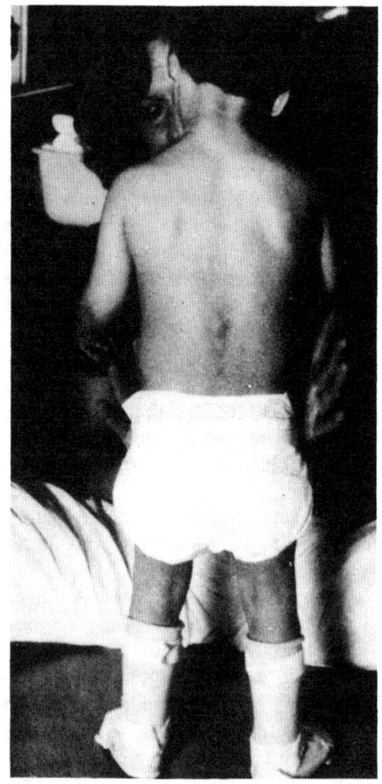

Fig. 2. Child wearing ankle-foot splint set in 5 degrees of dorsiflexion to reduce knee hyperextension using floor-reaction forces.

Children normally demonstrate a calcaneal valgus deviation of no more than 10 degrees through the age of 3 years and less than 5 degrees by the age of 6 years.[2,72] In early life, a measure of calcaneal valgus deviation can be attributed to the angled distal articulating surface (plafond) of the tibia, which inclines upward on the lateral aspect relative to the transverse plane.[8,11] The infant foot also reveals a forefoot varus of up to 10 degrees that gradually diminishes to 0 degrees in early childhood. This deviation can cause the foot to pronate as the varus forefoot seeks the ground (see article by Tiberio in this issue).[6,7]

In the child with bilateral hypertonus, however, the hypertonic forces imposed on the calcaneus and the inability to shift the body weight over the heel and the lateral segments of the foot threaten to overstretch the medial ligaments supporting the subtalar joint.[11,33] The result is an increase in lateral deviation (eversion) of the calcaneus into a valgus position, forming an angle with the tibia that exceeds the age-appropriate maximum.

Protection of the medial and plantar supporting ligaments, therefore, is the first concern of intervention for equinovalgus deformity.[2,7] In a well-built orthotic device for the ankle and foot, calcaneal valgus is prohibited within the structural limits of the talocrural joint configuration; the forefoot is prohibited from deviating into abduction; and the medial, lateral, and transverse arches are supported.[23] Ankle position is addressed only after the structures of the foot are aligned.[7,55] The improved alignment provided by designing an orthosis with these corrective features has been demonstrated on roentgenograms.[23]

Equinovarus. More than 90% of children with spastic hemiparesis demonstrate equinovarus, in which equinus is evident in heel raise while the posterior tibialis muscle forces the elevated calcaneus into medial deviation (supination). Upon initial stance, the foot supinates rather than pronates.[11] (This response differs from the compensation described by Tiberio [see his article in this issue] in which the foot has the necessary flexibility to compensate by pronating.) Because the supinated foot is relatively rigid compared with the flexible pronated foot, weight-bearing occurs on the lateral aspect of the forefoot, imposing a laterally-directed force on the loaded knee during stance. Because the problem of supination combines with contracture of the triceps surae muscle group, the weight-bearing knee might also compensate, either by flexing during stance, possibly to absorb shock, or by hyperextending, promoting elevation and retraction of the pelvis above, and limiting forward progression.[16] Both compensations limit stride length and stance duration on the affected side.

To reduce the deviations apparent in functional equinovarus deformity, the splint is built to align the calcaneus in the neutral position, prohibit adduction of the forefoot and lateral rotation of the tibia and fibula, and set the ankle in 5 degrees of dorsiflexion if necessary to overcome knee hyperextension.[23,26,41] If the equinovarus deformity is fixed, a series of casts might be instituted to regain mobility without surgical intervention. Any evidence of hamstring musculature contracture must also be reduced.[2]

Options in Splint Design for Hypertonicity

Management of deformities related to hypertonus should secure optimal biomechanical alignment of the structures of the foot and ankle. The treatment goal should be balanced, dynamic control of the ankle joint and the long and intrinsic muscles that control the foot and toes within the limits imposed by the severity of the neuromotor disorder.

In the past five years, the plastic-overlap, hinged AFO has been used in several children's rehabilitation facilities, although its originator is unknown. The availability of an articulating ankle within the structure of a total-contact AFO necessitates a review of the functional criteria for selecting AFOs.

In certain circumstances, despite the desire for dynamic systems, a solid ankle or a partial restriction of ankle motion is used to help the child achieve dynamic control of the ankle joint.[44] In other circumstances, a thin polypropylene supramalleolar orthosis (SMO) might be adequate. The SMO, also known as the Dynamic AFO,‖ is a very thin, low-cut AFO that applies the principles of the inhibitive footboard described by Duncan and Mott[47] as it secures the structures of the foot in neutral alignment. The SMO extends proximally to cover the dorsum of the foot and the malleoli.[53] The solid AFS and the hinged AFS are among the Aquaplast® splints commonly used to manage equinus-related foot deformities and are discussed below.

Splint Description and Development

Solid ankle-foot splint. The solid-ankle, total-contact AFO has become a standard prescription for the child with problems related to functional equinus deformity.[11,23,29] The AFO is usually designed with the ankle set at 90 degrees (neutral position). The solid AFS encases the ankle and the foot, excluding the dorsum, in a position of neutral subtalar and midtarsal joint alignment. The ankle, however, is usually positioned in slight dorsiflexion (up to 5°) in the solid AFS to simulate the normal position of the ankle in standing and in the stance phase in early walking and to facilitate a functional rather than hyperextended knee position.[2,69]

Solid-ankle devices are useful as protection for the medial ligaments of the feet of the nonambulatory, severely involved child who is positioned regularly in standing and as a distal stabilizing support for the child whose preambulatory skills are emerging or who has undergone surgical tendo Achillis lengthening or selective dorsal rhizotomy.

For the ambulatory child with functional equinus deformity, the solid AFS stimulates the function of the anterior tibialis muscle at heel-strike and of the soleus muscle as a stabilizing force on the tibia during stance, while it prohibits both desirable (normally occurring) and undesirable (abnormal) plantar flexion.[23,29,69] Velocity and stride length were shown to be enhanced in children with cerebral palsy after AFOs were applied.[23]

The solid-ankle device, however, also prohibits normal excursion of the tibia forward over the plantigrade foot during postural transitions (eg, squatting and rising to a standing position from a sitting position). In gait, the solid AFS also prohibits normal motion of the tibia over the plantigrade foot after midstance. The limitations of ankle motion imposed by the solid AFS, therefore, compete with its advantages for the child who is active and ambulatory.

Hinged ankle-foot devices. The total-contact hinged AFO or AFS features a free-hinge joint and plastic overlap stop that permit ankle dorsiflexion and prohibit a preset measure of plantar flexion (Fig. 3). The maximum angle of plantar flexion is determined by the contact between the shaft piece and the foot piece at the posterior aspect of their articulation.

Criteria for selecting hinged AFOs and AFSs are 1) a hypertonus that

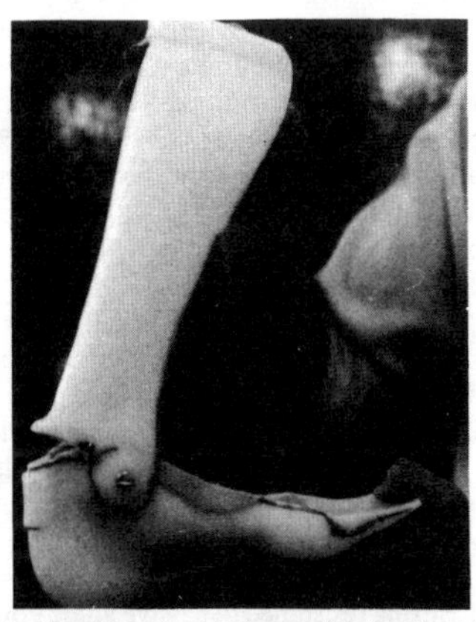

Fig. 3. Hinged ankle-foot splint allowing full ankle dorsiflexion. Posterior overlap prohibits plantar flexion. Total contact supports the foot.

‖ For further information on the Dynamic AFO, contact Nancy Hylton, c/o Children's Therapy Center, 26461 104th Ave SE, Kent, WA 98031.

causes equinus deformity and related problems at the foot and knee or 2) an equinus deformity that is functional rather than fixed (see article by Oatis in this issue).

Additional guidelines for using hinged devices include the following:

1. The hypertonic child is ambulatory. Most children with spastic diplegia and nearly all children with spastic hemiparesis become ambulatory by the age of 48 months, despite difficulties imposed by hypertonus.[11,34] Given adequate knee extension range, strength, and timing of action, the hinged device provides the opportunity to experience heel-strike. The hinged ankle also allows an extended period of plantigrade foot support during terminal stance before heel-off.
2. The hypertonic child is at a preambulatory functional level. The child spontaneously pulls to a standing position and cruises along furniture but exhibits equinus or a related deformity in the process.
3. Preambulatory activities are an important feature of the management program. Positional transitions (eg, squatting from a standing position and standing from a half-kneel position) are a focus of management. The hinged device could be implemented to maintain the equinus foot in a neutral plantigrade position during such transitions and to enhance frontal-plane stability (Fig. 4).

The same child, however, might demonstrate weakness or an inability to stabilize the ankles to stand alone or to walk, and flexion might result at the ankles and knees. The need for greater distal stability could then be addressed temporarily, either by adding an anterior shell to prohibit dorsiflexion or by adding a strap to the posterior aspects connecting the shaft to the foot piece until the child shows improved active distal stability (Fig. 5) (J. M. Carlson; personal communication; November 25, 1987).[73]

Contraindications for the hinged devices include the following abnormalities:

1. Fixed equinus deformity. The available range of unresisted passive ankle dorsiflexion, keeping the subtalar joint in neutral alignment, is limited to less than 5 degrees past neutral.[2,6,69]
2. Strong resistance to passive ankle dorsiflexion throughout the available range.
3. Crouch deformity.

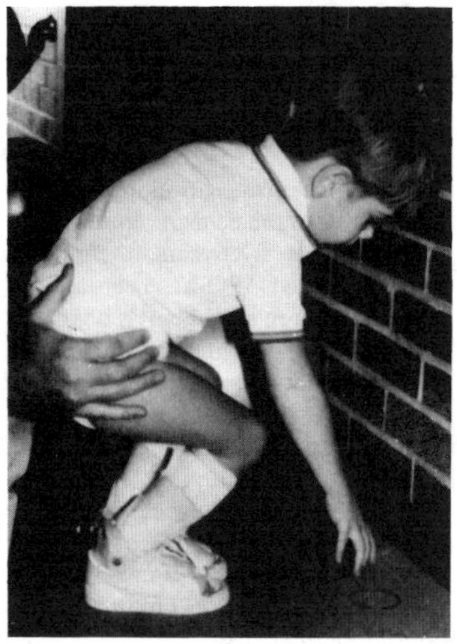

Fig. 4. Child wearing hinged ankle-foot splint to protect foot structures and maintain plantigrade foot position during postural transitions to and from standing.

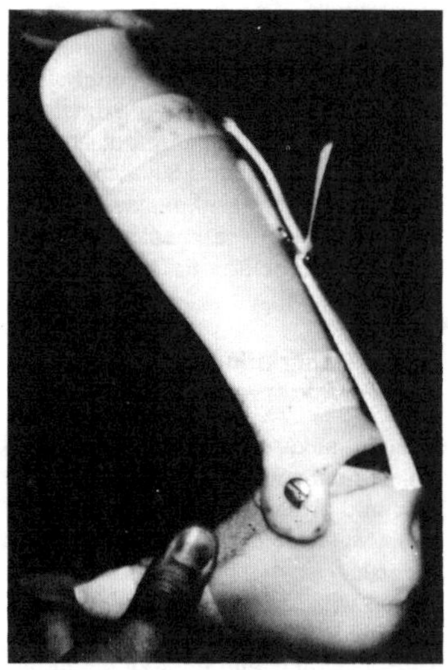

Fig. 5. Hinged ankle-foot splint with dorsiflexion strap stop combines elastic and nonstretch materials.

Weakness in Antigravity Muscles and Ligaments

Two deformities, crouch posture and flexible pes planus (pronation), will be discussed in this section. Crouch posture is noted in the standing position or during the stance phase of gait when the hips and knees flex excessively over the plantigrade foot (Fig. 6). Angles exceeding 30 degrees can occur at the hip, knee, and ankle joints.[68,74]

Although crouch posture is seen in

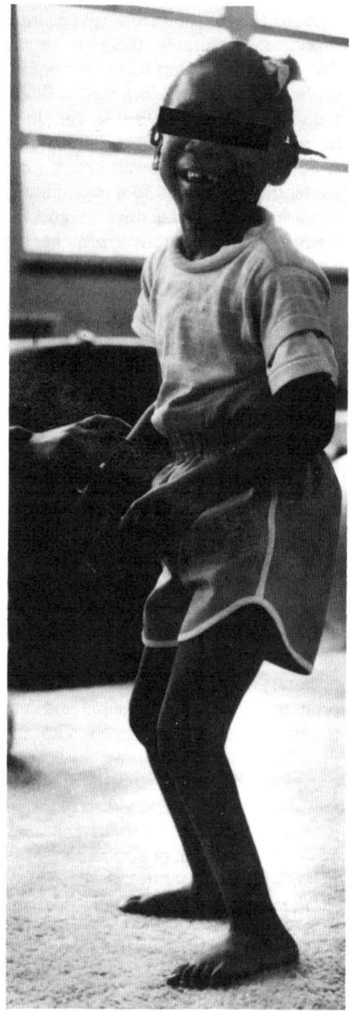

Fig. 6. Child exhibiting crouch posture. Primary source is weakness in triceps surae muscle group (ie, soleus muscle). Pronation is evident.

children 4 to 6 years of age, the posture often becomes distressing when the child approaches adolescence and complaints (eg, onset of knee pain, fatigue, or deterioration of posture or ambulatory capability) emerge. Other features are hip flexion contracture, hip internal rotation with adduction, femoral antetorsion, quadriceps femoris muscle weakness or overwork in the lengthened position, patella alta, hamstring muscle contracture, calcaneus deformity, hindfoot valgus and pronation, exaggerated arm swing, and increased vertical trunk displacement.[43,68,74]

Throughout the normal stance phase of gait, the knee joint is maintained within 20 degrees of flexion and the ankle within 15 degrees of dorsiflexion by the stabilizing activation of the triceps surae muscle group, assisted early in stance by the quadriceps femoris muscle.[24,74] After terminal stance, the triceps surae and posterior tibialis muscles continue to maintain the foot in supination as ankle plantar flexion of up to 20 degrees occurs between heel-off and toe-off, and body weight is transferred to the opposite foot.[67,68,75]

Weakness in the triceps surae muscle group, particularly in the soleus muscle, has been identified as the primary problem producing a crouched posture.[74] Excessive forward excursion of the tibia over the talus occurs in standing and results in knee flexion and progressive tightness of the hamstring muscles.[70,74,77]

Sutherland and Cooper[74] and Bleck[11] suggested that triceps surae muscle group weakness is caused primarily by surgical tendo Achillis lengthening that, if undertaken before reducing flexion contractures at the hips and knees, results in overlengthened heel cords. Two areas of postoperative management that can contribute to the development of crouch deformity are 1) inadequate immobilization using stabilizing AFSs or AFOs that can result in overstretching of the weakened plantar-flexor muscles with standing and walking activities and 2) a therapeutic exercise program that denies the opportunity and the need to regain strength in the weakened triceps surae muscle group. Given the needed mobility at the knee joint, therapeutic training after tendo Achillis lengthening should incorporate active and functional strengthening for the gastrocnemius and soleus muscles and for knee and hip extensors while maintaining mobility. Crouch deformity can also be attributed to factors such as hamstring muscles' overactivity and contracture[43] and pronation deformity in the foot. Pronation facilitates knee and hip flexion and adduction through the closed-chain biomechanics related to the rearfoot complex (see article by Oatis in this issue).[7]

Crouch Posture Intervention

The problem of effectively reducing crouch posture with orthotic interventions has not yet been solved. Typically, when the deformity threatens to defeat the child's efforts to continue ambulating, a desperate attempt to prevent such progression leaves the child lumbering around in a pair of knee-AFOs that are locked at the knee joint and are soon discarded as less useful than they are inconvenient. Within this decade, new orthotic designs have appeared that acknowledge the primary problem of weakness at the ankles, but no design before 1986 provided a sturdy guard against sinking into dorsiflexion while allowing plantar flexion to occur in gait.

If the ankle joint is rigidly supported against dorsiflexion, the brace that supports it functions as a first-class lever with the fulcrum, located at the distal end under the metatarsal heads, transferring the floor-reaction forces to the anterior aspect of the proximal tibia (Fig. 4).[22,29,42,43]

This concept was applied to the design of the AFRO.[43] The AFRO is built like a standard solid AFO in the area of the foot and ankle but sweeps anteriorly and proximally to cover the anterior surface of the proximal tibia. The proximal anterior band pushes backward on the proximal tibia as the child puts weight on the foot section.

Harrington et al, at Newington Children's Hospital in Newington, Conn, studied the criteria for favorable results using the AFRO, which they designed for crouch deformity. (The same criteria apply to the hinged crouch-control AFS discussed below.) The criteria they developed are 1) presence of some trunk balance or ability to use auxiliary walking aids, 2) a minimum grade of Fair quadriceps femoris muscle strength, and 3) flexion contractures at the hip and knee not exceeding 10 degrees. Of 11 children with crouch posture who were evaluated, all required elongation of the hamstring muscles, either by serial casting or surgery, before they could use the AFRO.[43]

The results of the Newington study were encouraging. All 11 children showed significant immediate reduction in the severity of crouch gait after AFRO intervention. Three children who underwent computerized gait analysis revealed improvement in the gait characteristics of single-limb support time and stability, stride length, walking velocity, and endurance. Although energy consumption (measured in joules per kilogram per meter) remained unchanged, stride length and velocity gains suggested that overall gait was more efficient.[43] The main limitation of the AFRO device was the rigid ankle, set at 90 degrees of flexion or in slight plantar flexion. When applied bilaterally, forward progression was prohibited until the ankle was adjusted into slight dorsiflexion, compromising a measure of alignment for function.

Parallel with, although unaware of, the development of the AFRO, I developed the solid crouch-control AFS (Fig. 7) late in 1982 with the assistance of CRC's orthopedic technician, Michael Smith. The primary aims for the crouch-control AFS were to align the joints of the foot and to mechanically prohibit excessive ankle dorsiflexion. In the ensuing years, we encountered the same limitations on function noted above, while the need for strengthening the plantar-flexor muscles became apparent both clinically and in the literature.[74,75]

In June of 1986, to address the problems of triceps surae muscle weakness and gait difficulty imposed by a bilateral rigid ankle support, I designed the hinged crouch-control AFS. Like the AFRO, the hinged crouch-control AFS uses floor-reaction forces, through a rigid sole and ankle dorsiflexion stop, to apply an extension force to the anterior aspect of the lower leg on weight-bearing. Close attention is paid to aligning the joints of the foot in a neutral position because this splint encompasses the foot like a rigid ski boot. The reduction of pronation is a factor in reducing crouch posture proximally.

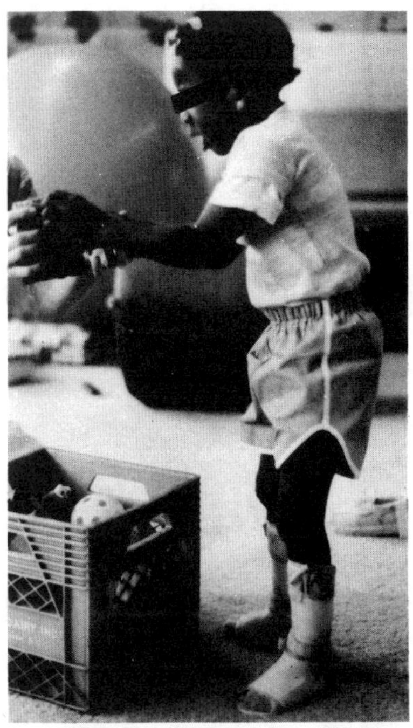

Fig. 7. Solid crouch-control ankle-foot splint applies anterior floor-reaction forces to reduce knee flexion while prohibiting pronation and ankle dorsiflexion.

The hinged crouch-control AES, however, allows plantar flexion to occur during the stance phase of gait 1) after heel-strike, when the foot can lower into full contact as a separate segment from the lower leg (Fig. 8), and 2) after mid-stance, during the push-off stage, which is more mechanical than active.[69,72,75]

The stress tolerance of Aquaplast® splinting material requires that the heavy forces of crouch posture be supported from the dorsum of the leg and foot. By contrast, the solid AFS and AFO buckle into ankle dorsiflexion, and both devices prohibit ankle plantar flexion. The hinged crouch-control AFS, by its dorsal approach to the foot and ankle, offers the falling tibia a reliable support and prohibits excessive elongation of the quadriceps femoris and triceps surae muscles.

Contraindications for using the hinged crouch-control AFS are 1) contracture of hip flexor muscles exceeding 10 degrees,[43] 2) hamstring muscle contracture resulting in a popliteal angle greater than 20 degrees with the same hip flexed to 90 degrees and the opposite hip extended,[11] 3) equinus (functional or fixed), 4) genu recurvatum or knee hyperextension, and 5) poor trunk control.

Research is needed to ascertain the effectiveness of the hinged crouch-control AFS in facilitating strengthening and timely activity of the ankle plantarflexor muscles in standing and gait. Individuals with normal neuromotor function who wear it describe a lever-type mechanism apparently related to the rigid fulcrum at the toe portion of the sole that seems to facilitate activation of the calf musculature as the body weight is carried forward in the stance phase. More research is needed to revise the design to minimize bulky excess. The flap-like extension of the foot piece up to the distal shaft piece could be reduced and reshaped considerably using high-temperature plastics.

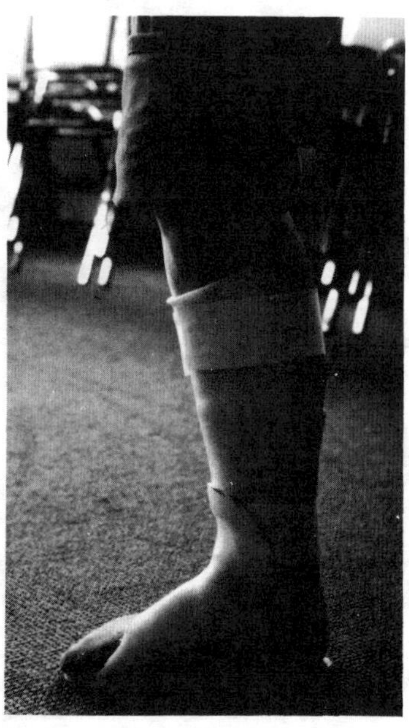

Fig. 8. Hinged crouch-control ankle-foot splint prohibits excess dorsiflexion and pronation. Plantar flexion can occur after heel-strike and mid-stance phases.

Flexible Pes Planus with Plantar-flexed Talus (Hypermobile Flatfoot or Flexible Pronation)

Pronation of the foot is the most common compensation for laxity in the supporting ligaments of the foot or for medial rotary weight-bearing forces imposed by other joints or structures in the leg and foot (see article by Tiberio in this issue).[2,6] In flexible pes planus, unlike equinovalgus, pronation occurs in weight-bearing and resolves off weight-bearing, but ankle mobility is full and unresisted by hypertonus.[6,7,30,73,74,78–80] Eventually, contracture can develop in the peroneal muscles and in the connective tissue structures on the lateral aspect of the foot and ankle.

On a standing lateral roentgenogram of the foot of a child between the ages of 18 months and 16 years, the average normal angle between the longitudinal bisection of the talus and the transverse plane is 26.5 degrees (s = 5.3).[30] Any increase in that angle indicates that the talus has plantar flexed on the calcaneus.

Instability of the subtalar joint is a common finding in children with neuromuscular disorders.[33,40] In the presence of hypotonia, or developmental delay, the potential for spontaneous correction of the valgus foot is limited by the lack of refinement of antigravity strength and control for weight shifts.[19,33,78,81,82]

Intervention with the stabilizing foot splint. The goal of intervention for flexible pes planus is to alleviate any deforming stresses on the structures within the foot itself, while remaining aware of the interrelationship between the foot and rotational forces from the superstructures (see article by Bernhardt in this issue).[2,6,7] Care in maintaining the normal neutrally aligned architecture of the foot is advised by some researchers throughout the period of bone maturation.[2,7,33]

The history of interventions with various combinations of corrective shoes; high-top orthopedic shoes; wedges at the heel or the heel and sole; and the insertion of arch supports, scaphoid pads, and navicular pads has shown that such interventions are ineffective in correcting flexible pes planus.[11,30,33,79,80]

The foot orthosis uses close conformity between the neutrally-aligned plantar surface of the foot and the inner contour of the device and implements floor-reaction forces with a well-built (usually athletic) outer shoe to stabilize the subtalar and midtarsal joints against collapse.[40,78–80]

In 1965, Bleck and Berzins undertook a 10-year prospective study of the effectiveness of the Helfet heel seat and the UCBL shoe insert.[30] They used these devices to treat "flexible pes valgus" (pes planus), apparently in children with normal muscle tone.[30] The mean age of the 71 children in the study group was 4.7 years. The mean duration of orthotic use was 14.5 months. The overall failure rate, in which no change in talar or talocalcaneal angles was noted radiologically, averaged 20%. The remaining 80% of the subjects showed either improved or corrected talar plantar flexion (within the authors' accepted maximum of 35° for children under 5 years of age). Correction was significantly greater when 1) the devices were used to treat children younger than 3 years, although they were effective up to the age of 8 years, and 2) the devices were implemented for longer durations, comparing treatment periods of 6 months or less with those that spanned a range of 24 to 46 months.[30]

Several other authors reported excellent results with the same or similar foot orthoses.[20,23,40,78–80] Rosenthal advised using the UCBL shoe insert for cerebral palsied children with associated problems of pes valgus, pes varus, and metatarsus adductus.[23]

The stabilizing foot splint (SFS) applies the same design concepts as the UCBL shoe insert, and the basic design is similar, cupping the calcaneus and extending under and alongside the tarsals and metatarsals. The main difference is that the heel is posted to prohibit rolling of the device within the shoe, because children with hypotonia usually demonstrate more severe problems of stabilization than children with normal muscle tone.

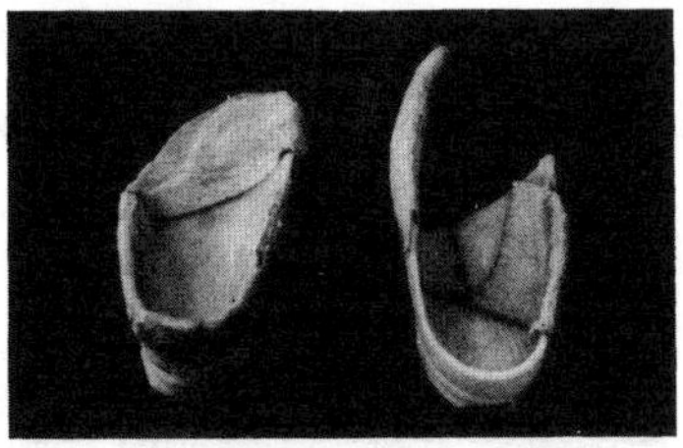

Fig. 9. Stabilizing foot splint. Basic design can be modified to address severity of pes planus: (L) medial forefoot varus post; (R) lateral extension to reduce forefoot abduction.

Trim lines for the SFS can be varied according to the child's need for support. For severe problems of flexible pronation, I frequently use one of the following modifications:

1. An extension of the plantar surface of the splint under the first metatarsal head, using splint material or a closed-cell, high-density padding material. This extension acts as a post to prohibit a varus forefoot from stressing the hindfoot into valgus as the forefoot lowers to the floor (Fig. 9).[6]
2. A padded extension of the lateral forefoot wall to the end of the fifth toe. This extension is useful if forefoot abduction is a significant feature of pronation and if the toe box of the shoe is roomy (Fig. 9).
3. Hylton's Dynamic AFO, or SMO, adds another dimension of control if these modifications fail and can be replicated using splint material.

Clinical evidence of the success of these modifications supports their continued use, but objective measures of their comparative effectiveness are not available, and research is recommended. When the severity of pronation overcomes these modifications of the SFS, I use a modified hinged AFS with no plantar-flexion stop to gain mediolateral stability without prohibiting sagittal plane motion at the ankle.

SUMMARY

Several factors associated with the development of normal foot alignment and function are beyond the scope of this article (see article by Bernhardt in this issue) and should be noted in the management of developmental neuromotor disabilities. They include research findings detecting evidence of anticipatory postural adjustment,[82] the possible influence of the tonic reflexes of the foot,[46,47] and the achievement of antigravity trunk control as a foundation for the development of dynamic stability in the lower extremities.[33,83,84]

With the availability of improved splinting materials, physical therapists' skills are expanding to include functional splinting for the lower extremity. The issues that must be addressed in the comprehensive management of neuromotor disorders in children include the provision of consistent systems of intervention that support the goals of deformity prevention and functional gain. Thoughtful application of the principles of lower extremity biomechanics, interwoven with a knowledge of the impact of motor development on the design and function of the developing foot and leg, can be expected to foster continued improvements in the functional and structural effectiveness of splints and orthoses as an adjunct to a general program of pediatrics therapeutic intervention. Research is needed comparing splints with similar orthotic devices and no orthotic device to determine radiologic evidence of the relative impact on alignment and the influence of splints on various features of gait (eg, stride length, velocity, and energy efficiency). Such findings would facilitate the creative process currently underway in this area of pediatric management.

REFERENCES

1. LeVeau BF, Bernhardt DB: Developmental biomechanics: Effect of forces on the growth, development, and maintenance of the human body. Phys Ther 64:1874–1882, 1984
2. McCrea JD: Pediatric Orthopedics of the Lower Extremity: An Instructional Handbook. Mount Kisco, NY, Futura Publishing Co Inc, 1985
3. Hensinger RN, Jones ET: Developmental orthopaedics: I. The lower limb. Dev Med Child Neurol 24:95–116, 1982
4. McDade W: Bow legs and knock knees. Pediatr Clin North Am 24:825–839, 1977
5. Phelps E, Smith LJ, Hallum A: Normal ranges of hip motion of infants between nine and twenty-four months of age. Dev Med Child Neurol 27:785–792, 1985
6. Root ML, Orien WP, Weed JH: Normal and Abnormal Function of the Foot: Clinical Biomechanics. Los Angeles, CA, Clinical Biomechanics Corp, 1977, vol 2
7. Jordan RP, Cusack J, Resseque B: Foot Function and Its Relationship to Posture in the Pediatric Patient with Cerebral Palsy and Other Neuromotor Disorders. Read at the Neurodevelopmental Treatment Association Symposium, Langer Biomedical Group, New York, NY, May 20–22, 1983
8. Bahler A: The biomechanics of the foot. Clinical Prosthetics and Orthotics 10(1):8–14, 1986
9. Bleck EE: Developmental orthopaedics: III. Toddlers. Dev Med Child Neurol 24:533–555, 1982
10. Engel GM, Staheli LT: The natural history of torsion and other factors influencing gait in childhood. Clin Orthop 99:12–17, 1974
11. Bleck EE: Orthopaedic Management in Cerebral Palsy. Philadelphia, PA, J B Lippincott Co, 1987
12. Banks HH: The foot and ankle in cerebral palsy. In Samilson RL (ed): Orthopaedic Aspects of Cerebral Palsy. Philadelphia, PA, J B Lippincott Co, 1975, pp 203–220
13. Perry J: Cerebral palsy gait. In Samilson RL (ed): Orthopaedic Aspects of Cerebral Palsy. Philadelphia, PA, J B Lippincott Co, 1975, pp 71–91
14. Molnar GE: Cerebral palsy. In Molnar GE (ed): Pediatric Rehabilitation. Baltimore, MD, Williams & Wilkins, 1985, pp 420–467
15. Levitt S: Treatment of Cerebral Palsy and Motor Delay, ed 2. Boston, MA, Blackwell Scientific Publications Ltd, 1982, pp 228–231
16. Bobath B, Bobath K: Motor Development in the Different Types of Cerebral Palsy. London, United Kingdom, Heinemann Medical Books Ltd, 1976
17. Goldner JL: Foot and ankle deformities in cerebral palsy (static encephalopathy). In Jahss MH (ed): Disorders of the Foot. Philadelphia, PA, W B Saunders Co, 1982, vol 1, pp 282–334
18. Fabry G, MacEwen GD, Shands AR: Torsion of the femur: A follow-up study in normal and abnormal conditions. J Bone Joint Surg [Am] 55:1726–1738, 1973
19. Rodgers MM, Cavanagh PR: Glossary of biomechanical terms, concepts, and units. Phys Ther 64:1886–1902, 1984
20. Cailliet R: Foot and Ankle Pain, ed 2. Philadelphia, PA, F A Davis Co, 1983
21. Smith EM, Juvinall RC: Mechanics of orthotics. In Redford JB (ed): Orthotics Etcetera, ed 3. Baltimore, MD, Williams & Wilkins, 1986, pp 21–51
22. Lehmann JF: Lower limb orthotics. In Redford JB (ed): Orthotics Etcetera, ed 3. Baltimore, MD, Williams & Wilkins, 1986, pp 278–351
23. Rosenthal RK: The use of orthotics in foot and ankle problems in cerebral palsy. Foot Ankle 4(4):195–200, 1984
24. Schafer RC: Clinical Biomechanics: Musculoskeletal Actions and Reactions, ed 2. Baltimore, MD, Williams & Wilkins, 1987
25. Deusinger RH: Biomechanics in clinical practice. Phys Ther 64:1860–1868, 1984
26. Cary JM, Lusskin R, Thompson RG: Prescription principles. In American Academy of Orthopaedic Surgeons: Atlas of Orthotics. St. Louis, MO, C V Mosby Co, 1975, pp 235–244
27. Arkin AM, Katz JF: The effects of pressure in epiphyseal growth: The mechanism of plasticity of growing bone. J Bone Joint Surg [Am] 16:1056–1976, 1956
28. Redford JB: Principles of orthotic devices. In Redford JB (ed): Orthotics Etcetera, ed 3. Baltimore, MD, Williams & Wilkins, 1986, pp 1–20
29. Bunch WH, Dvonch VM: Cerebral palsy. In American Academy of Orthopaedic Surgeons: Atlas of Orthotics, ed 2. St. Louis, MO, C V Mosby Co, 1985, pp 259–269
30. Bleck EE, Berzins UJ: Conservative management of pes valgus with plantar flexed talus, flexible. Clin Orthop 122:85–92, 1977
31. McCollough NC: Rationale for orthotic prescription in the lower extremity. Clin Orthop 102:32–45, 1974
32. McCollough NC: Biomechanical analysis systems for orthotic prescription. In American Academy of Orthopaedic Surgeons: Atlas of Orthotics, ed 2. St. Louis, MO, C V Mosby Co, 1985, pp 34–75
33. Salek B: Corrective Footwear in Young Children with Neuromuscular Disorders. Read at Northeastern Regional Conference, Neurode-

velopmental Treatment Association, Philadelphia, PA, November 7–8, 1981
34. Molnar GE: Orthotic management of children. In Redford JB (ed): Orthotics Etcetera, ed 3. Baltimore, MD, Williams & Wilkins, 1986, pp 352–387
35. Helfet AJ: A new way of treating flat feet in children. Lancet i:262, 1956
36. Lehneis HR: The use of modern materials in new design concepts in lower extremity orthotics. In Murdoch G (ed): The Advance in Orthotics. Baltimore, MD, Williams & Wilkins, 1976, pp 157–165
37. Redford JB: Materials for orthotics. In Redford JB (ed): Orthotics Etcetera, ed 3. Baltimore, MD, Williams & Wilkins, 1986, pp 52–79
38. Meyer PR: Lower limb orthotics. Clin Orthop 102:58–71, 1974
39. Henderson WH, Campbell JW: UCBL Shoe Insert: Casting and Fabrication. Technical Report 53. The Biomechanics Laboratory, University of California at San Francisco and Berkeley, August 1967
40. Carlson (misspelled as "Colson") JM, Berglund G: An effective orthotic design for controlling the unstable subtalar joint. Orthotics and Prosthetics 33(1):39–49, 1979
41. Rosenthal RK, Deutsch SD, Miller W, et al: A fixed-ankle, below-knee orthosis for the management of genu recurvatum in spastic cerebral palsy. J Bone Joint Surg [Am] 57:545–547, 1975
42. Saltiel J: A one-piece laminated knee-locking short leg brace. Orthotics and Prosthetics 23(2):68–75, 1969
43. Harrington ED, Lin RS, Gage JR: Use of the anterior floor reaction orthosis in patients with cerebral palsy. Orthotics and Prosthetics 37(4):34–49, 1983–1984
44. Westin GW, Dye S: Conservative management of cerebral palsy in the growing child. Foot Ankle 4(3):160–163, 1983
45. TE Groen JA, Domisse G: Plaster casts in the conservative treatment of cerebral palsy. S Afr Med J 38:502–505, 1964
46. Duncan W: Tonic reflexes of the foot: Their orthopedic significance in normal children and in children with cerebral palsy. J Bone Joint Surg [Am] 42:859–868, 1960
47. Duncan WR, Mott DH: Foot reflexes and the use of the "inhibitive cast." Foot Ankle 4(3):145–148, 1983
48. Hayes NK, Burns YR: Discussion on the use of weight bearing plasters in the reduction of hypertonicity. Australian Journal of Physiotherapy 16(3):108–117, 1970
49. Mohr JD: Neurodevelopmental (Bobath) Treatment Pediatric Certification Course (lecture notes). Massachusetts Chapter, American Physical Therapy Association, Boston, MA, 1974
50. Sussman MD, Cusick BD: Preliminary report: The role of short-leg, tone-reducing casts as an adjunct to physical therapy of patients with cerebral palsy. Johns Hopkins Medical Journal 145:112–114, 1979
51. Cusick BD, Sussman MD: Short leg casts: Their role in the management of cerebral palsy. Physical and Occupational Therapy in Pediatrics 2(2/3):93–110, 1982
52. Embry D: Preliminary report: Inhibitive tone casting used in conjunction with neurodevelopmental treatment. NDTA Newsletter, August 1982
53. Harris SR, Riffle K: Effects of inhibitive ankle-foot orthoses on standing balance in a child with cerebral palsy: A single-subject design. Phys Ther 66:663–667, 1986
54. Zachazewski JE, Eberle ED, Jefferies M: Effect of tone-inhibiting casts and orthoses on gait: A case report. Phys Ther 62:453–455, 1982
55. Jordan RP: Therapeutic considerations of the feet and lower extremities in the cerebral palsied child. Clinics in Podiatry 1:547–561, 1984
56. Ford C, Grotz RC, Shamp JK: The neurophysiological ankle-foot orthosis. Clinical Prosthetics and Orthotics 10(1):15–23, 1986
57. Carlson SJ: A neurophysiological analysis of inhibitive casting. Physical and Occupational Therapy in Pediatrics 4(4):31–42, 1985
58. Mills VM: Electromyographic results of inhibitory splinting. Phys Ther 64:190–193, 1984
59. Watt J, Sims D, Harckham F, et al: A prospective study of inhibitive casting as an adjunct to physiotherapy for cerebral-palsied children. Dev Med Child Neurol 28:480–488, 1986
60. Otis JC, Root L, Kroll MA: Measurement of plantar flexor spasticity during treatment with tone-reducing casts. J Pediatr Orthop 5:682–686, 1985
61. Bertoti DB: Effect of short leg casting on ambulation in children with cerebral palsy. Phys Ther 66:1522–1529, 1986
62. Tardieu G, Tardieu C, Colbeau-Justin P, et al: Muscle hypoextensibility in children with cerebral palsy: II. Therapeutic implications. Arch Phys Med Rehabil 63:103–107, 1982
63. Booth BJ, Doyle M, Montgomery J: Serial casting for the management of spasticity in the head-injured adult. Phys Ther 63:1960–1966, 1983
64. Cusick BD: Serial Casts: Their Use in the Management of Spasticity-induced Foot Deformity. Lexington, KY, Words at Work, 1988
65. Irwin-Carruthers SH, Davids LM, van Rensburg CK, et al: Early physiotherapy in selective posterior rhizotomy. South African Journal of Fisioterapie 41(2):45–49, 1985
66. Pathomechanics of stance: Clinical concepts for analysis. Phys Ther 64:1851–1859, 1984
67. Okamoto T, Kumanoto M: Electromyographic study of the learning process of walking in infants. Electromyography 12:149–158, 1972
68. Sutherland DH: Gait Disorders in Childhood and Adolescence. Baltimore, MD, Williams & Wilkins, 1984
69. Perry J: Kinesiology of lower extremity bracing. Clin Orthop 102:19–31, 1974
70. Tachdjian MO: The Child's Foot. Philadelphia, PA, W B Saunders Co, 1985
71. Brooks S: Joint Mobilization Applied to the Neurologically Involved Child (lecture notes of advanced course sponsored by Curative Rehabilitation Center, Wauwatosa, WI). Dallas, TX, August 12–16, 1985
72. Root ML, Orien WP, Weed JH, et al: Biomechanical Examination of the Foot. Los Angeles, CA, Clinical Biomechanics Corp, 1971, vol 1
73. Carlson JM: Double flexure designs for orthotic ankle joints. Abstract. Orthotics and Prosthetics 39(4):60, 1985–1986
74. Sutherland DH, Cooper L: The pathomechanics of progressive crouch gait in spastic diplegia. Orthop Clin North Am 9:143–154, 1978
75. Sutherland DH, Cooper L, Daniel D: The role of the ankle plantar flexors in normal walking. J Bone Joint Surg [Am] 62:354–363, 1980
76. Soderberg GL: Kinesiology: Application to Pathological Motion. Baltimore, MD, Williams & Wilkins, 1986
77. Lehmkuhl LD, Smith LK: Brunnstrom's Clinical Kinesiology, ed 4. Philadelphia, PA, F A Davis Co, 1983
78. Franco AH: Pes cavus and pes planus: Analyses and treatment. Phys Ther 67:688–694, 1987
79. LeLievre J: Current concepts and correction in the valgus foot. Clin Orthop 70:43–55, 1970
80. Rose GK: Correction of the pronated foot. J Bone Joint Surg [Br] 44:642–647, 1962
81. Gunsolus P, Welsh C, Houser C: Equilibrium reactions in the feet of children with spastic cerebral palsy and of normal children. Dev Med Child Neurol 17:580–591, 1975
82. Nashner LM, Shumway-Cook A, Marin O: Stance posture control in select groups of children with cerebral palsy: Deficits in sensory organization and muscular coordination. Exp Brain Res 49:393–409, 1983
83. Bly L: The Components of Normal Movement During the First Year of Life and Abnormal Motor Development. Birmingham, AL, Pathway Press, 1983
84. Scherzer AL, Tscharnuter I: Early Diagnosis and Therapy in Cerebral Palsy: A Primer on Infant Developmental Problems. New York, NY, Marcel Dekker Inc, 1982

Orthotic Devices for Ambulation in Children with Cerebral Palsy and Myelomeningocele

Children with cerebral palsy and children with myelomeningocele frequently require orthotic devices for standing and walking. The purpose of this article is to review the literature on orthotic devices for walking, present principles of lower-extremity orthoses, discuss designs of orthoses, and consider criteria for selecting orthotic devices. Although discussion of the devices is specific to children with myelomeningocele and to children with cerebral palsy, the orthoses can be used with children having other disabilities. The information presented should be of value to clinicians, educators, and researchers interested in reviewing orthotic applications for children with disabilities. [Knutson LM, Clark DE. Orthotic devices for ambulation in children with cerebral palsy and myelomeningocele. Phys Ther. 1991;71:947–960.]

Key Words: *Cerebral palsy, Children, Meningomyelocele, Orthoses, Orthotic devices, Physical therapy.*

Loretta M Knutson
Dennis E Clark

The prevalence of cerebral palsy (CP) at school entry is 2.0 per 1,000 live births.[1–3] The school-entry prevalence for myelomeningocele (MMC) may be slightly less than the MMC birth incidence of 1.0 per 1,000.[4] Collectively, approximately 3.0 children per 1,000 have one of these disabilities. Projecting from the statistics that 4,021,000 children were born in the United States in 1989,[5] over 12,000 children in a given year can be expected to be affected by one of these neurological disabilities. A majority of these children will have orthotic needs for which the attention of a physical therapist will be required. In a public health survey on payment for services, 54% of the 380 children with mixed diagnoses studied used braces.[6] Because so many children will use orthoses, physical therapists should be knowledgeable about orthotic programming.

The purpose of this article is to review contemporary practice in orthotic management, focusing on devices used for ambulation in children with CP and children with MMC. These two patient populations were chosen for four reasons. First, these children commonly need orthoses to walk. Second, their needs extend through and change during their lifetime. Third, their orthotic and gait training programs frequently fall under the direction of a physical therapist. Fourth, the orthotic management of these children can often be generalized to the care of children with other disabilities. This article is divided into sections organized to review the literature on orthotic devices for walking, present principles of lower-extremity orthoses, discuss orthotic design, and consider criteria for selecting orthotic devices according to patient needs.

Review of Literature

Although numerous references to and discussions of orthotic devices can be found in the literature, there are fewer reports of an investigative nature. Only recently have reports of studies been published on the effects of orthotic devices for children with disabilities. Table 1 summarizes key studies of pediatric orthotic use.

Cerebral Palsy

The use of orthoses in the management of children with CP has varied from the discussion by Little of "mechanical apparatus" in the mid-1800s and advocacy by Phelps and Deaver between 1930 and 1950 to avoidance

LM Knutson, PhD, PT, PCS, is Lecturer, Physical Therapy Graduate Program, and Senior Physical Therapist, Division of Developmental Disabilities, The University of Iowa, 2600 Steindler Bldg, Iowa City, IA 52242 (USA). Address correspondence to Dr Knutson.

DE Clark, BA, CPO, is Prosthetist/Orthotist and Owner of Dale Clark Prosthetics in Waterloo, Coralville, and Dubuque, Iowa. He is also on the Board of Directors of the American Board fo Certification in Orthotics and Prosthetics.

Table 1. *Original Investigative Studies in Pediatric Orthotics*

Orthosis	Investigator(s)	Subject Population			Variables Studied[b]
		Diagnosis[a]	N	Age (y)	
Foot orthoses	Wenger et al,[54] 1989	Flatfeet	129	1–6	Radiographs
	Penneau et al,[55] 1982	Pes planus	10	1.5–4.5	Radiographs
	Bordelon,[56] 1983	Flatfeet	50	3–9	Radiographs
	Bleck and Berzins,[57] 1977	Pes planus	71	1–12	Radiographs
	Mereday et al,[58] 1972	Pes planus	10	3.5–12.5	Radiographs
Supramalleolar orthoses	Embrey et al,[24] 1990	CP	1	2.7	Knee kinematics
Inhibitive casts and splints	Hinderer et al,[22] 1988	CP	1	. . .	Stride characteristics
	Bertoti,[25] 1986	CP	16	0.8–9	Stride characteristics
	Watt et al,[26] 1986	CP	28	1.5–5	Tone, motor skills, PROM, observational kinematics
	Mills,[27] 1984	HI (7), aneurysm (1)	8	10–22	EMG
Ankle-foot orthoses	Lough,[28] 1990	CP	15	3–12	EMG, walking velocity, foot radiographs, kinematics
	Mossberg et al,[10] 1990	CP	18	3–14	HR, walking velocity
	Thomas et al,[42] 1989	MMC	. . .	. . .	EMG, kinematics
	Brodke et al,[11] 1989	Nondisabled child	5	6–12	EMG, kinematics, kinetics, walking velocity
	Middleton et al,[21] 1988	CP	1	4.5	Kinematics, kinetics, walking velocity
	Harris and Riffle,[23] 1986	CP	1	4.5	Standing balance time
Knee-ankle-foot orthoses	Krebs et al,[43] 1988	MMC (12), upper motoneuron pathology (2), myopathy (1)	15	5–21	Gait kinematics, ADL, child and parent opinion
Reciprocating gait orthosis	Mazur et al,[37] 1989	MMC	3	. . .	Walking velocity, stride characteristics, EMG, kinematics
	Flandry et al,[41] 1986	MMC	8	4–19	HR, EE, walking velocity
	McCall and Schmidt,[49] 1986	MMC	37	1.3–1.6	Pulse rate, walking velocity
	Yngve et al,[48] 1984	MMC	3	3–16	Walking velocity
Hip guidance orthosis	Rose et al,[46] 1981	MMC	27	5.7–12.6	HR, walking velocity, ambulation status
Swivel walker	Stallard et al,[45] 1978	MMC	1	. . .	HR, walking velocity
	Davies,[44] 1977	MMC	. . .	. . .	HR
Parapodium	Lough and Nielsen,[47] 1986	MMC (9), SCI (1)	10	4–8	EE, HR, walking velocity

[a] CP=cerebral palsy, HI=head injury, MMC=myelomeningocele, SCI=spinal cord injury.

[b] PROM=passive range of motion, EMG=electromyographic activity, HR=heart rate, ADL=activities of daily living, EE=energy expenditure.

of orthotic devices, particularly full-control orthoses, during the peak of the neurodevelopmental treatment (NDT) era.[7,8] Today, a new enthusiasm for the use of orthoses has surfaced, specifically for below-knee devices used by children who are ambulatory.[9]

A 1985 report on a group of English children with CP born between 1970 and 1974 states that 50% to 75% of the children were ambulatory.[2] Because a majority of children with CP will use orthoses to assist walking, research that complements orthotic selection or adds to an understanding of orthoses is helpful. In one such recent study, Mossberg and colleagues[10] evaluated walking velocity and heart rate in 18 children with spastic diplegia walking with and without plastic ankle-foot orthoses (AFOs). Use of orthoses increased walking velocity and reduced the heart rate compared with walking without AFOs; however, the differences were not statistically significant.

Fifteen years ago, steel or aluminum braces with adjustable ankle joints were common. Although today metal braces are rarely used for children with CP, the purported advantages of polypropylene orthotic designs have not been well studied. Brodke and co-workers[11] evaluated five nondisabled children walking barefoot and using both traditional metal AFOs and fixed polypropylene AFOs. Walking speed and cadence were observed to decrease with either AFO compared with the barefoot condition; however, the decrease was more pronounced with the metal AFOs. The duration of quadriceps femoris muscle electromyographic (EMG) activity was greater with molded plastic AFOs than with metal AFOs and was greater for both braces than for barefoot walking. Changes in lower-extremity (ie, hip and knee), motion were not significantly different, but maximum knee extension during stance tended to be greater with polypropylene AFOs than with metal AFOs or barefoot walking. Both types of orthoses effectively limited ankle motion. The researchers concluded that metal AFOs impaired normal gait more than did polypropylene AFOs.

Polypropylene orthoses were first introduced in the 1960s.[12] Their use in children with CP did not become established until the mid- to late-1970s when clinical experience and satisfaction gradually dispelled views that plastic orthoses would increase spasticity (excessive contraction of the muscle and stiffness that prevents or opposes normal muscle lengthening) or would not be sufficiently strong to support the spastic (affected by spasticity) limb. The first designs of polypropylene orthoses, as described by Hoffer et al[13] in 1974, were strictly of the fixed design.

By the early 1980s, fixed polypropylene AFOs were being molded with features designed to hold the subtalar joint in neutral and inhibit spasticity.[14] The "subtalar-neutral" AFO was intended to oppose foot valgus or pronation during weight bearing, a problem that occurs frequently in children with spastic diplegia or quadriplegia.[15,16] The concept of subtalar-neutral alignment and "tone reduction," or reduction of the state of muscle contraction, was first introduced in inhibitive casts[17,18] and was later applied to orthoses.[14,19] Descriptive reports have been supplemented by case reports[20,21] and single-subject design research.[22–24] Hinderer and co-workers[22] found tone-reducing casts yielded a longer stride length than standard casts in two children under 6 years of age with CP.[22] Harris and Riffle[23] found inhibitive AFOs (right supramalleolar orthosis and left AFO) increased standing balance time in a 4½-year-old child with quadriplegia. Embrey and colleagues[24] demonstrated knee flexion could be reduced during gait in a 2½-year-old child who had hypotonia by the use of NDT and "ankle-height orthoses."

Early contoured AFO designs did not allow ankle motion. Recently, however, hinged polypropylene AFOs have been introduced and have received positive responses by physical therapy clinicians. Middleton and colleagues[21] reported the first comparison of fixed AFOs with hinged AFOs by studying a 4½-year-old child with spastic diplegia. The child's pattern of ankle dorsiflexion was more normal and the knee muscle moments were lower during the stance phase of gait with the hinged AFOs than with the fixed AFOs. The investigators concluded that hinged AFOs appear to be more effective than fixed AFOs for treating children who have spastic CP.

Without replication, the results of the case reports and single-subject studies cannot be generalized to other children. Some investigators, however, have studied groups of patients using inhibitive short leg casts,[25,26] splints,[27] and AFOs.[28] In studying two groups of children before and after 10 weeks of NDT, Bertoti[25] found the group of eight children wearing short leg casts had a 27% increase in stride compared with a 13% decrease in stride for the group of eight children who were uncasted. Watt and colleagues[26] examined the long-term effects of a 3-week treatment course involving inhibitive casting and NDT. Whereas improvements in passive ankle dorsiflexion and foot-floor contact when walking were seen 2 weeks after treatment, these changes were less evident after 5 months. Specifically, right ankle dorsiflexion showed an increase of 8.8 degrees 2 weeks after cast removal but only 3.6 degrees after 5 months. Right foot-floor contact was seen in 64% of the patients 2 weeks after casting and in 39% of the patients 5 months after casting. Mills[27] studied the EMG and range-of-motion (ROM) effects of inhibitive splints on eight adolescent and young adult subjects who had neurological insults. Compared with the presplint condition, no effects on integrated EMG activity during splint use were noted, but the ROM into extension increased. In a study by Lough,[28] the effects of no orthoses, fixed AFOs, and hinged AFOs were contrasted in 15 children with CP. Mean walking velocity increased by 5.6 cm/s, and ankle dorsiflexion increased during mid-stance of gait by 4.9 degrees for hinged orthoses compared with no orthoses. The EMG amplitudes were examined at 5% intervals across an ensemble average created for each of four muscles. Of 80 possible intervals of significant difference, only 3 were different—2 for the vastus lateralis muscle and 1 for the tibialis anterior muscle. No differences were found among the treatments for the medial hamstring or gastrocnemius muscles. The reduction in foot pronation, as determined from standing dorsoplantar radiographic measurements of the talonavicular angle, was significant for fixed AFOs (4.5° less) and approached significance for hinged AFOs (3.6° less) compared with no orthoses.

Myelomeningocele

The prognosis for ambulation by children with MMC is related to level of motor function. The effect of the spinal cord dysfunction level on energy expenditure was well documented in adults with paraplegia by Clinkingbeard and associates[29] and is in accord with reports of function for children with MMC.[30–38] Children with higher levels of spinal defect (eg, at and above L-2) require more extensive orthotic support and can be expected to expend more energy than children with defects below L-2. Table 2 summarizes reports on the status of and prognosis for ambulation in children with MMC. Consensus generally exists that the higher the level of defect, the smaller will be the percentage of the group who are ambulatory. Other factors influencing ambulation include mental retardation, muscle power within the level of defect, orthopedic deformities, hydrocephalus, and walking status at age 7 years.[30–39]

Whether children with high lumbar- and thoracic-level defects are provided early instruction for walking appears to be influenced by practice patterns of the geographic area. Although reports agree the majority of children with thoracic MMC who walk will later become nonambulatory, the study by Mazur and colleagues[37] supports the value of bracing and walking. Subjects who walked as children had fewer fractures and pressure sores, were more independent, and were better able to transfer than were patients who used a wheelchair from early in life. Sankarankutty et al[41] stressed the importance of effective bracing and suggested that modern orthoses can prolong ambulation in patients who otherwise may discard their devices. This notion was reinforced by Flandry et al[41] in their study, which demonstrated that the energy cost values for walking with the reciprocating gait orthosis (RGO) approximated those for wheelchair use.

Limited research has addressed the effects of orthotic designs on ambulation in children with MMC. In most practices, clinical experiences of the prescriber serve as guideposts in orthotic selection. A recent quantitative study by Thomas et al[42] revealed that children with MMC who wore AFOs showed reduced hip, knee, and ankle flexion; decreased muscle activation time; and decreased muscle coactivation during gait. Krebs and colleagues[43] found specific differences for children with MMC using metal versus polypropylene knee-ankle-foot orthoses (KAFOs); children preferred the polypropylene KAFOs and appeared to have better control of hip, knee, and ankle motion.

Studies in the 1970s and early 1980s at the Orthotic Research and Locomotor Assessment Unit (ORLAU) in Oswestry, England, measured velocity, heart rate, and ambulatory status with different orthoses used primarily for children with high-level spinal defects.[44–46] Descriptive results suggested improvements in all variables when children switched from previous bracing (ie, conventional hip-knee-ankle-foot orthosis [HKAFO] or swivel walker) to a hip guidance orthosis. In 1986, Lough and Nielsen[47] reported that children with MMC walked faster, but had higher energy expenditure and were less efficient, with their use of parapodiums than with their use of parapodiums adapted with a swivel-walker base.

Comparing the RGO used with different hip joint and cable configurations (normal reciprocal action, locked, or free motion), Yngve and colleagues[48] and McCall and Schmidt[49] favored the normal reciprocal mode based on patients achieving a faster walking velocity. Patients in both studies also reported preferring the reciprocal to the swing-through pattern of gait.

Principles of Lower-Extremity Orthoses

Several textbooks are available that provide a more comprehensive coverage of orthoses; each of these textbooks presents a list of principles, purposes, and goals of bracing.[50–53] Following are guiding principles that should be applied with the pediatric client.

1. *Prevent deformity.* Orthoses may be prescribed to prevent a deformity that is anticipated to occur or that might increase without treatment. Orthoses can also be used following surgery or serial casting to maintain correction of a deformity. Occasionally, orthoses are used to correct a deformity.

2. *Support normal joint alignment and mechanics.* Molded orthoses often have a greater chance of achieving this goal than do conventional metal devices because they provide total contact. Options in molded AFOs (solid, variable range, or free motion) can all support joint alignment. Even foot orthoses (FOs) can facilitate this goal as long as alignment includes the ankle joint, the subtalar joint, and other midfoot and forefoot structures. This principle is inherent in what some clinicians refer to as "tone reduction." Good alignment may be more important than the addition of extra pressure at selected sites in reducing tone.

3. *Provide variable range of motion when appropriate.* For ambulatory patients, restriction of some ROM is often necessary to assist weak muscles, oppose spastic muscles, enhance balance, protect certain soft tissues postsurgically, or improve the appearance of gait for the patient who lacks selective control to achieve a normal pattern. At the ankle, this may require restricting plantar flexion while allowing free dorsiflexion or allowing plan-

Table 2. *Studies Addressing the Status and/or Prognosis for Ambulation in Children with Myelomeningocele*

Investigator(s)	No. of Subjects[a]	Mobility Status	Factors Influencing Prognosis
Taylor and McNamara,[38] 1990	32—thoracic 32—lumbar 16—lumbosacral 1—sacral 6—unknown	58 wheelchair users; 23 community ambulators; 6 household ambulators	Level of neurological deficit and type of orthoses used
Mazur et al,[37,b] 1989	22—T10-12 14—L1-2	17 (47%) no longer walked; 12 (33%) were community ambulators; 7 (20%) were household ambulators	Those who had discontinued walking specified reasons including energy expenditure and ease
Samuelsson and Skoog,[39] 1988	163—total	0% of thoracic and L1-2, 54% of L-3, 67% of L-4, 80% of L-5, and 100% of sacral patients ambulate	Level of defect and associated neurological findings influence walking
Findley et al,[36] 1987	14—thoracic 4—L1-2 16—L3-4 19—L5-S1 24—sacral	20 not walking; 56 community ambulators, 26 of 56 occasionally used a wheelchair; 1 therapeutic ambulator	Walking outdoors independently and using a wheelchair by age 7 y was more predictive of adolescent ambulation than was neurologic level
Schopler and Menelaus,[35] 1987	109—total (sites of lesion not specified)	88% with grade 0–2 quadriceps femoris muscle strength exclusively used wheelchairs; 82% with grade 4–5 muscle strength were community ambulators; 89% with grade 3–5 muscle strength were at least household ambulators	Strong quadriceps femoris muscles predict good ambulation
Sankarankutty et al,[40] 1979	102—total 52—thoracic	5.7% were wheelchair users; 3 subjects over 15 y old (1 wheelchair user, 1 household ambulator, 1 therapeutic ambulator)	Level of defect important, but thoracic lesions do not prevent independence; improved orthotic design is needed
DeSouza and Carroll,[33] 1976	4—thoracic 19—upper lumbar 13—lower lumbar 32—sacral	1 of 4 with thoracic defects was a wheelchair user, 1 was a household ambulator, and 1 was a therapeutic ambulator	Level of defect, motor power, and orthopedic deformity influenced progress
Barden et al,[34] 1975	9—thoracolumbar 20—lumbar	2 of 9 with T12-L2 defects and 19 of 20 with L-3 defects still walked	Final hip position did not correlate with walking status
Hoffer et al,[13] 1974	10—thoracic 40—lumbar 6—sacral	52% were wheelchair users; all 10 with thoracic defects were nonambulators; all 6 with sacral defects were community ambulators	Factors other than level of spinal defect were age; presence of hydrocephalus, spasticity, and skeletal deformities; intelligence; and societal factors
Lorber,[31] 1971	134—total (sites of defects not specified)	1/3 limited to wheelchair use; 1/3 used calipers at least part time; 1/3 walked independently	. . .
Richings and Eckstein,[30,c] 1970	4—encephalocele 8—cervical 15—thoracic 5—thoracolumbar 51—lumbar 27—lumbosacral 15—sacral	7 (6%) used wheelchairs; 105 (94%) had some degree of mobility; 16 of 23 with complete paralysis of lower extremities achieved some mobility with braces	Improved orthotic design is needed

[a]When indicated, the total number of subjects was reduced according to the number of subjects for whom locomotor behavior was reported.

[b]Comparison study of early walking group (n=36) to matched early use of wheelchair group (n=36).

[c]Number at each level of defect was estimated from a figure.

tar flexion while restricting dorsiflexion. The plantar-flexion stop, for example, might be used for a child with CP who has an equinus deformity, whereas the dorsiflexion stop might be used to eliminate a crouched gait by stopping anterior motion of the tibia in the presence of an overlengthened heelcord. The dorsiflexion stop could also be used for the child with an MMC at L-5 who heel walks or has excessive ankle dorsiflexion. Various combinations of motion and restriction are possible.

4. *Facilitate function.* The orthotic device should not restrict the child, but should encourage function. The physical therapist is particularly important for assessing the fit and function of an orthosis. Changes in the orthosis may be needed as the patient's ability or muscle function changes, thus ensuring the device facilitates and does not restrain the patient's progress.

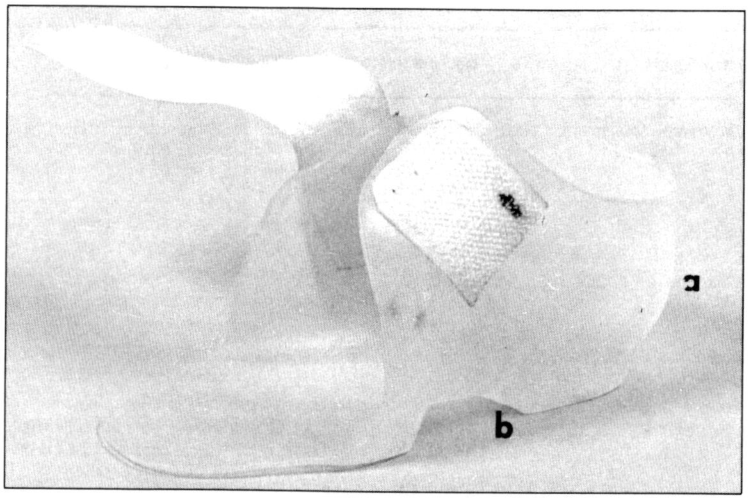

Figure 1. *Foot orthosis designed to oppose pronation by molding the heel cup to grasp the calcaneus firmly (a) and wedging, or posting, the heel medially (b).*

Orthotic Design

Foot Orthoses

With FOs (Fig. 1), attention must be given to achieving a close-contact fit that does not impinge on the medial or lateral malleoli. The distal trimline should extend just proximal to the metatarsal heads. The high medial and lateral walls should extend to the dorsum of the foot. Studies on FOs are reported in Table 1.[54–58]

Supramalleolar Orthoses

Supramalleolar orthoses (SMOs) (Fig. 2) have proximal trimlines that extend 30 to 50 mm above the malleoli. Although the malleoli are covered by the orthotic walls, the orthoses are trimmed anteriorly and posteriorly to allow plantar flexion and dorsiflexion.

Ankle-Foot Orthoses

Ankle-foot orthoses (Fig. 3) should be designed to extend 10 to 15 mm distal to the head of the fibula on the pediatric patient. All below-knee supports, whether AFOs (fixed or hinged AFOs), SMOs, or FOs, should incorporate supportive features to align the foot in a subtalar-neutral position. An anterior floor-reaction AFO is a variation on the design of an AFO used for children with excessive flexible knee flexion posture. This design has particularly been recommended for children with L-4 myelomeningocele and for children with CP who stand with knee flexion attributable to overlengthened heelcords. The polypropylene mold includes an anterior rather than a posterior shell only. An illustration of the floor-reaction AFO is shown in the article by Rose and colleagues in this issue. If the FO is cut low or supports only beneath the foot, it will not contain all key components of ankle and foot support.

Five Key Components of Ankle and Foot Support

Control of the subtalar joint. The AFO, SMO, and some FOs should grasp the calcaneus firmly (Fig. 1) to prevent medial and lateral motion with subsequent collapse of the heel into valgus and the subtalar joint into pronation. A medial heel post with slight wedging of the plantar surface will also oppose pronation and encourage normal alignment (Fig. 1).

Control of the midtarsal joint. The AFO, SMO, and FO must resist forefoot abduction or adduction. This can be accomplished by ensuring well-molded medial and lateral walls and borders of the orthosis (Fig. 2). At times, the medial or lateral trimlines may extend distal to the metatarsal heads (eg, in a child with MMC following treatment of clubfoot deformity). In this case, consideration should be given to the effect this extension will have on restricting toe extension late in the stance phase.

High (flexible) medial and lateral walls. If the walls of the AFO, SMO, or FO wrap over the dorsum of the foot, the force exerted by the walls will help restrain the heel for maximum control (Fig. 2). Additional benefits of the high walls are (1) control of forefoot abduction or adduction, (2) distribution of pressures over the foot for reducing unwanted stimulation, and, (3) assurance of constant contact with the orthosis during the entire gait cycle. A potential disadvantage is the lack of ease with which the child can don the orthosis. Some parents have reported their children have difficulty keeping the orthosis walls spread while sliding the foot into the device.

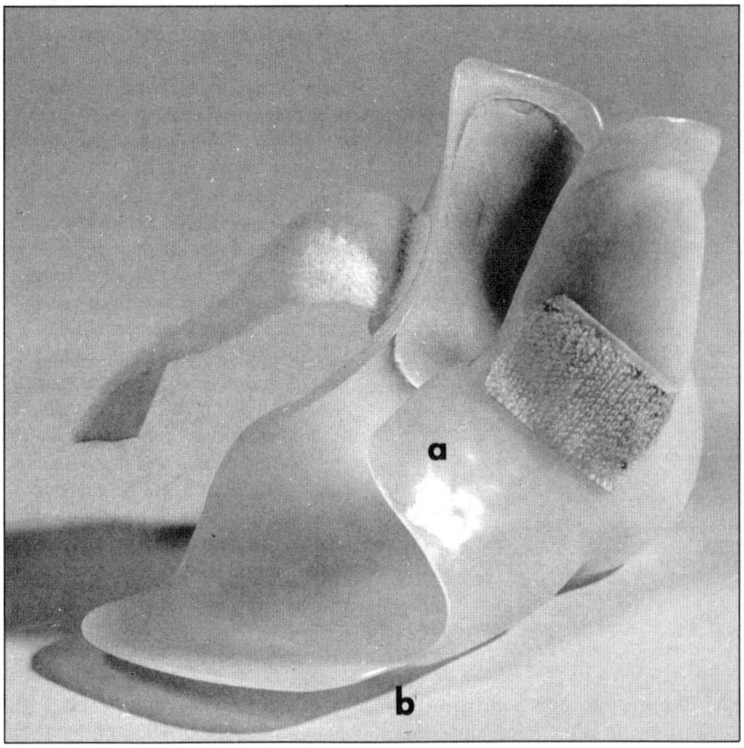

Figure 2. *Supramalleolar orthosis extending proximally to the malleoli. Well-molded medial and lateral walls that wrap over the dorsum of the foot (a) help control the midtarsal joint and keep the heel seated. Dorsal flaps also disperse pressure and may reduce sensitivity of the foot. Intrinsic toe elevation (b) can prevent stimulating the plantar grasp reflex.*

Toe elevation. Toe elevations may be intrinsic (ie, built into the plastic) (Fig. 2) or extrinsic (ie, removable and repositionable) (Fig. 3). Intrinsic toe elevations may shorten the life of the orthosis because the child's growth cannot be readily accommodated. By contrast, extrinsic elevations can be repositioned as the child grows. Additionally, the height of the elevations can be more easily increased or decreased.

Transmetatarsal arch. As with toe elevations, the transmetatarsal arch can be intrinsic or extrinsic. Caution must be taken to ensure appropriate placement of this feature so the child does not feel inappropriately positioned pressure. This feature has particularly been used with toe elevation for tone reduction.

Variable-Motion Ankle Joints

Until the past 5 years, the solid, molded, fixed orthosis was standard. Recently, however, hinged ankle joints have been introduced, in part, to encourage a more normal gait pattern. Hinged or variable-motion ankle joints can be used in KAFOs and AFOs. The following variable-motion ankle joints represent commonly used designs at the present time.

Overlap articulation. This joint is constructed from polypropylene or copolymer (Fig. 4). The overlap articulation design is the most widely used hinged ankle joint. When used alone, the joint allows free dorsiflexion or plantar flexion. When used in combination with other features of the brace, several possibilities for controlling motion emerge. Typically, the orthosis will be molded with a plantar-flexion stop at neutral. Modifications to the polypropylene, however, can place the stop in dorsiflexion or in plantar flexion. A plantar-flexion stop set in dorsiflexion is commonly used to restrict knee hyperextension. If the goal is to stop dorsiflexion, a posterior strap can be added. A further adaptation involves the addition of screws to restrict motion. A screw placed horizontally through the posterior overlap can stop all motion until the therapist is ready to allow dorsiflexion. A posteriorly placed vertical screw will allow variable ROM. Turning the screw adjusts the plantar flexion.

Gillette joint. The Gillette joint* is made of rubber vacuformed into polypropylene (Fig. 5). This hinge is normally used to provide a

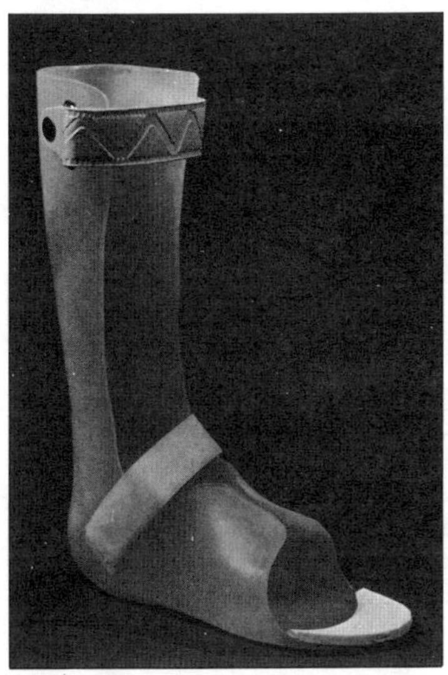

Figure 3. *Fixed molded ankle-foot orthosis with an ankle strap to restrain the heel. Extrinsic toe elevation to unload the metatarsal heads is optional.*

*Becker Orthopedic Appliance, 635 Executive Dr, Troy, MI 48083-4576.

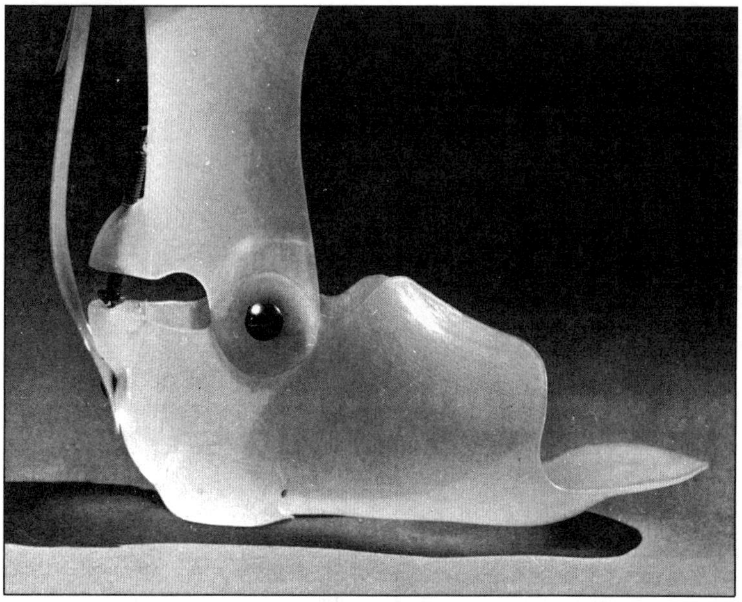

Figure 4. *Overlap articulation joint used in a hinged, variable-motion ankle-foot orthosis showing the posterior strap and the vertical screw.*

plantar-flexion stop and free dorsiflexion. By grinding the plastic posteriorly, some increased plantar-flexion ROM is possible.

Gaffney joint. This joint[†] is made of stainless steel vacuformed into the polypropylene (Fig. 6). Seven sizes of hinges are available. This design of hinged ankle joint is normally used to provide a plantar-flexion stop and unrestricted dorsiflexion.

Select joint. These joints[‡] are made of color-coded aluminum disks vacuformed into plastic (Fig. 7). Two sizes of disks are available. Within each size, five variations in disks allow the therapist to insert different disks and change selectively the ROM allowed at the ankle. Because each color-coded disk has its ROM stamped on it, the changes are easy to document. One drawback is the joint's lack of durability. Both the inserts and the plastic forms housing them are subject to wear. The anterior stops seem particularly susceptible to the forces imposed on them during active, forceful walking and may yield to increased ROM. A second drawback is that the metal hinges must be mechanically aligned and thus are not anatomically aligned. Generally, anatomic alignment is used for joint placement, because cosmesis and function are assumed to be better when the brace's joint overlies the true (ie, human or anatomic) joint. A third disadvantage is the bulk of the brace. The bulk of the brace makes it difficult to place a shoe over the hinge and reduces the cosmesis of the device. Some difficulty may also be encountered by the child clicking his or her ankles together.

Oklahoma ankle joint. This joint* is made from polypropylene vacuformed in plastic (Fig. 8). Five sizes, pediatric to adult, are scheduled to be available commercially in 1991. This hinge joint allows all the flexibility of the plastic overlap joint.

Knee-Ankle-Foot Orthoses

The proximal medial aspect of the thigh portion of a KAFO (Fig. 9) should extend to within 45 mm of the perineum on the medial side and to within 75 mm of the greater trochanter on the lateral side. Various knee joints can be used, and the reader is referred to other references for coverage of the options available.[50–53] The knee joint must be aligned in all three planes—sagittal, coronal, and transverse. In the sagittal plane, the joint should be one half the distance between the posterior aspect of the patella and the posterior aspect of the leg. From the coronal plane, the joint should be at the midpoint of the patella. In the transverse plane, the joints must be aligned with the line of gait progression.

Hip-Knee-Ankle-Foot Orthosis

Conventional metal HKAFOs are rarely used today by children with CP or children with MMC. If these devices are prescribed, however, their fit must be examined in the sitting and standing positions. If the patient is being fitted bilaterally, the critical fitting is done in a sitting position. Ideally, the hip joint should be positioned 10 mm superior to the greater trochanter.

Special designs of HKAFOs (parapodium, swivel walker, and RGO) are described in the next section. Only the Rochester HKAFO, which is not used for walking, is mentioned here. This orthosis is mainly used by the very young child with MMC as a nighttime sleeping brace. The orthosis can also be helpful to encourage early weight bearing in the child under 15 months of age who has a high lumbar- or thoracic-level MMC. Parents are instructed to support and supervise their child in standing with this device. A belt across the chest, and thigh and calf straps, help restrain body position for standing.

[†]Gaffney Technology, 2575 NE Kathryn St, #26, Hillsboro, OR 97124.

[‡]United States Manufacturing Co, 180 N San Gabriel Blvd, Pasadena, CA 91107-3488.

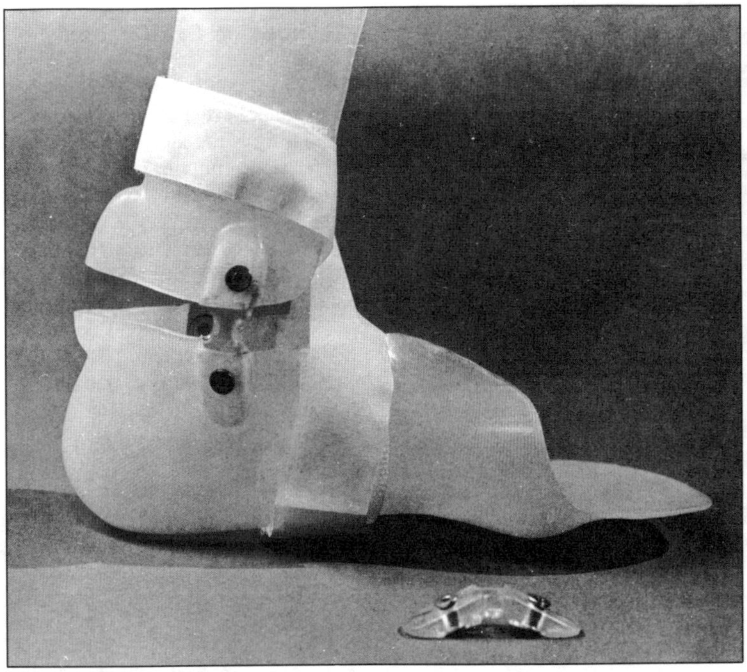

Figure 5. *Ankle-foot orthosis (AFO) with Gillette joint vacuformed in polypropylene. Joint shown in foreground is freestanding. Self-adhesive fastener adhered to the AFO is configured for a figure-eight ankle strap.*

Parapodium

The Toronto parapodium (Fig. 10) has one lock for both hip and knee joints, whereas the Rochester parapodium has separate hip and knee joint locks.[59,60] With the child standing, the parapodium should fit such that the center of the chest pad is at the xiphoid, the knee pad is across the patellae, and the metal portion of the trunk support clears the axillae by one to two fingers. If the metal expends too proximally, the brace may restrict arm use. If too low, the child may outgrow the appliance quickly. From the side, alignment of the trunk, hips, knees, and ankle joints should be checked. Cutouts on the knee pad should neither be so minimal they cause knee hyperextension nor so extreme they allow excessive knee flexion. The foot mold should align the malleoli slightly posterior to the knee. The final step of a parapodium fit check involves determining whether the child's pelvis rotates excessively to one side of the pelvic support when the child moves. This check can be performed after the child has been rolling, pushing to a standing position, or walking in the brace. If excessive rotation occurs, increasing the anterior-posterior depth and the tightness of the pelvic support across the greater trochanters may help prevent the shifting.

Swivel Walker

The first swivel walker (Fig. 11) was designed at ORLAU in the 1970s as a modification of an earlier prosthetic device used for children affected by the thalidomide crisis in the 1960s.[61] The fit considerations of the swivel walker parallel those of the parapodium, except for the unique point of spacing for the swivel-walker footplates. Based on a case report, recommendation has been made for the spacing to be one-fifth of body height.[62] The crutchless mode of walking is characteristic of this brace. A modification merging the parapodium with the base and footplate assembly of the swivel walker was used

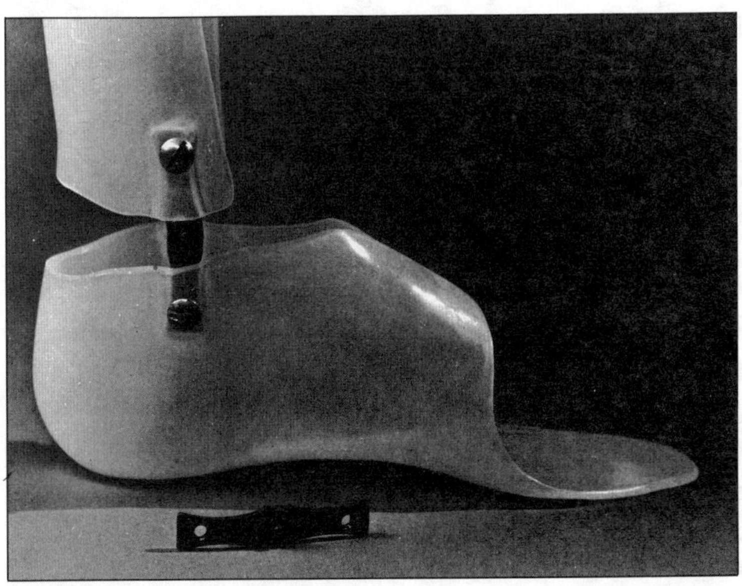

Figure 6. *Lateral view of the ankle region of a hinged ankle-foot orthosis displaying the Gaffney joint. The joint is shown freestanding in the foreground.*

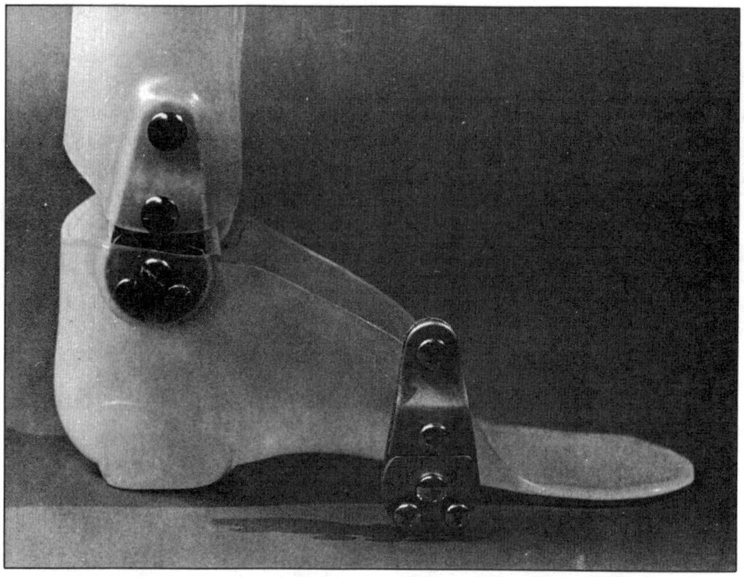

Figure 7. *Medial view of the lower portion of an ankle-foot orthosis with a Select joint inserted at the ankle. Another disk is freestanding in the foreground. Numbers impressed into the metal designate the degrees of motion possible; for example, the disk shown prevents motion.*

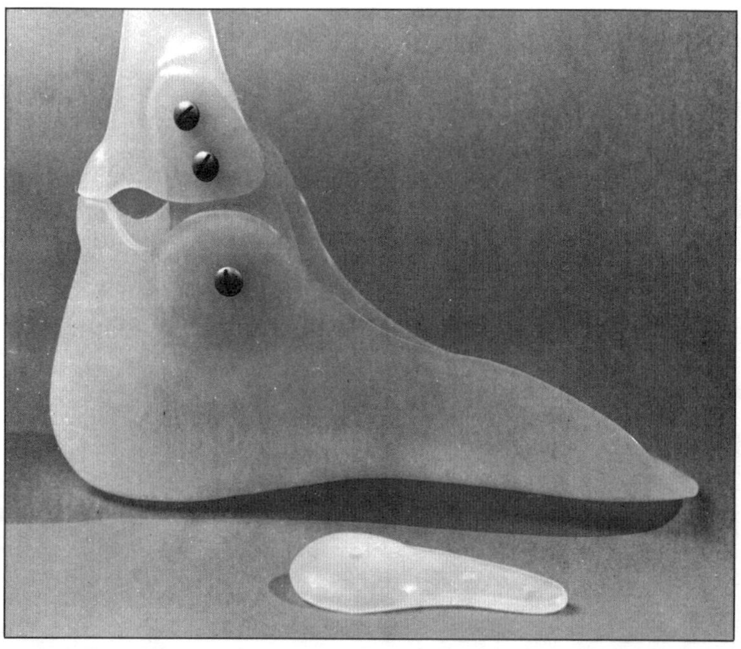

Figure 8. *Medial view of the lower portion of a hinged ankle-foot orthosis designed with an Oklahoma joint. The joint is shown freestanding in the foreground.*

by Lough and Nielsen[47] to contrast swing-to walking with swivel walking.

Reciprocating Gait Orthosis

The RGO (Fig. 12) has extensions that extend superiorly above the hip joints to the level of the xiphoid with a circumferential strap that extends around the torso at the level of the xiphoid. A wide pad is also placed at the level of the hip joints to hold the pelvis into the control of the butterfly-shaped pelvic band and thus maximize the reciprocal action created by the cable system. The cable system couples flexion of one hip with extension of the opposite hip. Release of the cables on both sides allows bilateral hip flexion for sitting. A modification to the RGO that includes muscle electrical stimulation and a new hip joint release mechanism has been designed, but evaluation has only been reported in adults with paraplegia.[63]

Selection of Orthotic Devices

Although generalizations can be made regarding the best orthosis to use according to the child's age, disability type, and degree of motor impairment, unique features about the child and his or her family and community should be considered. The following information provides general guidelines only and assumes good clinical judgment will be used when making orthotic choices for specific patients.

Cerebral Palsy

Children with hemiplegia, diplegia, or mild to moderate spastic quadriplegia can all benefit from the orthotic devices discussed in this article. Although children with severe quadriplegia are not likely to ambulate, a number of the orthoses mentioned may be appropriate for preventing deformity and assisting postural support in sitting.

In the United States today, neither HKAFOs nor KAFOs are commonly prescribed for children with CP. As mentioned earlier, this may have stemmed from a shift in the 1950s and 1960s to an NDT philosophy and a departure from the previous orthopedic approach described by Deaver and Phelps in which extensive bracing was common.[7,8] Because new orthotic materials have been introduced, reconsideration of the present philosophy may be warranted.

The use of AFOs has remained a standard treatment because of their usefulness in preventing equinus contractures. Some clinicians have recommended a progression from casts before the child walks to AFOs once walking begins. Although debate continues over the relative advantages of hinged versus fixed AFOs, studies by Middleton et al[21] and Lough[28] have favored hinged AFOs. Because specific guidelines for selecting the style of hinged ankle joint do not exist, the choice should be made jointly by members of the treatment team consisting of physician, physical therapist, and orthotist.

Issues related to orthotic prescription for children with hypotonia or athetoid (dyskinetic) CP have not been well addressed in the literature. Many clinicians believe children with hypotonia are more stable with molded FOs, SMOs, or AFOs. By contrast, children with dyskinesia frequently have difficulty with molded orthoses because of friction irritation created by writhing movement. Partial or full lining of the orthosis may reduce the irritation.

The selection of an AFO for a child with CP will change depending on age, nature of the disability, associated findings, and surgical history. The following recommendations are based on reports in the literature, as well as personal clinical and research experience.

1. The preambulatory child under 30 months of age who appears to be at risk for plantar-flexion contracture should begin with a fixed AFO or an "inhibitive cast." Hinged AFOs are more complex and should be postponed until the second fitting. Ankle straps or high medial-lateral walls will help secure the heel.

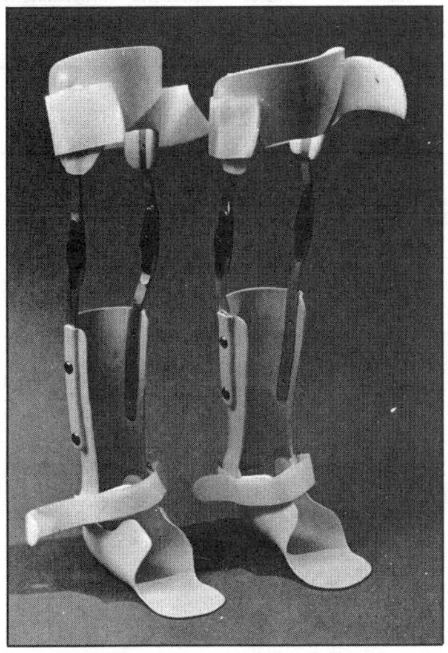

Figure 9. *Oblique view of knee-ankle-foot orthoses with an anterior thigh cuff.*

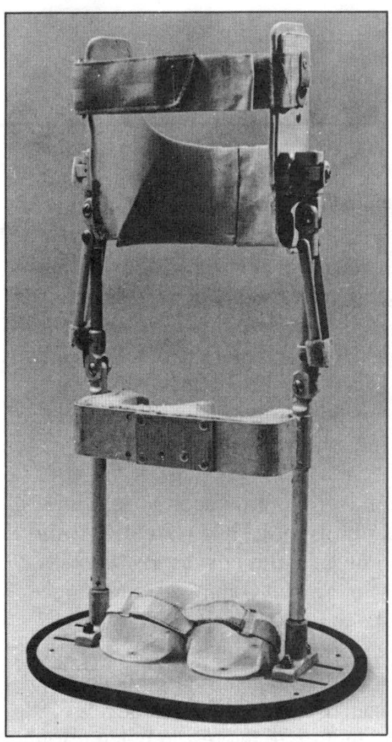

Figure 10. *Front view of the Toronto parapodium.*

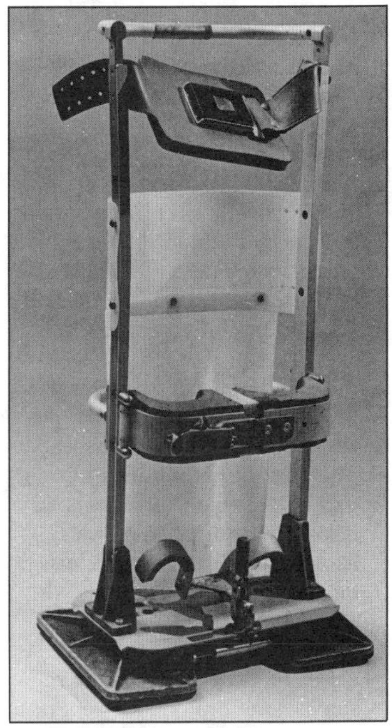

Figure 11. *Front view of the Orthotic Research and Locomotor Assessment Unit (ORLAU) swivel walker.*

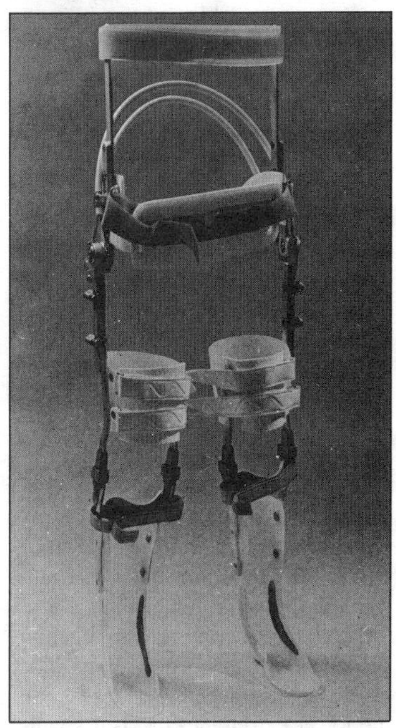

Figure 12. *Front view of a reciprocating gait orthosis (RGO).*

2. The child who walks in equinus will likely require restriction of plantar flexion to neutral. This can be accomplished with a hinged AFO or a fixed AFO. The hinged AFO will facilitate a more normal gait pattern.

3. When genu recurvatum is present, an AFO that blocks plantar flexion at 5 degrees of dorsiflexion should create a knee flexion moment at the onset of stance phase that will counter the hyperextension.

4. If the child with CP responds well to a hinged AFO that restricts plantar flexion, gradual reintroduction of a small range of plantar flexion may be possible. When this is anticipated, the Select joint, which allows several joint settings, may be the best choice.

5. The child who is heavy or large, is extremely active, or does not reside near an orthotist may not be a good candidate for the Select joint because of the potential for earlier wear with this type of hinge.

6. For a child with very mild hypertonia and medial-lateral instability, but not equinus, a free-motion hinged AFO or SMO may suffice. Caution is needed to identify increasing plantar-flexor tightness, which would indicate the need for an AFO that restricts plantar flexion.

7. A child with weak plantar flexors because of surgical lengthening or selective posterior rhizotomy should have an AFO that restricts dorsiflexion.

Myelomeningocele

The type of orthosis prescribed for a child with MMC is influenced by the child's level of motor function. The physical therapist should assume a key role in clarifying muscle function before an orthosis is prescribed. If a child demonstrates muscle activity in the lower extremities that is not willful or strong, or is reflective, a judgment about "functional motor level" should be made. We believe that the functional motor level reflects the child's ability to use muscles for skilled activities rather than the muscles innervated. When a discrepancy exists between the functional motor level and the motor level represented by the muscle activity present, the functional motor level should guide selection of the orthosis.

Table 3. *Factors Limiting Ambulation Progress in Young Children with Myelomeningocele*

Limitations to Progress	Guidelines/Suggestions
1. Developmental delay (in mental, language, social, or fine motor areas)	Begin experiences according to the child's developmental readiness unless structural benefits warrant attention earlier; 18 months is usually the upper limit of chronological age for beginning upright experiences
2. Upper-extremity dysfunction	Children having dysfunction of one or both hands may have difficulty learning to use a walker or crutches; an orthosis that does not require use of a walking aid (eg, a swivel walker) may be the best choice for children with high lesion levels
3. Structural limitations such as congenitally dislocated hips, clubfoot deformity, extremity contractures, or gibbus (convex spine)	Casting or surgical correction may be needed first; persisting deviances, such as a leg-length discrepancy, may restrict use of some orthoses (eg, a reciprocating gait orthosis)
4. Health issues necessitating focus in other areas or resulting in hospitalization, surgery, casting, and so forth	Once issues are managed, the work on ambulation can be resumed; the timetable for sequencing changes in braces may be slower than for other children
5. Visual status (acuity and perception)	Progress beyond standing in an orthosis may come slowly or not at all if visual acuity is very impaired
6. Social-environmental restraints	Time spent learning to use a brace may be longer and rate of progress slower than expected

An early consideration in selecting an orthosis for a child with MMC is the timing for the first device. Whereas Drennan[64] recommended bracing at the neurodevelopmental age when children normally learn to stand and walk, Carroll[65] advocated beginning standing when the child begins to demonstrate interest in being upright. Based on Drennan's recommendation, an orthosis would be prescribed when a child is 9 to 12 months old. Carroll's recommendation appears preferable, because it encourages adjustment for individual differences in social or cognitive developmental readiness. If the developmental readiness guideline is used, however, an exception becomes necessary for orthopedic benefits when the child reaches 20 to 24 months of age but remains below the 9-month level developmentally. In such cases, an orthosis should be ordered and the parapodium may be the best choice for a first device, even if the child has a low lumbar MMC.

A further consideration related to orthotic selection is that the types of orthoses used by children with MMC typically change with age. Changes are particularly common during the first 6 years of life, and families should be assisted in planning for these changes. Before changing from the current orthosis to a more sophisticated design, a child should be able to walk with the current device. Table 3 presents guidelines for responding to factors that may impede walking progress in young children learning to use their first orthosis. Minor changes may be indicated within 6 months of initiating orthotic use. Such changes could include addition or removal of a swivel base to the bottom of a parapodium or addition of an above-knee component of AFOs.

Based on clinical reports, personal experience, and research, the following guidelines for initial to later orthotic devices are provided.

1. A child with an S-2 motor level may begin standing and walking without an orthosis but may later benefit from FOs.

2. A child with an L4-5 motor level may ambulate throughout life with AFOs or SMOs. Rarely would a parapodium be needed as a first device.

3. A child with an L3-4 motor level will benefit from the postural support and stability provided by a parapodium used as a first standing and walking orthosis. Although some reports[48,49] have cited the use of an RGO at this motor level, the child should eventually ambulate with AFOS, AFOs attached to twister cables or a single lateral upright and pelvic band, or standard KAFOs.

4. A child with a motor level above L-2 will likely require an HKAFO as a first and later device. The child may begin with a parapodium on a swivel walker, then switch to an RGO. Transition from a parapodium to an RGO is not recommended before 30 to 36 months' developmental age. The likelihood of a child with high spinal-level MMC using only a wheelchair after age 15 years is great; however, factors including the orthosis used, the philosophy of the program, and personal characteristics of the child and family can influence outcome.

5. A child with discrepant motor and "functional motor" levels, should be fitted with an orthosis according to the functional motor level. For example, a child having some muscle activity through the L-5 level, who belly crawls rather than creeps, does not pull to stand or support body weight in vertical, and uses mainly hip flexors, should be considered to have a functional motor level of L-2. A parapodium or standing frame would be more appropriate than AFOS for a first device. Changes can be made as indicated with age.

Summary

This article has provided a summary of research on orthoses used for children with CP and children with MMC. Principles of orthotic application and guidelines for orthotic selection have been presented. Each child needs to be assessed individually, with consideration given to functional ability, management goals, and orthotic options. Although progress has been made in the development of orthoses and in the understanding of how the orthoses affect gait variables, further research will be needed as advances in material properties and designs are made available. Additionally, physical therapists should give further consideration to such matters as critical timing for introducing or progressing gait and methods for gait and other functional skill training with orthoses. The issue of using a total-mobility approach, which represents a combined program of seated mobility and ambulation versus either mobility mode used exclusively, also warrants attention from clinical researchers.

References

1 Paneth N, Kiely N. The frequency of cerebral palsy: a review of population studies in industrialized nations since 1950. In: Stanley F, Alberman E, eds. *The Epidemiology of the Cerebral Palsies.* Philadelphia, Pa: JB Lippincott Co; 1984:46–56.

2 Evans P, Elliott M, Alberman E, Evans S. Prevalence and disabilities in 4 to 8 year olds with cerebral palsy. *Arch Dis Child.* 1985; 60:940–945.

3 Kudrjavcev T, Schoenberg BS, Kurland KT, Groover RV. Cerebral palsy: survival rates, associated handicaps, and distribution by clinical subtype (Rochester, MN, 1950–1976). *Neurology.* 1985;35:900–903.

4 Shurtleff DB, Lemir RJ, Warkany J. Embryology, etiology, and epidemiology. In: Shurtleff DB, ed. *Myelodysplasias and Extrophies: Significance, Prevention, and Treatment.* New York, NY: Grune & Stratton Inc; 1986:39–64.

5 Wegman ME. Special article: annual summary of vital statistics—1989. *Pediatrics.* 1990; 86:835–847.

6 Walker DK, Palfrey JS, Butler JA, Singer J. Use and sources of payment for health and community services for children with impaired mobility. *Public Health Rep.* 1988;103:411–415.

7 Wolf JM, ed. *The Results of Treatment in Cerebral Palsy.* Springfield, Ill: Charles C Thomas, Publisher; 1969:18–26.

8 Bleck EE. *Orthopaedic Management in Cerebral Palsy.* London, England: MacKeith Press; 1987:142–183.

9 Cusick BD. *Progressive Casting and Splinting for Lower Extremity Deformities in Children with Neuromotor Dysfunction.* Tucson, Ariz: Therapy Skill Builders; 1990.

10 Mossberg KA, Linton KA, Friske K. Ankle-foot orthoses: effect on energy expenditure of gait in spastic diplegic children. *Arch Phys Med Rehabil.* 1990;71:490–494.

11 Brodke DS, Skinner SR, Lamoreux LW, et al. Effects of ankle-foot orthoses on the gait of children. *J Pediatr Orthop.* 1989;9:702–708.

12 Yates G. Molded plastics in bracing. *Clin Orthop.* 1974;102:46–57.

13 Hoffer MM, Garrett A, Koffman M, et al. New concepts in orthotics for cerebral palsy. *Clin Orthop.* 1974;102:100–107.

14 Rosenthal RK. The use of orthotics in foot and ankle problems in cerebral palsy. *Foot Ankle.* 1984;4:195–200.

15 Banks HH. The management of spastic deformities of the foot and ankle. *Clin Orthop.* 1977;122:70–76.

16 Bennet GC, Rang M, Jones D. Varus and valgus deformities of the foot in cerebral palsy. *Dev Med Child Neurol.* 1982;24:499–503.

17 Cusick BD, Sussman MD. Short leg casts: their role in the management of cerebral palsy. *Physical and Occupational Therapy in Pediatrics.* Binghamton, NY: The Haworth Press Inc; 1982;2:93–110.

18 Duncan WR, Mott DH. Foot reflexes and the use of the "inhibitive cast." *Foot Ankle.* 1983;4:145–148.

19 Jordan RP. Therapeutic considerations of the feet and lower extremities in the cerebral palsied child. *Clin Podiatr Med Surg.* 1984;1:547–561.

20 Selby L. Remediation of toe-walking behavior with neutral-position, serial-inhibitory casts: a case report. *Phys Ther.* 1988;68: 1921–1923.

21 Middleton EA, Hurley GRB, McIlwain JS. The role of rigid and hinged polypropylene ankle-foot-orthoses in the management of

cerebral palsy: a case study. *Prosthet Orthot Int.* 1988;12:129–135.

22 Hinderer KA, Harris SR, Purdy AH, et al. Effects of "tone-reducing" vs standard plaster-casts on gait improvement of children with cerebral palsy. *Dev Med Child Neurol.* 1988;30:370–377.

23 Harris SR, Riffle K. Effects of inhibitive ankle-foot orthoses on standing balance in a child with cerebral palsy: a single-subject design. *Phys Ther.* 1986;66:663–667.

24 Embrey DG, Yates L, Mott DH. Effects of neuro-developmental treatment and orthoses on knee flexion during gait: a single-subject design. *Phys Ther.* 1990;70:626–636.

25 Bertoti DB. Effect of short leg casting on ambulation in children with cerebral palsy. *Phys Ther.* 1986;66:1522–1529.

26 Watt J, Sims D, Harckham F, et al. A prospective study of inhibitive casting as an adjunct to physiotherapy for cerebral-palsied children. *Dev Med Child Neurol.* 1986;28: 480–488.

27 Mills VM. Electromyographic results of inhibitory splinting. *Phys Ther.* 1984;64:190–193.

28 Lough LK (Knutson LM). *The Effects of Fixed and Hinged Ankle-Foot Orthoses on Gait Myoelectric Activity and Standing Joint Alignment in Children with Cerebral Palsy.* Iowa City, Iowa: The University of Iowa; 1990. Doctoral dissertation.

29 Clinkingbeard JR, Gersten MW, Hoehn D. Energy cost of ambulation in the traumatic paraplegic. *Am J Phys Med.* 1964;43:157–165.

30 Richings JC, Eckstein HB. Locomotor and educational achievements of children with myelomeningocele. *Ann Phys Med.* 1970;10: 291–298.

31 Lorber J. Results of treatment of myelomeningocele: an analysis of 524 unselected cases, with special reference to possible selection for treatment. *Dev Med Child Neurol.* 1971;13:279–303.

32 Hoffer MM, Feiwell E, Perry R, et al. Functional ambulation in patients with myelomeningocele. *J Bone Joint Surg [Am].* 1973;55: 137–148.

33 DeSouza LJ, Carroll N. Ambulation of the braced myelomeningocele patient. *J Bone Joint Surg [Am].* 1976;58:1112–1118.

34 Barden GA, Meyer LC, Stelling FH. Myelodysplastics: fate of those followed for twenty years or more. *J Bone Joint Surg [Am].* 1975; 57:643–647.

35 Schopler SA, Menelaus MB. Significance of the strength of the quadriceps muscles in children with myelomeningocele. *J Pediatr Orthop.* 1987;7:507–512.

36 Findley TW, Agre JC, Habeck RV, et al. Ambulation in the adolescent with myelomeningocele, I: early childhood predictors. *Arch Phys Med Rehabil.* 1987;68:518–522.

37 Mazur JM, Shurtleff DB, Menelaus MB, Colliver J. Orthopaedic management of high-level spina bifida: early walking compared with early use of a wheelchair. *J Bone Joint Surg [Am].* 1989;71:56–61.

38 Taylor A, McNamara A. Ambulation status of adults with myelomeningocele. *Z Kinderchir.* 1990;45:32–33.

39 Samuelsson L, Skoog M. Ambulation in patients with myelomeningocele: a multivariate statistical analysis. *J Pediatr Orthop.* 1988; 8:569–575.

40 Sankarankutty M, Rose GK, Stallard J. The effect of orthotic treatment on spina bifida patients. *Spina Bifida Therapy.* 1979;1:187–196.

41 Flandry F, Burke S, Roberts JM, et al. Functional ambulation in myelodysplasia: the effect of orthotic selection on physical and physiologic performance. *J Pediatr Orthop.* 1986; 6:661–665.

42 Thomas SE, Mazur JM, Child ME, Supan TJ. Quantitative evaluation of AFO use with myelomeningocele children. *Z Kinderchir.* 1989;44:38–40.

43 Krebs DE, Edelstein JE, Fishman S. Comparison of plastic/metal and leather/metal knee-ankle-foot orthoses. *Am J Phys Med.* 1988;67:175–185.

44 Davies JB. Use of heart rate in assessment of orthoses. *Physiotherapy.* 1977;63:112–115.

45 Stallard J, Rose GK, Farmer IR. The ORLAU swivel walker. *Prosthet Orthot Int.* 1978;2: 35–42.

46 Rose GK, Stallard J, Sankarankutty M. Clinical evaluation of spina bifida patients using hip guidance orthosis. *Dev Med Child Neurol.* 1981;23:30–40.

47 Lough LK (Knutson LM), Nielsen DH. Ambulation in myelomeningocele: parapodium versus parapodium with ORLAU swivel modification. *Dev Med Child Neurol.* 1986;28: 489–497.

48 Yngve DA, Douglas R, Roberts JM. The reciprocating gait orthosis in myelomeningocele. *J Pediatr Orthop.* 1984;4:304–310.

49 McCall RE, Schmidt WT. Clinical experience with the reciprocal gait orthosis in myelodysplasia. *J Pediatr Orthop.* 1986;6:157–161.

50 Bunch WH, Keagy RD. *Principles of Orthotic Treatment.* St Louis, Mo: CV Mosby Co; 1976.

51 Rose GK. *Orthotics: Principles and Practice.* London, England: William Heinemann Medical Books Ltd; 1986.

52 Redford JB, ed. *Orthotics Etcetera.* 3rd ed. Baltimore, Md: Williams & Wilkins; 1986.

53 Shurr D, Cook T. *Prosthetics and Orthotics.* East Norwalk, Conn: Appleton & Lange; 1990.

54 Wenger DR, Mauldin D, Speck G, et al. Corrective shoes and inserts as treatment for flexible flatfoot in infants and children. *J Bone Joint Surg [Am].* 1989;71:800–810.

55 Penneau K, Lutter LD, Winter RD. Pes planus: radiographic changes with foot orthoses and shoes. *Foot Ankle.* 1982;2:299–303.

56 Bordelon RL. Hypermobile flatfoot in children: comprehension, evaluation, and treatment. *Clin Orthop.* 1983;181:7–14.

57 Bleck EE, Berzins UJ. Conservative management of pes valgus with plantar flexed talus, flexible. *Clin Orthop.* 1977;122:85–94.

58 Mereday C, Dolan CME, Lusskin R. Evaluation of the University of California biomechanics laboratory shoe insert in "flexible" pes planus. *Clin Orthop.* 1972;82:45–58.

59 Motloch WM. The parapodium: an orthotic device for neuromuscular disorders. *Artificial Limbs.* 1971;15:36–47.

60 Kinnen E, Gram M, Jackman KV, et al. Rochester parapodium. *Clin Prosthet Orthot.* 1984;8(4):24–25.

61 Rose GK, Henshaw JT. Swivel walkers for paraplegics: considerations and problems in their design and application. *Bull Prosthet Res.* 1973;10-20:62–74.

62 Stallard J, Rose GK, Tait JH, Davies JB. Assessment of orthoses by means of speed and heart rate. *J Med Eng Technol.* 1978;2:22–24.

63 Solomonow M, Baratta R, Hirokawa S, et al. The RGO Generation II: muscle stimulation powered orthosis as a practical walking system for thoracic paraplegics. *Orthopedics.* 1989; 12:1309–1315.

64 Drennan JC. Orthotic management of the myelomeningocele spine. *Dev Med Child Neurol.* 1976;18(suppl 37):97–103.

65 Carroll N. The orthotic management of the spina bifida child. *Clin Orthop.* 1974;102: 108–114.

Part III: Measurement and Assessment

A Shorter Method to Record Progress of Spastic Cases

Jacob Sirkin, M.D., and Lois A. Whitfield[1]

In the treatment of spastic cases it is most essential to have adequate records in order to have a complete story concerning the progress of each patient. Due to the fact that treatment of these cases covers a prolonged period of time, i. e., several years, it is quite difficult to show in a clear concise manner, the progress made by the patient, in ordinary detailed reports which are made at intervals.

Most records in this type of case consist of either written notes, which of necessity must be detailed and

1. Chief Physical Therapist, Newark State School, Newark, New York.

NEWARK STATE SCHOOL, NEWARK, NEW YORK

Department of Physical Therapy

NAME D■■■, John ADMITTED April 1, 1933

FIRST EXAMINATION: Aug. 1, 1933 EXAMINER: Dr. Severance

AGE	I. Q.	SUBSEQUENT I. Q.	Aug.'34	Oct.'35	June '36	
3 yrs. 9 mos.	29		41	64	...67.	......

HISTORY OF BIRTH AND INFANCY: Apparently normal delivery. Mother had severe uterine hemorrhage during pregnancy. Patient cried a great deal. Crawled at 1 yr.

DIAGNOSIS: Considerable spasticity and apparent athetosis.

TREATMENT RECOMMENDED:

- MUSCLE RELAXATION ✓
- MUSCLE TRAINING ✓
- MUSCLE STRETCHING
- OPERATIVE

DURATION OF TREATMENT: Approximately 2 - 5 yrs.

PROGNOSIS: Possibility of nearly complete recovery.

Fig. 1

CAPABILITIES	Aug. 1, 1933	Jul. 17, 1934	Nov. 24, 1934	Apr. 9, 1935	Jun. 1, 1936
Lies quietly			+	+	+
Disturbed by extraneous noises	+	+			
Purposeful movements	+	+	+	+	+
Rolls over alone		+	+	+	+
Sits in chair alone	+	+	+	+	+
Sits on stool with pelvic fixation			+		
Sits on stool alone				+	+
Balances self with assistance	+	+			
Balances self standing alone			+		
Walks assisted	+	+	+		
Walks in walker		+	+		
Walks alone				+	+
Drools	+				
Speech - none	+				
Speech - monosyllables		+			
Speech - single words			+		
Speech - sentences				+	+
Speech plain					
Speech - gutteral		+	+	+	+
Dresses self with assistance		+	+		
Dresses self alone				+	+
Feeds self with assistance	+				
Feeds self alone		+	+	+	+
Continent		+	+	+	+
Grasping left hand - supination	Partial	Partial	+	+	+
Grasping left hand - pronation	+	+	+	+	+
Grasping right hand - supination	Partial	Partial	+	+	+
Grasping right hand - pronation	+	+	+	+	+
Straight leg raising - left	25°	90°	90°	90°	90°
Straight leg raising - right	25°	70°	90°	90°	90°
Overflow	4+	3+	2+	2+	2+

Fig. 2. Blank space indicates negative capability, "+" sign indicates positive capability. When patient advances from "walks assisted" to "walks alone," the former is left blank. Other improvements are treated in the same way.

lengthy, or motion pictures taken at intervals, usually six months apart. We still make use of both of these types but have felt the need for a short concise summary which could be used conveniently without pouring over lengthy records or showing moving pictures.

It seems to us that records which can be visualized at a glance by the examiner are advisable, in order that clarity as well as brevity may be incorporated in them.

In order to do this, we devised, at the suggestion of Dr. R. D. Severance, who is Consulting Orthopedist at the Newark State School, a card system which we feel might be of interest and help to others working in this field. As figures 1 and 2 show, not a great deal has to be written, yet the progress of a patient over a period of years may be noted at a glance. Also we have the history of the patient summarized along with diagnosis, treatment recommended, and the prognosis at the time of the first examination.

Another advantage of the card is that the physician, when making his periodic examination, is able to have before him the items which should be mentioned in his report. Occasionally when the physician checks on his records of previous examinations, he is unable to find mention of a detail which he had not intended to omit. The card system thus is an aid both to physician and technician in the recording of progress notes.

We realize that in other places a modification of the card system might be advisable, but it is offered as a basis upon which to work, or it may be used as it is, since we have found it satisfactory for our needs.

Vol. 19, No. 4 The Physiotherapy Review 187

The Examination and Treatment of the Spastic Patient:

The Role of Performance and Muscle Tests

May L. Watrous, M.S.,* and Roscoe D. Severance, M.D.**

Some years ago it was customary to treat a spastic patient by giving him a more or less stereotyped series of rhythms and exercises. Little if any interest was shown in the types of disability present in his muscles.

*Physical Therapist, Syracuse Department of Health and Syracuse Free Dispensary, Syracuse, New York.

**Orthopedic Surgeon, Ithaca Reconstruction Home and Newark State School; District Orthopedic Surgeon, New York State Department of Health; Associate Professor of Orthopedic Surgery, Syracuse University Medical College and Hospital, Syracuse, N. Y.

Recently Dr. Winthrop Phelps,[1] among others, has stressed the need for a differential muscle examination as an aid in planning exercises for such a patient. He has also pointed out the need for special consideration of non-spastic athetoid and incoordinate types, as distinguished from the spastic cases discussed in this paper.

In line with these new trends, a study was made to determine what would constitute an adequate muscle examination for a spastic patient. For experimental purposes a four-way muscle test and a simple code for recording results were devised. The test recorded the following information on each muscle examined: (1) the range of active motion; that is, how far the individual could move the joint without assistance; (2) the degree of spasticity; (3) the strength of the muscle; and (4) the amount of relaxation. Records were kept during a period of a year and one-half on modified muscle test blanks similar to those used for anterior poliomyelitis.

The four-way muscle test proved to be valuable for treatment planning. However, it was time-consuming, fatiguing, and it failed to give all the information desired.

THE PERFORMANCE TEST

During the period that the muscle examination was used it became increasingly clear that another type of test was needed to supplement it. The muscle test gave information concerning every important muscle in the body but no information as to which necessary acts of life the individual could or could not perform. For example could he button his coat, step up or down on a curb, cut his meat?

There was therefore a fundamental question: Are we trying to educate a single muscle to do its duty, or are we trying to educate the spastic as an individual to lead a useful independent life?

Desirable as this latter aim is, the physical therapist is likely to take refuge in the simpler, more specific muscle goal. The muscle test used alone encouraged such an attitude, for it focused the attention on efficient joint motion with all manipulative activity subordinated to that end.

In our opinion, the accomplishment of the necessary or useful "life skills" should be the treatment goal, with skills that the individual fails to perform, or simpler ones of a preparatory nature, selected and included as an integral part of each treatment. A treatment made up of instruction in these skills alone, however, would be inadequate. If the muscle test shows there is marked muscle weakness, inability to move a joint, or other limitations, suitable exercises should be planned for these conditions with the orthopedic surgeon's advice. On the other hand, a treatment consisting solely of rhythmic or resistive exercises may be limited in usefulness as well as aim.

To secure information as to which habits of life an individual can perform and which ones he cannot, a performance test was devised. The test includes over one hundred items, such as to open the door, to pull a light cord overhead, to pick up a coin (or pin) with the thumb and first finger, to blow a whistle, to put on shoes, to balance on one foot. The items in the test are graded from the easiest act (usually involving the shoulder joint alone, or the trunk) to the more difficult (such as sewing and hopping). The scoring is simple and objective. *"V"* is used if the child can perform the act; *"O"* if he fails to do it; *"I"* to indicate incomplete performance; that is, if he does the act but needs further training for smoother or more adequate performance.

The performance test has been found to be useful in planning a program for clinic and home. In addition it furnishes an objective record of improvement and accomplishment understood and appreciated by the parent and others.

DISCUSSION OF THE MUSCLE TEST

Over a period of a year and one-half muscle examinations were made by one examiner on twenty-five spastic patients, approximately three-fourths of whom were children. The figures in the following charts represent the averages of all the gradings on involved muscles that were available for study during the period specified in the charts. The same individuals are not necessarily included in all groups.

How often should a muscle examination be given?

To answer this question it was essential to know how much change could be expected to take place in the range of voluntary (active) motion in the joints and in strength.

The tables do not attempt to show the improvement of an individual or a group; they show the average amount of "change" (improvement or loss) in a given length of time. Loss in the range or strength of a muscle rarely occurs with cooperative patients. "No change" in a muscle is a frequent finding, for it may be that all attention is centered on control of proximal joints. If it were desired to show improvement, all gains in the range of motion and strength of muscles should be summed, not averaged.

TABLE I

CHANGE IN THE RANGE OF ACTIVE MOTION* IN THE JOINTS OF SPASTIC PATIENTS DURING A TWELVE-MONTH PERIOD

	3-mo. period	6-mo. period	9-mo. period	12-mo. period
Average amount of change in tenths.	2.18	2.88	2.80	3.05
Number of muscles studied	237	125	103	137
Number of individuals studied ...	16	9	9	8
Number of muscles changing from "O" to normal ..	2	8	3	11

* The range of active motion was measured in tenths from "O" (no motion) to 10 (complete range of motion). It will be noted that the average amount of change in the range of active motion of all joints examined was approximately three-tenths during the year's time.

Conclusion: For the purpose of exercise planning for spastic cases, a year's interval between examinations should be adequate. This conclusion is supported further by examination of the following table:

TABLE II

CHANGE IN THE STRENGTH OF MUSCLES GRADED BY POLIOMYELITIS MUSCLE TESTS IN SPASTIC CASES DURING A TWELVE-MONTH PERIOD

	3-mo. period	6-mo. period	9-mo. period	12-mo. period
Average amount of change in strength in 10 arbitrarily chosen units	1.50	1.64	1.70	1.66
Number of muscles studied	262	156	103	112
Number of individuals studied ...	15	10	8	10

* The units chosen as an index of strength range from "O" (no trace felt) to 10 (normal strength). They were as follows: O, P—, P, P+, F—, F, F+, G, G+ N. It will be seen the average change of all muscles tested was not quite two of these units in a year's period.

Are all four measurements necessary on a muscle examination?

The amount of spasticity was measured in three degrees with a O (or no spasticity) determination. To determine spasticity the joint was passively manipulated; if contraction occurred consistently when the muscle was stretched rapidly, it was said to be spastic. In hemiplegic cases the presence of spasticity was checked by comparison with the normal leg or arm. This record was found to be interesting and sometimes useful in planning a program, but it was unreliable, reflecting the temporary condition of the patient.

The degree of variation in the amount of spasticity from one examination to another on the same muscles can be judged from the following study. These measurements were made from the muscle examinations of two representative adults and three cooperative children chosen from the group.

	Percentage	No. of muscles studied
Alike on two examinations out of four	75	199
Alike on three examinations out of four	43	144
Alike on four examinations out of four	24	84

The question is raised whether or not it is necessary from the point of view of exercise planning to note if the muscle is spastic. It is sometimes found that both flexors and extensors of a joint are spastic, with or without a difference in the degree of the spasticity. The information needed, in these cases as well as in cases where only the antagonist is spastic is the extent of voluntary movement in the joint, the amount of strength and the effectiveness of the movement.

The determination of "no spasticity" was not found to be uniformly consistent for a given muscle under the conditions of a muscle test. Study over the period of a year disclosed that at the time of one examination a certain muscle would show spasticity which at another examination would be found not to be spastic.

The number of muscles graded as showing "no spasticity" which showed spasticity in subsequent examinations can be judged from the following percentages. The examinations were spaced at three-month intervals. No muscles were included from normal extremities.

	Percent
Muscles showing "no spasticity" on four tests out of four	52
Muscles showing "no spasticity" on three tests out of four	22
Muscles showing "no spasticity" on two tests out of four	8
Muscles showing "no spasticity" on one test out of four	17

The notation of the degree of relaxation was found to be of interest, but in actual practice it was seldom used in planning an exercise program. The range of active motion, while not identical, at least gave enough information as to the degree of relaxation to raise the question whether or not such a record was worth the time involved. The degree of relaxation was determined by passive manipulation of the joint and instruction or suggestion to encourage the patient to relax. The range in tenths, 0 (no relaxation present) to 10 (complete relaxation) through which the joint could be moved passively before the muscle could be felt to contract, was taken as a measure of the degree of relaxation.

Conclusions: The range of active motion in joints and the degree of strength of muscles were found to be the measures that were used almost exclusively in making up an exercise program. In our experience the muscle examination could be limited to these two measures plus a notation to indicate confusion, unsteadiness and contractures. A simple symbol to record confusion is a circle drawn around the figure which indicates the range of active motion: a partial circle indicates mild confusion; a complete circle indicates extreme confusion. The letter "u" can indicate unsteadiness when present. These symbols reduce notes of a general nature to a minimum.

How should the performance test be used, and what relation should it bear to the muscle examination?

It has been stated before that the performance test supplements the muscle examination. In addition it is useful in other ways. The problem of maintaining the patient's interest is facilitated by selecting acts from the test for use in the treatment period. The patient is quick to appreciate that these skills are necessary in his struggle for independence, but more than this, he enjoys manipulating objects or placing himself in some relation to objects. The mother (or attendant, if the child is institutionalized) is an invaluable aid in teaching these complex skills, and the physical therapist in school, as well as in clinic, should gain her cooperation. A chart of immediate goals can be made up from the performance test for use at home. While not the most desirable device, awarding a gold star to a child for a skill learned is far better than constant reminding or nagging. Such a simple stimulus may serve as a start towards encouraging the mother to plan goals neither too easy or too hard, so that the child gains satisfaction through success.

In view of the fact that these tests have been used only two years, conclusions necessarily must be tentative.

SUMMARY OF CONCLUSIONS

1—Performance and muscle tests should be used in planning an exercise program for the spastic patient and also as valuable objective records for determining the progress of the patient and the efficacy of any type of treatment.

2.—A yearly interval between examinations is adequate for purposes of exercise planning unless some gross change is noted.

3—The muscle test should determine: (a) the range of active motion in the joints, (b) the strength of the muscles, (c) the degree of the contractures, and (d) the motor peculiarities, (confusion, unsteadiness, etc.).

4—Under the condition of a muscle test the degree or absence of spasticity was found to be too variable to serve as a reliable measurement.

5—The records of the degree of spasticity and the degree of relaxation were found to be of little value in making up an exercise program; experience suggests that they need not be included in a muscle examination.

REFERENCES

1. Phelps, Winthrop M.: Birth Injuries, Physio. Review, Jan.-Feb. 1937, Vol. 17, No. 1.

2. Legg, A. T., and Merrill, J. B.: Physical Therapy in Infantile Paralysis, W. F. Prior Co., Hagerstown, Md., 1932.

Developmental Diagnosis and Guidance

for the Palsied Child

Arnold Gesell, M.D.

To understand any child whether normal or handicapped, we must understand his capacities of growth. This is peculiarly true of the child who is handicapped by a cerebral injury, whether that injury occurred before, during or after birth. Was the injury slight or grave? Is the damage selective or devastating? Within what limits will the child respond to physical therapy?

A knowledge of normal development is needed to answer such questions. Indeed, certain forms of cerebral injury cannot even be diagnosed early without appreciation of the normal stages and sequences of development as manifested in the infant's behavior patterns.

Behavior is the most comprehensive index of a child's maturity and well being. Behavior assumes patterns which can be objectively tested and observed. These patterns change with age; they can be clinically diagnosed. *Developmental diagnosis is a diagnosis of maturity status. Specifically, the developmental diagnosis of infants is the application of graded functional tests of behavior to determine the maturity and the integrity of the central nervous system.* Such tests are significant for all types of children, normal as well as defective and handicapped.

The body grows; behavior grows. The infant is a growing action system. He comes by his mind in the same way in which he comes by his body, that is, through processes of development which create maturing patterns of behavior. Medically considered, his mind indeed is a complex of growing behavior patterns.

In our method of developmental diagnosis at the Yale Clinic, we use simple test objects to elicit characteristic patterns of behavior—patterns which are symptomatic of stages and degrees of maturity. For example, one of our test objects is a red, one-inch cube. The newborn infant is so immature that he cannot perceive the cube, but he does clasp it with a reflex grasp when it is pressed into his palm. At *sixteen weeks,* when the infant is held in a supported sitting position, he perceives a nearby cube and fixates his eyes upon it. His nervous system is growing at a prodigious rate. At *twenty-four weeks* he can coordinate eyes and hands; he seizes a cube on sight. It is a crude palmar grasp. At *twenty-eight weeks* the radial digits come more prominently into play. New behavior patterns are taking shape as the nervous system undergoes its progressive organization. Having seized a cube, he can transfer it from one hand to another. At *forty weeks* he grasps the cube deftly by thumb opposition. At *twelve months* he can release the cube on intent. At *eighteen months* he builds a vertical tower of three cubes. At *two years* he builds a horizontal wall of three cubes, at *three years* a bridge of three cubes, and at *five years* he builds a staircase of six cubes.

These are lawful sequences of growth, only secondarily influenced by cultural factors. They are so fundamentally determined by intrinsic growth factors that they may be used as criteria for appraising the maturity and integrity of the nervous system. All psychologic development, even in the sphere of intelligence and emotions, is subject to similar maturity sequences. These growth sequences and these patterns of behavior are identified and appraised through the method of developmental diagnosis.*

The method is based upon a systematic investigation of the behavior growth of a large group of normal infants whose development was followed at periodic intervals from birth through the first five years. The infants were examined under controlled but home-like conditions, with the full cooperation of the parents. Great care was taken to secure natural and optimal behavior. Extensive cinema records were made at lunar month intervals during the first year of life and at lengthening intervals later. These records were subjected to minute inspection and analyzed as so many anatomic cross sections of behavior patterns. The home behavior of the infants also was explored. On the

Director, The Clinic of Child Development, School of Medicine, Yale University, New Haven, Conn.

*Gesell, Arnold, and Amatruda, Catherine S.: Developmental Diagnosis: Normal and Abnormal Child Development. Clinical Methods and Pediatric Applications (New Enlarged Second Edition). Paul B. Hoeber, Inc., New York, 1947.

basis of these periodic observations, it was possible to define the behavior characteristics typical of a series of advancing age levels; four, sixteen, twenty-eight and forty weeks; twelve and eighteen months; two, three, four and five years.

Four major fields of behavior were embodied in these norms of development as follows:

Motor Behavior: Posture and locomotion; prehension and manipulation; gross and fine motor coordination

Adaptive Behavior: Self-initiated and induced behavior; learning; resourcefulness in adjusting to new situations; exploitive behavior

Language Behavior: Vocalizations; vocal signs; words; gestures; comprehension

Personal-Social Behavior: Reactions to persons; response to gesture and speech; socialized learning; habits of self help

It should be emphasized that developmental diagnosis is not intelligence testing in a narrow sense. Developmental diagnosis is a clinical method designed to assess the child's behavior equipment in the four major fields. It aims to analyze the developmental status of the child—to interpret the assets and deficiencies of his action system in terms of his maturity and his total personality make-up.

No handicap is more in need of intelligent understanding than cerebral palsy. No handicap takes as many variegated forms. At one extreme, we have the devastating type in which all growth potentials are abolished. At the other extreme the handicap is minimal. It may even escape notice in infancy and yet it can be discovered by methods of developmental diagnosis which bring the deviating behavior patterns into view. Atypical motor signs show themselves in incoordination of eye movements, in sucking, swallowing and other feeding reactions, in reaching, in hand, arm, and finger postures, in delays and deformations of speech. Sometimes, also, there are deficits in vision and in personality organization.

Between the two extreme types lie a vast group of selective cerebral palsies in which the motor disabilities may be moderate or severe. They may be so severe as to suggest that the child is mentally deficient. But again discriminating developmental diagnosis of behavior may reveal a relatively normal intelligence and personality. The motor disabilities manifest themselves in the fields of prehension, manipulation, locomotion, speech and emotional control. Just as blindness and deafness are sensory handicaps, so spasticity and athetosis are essentially motor handicaps. The symptoms are extremely diverse, and for this reason each case requires careful and periodic diagnostic study. In this type of handicap, a careful explanation of the meaning of the symptoms is especially important. Such explanations will help the parents to understand the nature of the handicap, the purpose of the training, the rationale of the orthopedic measures. A palsied child is not a sick child, but a crippled child. He does not need overprotection. He needs understanding and opportunity suited to his disabilities. But he cannot get such understanding unless parents are enlightened through interpretive guidance.

Some Problems of the Physical Therapist in Testing Cerebral Palsied Children*

Shirley J. Francis, B.S.

The diagnosis of cerebral palsy is based primarily on the neurological findings, but testing must be carried out in many areas before a fair assessment can be made of the child's potential for habilitation. As a member of the "team" responsible for evaluation of the cerebral palsy patient, the physical therapist is in the peculiar position of having no standardized examination such as the manual muscle test. This lack is partly due to the nature of cerebral palsy, which precludes the administration of an ordinary manual muscle test because of the child's inability, except in very mild cases, to elicit isolated muscle action; and partly due to the fact that in dealing with brain damage, we find not only motor dysfunction but other deficits which influence motor function and may alter the child's total physical performance. Because cerebral palsy is generally complex, testing involves the evaluation of a series of problems of varying degrees, each interacting with the other. Before beginning a physical evaluation, the physical therapist should be acquainted with as many findings as are available through examinations by other members of the "team."

One of the most important areas tested is the psychological. The therapist should know if the child is old enough to be treated. In this instance, "old enough" means not only in chronological age and mental age, but socially mature enough to cooperate in treatment. The psychological report will also indicate areas of special learning difficulty. The "brain-injured" child [1] is particularly trying to test or to treat because of distractibility, tendency for motor perseveration, and perceptual and conceptual problems. "Old enough" may also be partially determined by studies which have been done to ascertain that the child has sufficient skeletal maturation for weight bearing and can tolerate braces locked in straight alinement.

Testing in the sensory areas is equally important. The audiometric report may show that the child has a hearing loss which may be a true central deafness, or that he has a mild to severe pitch cutoff type of hearing loss generally associated with athetosis due to Rh incompatibility.[2] If the child is wearing a hearing aid, it should be worn during testing, but with the young child, too much reliance should not be placed on the aid to bring the hearing up to normal. Many young children have not adjusted to their aids and are still somewhat dependent upon lip reading and visual clues for directions. It becomes an important and often lengthy procedure, therefore, to keep a face-to-face relationship with either the deaf or hard-of-hearing child and to give him directions in a loud voice supplemented with gestures or demonstrations.

Dr. Perlstein[3] and others have found that approximately 50 per cent of cerebral palsied children have visual problems which range from total blindness to a mild strabismus. Lack of sight or the inability to focus properly causes a child to be insecure in attempting postural balance work, and once he becomes ambulatory he has the large problem of spatial orientation and dealing with obstacles. Blind children are difficult to test because of this marked insecurity. A little boy we have treated brought so many small pillows with him as security props, that in testing him, it first became a challenge to get rid of the pillows long enough to see if he could support his weight with his hands. We made the mistake of trying to orient this child to the building after he had begun crutch walking; he would have learned faster if he had covered the same ground first on hands and knees which was his previous method of exploration.

Another problem encountered on the sensory level may be the presence of astereognosis, especially for form perception, which has been found to be of particularly high incidence in patients with infantile hemiplegia.[4, 5] The young child with a handicapped hand does not willingly attempt to use it, but with training he may gain some degree of skill and perception. On initial testing, especially with spastic quadriplegics who

Rehabilitation Therapy Supervisor, The Moody State School for Cerebral Palsied Children, Galveston, Texas.

* Presented at a Workshop on Testing Procedures of the Texas Southeastern District, APTA, February, 1959.

are not using either hand, the physical therapist cannot tell if the child has had a poverty of experience or if he has true sensory loss.

A most interesting and challenging problem is the child who is neither deaf, ataxic, nor apparently "brain injured," but who does not comprehend simple directions. His problem may be related to the experience level in a home environment where he is the only child. He may have been so overprotected that he has never had the chance to learn changes in body position and doesn't know where "up" is—or "down" —or "sideways." Or this child may have been braced continuously at such an early age that the normal, exploratory experiences (beginning on the floor) have been denied him. (The Harris County Treatment Center[6] in Houston, Texas, has been combining floor play and use of a "tumble bug" with their nursery school group to give some of the very young children this experience in changing body positions. The consulting psychologist at the Center, Dr. Willie Mae Verniaud, says that the children enjoy the floor play very much.)

The child's record should be studied for any notation concerning previous convulsions or EEG readings which indicate a potential for convulsions. A child who suddenly stops and stares blankly or whose attention wanders is difficult to test. These children are suspected of having petit mal seizures which are nearly imperceptible, are of brief duration, but which may occur at frequent intervals during the day. If a child is an epileptic and medications are being administered for control, the examination of motor abilities may not give a true picture since certain drugs tend to make the child lethargic and slow in response.

The medical history should be noted also for X-ray reports which may show congenital or acquired deformities that may indicate precautionary measures in testing. The strangest one of this type we have known was a girl with athetosis and osteogenesis imperfecta. Needless to say, testing was carried out with extreme caution. Any abnormality of the heart may also call for limitation of physical activity, and the child's tolerance might be such that testing cannot be accomplished in one or two sessions but may take several sessions.

TESTING BY THE PHYSICAL THERAPIST

After learning as much as possible about the child in the areas just discussed, the therapist is ready for testing. In general, we find that the spastic child is blocked in his attempts at movement through normal ranges; the athetoid child is too unstable to perform isolated muscle action; and the ataxic child lacks primary coordination. Testing, therefore, becomes an analysis of the child's ability or inability to perform normal functions. Following are some of the specific factors which enter into testing by the physical therapist.

1. *Tonic neck reflex*

When a child has a hyperactive tonic neck reflex maintaining his head toward one side so that he cannot actively turn his head, the extremities on the side to which his head is turned will be extended and his opposite extremities will be held in flexion. This child is hard to test for sitting balance because he is drawn backward and to the side of the extended leg; in attempting standing balance and ambulation, he has trouble in placing both feet on the floor and generally lacks reciprocation. He may have the mental concept of these activities and the muscle power to accomplish them if the TNR could be controlled but, unless he can reverse his TNR at will, or utilize it for specific functions, it is impossible to test sitting, standing balance, or walking.

2. *Cerebral zero muscles—actual or apparent*

Flaccid paralysis is perhaps one of the best known disturbances and results in lack of muscle function. In the spastic, it may be noted in testing that there are nonfunctioning muscles. The problem in testing is to determine if these muscles are truly "cerebral zero" muscles. Mentally defective children and some brain-injured children are incapable of performing on command and are prone to show apparent flaccidity. With patient and continued observation of play, it may be possible to note muscle function which at first did not seem to be present.

3. *Spastic muscles on all sides of a joint*

In this problem, flexion is prevented by spastic extensors, and hyperactive flexors inhibit attempts to extend. In this type of child, movement is blocked in either direction. His true strength cannot be estimated and reciprocal action is not possible. After a training period, he may "break through" the blocking with one leg, only to show crossed overflow in the opposite extremity. Spasticity on all sides of the joints may also be found in the upper extremities and resembles rigidity, so that there may be some confusion in differential diagnosis.

4. *Gravity*

The force of gravity becomes an important factor when a spastic child attempts to move against it. Spasticity is most commonly found in the flexor muscles. The extensor antagonists are thus at a disadvantage when the child tries to maintain the body in the upright position. The impression of muscle strength of a spastic patient as seen on the treatment table is not valid generally and may be disappointing when he is placed in the weight-bearing position. This problem is particularly noted in the hips and knees.

5. *Measurement of contractures and leg length*

In these two areas of measurement, there are particular problems in positioning the child. The athetoid child has tense, frequently bizarre involuntary movements, and the spastic child is difficult to hold in straight alinement at the limit of his range of passive motion. The therapist working alone really has a problem with this and, if it is at all possible, should get someone to assist in holding the child during the measuring process.

6. *Mixed types of cerebral palsy*

Children with a diagnosis of one or more types of cerebral palsy are difficult to test in that it cannot always be ascertained by the therapist which neuromuscular problem is causing the greatest loss of functional ability. Mixed types which may be seen are athetosis combined with underlying spasticity; spasticity with overlaid athetosis, tremor or ataxia; tremor with ataxia; and rigidity with tremor. To illustrate this problem: Anne, aged 7, had a diagnosis of spasticity with overlaid athetosis; her knee flexion was 45 degrees on admission. After three months of therapy which was aimed at improving the range of knee extension, no gains had been made and surgery was discussed. Anne was taken from school to a hospital for tests given in this order: Thorazine, light anesthesia, and hypnosis. Under anesthesia, she demonstrated the desired relaxation and it was found that true contractures were 10 degrees on the right and 15 degrees on the left. Following a bilateral hamstring release, this child is ambulatory.

As stated in the beginning, we have no standardized test. One test which is gaining approval and use is the Motor Age Test[7] which grades the child on the basis of functional ability. The score is given in months according to the Gesell Scale for average motor development. Through this test, we may find ourselves confronted with a child who is 5 years old chronologically, 3 years old mentally, and who has a motor quotient level of 7 months. By a comparison of the age levels, this test gives a good index to the approach to motivation of the child in treatment. The test is also considered valuable as an objective determination of motor development and as a means of recording progress through retests at 6 month intervals. For instance, it may show that in 6 months time, the child has gained 4 months in motor development. The Motor Age Test, in my opinion, is the most logical approach to evaluation of the motor abilities of the cerebral palsied child—for all types and regardless of age. The need for standardized and valid testing procedures may be partially fulfilled by universal use of the Motor Age Test.

REFERENCES

1. Strauss and Lehtinen: Psychopathology and Education of the Brain Injured Child, New York, Grune & Stratton, Inc., 1947, Pp. 28-53, 75-95.
2. Aberson, Neva: The relation of the Rh factor to cerebral palsy, Cerebral Palsy Rev., 14:7:3-6.
3. Perlstein, M. A.: Cerebral palsy: medical and educational implications, Am. J. Ment. Defic., 60:1:116, 1953.
4. ———and Hood, P. N.: Infantile spastic hemiplegia, Am. J. Phys. M., 34:391, 457, 1955.
5. Hohman, L. B., Baker, L., Reed, Ruth: Sensory disturbances in children with infantile hemiplegia, triplegia and quadriplegia, Am. J. Phys. M., 37:1-6, 1958.
6. The Harris County Treatment Center for Crippled Children, 1415 California, Houston, Texas.
7. Johnson, M. K., Zuick, F. N., Wingate, Kathleen: The motor age test: Measurement of motor handicaps in children with neuromuscular disorders such as cerebral palsy, J. Bone Surg. Am. Vol., 33-a:3:693-707, 1951.

Developmental Analysis in Evaluation and Treatment of Cerebral Palsy*

Dorothy Page, B.S.†

Motor manifestations of cerebral defect are but a part of a broader problem. At the Cerebral Palsy Treatment Center we think of cerebral palsy in terms of changing and broadening concepts; not as a single diagnostic entity but as a multiple handicapping condition. In a recent publication, Denhoff and Robinault[1] emphasize the need for considering those patients with neuromotor dysfunction as only a part of the group of neurologically-impaired subjects. Studies of "syndromes of cerebral dysfunction," which include cerebral palsy, mental retardation, epilepsy, hyperkinetic behavior disorders and perceptual or sensory defects, show similar etiology.

Sequential Development

With this understanding, a treatment approach based on sequential and integrated development has been gradually emerging for several years. We are more careful to seek the basic reasons which limit natural, orderly development, rather than to accept the most obvious motor dysfunction as the point of primary emphasis. The carefully documented observations of infant behavior by Dr. Gesell and his colleagues[2] provide us with fundamental information.

We realize that efforts in this direction are not unique at our center. However, we have tried to consider the absolute necessity to relate carefully and systematically all information available from diverse sources, to consider disturbances of perception, or the abnormal reception or interpretations of the sensations of vision, hearing, touch, taste and smell. Observing an infant with an intact neurological system, we can see the effect of reactions to stimuli with which the infant is not yet familiar. As the nervous system becomes integrated and learning takes place, there is a greater selectivity of response. Where there is a neurological deficit there is a prolongation of the infantile reactions, inappropriate responses, or delays in learning. As an example, we can observe strabismus. We may be told that, in spite of it, there is normal visual acuity. What effect does the lack of binocular fusion have on motor behavior? The effects of disturbances of tactile sensation are receiving considerable attention,[3] but there is still much more to be learned.

If we disregard perceptual disorders, or are not aware of them, we are forcing the individual into stress situations, or putting him into "deep water" before he is ready. We appreciate that there are individual variations in ability to tolerate stress; we all have defenses for these situations. The child does also, although these are not always identified as such stress reactions.

A closely related and an equally significant area is that of emotional development and the child's relationships to parents, siblings and peers. The variables here are innumerable; without an appreciation of them and an effort to modify detrimental situations, the effectiveness of any program will be lost. Disturbing relationships may not be immediately apparent, but may be the cause for later failures and regressions.

Obviously, the level of intellectual functioning cannot be overlooked. A careful evaluation by a clinical psychologist identifies the areas of perceptual impairment, or an assessment of the child's ability to relate and respond to his environment. Discrepancies of performance levels between verbal and motor skills give indications of the presence or absence of sensory impairment. Mental retardation may be the major factor suppressing total development; therefore, it is important to relate this to the level of activity expected of the child.

We must continually be looking for the reasons for retardation of motor development, rather than merely observing that it is present and noting to what level the child has progressed. Our emphasis should be on the orderly, integrated development of the child in all spheres of behavior—motor, adaptive, language and personal-social.

Analysis of Motor Behavior

Again relying on the work of Dr. Gesell and his colleagues, we know that early behavior is

* Read at the Annual Conference of the American Physical Therapy Association, Chicago, July 1961.

† Director, Cerebral Palsy Treatment Center, Albany Medical Center Hospital; Instructor, Russell Sage—Albany Medical College, Division of Physical Therapy, Albany, New York.

essentially a gross motor response to stimuli. Physical therapists must concern themselves with the basic activities in the developmental sequence. In past efforts, our tendency has been to estimate a child's highest level of accomplishment and to plan our treatment program from that point. In pursuing such a course we fail to consider total development.

A careful analysis of a child's abilities to perform the basic motor activities which a two to four month-old infant is capable provides the basis for a physical therapy program. A child demonstrating inefficient life-sustaining functions and abnormal gross motor patterns will be unable to meet the demands required for learning more refined skills. In a careful analysis, questions to be asked and observations to be made include the following: Is the pattern of respiration still at an infantile level? Is sucking and swallowing adequate? Does the child show symmetrical posture in prone and supine position? Is he able to follow with his eyes to and beyond the mid-line? Is he able to oppose his hand at the mid-line? What is his response to auditory stimuli? Is he capable of attaining and maintaining a position of total flexion? In this position is there a lag of one body segment? Is he capable of attaining and maintaining a position of total extension? In prone lying, can the elbow-holding position be achieved, and is the head stable in the mid-position? Can he move forward and backward using upper extremity flexion and extension? More specifically, is there weakness or inactivity of lateral abdominal musculature? What effect does this have on the action of the hip musculature? In the total flexion pattern, is ankle dorsiflexion complete? If not, the ankle will be unable to function adequately at more advanced levels, when reverse action is required for anteroposterior balance in the squat position or in upright stance. In the total extension pattern, are the hamstrings flexing the knees while the hips are extended? If they are unable to function in this position, the hamstrings will also be incapable of normal function in upright stance. A child who may crawl in some fashion, but lacks sufficient control to stabilize the head is going to demonstrate poor patterns of posture and locomotion if we accept the crawling as an adequate accomplishment and press forward to the next milestone. If control of the head and trunk is not sufficient to stabilize in the sitting or upright posture, respiration will be inadequate for more advanced activities. Such factors are paramount in program planning, regardless of the age of the patient.

Further investigation of the child's functional level and perceptual areas may be necessary, particularly of those children who have kept a nearly normal pace in development but when reaching higher levels of motor skills show awkwardness, stumbling or insecurity. In the case of the child with minimal motor handicap, the answer may be found by a careful evaluation of the co-ordinate function of the eyes. The child who may be delayed in learning finer manual skills may show disturbances in reception of tactile sensations.

From a neurological examination and our own analysis of these functions, we should understand whether the deficiencies noted are a result of pyramidal or extra-pyramidal tract disorders or possible combinations of both. We should understand whether the dysfunction is a result of over-response or diminished response to a sensory stimulus.

Treatment Program

The analysis of motor behavior which has been recorded serves not only as a base for future comparison but also as a guide to treatment planning. Therapy is directed toward assisting the patient to increase his level of function in natural sequence. It is an attempt to correct the basic and most proximal deficiencies, or those activities which are predecessors to higher levels of activity.

Methods of neuromuscular facilitation are used in the treatment program.[4, 5] These methods rely on application of appropriate sensory stimuli or physiological demands and must be selected for each individual patient with the primary problem in mind. The application requires that a therapist have knowledge of the underlying neurophysiological principles.

Total patterns of function are used in efforts to correct weaknesses and abnormal motions. Selected sensory stimuli are applied to facilitate an increased response in the deficient part of the pattern. Activities which are normally learned at a subconscious or reflex level are approached in this manner.

At the Center, children who were able to walk with the aid of braces and crutches with considerable effort have been participating in this type of program. Assistive devices which they could not manage independently and efficiently were avoided. In addition to the formal or attended activities, they have been allowed and encouraged to move about in the easiest and safest manner. The emphasis has been on a frequent change of position and permitting activities requiring a minimum of assistance. Regardless of previous levels of accomplishment, it has been our experience that we have improved that level by using a careful analysis of basic skills and planning the therapy program in keeping with the primary deficiencies.

Parent Participation

Parental understanding and participation in any program is of great importance. With children beginning treatment, the parents are included in the evaluation process, and procedures and program planning are interpreted to them. In the case of older children, with whom we wished a redirection of emphasis, other means were employed. Group meetings were held with the parents. They were invited and encouraged to discuss their understanding and feelings toward various procedures which had been used. With assurance that we shared many of their questions, it was then possible to discuss in positive terms the need for a reassessment of our procedures. In addition to the group discussions, individual conferences were held for further clarification, demonstration and instructions.

With only two exceptions, parents of patients known to us for six to eight years have been able to adapt to the change of procedure and are more willing and better able to follow through with a program at home. In the two situations in which there has been a reluctance on the part of the parents to relate to this, the program has been regarded as a regression or as a return to infantile levels. In these situations, we are and have been aware of other factors influencing their attitudes toward any therapy, such as their unresolved psychological conflicts about having a handicapped child.

On the whole we find that the parents are able to relate very quickly to this type of program, particularly those parents with the younger children. With early concentrated analysis, program planning and interpretation and instructions, it has been possible to delegate more quickly the responsibility for training activities to the parents.

Observations

With regard to the children, we have observed the following positive results. There has been less fatigue and prolongation of task interest. Without the aid of braces or other supportive apparatus, there has been an increase in functional range of motion and decreasing deformities. There has been less fear and a greater willingness to move about independently, by whatever means are available. Once gross patterns have become more firmly established, there has been a corresponding improvement in finer skills without directing voluntary effort toward that goal. In children demonstrating visual-perceptual difficulties, with a retraining program, we have seen concurrent improvement in scholastic achievement and a reduction of reactions of over-stress. Reviewing the results of motor-age tests given prior to this change of emphasis, wide variations in rates of development were noted. In the past, as spurts of growth occurred, it was not unusual to observe regression as reported by these tests. Present observations seem to indicate a more consistent rate of development.

Summary

The importance of a better understanding of early development and the effects of sensory impairment upon integrated functioning of the child with manifestations of cerebral dysfunction is discussed. To understand the needs of each patient demands a careful analysis to determine the base level of efficient and integrated function. It is only then that we have a foundation for establishing a training program, a program which pays heed to all avenues of learning and enhances the rate of development in an orderly sequence.

References

1. Denhoff, E., and Robinault, I.: Cerebral Palsy and Related Disorders, A Developmental Approach. McGraw-Hill Book Co., New York, 1960.
2. Gesell, A., and Armatruda, C. S.: Developmental Diagnosis, Ed. 2. Paul B. Hoeber, Inc., New York, 1954.
3. Cruthers, B., and Paine, R. S.: The Natural History of Cerebral Palsy. Harvard University Press, Cambridge, Massachusetts, 1959.
4. Rood, M. S.: Neurophysiological reactions as a basis for physical therapy. Phys. Ther. Rev., 34: (9), 1954.
5. Knott, M., and Voss, D. E.: Proprioceptive Neuromuscular Facilitation. Paul B. Hoeber, Inc., New York, 1958.

SPECIFIC TESTS AND EVALUATION TOOLS

for the Child with Central Nervous System Deficit

SARAH SEMANS, M.A.

WHAT SHOULD BE ASSESSED?

To keep in focus the most important aspects of the problems to be assessed in the child with central nervous system deficit, it is well to keep in mind a broad view of the child's difficulty and its significance for him. A disorder in the brain may present a wide variety of behavioral difficulties. A child with such disorder has—in fact, has had from birth—problems of coping with his environment and interacting with it. Physical therapists must find out how they best can help him to function to the fullest extent of his potential, be it great or small.

Adapted from a paper presented at the Symposium on The Child with Central Nervous System Deficit, September 28–October 2, 1964, at The University of Pennsylvania, Philadelphia.

The author is Assistant Professor, Division of Physical Therapy, Stanford University School of Medicine, Palo Alto, California.

His problem has many aspects, some of which can be dealt with more effectively by other specialists. Certain aspects, however, can be most effectively handled by physical therapists. A rigid division of labor between therapists is unwise. Depending upon individual training and competence, the traditional roles of the physical, occupational, and speech therapist may overlap. Most physical therapists, however, will be chiefly concerned with the basic gross motor adaptations of the child to his environment. All specialists are concerned with maturation and learning.

Effort may be required to focus on those aspects of motor behavior which are of most concern and which must be evaluated. Because the distal parts of the child are most visible and because the physical therapist's training conditions him to look at muscles and joints, it is sometimes difficult to observe total patterns of motor behavior. It is important to learn to look at patterns of posture and movement in relation to central nervous system deficit in order to explore ways of altering such patterns in useful directions by stressing one or another pattern of input. To form an idea of the child's potential, the physical therapist needs to assess the extent and severity of the handicap coupled with the learning already accomplished. It is also necessary to know how well the child is responding to physical therapy procedures and his rate of progress.

A battery of tests is required, including motor ability, perceptual and intellectual status, and, when appropriate, prevocational and vocational aptitude. The present discussion will be concerned with assessment in the motor sphere. However, increasing recognition of the role of perception in learning should alert us to the need for testing in this area. Attention is called to the Perceptual Motor Test Battery prepared in 1964 by Dr. Jean Ayers.[1] It includes twenty-five tests, some of which are standardized psychological tests and some originally designed. In the book *Psychological Evaluation of the Cerebral Palsied Person* by Allen and Jefferson available tests are reviewed for intellectual, personality, and vocational assessment.[2]

Within the motor sphere three main areas are to be investigated: (1) developmental, (2) pathological, (3) adaptive.

DEVELOPMENTAL TESTS

One aspect of developmental evaluation has been very well worked out; that is, determination of the level of operation of the child or the milestones reached, based on the developmental scales of Gesell.[3] This information will be of value in several ways:

1. It will indicate where to start and what to strive for next in working with the child.

2. Translated to the parents, it will help them in understanding the child's limitations—what can and cannot be expected of him; it will establish agreement on the next step as immediate goal and it may help them in planning for the future.

3. Since there is usually a spread in level of achievement in different areas—more advance in some areas than others—it will indicate where to go trouble-shooting to find what is causing the delay. For instance, one may find a total flexion pattern in the arms interfering with development of prehension, or a persistent Moro reflex interfering with sitting balance. If one can remove the delaying factors, the child can develop on a broad front.

4. By charting successive examinations on a graph, the rate and general trend of development can be ascertained.

Although Gesell's norms and the developmental scales are standardized, the majority of tests derived from them for evaluation of the child with neurological deficit are not standardized. Reliability studies are lacking; instructions for administration of test items and criteria for successful accomplishment are not always clear or are lacking. Footh and Kogan, having noted such inadequacies, have overcome them in their General Motor Development Test.[4] The instructions and criteria for each item are quite clear, and their reliability in scoring is excellent.

In other tests reviewed, some items selected are not valid for cerebral-palsied children and in some tests, significant items are not included. For example, the item "takes full (or partial) support when placed on the feet" may not be valid for such children because the test procedure is likely to elicit pathological rigidity in the legs rather than showing the normal accretion of support tonus in the limbs which the test is intended to indicate. Tests of eye control and the breakdown in various levels of prehension are sometimes lacking.

The Developmental Screening Instrument of Dr. Hilda Knoblock has clear and specific instructions and sufficient detail.[5] The test items are grouped in five categories: adaptive, gross motor, fine motor, language, and personal-social. This division has the virtue of indicating the specific area of retardation. For instance, a child might have well-co-ordinated, discrete finger movements (fine motion) and yet not know how to use them for a useful purpose (adaptive).

Dr. Margaret Jones' *Appraisal of Progress in the Cerebral Palsied Child* has similar categories based on Gesell's norms, but is less detailed and lacks specific instructions.[6] The graphic summaries with these tests compare rates of physical growth and development in each area.

The Doman-Delacato Developmental Profile has the virtue of being brief—on one page—and includes a graphic summary.[7] A numerical score is derived from six categories at seven developmental stages. The categories are mobility, language, and manual, visual, auditory, and tactile competence. Instruction manuals are available for the mobility and language categories. The validity of the sample of mobility test items might be questioned because reciprocal organization and cerebral dominance are emphasized to the exclusion of some other aspects of motor development which may be of equal importance.

Another published developmental scale, the Blum-Fieldsteel Developmental Charts, includes a test for motor activities and a test for functional activities with a cumulative record for each.[8] It is well set up to show rate of development but it is impractical for any except the most mildly involved children since the early level items with which the physical therapist would be concerned over long periods are crowded together in the bottom of the record. Also, finer gradations of levels during the first eighteen months are needed.

The Motor Age Test of Johnson, Zuck, and Wingate is objective, reproducible by different testers, and gives a separate numerical score for upper and lower extremities.[9] Although useful for mildly involved children, it lacks discriminating items at the lower developmental levels.

Ingram, Withers, and Speltz [10] developed a similar test based on the Gesell developmental schedule and modification of the Johnson, Zuck, and Wingate tests. It ranges from four weeks to five years and yields a motor quotient and a social quotient.

The Dallas Motor Development Test is predominantly one of motor development of the trunk and extremeties as a whole.[11] It is geared toward the lower developmental levels and extends through the six-year age level. It has been used on 2,500 children over a ten-year period, but has not been tested for reliability, and criteria for some of the test items are not clear.

A Code Method for Evaluating Function in Cerebral Palsy developed at the Detroit Orthopedic Clinic is not strictly a developmental test.[12] There are four charts of function in speech, hand facility, balance and locomotion, and maturity. The test items are grouped according to developmental sequence in each. Some items are derived from Gesell's developmental schedules and some are from other sources. "The combined charts will convey a profile of the functional activity level of the child, expressed in a numerical code." The instructional manual and charts are well set up and the test items clearly described.

A number of other institutions have developed their own tests based on Gesell's developmental schedules.

A good standardized test form based on Gesell's norms should be available for physical therapists. It should have the majority of items from the period of birth to eighteen months, since this is the period of basic motor development. Items should be carefully selected and described. A companion test for finer skills should also include very early items such as visual control, but should extend into later chronological age periods. Questions arise, such as should one person administer all categories of the development test in a combined form? Should the physical therapist be trained to do this? Or, should each of the different categories be tested separately by a different specialist?

Although it is of great interest and will undoubtedly be worth while to try to correlate behavior patterns with specific brain mechanisms, present knowledge of central nervous system integration does not warrant the assignment of specific behavioral patterns to certain geographic levels of the brain in tests of this kind.

Mechanisms of Development

Missing in the type of developmental test described above, based on the achievement of milestones, is information about the developmental processes themselves which bring about the achievement of these milestones. The lack of tests in this area reflects the meager information which has been available concerning these important neurophysiological processes. These include those well-organized, mostly subcortical and automatic mechanisms which pattern most of the early behavior as well as the adult posture and movement patterns which are not consciously directed. They have been described as orientation or righting reactions, equilibrium reactions, reactions to progressive movements, approach and avoidance responses, defense and attack, other bodily expressions of emotion, and the somatic components of vegetative functions, *e.g.*, sucking, licking, spitting, chewing, defecating. (A number of these mechanisms are described in papers by Twitchell in this issue.[13, 14])

As André-Thomas points out, such responses are like reflexes but more complex and inconstant and their appearance depends upon the general state.[15] Although inborn, relatively few of these responses are present at birth but emerge in an organized sequence first in primitive form and gradually modified to the mature form.

Upright walking movements, for example, go through several stages. After inhibition of primary walking ("reflex stepping"), the hips flex in weight bearing and the feet drag if propelled along; then, an extensor phase begins, at first intermittent when the child beats or stamps a foot and bounces; gradually he begins to make steps again if pulled along, jerky and unpatterned, toes touching first.[15] Further progress awaits equilibrium, which, having gone through several stages in horizontal and sitting positions, is developed in standing by cruising laterally. The mechanisms of cruising (variously called "stembein," "d'arc-boutement," "protective extension," "propping," and "hopping" reactions) must be assessed. This same cruising pattern is then used in the child's first independent locomotion forward as a toddler with wide abduction of arms and legs, exaggerated lifting of legs, and lateral shift. Similar walking progressions of the arms precede those of the legs. Propping reactions of the arms develop in three recognized stages: in front at six–seven months, laterally at eight months, and posteriorly at ten–twelve months.[15]

It is even more important to assess mechanisms underlying the progressive development of prehension (see pages 419–423).[16]

Several aspects of the evolution of movement must be mentioned:

1. The progressive selectivity of movement from proximal to distal segments.

2. Co-ordination of compensatory trunk balance reactions with prehension, each assisting the other, *e.g.*, leaning forward with reaching up.

3. Equilibrium reactions of arms and legs which

combine with compensatory trunk reactions to secure sitting and standing.

4. Achievement of manipulative skills by co-ordination of the segregated wrist and finger movements with developing visual and tactile perception.

These and other components of co-ordinating mechanisms should be included in testing the underlying mechanisms of sensory-motor development. An increasing number of sources of information on mechanisms of development are available.[15, 17–23]

Equilibrium Reactions

Detailed studies of the equilibrium reactions [24–26] had not been utilized to any great extent nor their value appreciated until they were brought to our attention by the Bobaths.[27] Rademaker and Zador studied in detail with cinematographic records the patterns of these responses in animals and man, their maturation in the human infant from brief beginnings at four to six months to the mature forms at about six years.[24, 25] They also studied the effects on the equilibrium reactions of lesions of different parts of the central nervous system. Rademaker had found the receptors for equilibrium reactions to be the labyrinths and the limb proprioceptors. The brain stem from the 8th nerve to thalamus was required but not the cerebellum nor the striatum, nor was the cortex required for those in horizontal positions. The cortex is required for these responses in the upright positions in man. The responses are all present but exaggerated and poorly controlled in cerebellar ataxia. In athetoid children, the equilibrium responses are lively but often distorted.

Testing of these basic mechanisms of developing equilibrium would appear to be of particular importance to the physical therapist for treatment planning. In the manual on *Reflex Testing Methods* by Mary Fiorentino some of these reactions are included as well as some of the righting reactions.[28]

In a recent study by Ruth Ladue at Stanford University, a group of supposedly normal children between six and eight years were given, as part of a more extensive evaluation, some of these equilibrium tests.[29] A few of these children still showed the transitional form of the reactions characteristic of the three- and four-year levels. This entire test which included the later stages of gross motor development and elements of motor function was designed to test minimal cerebral dysfunction.

PATHOLOGICAL ASPECTS

As often pointed out, evaluation of the child with neurological deficit should include not only *what* he can do but how he does it. The developmental activities and their underlying mechanisms just discussed, as well as activity of a more volitional or planned nature, are distorted, delayed, or blocked completely by the effects of the brain injury or defect. Assessment of the child should indicate in some way the nature and extent of the interference. Tonic brainstem and spinal reflexes may be released by lesions of those higher centers which normally reorganize them. These prevent selectivity of movement and adaptation of posture as the Bobaths have shown.[27] As Denny-Brown has pointed out, the abnormal motor manifestations resulting from brain injury are expressions of disequilibrium of conflicting elements of behavior at various levels of integration.[30] One or the other type of primitive conflicting responses (avoidance or reaching out) may dominate, or they may fluctuate from one to the other without being resolved, as observed in athetoid and dystonic postures and movements. A distinction should be made if possible between the frankly pathological posture and movement responses and those of a normal but immature nervous system which may resemble them. This requires clinical judgment based on familiarity with normal infants.

Tests for some of these abnormal postural reflexes are illustrated in Fiorentino's manual.[28] Others can be found among the tests used in neurological examinations of infants. Another way of assessing abnormality is illustrated in the Cerebral Palsy Assessment Chart for Basic Motor Control tests reported here (pages 463–468) which was constructed to indicate degree of freedom from these abnormal influences.[31]

The state of muscle tone is recorded routinely in neurological examinations. The French neurologists consider several aspects of tone. André-Thomas [15] distinguishes three components: (1) consistency, tested by palpation, (2) extensibility, tested by range of muscular lengthening, and (3) passivité, tested by resistance to passive stretching. Tardieu in the French manual on Cerebral Palsy, *I.M.C.*, has a range-of-motion chart in which these components of tone are recorded.[32] The same manual contains an interesting code method of assessing the various aspects of athetosis.

ADAPTIVE ASPECTS

Functional activities or achievement tests have long been used in evaluating children with cerebral palsy. Most institutions have evolved a suitable test of activities of daily living, many adapted from the original test by Brown.[33] Tests which block in successful achievements with color are easy to see at a glance and are favored by therapists and children. Such tests are often joint projects of physical and occupational therapists. As bracing and special equipment are becoming less frequently used in training programs, items such as getting in and out of braces and managing special equipment are being deleted. Wheel chair management and use of crutches in postsurgical cases should be included where appropriate. It is important to continue testing competence in everyday activities.

THE ASSESSMENT CHART OF MOTOR ABILITIES

The Assessment Chart of Motor Abilities is intended as one of a battery of tests.[31] It is concerned with basic postural controls which underlie functional activities. It contains prerequisites for arm use, moving about, control of body segments relative to gravity, getting up and down, and the stance phase of walking. Movement proceeds from posture which is not static but variable with the movement it supports.

A series of test postures adapted from those originally developed by the Bobaths are utilized.[34] Each of the test postures constitutes a patterned, measured input stimulus which is applied, and the response is graded with reference to that of a normal child. The test is operational in that specific behavioral responses are utilized to reveal presence of or freedom from the pathological processes which would interfere with their accomplishment. Thus, freedom from hypertonus is measured by the ability to be placed and remain in a position which is the reverse of the tonic pattern. The full range of motion demanded also indicates presence or absence of adaptive shortening. If the test posture cannot be attained initially, maneuvers to release tension are used to determine whether the limitation is a result of hypertonus or contracture. Tardieu found in his joint range tests that such maneuvers were as effective as curare in differentiating these limiting factors.[32]

Lack of sufficient tone or flaccidity is indicated by failure to maintain the required antigravity positions.

To grade the quality of active movement, the child is asked to assume the test posture independently, and is graded 3, 4, or 5 according to the manner of accomplishment. Thus, the influence upon movement of dyskinesia and fluctuating tone, as in conflicting athetoid postures, would be indicated by the grade. Minor states of spastic hypertonus which slow movement or necessitate effort are also indicated by less than normal grade even if the test item is accomplished.

The individual items are designed to show degree of freedom from the abnormal posture and movement patterns which would prevent or distort assumptions of the test postures. The items are grouped in supine, prone, sitting, kneeling, and standing postures.

Aspects of the child's problem which are measured include:

1. Automatic postural adjustment to the imposed position.
2. Inhibition or control over abnormal postural reflexes.
3. Limitations of range of movement.
4. Capacity for motor learning (reproducing the postural pattern).
5. Readiness for specific developmental activities.
6. Rate of progress.

Development of the Assessment Chart

The Assessment Chart of Motor Abilities was developed by a group of physical and occupational therapists in Northern California—supervisors in state and county programs for physically handicapped children and physical therapy school instructors. Two motivating factors underlay the project. First was the need to replace the outmoded "Basic Motor Abilities Test" in current use in the school program. This test was considered unsatisfactory because its construction was based on inadequate understanding of the neurophysiology involved. The second motive grew out of the Bobaths' visit to the United States and their course at Stanford University in 1958. The course, under the joint auspices of Stanford University and the State Crippled Children's Services, was sponsored by The Children's Bureau which requested a follow-up evaluation of the treatment methods introduced. Such an evaluation seemed a reasonable request at the time; a committee was established for this purpose and proceeded to search for a suitable instrument for evaluating the results of treatment. Several alternative test forms were considered.

The need for determining developmental status of the child was recognized, but a developmental test alone failed to indicate the pathological aspects of the child's motor behavior and the subsequent changes in respect to such abnormal influences. Qualitative testing of posture and movement responses at each developmental level proved too cumbersome. A modified form of Bobaths' Assessment Chart was finally chosen as being most suitable.[34]

The grading system was changed from six to five grades, some items were eliminated, and the wording of other items was changed to make the test items as objective as possible and to increase the reliability of the test as a whole.

Revisions were made following each of several field trials. With forty-six examiners, there was 61 per cent agreement on a choice of six grades (0-5); 85 per cent agreed within one grade, 96 per cent within two grades, and 99 per cent within three grades. This agreement among examiners was comparable to that among those giving manual muscle tests for poliomyelitis during the Salk vaccine field trials [35] and was considered adequate for the purpose.

A further study of the test was made to compare the test scores to scores on a developmental test given the same group of children and also to relate the test scores to certain functional activities.[36]

Comparison of test scores on the Assessment Chart with those on the Dallas Developmental Test showed a coefficient of correlation of .87. In relating the assessment scores to specific activities, it was found that early activities such as prone support on forearms with trunk extension and face vertical and secure sitting could be predicted within narrow limits. Independent walking, however, showed a wide spread of scores, which may result from the grading system which indicates quality of the performance.

In revising the Assessment Chart, a number of the original test items were omitted because of difficulty in applying the grading system to them. These were "moving" tests, mostly automatic in nature involving righting and equilibrium responses. Since these developmental mechanisms are important to assess both for treatment planning and recording progress, a supplement to the present test is being developed in which such automatic responses can be checked plus or minus. In addition to protective and equilibrium reactions of trunk and limbs, patterns of turning over, getting up, and reciprocal organization in locomotion can be included.

The Assessment Chart has proved useful in analysis of the child's motor problem, in guiding treatment, and in checking progress. The numerical score in the form of a motor quotient can be used in a graph along with the results of other types of tests to give an over-all picture of progress.

The original purpose of evaluating a new system of treatment turned out to be impractical and invalid. First, the training of physical therapists in the special skills involved time off for special training. Then, orientation of the treatment "team" (including parent training) was necessary for consistency of approach. Difficulties arose in a public school program. Since many of the programs were orthopedically oriented, it was difficult to find a group of children who could be followed for several years without the complication of bracing or surgery. Since public school physical therapists do not go into the homes and parents could not be present for treatment, and since it is generally agreed that the skill of the parent in handling the child and other outside activities have a much greater influence on the child than the half-hour periods with the physical therapist, this variable seemed uncontrollable.

Finally, and most important, the various "systems" of treatment which are neurologically oriented have much in common and utilize many of the same principles and procedures. A good physical therapist who understands the motor problem probably would use similar procedures to attack the same problem regardless of the system in which he was trained. It is quite possible that two physical therapists following one system might vary in their approach to the child as much as two trained in different systems. These many uncontrolled variables make it useless to attempt to compare one person's "system" of procedures with another's system.

However, it might be worth while to compare the effectiveness of specific procedures, *e.g.,* to combat the problem of hip flexion and internal rotation in diplegia. Or one might compare the results of teaching a patient to walk with braces and crutches with the standard methods used for lower motor neuron disorders and of teaching a patient a developmental program emphasizing facilitation of righting and equilibrium reactions or reciprocal patterning. One could compare in a state mental hospital the advantages of an S.O.S. (Stimulation of Senses) program over one of routine nursing care. In a day-care center, one could assess the value of a developmental program in comparison to one purely diversional. With a large group of hemiplegic children, the relative effectiveness of tactile stimulation with prehensile activities and a program emphasizing the postural supportive function of the arm might be compared. One might determine whether the improvement in a program of motor co-ordination would be reflected in the school work or social adjustment of children with "minimal brain damage." Many other pressing problems will occur to those working with children with neurological deficit for which the effectiveness of suggested procedures or types of management can be evaluated with appropriate testing instruments.

SUMMARY

Some specific tests to determine how well the child with neurological deficit can interact with his environment in the motor sphere have been reviewed. These included assessment of the developmental, pathological, and adaptive aspects of his problem. A standardized developmental test with emphasis on the early stages is needed. Further work is needed to devise tests of the inborn, automatic mechanisms underlying motor adjustment to the environment. Possible uses of evaluation tools in determining effectiveness of specific procedures and types of management were discussed.

REFERENCES

1. Ayres, A. J.: Perceptual Motor Test Battery. In Ayres Space Test. Los Angeles: Western Psychological Services, 1962.
2. Allen, R. M., and Jefferson, T. W.: Psychological Evaluation of the Cerebral Palsied Person. Springfield, Illinois: Charles C Thomas, 1962.
3. Gesell, A., and Amatruda, C.: Developmental Diagnosis. New York: Paul B. Hoeber, 1947.
4. Footh, W. K., and Kogan, K. L.: Measuring the effectiveness of physical therapy in the treatment of cerebral palsy, J. Amer. Phys. Ther. Ass., 43:867–873, December 1963.
5. Knoblock, H.: Developmental Screening Instrument. Columbus, Ohio: Child Development Service, The Children's Hospital, 1963. (Mimeographed.)
6. Jones, M. H.: Appraisal of progress in the cerebral palsied child. In Proceedings, Fourth Symposium on

Cerebral Palsy by the Research Council. United Cerebral Palsy Association, Inc., New York Academy of Medicine, November 15, 1952. Pamphlet published and distributed by United Cerebral Palsy Association of Los Angeles County.

7. Doman, G. J., Delacato, C. H., and Doman, R. J.: The Doman-Delacato Developmental Profile; and Doman, G. J., and Moran, P.: The Doman-Moran Graphic Summary. Philadelphia: The Institutes for the Achievement of Human Potential, 1964.
8. Blum, L. H., and Fieldsteel, N. D.: Blum-Fieldsteel Developmental Charts. New York: World Book Company, 1952.
9. Johnson, M. K., Zuck, F. N., and Wingate, K.: The motor age test: Measurement of motor handicap in children with neuromuscular disorders such as cerebral palsy, J. Bone Joint Surg. (Amer.) 33:693–707, July 1951.
10. Ingram, A. J., Withers, E., and Speltz, E.: Role of intensive physical and occupational therapy in the treatment of cerebral palsy: Testing and results, Arch. Phys. Med., 40:429–438, October 1959.
11. Dallas Society for Crippled Children: The Dallas Motor Development Test. 1963. (Mimeographed.)
12. Anderson, R., Bargowski, E., and Blodgett, W. H.: A Code Method for Evaluating Function in Cerebral Palsy. Detroit: Detroit Orthopaedic Clinic, 1961.
13. Twitchell, Thomas E.: Attitudinal reflexes, J. Amer. Phys. Ther. Ass., 45:411–418, May 1965.
14. Twitchell, Thomas E.: Variations and abnormalities of motor development, J. Amer. Phys. Ther. Ass., 45:424–430, May 1965.
15. André-Thomas, Chesni, Y., and Saint-Anne Dargassies, S.: The Neurological Examination of the Infant. Little Club Clinics in Developmental Medicine, No. 1. London: National Spastics Society, 1960.
16. Twitchell, Thomas E.: Normal motor development, J. Amer. Phys. Ther. Ass., 45:419–423, May 1965.
17. Peiper, A.: Cerebral Function in Infancy and Childhood. New York: Consultants Bureau, 1963.
18. Twitchell, Thomas E.: On the motor deficit in congenital bilateral athetosis, J. Nerv. Ment. Dis., 129:105–132, August 1959.
19. Paine, Richmond S.: The immediate value of neonatal neurological examination. In Child Neurology and Cerebral Palsy. Little Club Clinics in Developmental Medicine, No. 2. London: National Spastics Society, 1962, pp. 62–68.
20. Illingworth, R. S.: An Introduction to Developmental Assessment in the First Year. Little Club Clinics in Developmental Medicine, No. 3. London: National Spastics Society, 1962.
21. Prechtl, H., and Beintema, D.: The Neurological Examination of the Full-Term Infant. Little Club Clinics in Developmental Medicine, No. 12. London: The Spastics Society Medical Education and Information Unit, William Heinemann Medical Books, Ltd., 1964.
22. Films: Neurological Examination of the Newborn Infant and Neurological Examination of the 1-year-old Infant. Narrated by Richmond S. Paine. Available on loan from United Cerebral Palsy Association, Inc., 321 East 44th Street, New York, New York 10036.
23. Film: Neurological Examination of Infants. Paul Ellwood. 28 minutes, sound. Available on loan from Kenny Rehabilitation Institute, Minneapolis 4, Minnesota.
24. Rademaker, G. G. J.: Reactions Labyrinthiques et Equilibre. Paris: Masson et Cie., 1935.
25. Zador, J.: Les Reactions d'Equilibre Chez l'Homme. Paris: Masson et Cie., 1938.
26. Weisz, S.: Studies in equilibrium reactions, J. Nerv. Ment. Dis., 88:150–162, 1938.
27. Bobath, B.: A study of abnormal postural reflex activity in patients with lesions of the central nervous system, Physiotherapy, 40:259–267, 295–300, 326–334, 368–373, September, October, November, December 1954.
28. Fiorentino, M. R.: Reflex Testing Methods for Evaluating C.N.S. Development. Springfield, Illinois: Charles C Thomas, 1963.
29. Ladue, R. A.: Evaluation of basic motor abilities for patients with neuromuscular dysfunction, unpublished Master's thesis, Stanford University.
30. Denny-Brown, D.: The Basal Ganglia and Their Relation to Disorders of Movement. New York: Oxford University Press, 1962.
31. Semans, Sarah, et. al.: A cerebral palsy assessment chart, J. Amer. Phys. Ther. Ass., 45:463–468, May 1965.
32. Tardieu, G.: Bilan et caracteres distinctifs des diverses raideurs d'origine cerebrale. Les Feuillets de l'Infirmite Motrice Cerebrale, Volume II. Paris: Association Nationale des Infirmes Moteurs-Cerebraux.
33. Brown, M. E.: Daily activity inventories of cerebral palsy children in experimental classes, Phys. Ther. Rev., 30:415–421, October 1950.
34. Bobath, K.: The long-term results of treatment. In Child Neurology and Cerebral Palsy. Little Club Clinics in Developmental Medicine, No. 2. London: National Spastics Society, 1960.
35. Lilienfeld, A. M., Jacobs, M., and Willis, M.: A study of the reproducibility of muscle testing and certain other aspects of muscle scoring, Phys. Ther. Rev., 34: 279–289, June 1954.
36. Mosser, D. A.: An evaluative study of a cerebral palsy assessment chart, unpublished Master's thesis, Stanford University.

A Cerebral Palsy Assessment Chart

Instructions for Administration of the Test

SARAH SEMANS, M.A., ROSALYN PHILLIPS, B.A., MADELINE ROMANOLI, R.N., RUTH MILLER, B.S. and MARY SKILLEN, B.A.

SOURCE AND BASIS OF SELECTION OF TEST ITEMS

The test items were selected and adapted from the Asssesment Chart developed by Karel Bobath, M.D., and Berta Bobath, F.C.S.P.[1] The general arrangement follows that of the original tests.

The decision to use the series of test postures for assessment of motor ability was based on the following considerations. Movements, which evolve into functional activities, can serve no practical purpose unless they can be supported and controlled by the appropriate postures which render them effective. Lacking their underlying postural control, attempted movements are haphazard and cannot be sustained to reach their goal. Well-defined postural patterns appear in an orderly sequence as the child develops. By selecting characteristic postural patterns simple enough for accurate observation, the assessment can be reasonably objective. The progress sequence from hori-

From the Division of Physical Therapy, Stanford University School of Medicine, Palo Alto, California, and the Department of Public Health, Bureau of Crippled Children's Services, State of California, Berkeley.

TABLE 1

CEREBRAL PALSY ASSESSMENT CHART
BASIC MOTOR CONTROL

Name:________________________Birthdate:________________Diagnosis:________________

Examiner:		Name:		Name:		Name	
Test Postures and Movements		Date	Remarks	Date	Remarks	Date	Remarks
Supine 1. Hips and knees fully flexed, arms crossed, palms on shoulders.	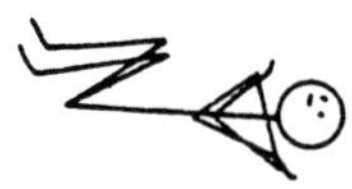						
2. Hips and knees fully flexed. (a) Extend right leg. (b) Extend left leg.	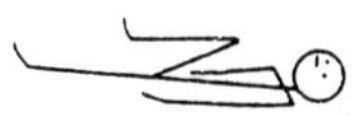	R. L.		R. L.		R. L.	
3. Head raised.	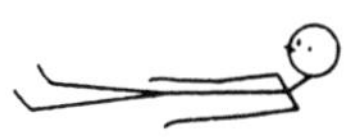						
Prone 4. Arms extended beside head. Raise head in midposition.	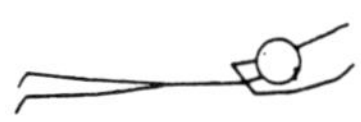						
5. Arms extended beside body, palms down.	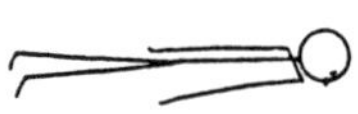						
6. (a) Flex right knee, hips extended. (b) Flex left knee, hips extended.	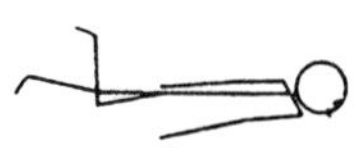	R. L.		R. L.		R. L.	
7. Trunk supported on forearms, upper trunk extended, face vertical.	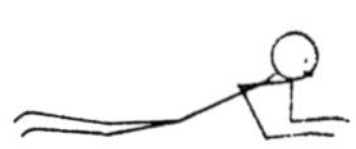						
8. Trunk supported on hands with elbows and hips extended.	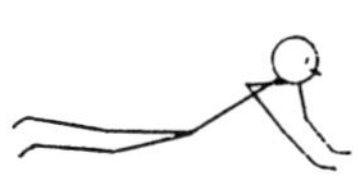						
Sitting erect 9. Soles of feet together, hips flexed and externally rotated to at least 45°.	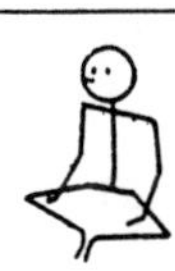						
10. Knees extended and legs abducted; hips 90°–100°.	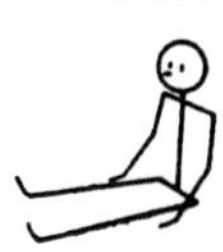						

TABLE 1—Continued

CEREBRAL PALSY ASSESSMENT CHART
BASIC MOTOR CONTROL

Name:________________ Diagnosis:________________ Birthdate:________________

Examiner:		Name:		Name:		Name:	
Test Postures and Movements		Date	Remarks	Date	Remarks	Date	Remarks
11. Legs hanging over edge of table. (a) Extend right knee. (b) Extend left knee.	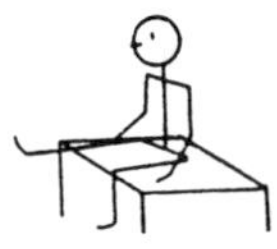	R. L.		R. L.		R. L.	
Kneeling 12. Back and neck straight (not hyperextended). (a) Weight on knees. (b) Weight on hands.	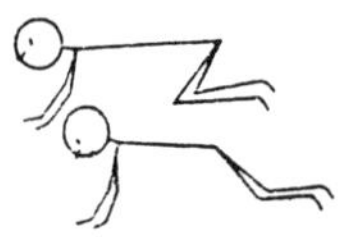	a b		a b		a b	
13. Side sitting, upper trunk erect, arms relaxed: (a) On right hip. (b) On left hip.	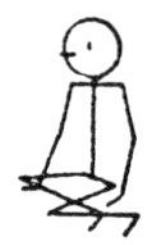	R. L.		R. L.		R. L.	
14. Kneeling upright, hips extended, head in midposition, arms at sides.	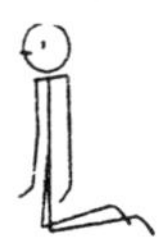						
15. (a) Half kneeling: weight on right knee. (b) Half kneeling: weight on left knee.	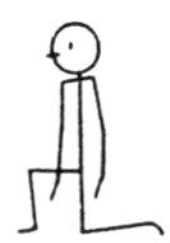	R. L.		R. L.		R. L.	
Squatting 16. Heels down, toes not clawed, knees pointing in same direction as toes, hips fully flexed, head in line with trunk.	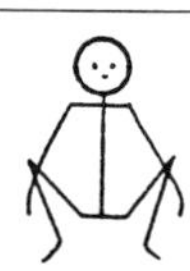						
Standing and components of walking 17. Standing, correct alignment.	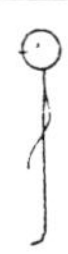						
18. Pelvis and trunk aligned over forward leg. Both knees extended. (a) Right leg forward. (b) Left leg forward.	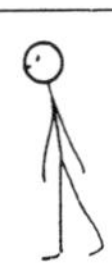	R. L.		R. L.		R. L.	
19. Bear weight on one leg in midstance. (a) Shift weight over right leg. (b) Shift weight over left leg.	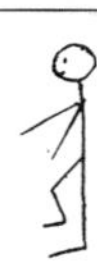	R. L.		R. L.		R. L.	
20. Heel strike. Rear leg extended and externally rotated, heel down. Both knees straight: (a) Right heel strike. (b) Left heel strike.	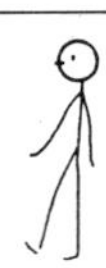	R. L.		R. L.		R. L.	

zontal to upright postures indicates how far the child has come in his development of postural control.

Information Yielded by the Test

In cerebral palsy, the state of muscle tone and abnormal patterns of movement interfere with the orderly sequence of motor development. The test postures selected show the nature and extent of this interference. Ability to sustain a test posture not previously possible indicates a freedom from that pathological state which had prevented its achievement. The significance of such newly gained freedom is that it makes possible the learning of new skills. For example, when a child achieves postural support on the arms, indicating a freedom from hypertonus of the flexor muscles, he can learn hand skills which persistent flexion would not have permitted. Thus, the various items representing basic postural controls which underlie support and alignment of the body with respect to gravity, hand use, and locomotion indicate whether or not there is sufficient freedom from pathological influences to develop useful skills in each of these areas. In the early tests, attention is focused on control of proximal parts; in later tests, greater individuation and segregation from the total limb synergies is required.

By noting limitations in range of motion which prevent passive positioning in the test postures, the assessment can also serve as a range-of-motion test.

Ease and quality of movement are indicated by the numerical grade for the active movement when the child is asked to assume the test position.

Since each of the test items has some developmental significance and since total scores were found to correlate closely with developmental test scores, the assessment yields information regarding developmental status of the child.

The initial test serves as a guide in planning treatment procedures by indicating areas of needed emphasis. Increase in total score may represent the effects of maturation, or treatment, or a combination of both factors. Changes in either a negative or positive direction in specific areas may reflect the relative effectiveness of treatment.

Explanation of Testing Procedures

Throughout the testing, the therapist should insure maximal freedom from emotional and physical tension through proper handling. In all tests, the therapist should first place the child in the test position. Physical manipulation to reduce tension should be used if this factor interferes with placement. If the therapist is unable to place the patient, inability to relax tension or the presence of contractures or structural deviations are indicated. Secondly, after being placed, the child is asked to stay in the test position. As a third step, he is asked to *move into* the test position independently.

Grading Through Use of a Key

A grading system with values from 0 to 5 is used as follows:

0—Cannot be placed in test posture.

1—Can be placed in test posture, but the position cannot be held.

2—Can hold test posture momentarily after being placed.

3—Can assume an approximate test posture unaided, in any manner.

4—Can assume and sustain test posture in a near normal manner (note any abnormal detail).

5—Normal.

Interpretation of Use of Key in Grading

Grades 0 to 2 indicate the severity of the handicap as tested by resistance to passive motion, by limitation of joint range, or by ability to maintain posture. These are static tests. *Grades 3 to 5* indicate the quality of movement when performed actively by the patient. *Grades 3 to 5 would not be given when grades 1 and 2 cannot be attained.*

If for any reason the child cannot be placed, he is given a grade of 0 and a note is made to explain, under appropriate REMARK column, why, *e.g.*, a child with an elbow flexion contracture, even though he can assume a posture normally except for the use of the elbow, would be graded 0 on all test postures requiring complete elbow extension.

For a *grade of 2,* it is only necessary to maintain the test posture momentarily. This indicates some control over the disabling factors.

For *grades of 3 to 5,* it is important that the child understands what is expected of him when he is asked to move into the test position. Proper placing will usually be sufficient, but visual cues such as a demonstration by the therapist or the use of dolls or stick figures or assistance given preceding the test may be helpful.

Grade 4 requires the child to *assume* and *sustain* the test position, but allows for slight abnormality of movement, or a lack of a very few degrees from the test posture into which he could be placed passively. For example, a spastic child may not be able to achieve the same degree of extension of the thoracic spine in the sitting position as he could in the supine or prone positions, or he may have slower than normal movement; the athetoid child may perform the complete movement, except for tension or extraneous movement in some distal part.

To obtain a *grade of 5,* each test should be exactly as indicated.

In judging whether a movement is normal, the following qualities should be considered: normal movement—smooth, easy, free, and in the line of movement; abnormal movement—jerky, tremorous, sluggish, labored, or deviating from the line of movement.

Testing Hemiplegia

In hemiplegia, the primary consideration should be that of evaluating the affected side.

SPECIFIC INSTRUCTIONS FOR ADMINISTERING THE TEST ITEMS

Each item in the test represents a necessary postural control for various functional activities. For instance, the arm position in Test 1 is a prerequisite for engaging the hands in front of the body and for later self-help activities. Other test positions will be recognized as stages of postural control preparatory to creeping, sitting, standing, and walking. It is helpful to keep in mind the functional significance of each test while administering it in order to observe the most critical aspects contributing to the test score. The following groups are arranged in the approximate order of normal developmental sequence.

Supine

Test 1

Purpose. To test freedom from extensor hypertonus in the supine position. Emphasis in this test is on proximal joints.

Bring knees, one after the other, to chest with enough external rotation at hips to point knees toward axillae. This is needed to get complete flexion; if not attained, there is probably not full range of hip flexion. Steady knees in position with your body while placing child's arms as follows: Pull arms forward at shoulders, abducting the scapulae, and fold across chest so that open palms cup shoulders; arms should be up, away from chest wall; head should remain in a neutral position; feet should be relaxed in plantar flexion. If child assumes position except for dorsiflexed feet or incompletely relaxed hands, grade 4 should be given.

Test 2

Purpose. To test ability to flex or extend one leg at a time through full range.

Starting with hips and knees fully flexed, arms across chest or relaxed at side, bring right leg down to table in an extended position, avoiding internal rotation. Back should not arch. Return to starting position and repeat with left leg.

Test 3

Purpose. To test ability to raise head.

Place in a symmetrical supine position with legs extended and arms at sides. Raise head by flexing at the atlanto-occipital joint and in the cervical spine. The shoulders remain relaxed. If the child can raise the head but protracts the shoulder, a grade of 3 is given.

Prone

Test 4

Purpose. To test freedom from flexor hypertonus in prone position.

Place prone, lift under shoulder to free arm; place arms overhead one after the other, elbows and wrists extended, palms down, legs extended and relaxed. Head is raised in midposition. Replace arms below shoulder level before asking child to move into test position.

Test 5

Purpose. To test freedom of arms and shoulders from flexor hypertonus in prone position.

Place prone, arms beside body, palms down. To extricate arms from under the body, lift the shoulder and externally rotate arm. Place hands out a short distance from the body so that arms are not pressed against the thorax. To assume position actively, start with arms at shoulder level or above. Note any change of tension resulting from turning head from one side to the other.

Test 6

Purpose. To test selective control of hip and knee.

Place prone, arms relaxed beside head or at sides. Flex right knee to 90 degrees without flexion at hip. The foot should not dorsiflex; other leg should remain relaxed. Repeat with left leg. For grade 4 or 5, there should be no appreciable motion in the hip.

Test 7

Purpose. To test postural control in spinal extension.

This is important for beginning locomotion (crawling), erect sitting, and beginning use of hands. Place prone, extend thoracic spine, and place arms one after the other in at least 90 degrees shoulder flexion and slight abduction, supported on forearms. Head is raised with face vertical. Arms point straight ahead and hands are open.

Test 8

Purpose. To test ability to support weight on extended arms.

Start from test position 7. Lift child's head giving gentle traction on cervical spine so that support is on extended arms and heel of open hand; entire spine and hips are fully extended. Alternate method: Lift under shoulders or under chest. This position is often difficult to attain but is necessary for creeping.

Sitting Erect

Test 9

Purpose. To test control of hips in flexion, abduction, and external rotation.

Place in erect sitting position with legs abducted, flexed, and externally rotated to at least 45 degrees; soles of feet together, arms relaxed. For grades 3 to 5, start in any sitting position on flat surface.

Test 10

Purpose. To test erect sitting with legs straight.

Place in erect sitting position with thighs abducted without internal rotation, and with knees extended; angle at hip should be 90 to 100 degrees, arms relaxed.

Test 11

Purpose. To test selective control of hip and knee.

Place in erect sitting position, angle at hip 90 to 100 degrees, legs hanging vertically. Extend knee fully without further extension of hip. Other leg and arms should remain relaxed. (a) Right knee extended; (b) left knee extended.

Kneeling

Test 12

Purpose. To test weight-bearing and balance control on knees and heels of open hands.

Start in four-point kneeling, back and neck straight (not hyperextended), legs parallel, elbows extended, hands pointing forward. (a) Weight predominantly on knees; (b) weight predominantly on hands.

Test 13

Purpose. To test ability of trunk to adapt to gravitational changes.

Place in side sitting from four-point or upright kneeling by lowering the hips to one side of feet. Head and upper trunk should be erect; arms free. (a) On right hip; (b) on left hip.

Test 14

Purpose. To test anterior-posterior control of pelvis and trunk on thighs.

Place in upright kneeling position, hips extended, legs parallel, trunk and head erect, head in midposition, arms relaxed.

Test 15

Purpose. To test control of rotation at hip.

Place in half-kneeling position from upright kneeling. The other foot is placed on floor in front and to the side for adequate supporting base. Hip, knee, and ankle of forward leg at 90 degrees, toes not clawed. Pelvis and trunk face forward, knee slightly outward.

Squatting

Test 16

Purpose. To test control of extensor spasticity.

Place from squat sitting, *i.e.,* legs and hips fully flexed and outwardly rotated, feet flat on floor, toes not clawed, knees pointing in same direction as toes, arms forward for balance. Shift weight forward over feet into squatting position. Older child can be placed from a low stool. It is easier to assume this position if the legs are spread wide apart.

Standing and Components of Walking

Test 17

Purpose. To test normal distribution of tone in standing.

Place in standing position with body segments in normal alignment with relation to the line of gravity in midcoronal and midsagittal planes, *i.e.,* weight evenly distributed over both feet, legs in midposition of rotation, and so on. Points of control might be the hip of one side and the knee of opposite side, or hip and opposite arm. A lift may be used to equalize leg length.

Test 18

Purpose. To test the ability to shift weight forward onto stance leg with rear leg extended ready for push off.

Place in forward step position. Shift weight over forward leg with trunk, pelvis, thigh, and leg correctly aligned over foot. Rear leg should be extended, outwardly rotated at hip, and resting on the normal roll-off point (the head of the first metatarsal); arms should be relaxed. For grades 2 to 5, the therapist may steady child by holding one hand.

Test 19

Purpose. To test the ability to support the body over one leg (absence of Trendelenberg sign).

From a symmetrical standing position, shift weight laterally over one leg and lift the other free of the floor, as for the swing phase of walking. Trunk should remain erect. For grades 2 to 5, therapist may steady child by holding one hand.

Test 20

Purpose. To test heel strike.

One foot is advanced in dorsiflexion and heel placed on the floor. Weight is supported mainly on rear leg, hip extended, both knees straight. Ankles remain at approximately 90 degrees. Arms should be relaxed. For grades 2 to 5, therapist may steady child by holding one hand.

REFERENCE

1. Bobath, K.: The long-term results of treatment. In Child Neurology and Cerebral Palsy. Little Club Clinics in Developmental Medicine, No. 2. London: National Spastics Society, 1960.

A Preliminary Report

Use of a Developmental Inventory as a Chart of Progress

M. ANN WILLSON, B.A.

Because increased knowledge and improved techniques make possible earlier diagnosis so that physical therapists see patients earlier and try to avoid defective patterns of motor behavior, contractures, and other deformities, "The Inventory of Development" can offer guidelines and documentation of progress made during the course of physical therapy. The "Inventory" is based on patterns of development, care, and the handling of children from the time of birth.

THIS PAPER ADVANCES the premise that records intended to report the effect of physical therapy on a child with a congenital disorder must include an assessment of that child's development compared with normal development. Correlatively, "normal" should be represented by the most reliable standard available. The standard suggested here is the chronology of behavioral development presented in the works of Gesell,[1] Illingworth,[2] and Knobloch.[3]

From the Division of Maternal, Child, and Crippled Children's Services, Delaware State Board of Health, Dover 19901.

Adapted from an original paper presented at the Forty-fifth Annual Conference of the American Physical Therapy Association, Chicago, Illinois, June 30–July 5, 1968.

The purpose of this paper, therefore, is to describe the preparation and use of an inventory of development as a chart of progress.

No amount of argument in favor of use of a test is as persuasive as the opportunity to administer that test and utilize the results. While at the Children's Hospital of Philadelphia, the author had the good fortune to be included in a collaborative effort with an occupational therapist and speech pathologists administering a developmental inventory for screening purposes. More recently, with the staff of the Delaware State Board of Health, the inventory form has been revised for use as a record of progress. Review of the literature during the revision process revealed that administration of the entire Gesell Schedules (a lengthy process) is usually carried out by psychologists, but shorter forms have been adapted to aid in diagnosis, prognosis, and evaluation of effects of treatment.[4–10] The terminology is becoming widely used and understood by all who deal with children, even their parents. Developmental assessments are recommended for use by nurses in casefinding,[4, 5] and by physicians, educators, and others for screening.[6–10] It follows on the continuum of medical management for children who deviate from normal motor development that physical therapists should utilize developmental schedules to chart progress of those children toward normal.

The author does not suggest abandonment of special tests that have been developed by physical therapists for evaluation of a patient's clinical course based on the diagnosis or treatment rationale. However, such tests are valid only insofar as they take into account changes that occur normally with growth and development of the human body. Three examples that bear out this point are:

1. Manual muscle testing, using the parameters of flexibility and strength, gives useful information about the extent of disability or recovery of muscle function in patients with neuropathies and myopathies and provides a basis for a program of exercise. Obviously strength usually increases with growth, and we are all well aware of the difficulties in determining what is normal strength for an infant. Age-level variations in flexibility are more subtle (and usually show a decrease in contrast to strength changes), but flexibility variations affect the very bases of performing muscle tests. "Accurate data regarding . . . normal flexibility . . . should constitute a guide in determining whether individual ability to accomplish certain movements is normal or abnormal." [11]

2. Records of patients' achievements in activities of daily living (ADL) extend the meaning of loss, recovery, or improvement of function in terms of level of independence. ADL tests are useless for application to children unless they take into account the chronological age at which achievement is to be expected. This touches on the effect of maturation.

3. Tests of response to body position in space and manipulation (tactile and proprioceptive stimulation) [12–14] yield information about *development* of control over primitive reflexes and postural mechanisms so that the effect of maturation is built into the test.

Postnatal maturation is dependent upon integrity of embryonic development, genetic inheritance, and metabolism. Effectiveness of physical therapy must be influenced by rate and degree of maturation, especially of musculoskeletal and central nervous systems. The Gesell scales are composed of behavioral manifestations of the integrated functioning of the musculoskeletal and nervous systems as well as the visual and auditory apparatus.

Developmental Tests in Use

The idea of use of developmental tests by physical therapists is not new. Phelps pointed out the importance of following a developmental scale in planning a therapeutic program for children with cerebral palsy such that activities would be (presented and) learned in the proper order without missing fundamentals. He presented a scale of twenty-five items listed in sequential order according to the chronology of normal development.[15]

In 1964 Semans recommended construction of a developmental scale for use by physical therapists in evaluation of children with central nervous system deficits.[16] She enumerated some uses of information gained from tests based on the developmental scales of Gesell as:

1. Indication of baseline and goals.

2. Statement of treatment goals in language suitable for explanation to parents (and this author adds, for discussion with professional colleagues).

3. Localization of factors delaying motor development by examination of a child's level of behavior in several areas.

4. Recognition of rate and general trend of development by compiling serial test results.

Semans also provided a valuable review and critique of developmental scales that had previously been reported in use by physical therapists. She found among them some common problems, such as lack of studies of reliability for application to this special population, inadequate instructions for administration, undefined criteria for accomplishment of items, inclusion of inappropriate items, and exclusion of pertinent items.

The developmental tests of Gesell are divided into four areas of behavior: motor, adaptive, language, and personal–social. Tests that have been adapted from the Gesell Schedules for use by physical therapists have usually been confined to the behavioral areas specifically defined as motor development. The Dallas Motor Development Test [17] is limited to development of posture and locomotion. A similar test was reported from the New York State Rehabilitation Hospital at West Haverstraw [18] with a companion test for motor development of the upper extremities to be used by occupational therapists. The Edith Hartwell Clinic Motor Age Examination [19] is also comprised of two sections: One of lower-extremity motor development and the other of upper-extremity motor development, with the addition of the Oseretsky

Tests [20] to the latter for items in chronological age levels above six years. The Cerebral Palsy Activity Record reported in use at the Campbell Clinic and Crippled Children's Hospital School in Memphis, Tennessee,[12] includes items of motor and social behavior from four weeks to five years. The (Seattle) Preschool Functional Activity Test [22] provides a detailed examination of walking skill, presented in the developmental sequence from the most primitive activities that precede walking to refinements and variations like hopping and kicking a ball. It also includes some activities of self-care, although they are not arranged in developmental sequence.

The above tests were reviewed in order to avoid redundancies and to provide a basis on which to build the test under discussion. Four of the authors [17, 19, 21, 22] were queried (by mail) if they had acquired more recent data, whether the test was still being used in the same or a revised form or the reason for discontinuation of its use, if that were the case.* The Dallas Society for Crippled Children indicated that the Dallas Motor Development Test is still in use by them.[23] The Edith Hartwell Clinic responded that a five-year follow up of the Motor Age Examination is now under way, with some revision of procedure, but no revision of items.[24] The Seattle Spastic Children's Clinic and Preschool replied that their test is not now used regularly, probably because of its excessive length.[25] Although no reply was received from the Memphis group, it should be noted that their test had been in use for seven years when it was reported, and some contemplated changes were mentioned in the report.[21]

The Preschool Functional Activity Test [22] was judged lengthy to administer both because of its inclusiveness, and its concern with the details of deviations from normal method and degrees of assistance that are to be allowed in scoring gross motor activities. For example:

The activity, *Rolls from supine to prone toward left.* Positioning and assistance: (a) Flex right leg, (b) right arm across body, (c) head turned left, (d) right leg crossed to the left, (e) left arm tucked close to left side, (f) therapist assisting by pushing right hip and shoulder, (g) arm placed over head. (Scoring choices:) (1) If given the advantage of positioning and assistance, and no sign of accomplishment is shown; (2) maximum—two or more forms of assistance or positioning; (3) Minimum—any one of the positionings, no assistance; (4) Great deal of effort, time lag, bizarre; (5) Smooth, fast, and without effort.

Furthermore, it was disturbing to this author, having labored to arrive at an accurate score for the first forty-three items of General Motor Growth (locomotion), to find that a patient who had achieved a fairly respectable number on Part I achieved a total score of "0" on the remainder of the test where the choices were "can" or "cannot" perform the activity. It was especially disturbing because the latter items were more direct measures than the former of independence in activities of daily living and ability to participate in peer group activities. If I were to use the same test again, I would administer the last section first and then be more selective in use of the items from Part I to work out the needs and methods for remedial work. This is essentially what I have done recently, using first an Inventory of Development and then the Basic Motor Control Chart after Bobath as described by Semans.[16]

The Cerebral Palsy Activity Record [21] has items grouped in eleven "zones." These chronological divisions, at first glance, match the "Key Ages" of the Gesell Schedules,[26] with one addition: a fifteen-month zone. However, the age designation of each zone marks the end of a period of development rather than indicating the average age of achievement for each of the items within the zone. Apparently some item-time shifts were made in order to include a maximum number of items with pertinence to habilitative treatment, as in this example:

In the 28-week zone, motor activities are listed as:

Rolls to prone from supine.†
Sits, leaning forward.
Bounces actively in supported standing.
Grasps cube, rakes at pellet.

This procedure strengthens the zone in terms of item numbers, but weakens the sequential component. Usually a child rolls from supine to prone before he sits, but in the above example he is credited with the same level of development for either.

* A copy of the fifth of the above-mentioned tests and an accompanying reprint were obtained on a visit by the author to the New York State Rehabilitation Hospital at West Haverstraw in August 1967.

† The activity of rolling supine to prone is an important one, but is listed on the Gesell Schedules [26] at twenty-four weeks. It occurs too late to be included in the next previous zone on the Cerebral Palsy Activity Record, which is sixteen weeks, so it is logical to include it in the twenty-eight-weeks zone.

——Developmental Inventory as a Chart of Progress——

Proposal for a "New Inventory of Development"

The Inventory of Development proposed here is composed of four sections that closely follow the divisions made by Gesell.[1] They are: Gross Motor, Fine Motor (Adaptive [1]), Communication (Language [1]), and Personal–Social. (*See* Tables 1–4). The physical therapist will be primarily interested in motor development when planning treatment, but in order to teach the desired skills, the therapist will need to recognize a child's ability to perceive, interpret, and reproduce the spoken word, and in order to set realistic goals will need some measure of the child's effectiveness in handling some basic requirements of social living (self-care, concept–formation, and generalization). Moreover, a chart of progress should encompass not only basic skills learned

TABLE 1
DIVISION OF MATERNAL, CHILD AND CRIPPLED CHILDREN'S SERVICES
Delaware State Board of Health
INVENTORY OF DEVELOPMENT—GROSS MOTOR

Patient's Name ______________ Diagnosis ______________ Birthdate ______________

Scoring Key: O=Observation H=History

Gross Motor: Posture and Locomotion	Average Age	Date	Date	Date	Date	Date	Date
Lifts head briefly (prone)	4 wks						
Head comes up from ventral suspension	8 wks						
Up on forearms (prone)	12 wks						
Head erect, steady if held sitting	16 wks						
Lifts head and chest (prone)	20 wks						
No head lag if raised from supine	20 wks						
Rolls over both ways	24 wks						
Lifts head from supine	28 wks						
Sits erect momentarily	28 wks						
Sits erect 1 minute	32 wks						
Stands briefly, hands held	32 wks						
Stands holding a rail	36 wks						
Sits indefinitely (gets to and from)	40 wks						
Crawls on abdomen	40 wks						
Pulls to stand	40 wks						
Creeps, hands and knees or scoots, sitting	44 wks						
Cruises sideways holding onto furniture	48 wks						
Walks, one hand held	12 mos						
Walks, hands and feet	12 mos						
Walks, alone	14 mos						
Stoops and recovers	15 mos						
Kneels, alone	15 mos						
Creeps up stairs	15 mos						
Walks up stairs, one hand held	18 mos						
Walks fast or runs stiffly	18 mos						
Squats in play	21 mos						
Walks backward	21 mos						
Runs well (no falling)	2 yrs						
Walks up and down stairs alone	2 yrs						
Picks up object from floor without falling	2 yrs						
Kicks ball without losing balance	2 yrs						
Jumps, both feet	2½ yrs						
Walks on tiptoes (good balance)	2½ yrs						
Rides a tricycle	3 yrs						
Stands on one foot momentarily	3 yrs						
Stands on one foot two seconds	3½ yrs						
Up and down stairs, alternate feet	4 yrs						
Hops on one foot	4 yrs						
Stands on one foot over eight seconds	5 yrs						

TABLE 2

DIVISION OF MATERNAL, CHILD AND CRIPPLED CHILDREN'S SERVICES
Delaware State Board of Health
INVENTORY OF DEVELOPMENT—FINE MOTOR

Patient's Name ________ Diagnosis ________ Birthdate ________

Scoring Key: O=Observation H=History

Fine Motor: Eyes, hands	Average Age	Date	Date	Date	Date	Date	Date
Follows object 90°	4 wks						
Follows past midline	8 wks						
Retains toy briefly	8 wks						
Holds toy minutes	12 wks						
Follows 180°	12 wks						
Looks at pellet (focus and convergence)	16 wks						
Mouthing of objects	16 wks						
Crude grasp	20 wks						
Resecures dropped object	24 wks						
Transfers objects, 1 hand to other	28 wks						
Definitely shakes rattle	28 wks						
Holding 1 toy grasps another	32 wks						
Hits objects together	36 wks						
Manipulates string	36 wks						
Index finger approach	40 wks						
Grasp release	40 wks						
Removes block from cup	44 wks						
Neat pincer grasp	48 wks						
Casts ball imitatively	15 mos						
Builds tower of 2 blocks	15 mos						
Hurls ball on request	18 mos						
Tower of 3 or 4 blocks	18 mos						
Scribbles spontaneously (pencil in fist)	18 mos						
Turns 2–3 pages	18 mos						
Tower of 6 or 7 blocks	2 yrs						
Turns pages singly	2 yrs						
Turns doorknob	2 yrs						
Unscrews lid	2 yrs						
Imitates vertical stroke on paper	2 yrs						
Imitates circular stroke on paper	2 yrs						
Copies a circle	3 yrs						
Tower of 9 blocks	3 yrs						
Traces a square	3 yrs						
Imitates 3 block bridge □ □□	3 yrs						
Imitates block train □ □□□	3 yrs						
Picks longer line II (3 of 3 tries)	4 yrs						
Copies a cross	4 yrs						
Imitates a square	4 yrs						
Imitates a 5 block gate □ □□ □□	4 yrs						
Scissors to cut a picture	4 yrs						
Holds a pencil like adult	4 yrs						
Copies a square	5 yrs						
Draws a recognizable man	5 yrs						
Copies a diamond	6 yrs						
Copies printing	6 yrs						
Builds a straight tower of blocks	6 yrs						

——Developmental Inventory as a Chart of Progress——

("neat pincer grasp," Table 2), but the usefulness of the achievement ("buttons front buttons," Table 4). Progress, or the lack of it, may be evident at an equal rate in all areas. If so, recognition of the effect of maturation (although the rate may be depressed) can eliminate unnecessarily intensive exercise programs or the frustration of attempting to learn an activity for which the organism is simply not ready. On the other hand, progress may be limited to one or two of the behavioral areas,

TABLE 3

DIVISION OF MATERNAL, CHILD AND CRIPPLED CHILDREN'S SERVICES
Delaware State Board of Health
INVENTORY OF DEVELOPMENT—COMMUNICATION

Patient's Name ______ Diagnosis ______ Birthdate ______

Scoring Key: O=Observation H=History

Communication: Speech production, hearing, and language	Average Age	Date	Date	Date	Date	Date	Date
Reflexive sounds, mostly vowels	4 wks						
Sucks and swallows well	4 wks						
Changes facial expression and/or vocalizes when talked to	8 wks						
Turns head to (not necessarily toward) sound	12 wks						
Laughs aloud	16 wks						
Turns head toward speaking voice	20 wks						
Babbles several sounds on 1 breath	24 wks						
Imitates cough	24 wks						
Imitates protrusion of tongue	24 wks						
Chewing motion in response to feeding	26 wks						
Single syllables, such as "ba," "da," "la"	32 wks						
"Ma-ma," "da-da" form of babbling	32 wks						
Responds to "no-no"	40 wks						
Responds to and understands name	44 wks						
Listens to & imitates sounds ("mama," "daddy," "choo-choo," "rrr" (Motor))	48 wks						
Says 1 word with meaning	48 wks						
Obeys "Give it to me"	12 mos						
Drooling or slobbering virtually controlled (in relation to food)	12 mos						
Says 2 or 3 words meaningfully	12 mos						
Uses vocabulary of 5–10 words	18 mos						
Uses 2-word phrases	18 mos						
Identifies objects by pointing	18 mos						
Eats table foods, including chewy meats	2 yrs						
Follows 1-step directions	2 yrs						
Answers single questions (Name?, "Where's Mommy?")	2 yrs						
Says 2–3 word sentences (with nouns, verbs, & some pronouns)	2 yrs						
Identifies use of many things in pictures ("Show me the one you wear . . . eat . . . drink from")	3 yrs						
Describes use of ball, cup, pencil [a]	3 yrs						
Names 1 color	3 yrs						
Follows 2-stage commands	4 yrs						
Has number concept of 2 or 3	4 yrs						
Speaks in complete sentences (including articles)	4 yrs						
Follows 3-stage commands	5 yrs						
Repeats all consonant sounds correctly	5 yrs						
Correct usage of all parts of speech (appropriate to cultural background)	5 yrs						
Tells stories about pictures	5 yrs						

[a] Only verbal response is acceptable.

TABLE 4
DIVISION OF MATERNAL, CHILD AND CRIPPLED CHILDREN'S SERVICES
Delaware State Board of Health
INVENTORY OF DEVELOPMENT—PERSONAL-SOCIAL

Patient's Name ______ Diagnosis ______ Birthdate ______

Scoring Key: O=Observation H=History

Personal-Social: Self care, play and social interaction	Average Age	Date	Date	Date	Date	Date	Date
Follows moving person	8 wks						
Hand regard	12 wks						
Spontaneous social smile	16 wks						
Smiles at mirror image	20 wks						
Discriminates strangers	24 wks						
Pats mirror image	28 wks						
Reaches persistently for toys	32 wks						
Feeds self cracker	36 wks						
Holds own bottle	36 wks						
Pat-a-cake	40 wks						
Bye-bye	40 wks						
Plays Peek-a-boo	40 wks						
Extends object to examiner on request. No release	44 wks						
Repeats performance laughed at	48 wks						
Cooperates with dressing	12 mos						
Points and vocalizes wants	15 mos						
Feeds self, spills, using spoon	18 mos						
Pulls a toy	18 mos						
Asks for food and drink	21 mos						
Asks for toilet (does not necessarily follow through)	21 mos						
Handles cup well	21 mos						
Removes shoes, socks	2 yrs						
Points to 4 body parts (nose, eye, mouth, hair)	2 yrs						
Plays with dolls or cars appropriately	2 yrs						
Helps put things away	2½ yrs						
Pushes toy with good steering	2½ yrs						
Feeds self	3 yrs						
Puts on socks	3 yrs						
Undresses rapidly and well	3 yrs						
Recognizes 3 colors	4 yrs						
Washes, dries face and hands	4 yrs						
Knows front from back	4 yrs						
Laces shoes	4 yrs						
Dresses completely	5 yrs						
Buttons front buttons	5 yrs						
Complete independence in toileting	5 yrs						
Names 3 out of 4 coins given in order of: nickel, penny, quarter, dime	6 yrs						
Knows right from left	6 yrs						
Knows number of fingers	6 yrs						
Ties bows on shoes	6 yrs						

in which case it is desirable to recognize and capitalize on a patient's strengths and avoid undue frustrations in attempting to improve upon his deficiencies.

Selection of Items

The basis we used for item selection was similar to that described by the group from West Haverstraw as follows: "The test items have been chosen so that progressive steps are provided which lead to independent locomotion (and) independent performance in the areas of hand use, feeding, dressing, grooming, and pre-writing." [18] (We feel that inclusion of the entire area of "communication" is essential to the prewriting skills.)

Item content and distribution are approximately the same in the tests from West Haver-

——Developmental Inventory as a Chart of Progress——

straw, Dallas, and the Edith Hartwell Clinic, and in all of them, items are grouped (for scoring purposes) wherever more than one activity is expected at the same age.

The items on the Developmental Inventory of the Delaware State Board of Health are ungrouped beyond their distribution among the four behavioral areas. Within each area they are simply listed chronologically according to age of expectation. For consistency, where the authorities [1–3] differed on age of expectation for an item, the uppermost age was assigned to the item.

Item selection for the "Inventory" has also been influenced by practicality for administration. For example: "Sits indefinitely, gets to and from" (Table 1) is an important basis for work on creeping, standing, and walking and is straightforward to observe. Skipping, on the other hand, seems straightforward, but a pediatrician who reviewed the "Inventory" questioned the generality of ability to skip in the general population at large. The author then observed 103 children in public kindergarten and 100 children in the first grade of public school. Each child was asked to hop on one foot, skip on one foot (skip-step-skip-step), and skip with both feet. Any child who did not respond appropriately to verbal instructions was asked to imitate a demonstration of the activity. The results are summarized in Table 5. An additional factor for consideration is that the kindergarten teachers stated that they had spent time with their classes on rhythm games and dances which included skipping and had attempted to teach the activity to any child who could not do it initially. The first grade children were in a district which did not provide public kindergarten.

The following decisions were made on the basis of this study:

1. One hundred per cent of children observed could hop on one foot by age six years. Gesell states that the activity is learned by the average by the age of four years. This item was used as a control.

2. Twenty-three per cent of children in regular kindergarten (with benefit of special training) and 21 per cent of children in regular first grade were unable to skip. Furthermore, the author could not defend the activity as one essential to daily living. The item was eliminated.

3. Very few children skipped on one foot instead of regular skipping when the latter was the verbal command. These same children were unable to skip with two feet. Children who could skip well (co-ordinated movement with little effort apparent) had no difficulty imitating skipping with one foot. Those children who skipped hesitantly, awkwardly, or

TABLE 5
SURVEY OF SKIPPING ABILITY AMONG KINDERGARTEN AND FIRST GRADE CHILDREN IN PUBLIC SCHOOLS

	Age (Range)	Sex	Number of Children Tested	Hopped on 1 Foot Satisfactory Response Number(%)	Skipped on 1 Foot Response to Command to Skip Number(%)	Skipped on 1 Foot Imitated Number(%)	Skipped Both Feet Satisfactory Response Number(%)
Kindergarten	5 years (5+6–5+11)	M	28	28(100)	1(4)	1(4)	16(57)
	5 years (5+6–5+11)	F	23	23(100)	0(. .)	17(74)	19(82)
	6 years (6+0–6+ 5)	M	25	25(100)	3(12)	8(32)	21(84)
	6 years (6+0–6+ 5)	F	27	27(100)	2(7)	13(48)	24(88)
	Totals		103	103(100)	6(6)	39(38)	80(77)
First Grade	6 years (6+4–6+11)	M	36	36(100)	2(6)	9(25)	22(61)
	6 years (6+4–6+11)	F	24	24(100)	2(8)	12(50)	20(83)
	7 years (7+0–7+10)	M	22	22(100)	0(. .)	12(55)	20(80)
	7 years (7+0–7+ 3)	F	17	17(100)	0(. .)	3(17)	17(100)
	8 years (8+3)	M	1	1(100)	0(. .)	0(. .)	0(. .)
	Totals		100	100(100)	4(4)	36(36)	79(79)
Combined	5 years (5+6–5+11)	M-F	51	51(100)	1(2)	18(35)	35(68)
	6 years (6+0–6+11)	M-F	112	112(100)	9(8)	42(37)	87(78)
	7 years (7+0–7+10)	M-F	39	39(100)	0(. .)	15(38)	37(95)
	8 years (8+3)	M	1	1(100)	0(. .)	0(. .)	0(. .)
	Totals		203	203(100)	10(5)	75(37)	159(78)

with apparent need for mental concentration and effort were unable to imitate skipping with one foot.

Some general inferences were drawn which led to elimination of the item from the inventory:

1. Skipping on one foot appeared very rarely as an apparent transition from hopping to skipping.
2. Skipping on one foot is more difficult than skipping with both feet, once the latter has been learned.

In the developmental scales used as sources for the items on the "Inventory," gross motor activities are scarce at the five- and six-year levels. The work of Kephart [27] points to a dependent relationship between concept formation and learning of motor patterns. One would assume that learning of increasingly complex motor skills would enhance learning on a symbolic or conceptual level. Illingworth provides evidence for questioning this assumption in his statement that "the mentally retarded child is retarded in all fields of development except occasionally gross motor development." [2]

We should not overlook the effect of motor dysfunction on tests that require manipulation or writing, nor should we regard inability to deal with symbols or concepts purely as a manifestation of motor dysfunction. Observations such as those of Piaget [28] and specialized tests of perception [29–31] take the behavioral approach to study the relationship between sensory stimulation and motor performance. We lack sufficient knowledge for measurement of the neurophysiological basis of conceptual learning.

When the "Inventory" was in early preparatory stages, there was no cut-off point for test administration in terms of items missed. It was noted that in the personal-social area there were some items at the six-year level (for example, "blows–cleans nose" borrowed initially from the West Haverstraw test) which could be performed successfully by children who failed at all other tasks above the two-year level. Any items which were thus suspect were removed for further assessment of level of difficulty, and we have subsequently adopted the procedure of terminating the test in a given area when five *consecutive* items have been missed.

Scoring consists simply of "can" or "cannot" perform the item. We have elected not to define performance in terms of time required for the task, although we recognize that time is a determining factor and probably the easiest one to measure. We feel a necessity to insist that the judgment remain subjective on the part of the examiner, and this places the burden upon anyone using the test to be intimately familiar with behavior of normal children. The determination that a child "can" be credited with an activity will mean that he does it in a manner which is competitive or at least compatible with a normal child at that stage of development. This involves considerations of ability to duplicate the performance, the satisfaction he derives from it, whether he initiates the behavior because of a specific stimulus presented or follows verbal instructions, whether he alters the performance appropriately in the presence of extraneous stresses, and whether his interest and attention to the task indicate that it is established firmly enough to be built upon for more complex skills.

Comparison with Other Developmental Tests

Factor analysis of test results from the Bayley Scales of Infant Development yielded the following picture:

> Factor I, the sensory motor, is dominant in the first year, with its highest loading around eight months. Factor II is dominant in the second and third years, with its highest loading around 30 months, and seems to be related to something like persistence or goal-directed behaviors. Factor III, which is not present at all during the first eight months, becomes dominant at about four years, and after six years—when the I.Q.'s become stable—it appears to be the only one operating. . . . This factor III seems to be the "intelligence" which Binet was measuring.[32]

The "Inventory" presents some items which include very elementary utilization of symbols and concepts, but we have made no attempt to extend it beyond the six-year level. We feel that another type of test is needed for activities above the six-year level.

The authors of the Cerebral Palsy Activity Record proposed addition of reflex activities to their test in order to "orient it toward diagnosis of neurological age." [21] The "Inventory" proposed here has been constructed for use as a chart of progress, not as a diagnostic or screening instrument, and primitive reflex patterns have not been included in the gross motor area.* We offer the following additional con-

* For a historical review of the study of tonic neck reflexes from animal preparations through brain-damaged human beings and normal neonates to normal adult hu-

—Developmental Inventory as a Chart of Progress—

siderations as justification for excluding primitive reflexes from the "Inventory":

1. Questionable inter-examiner reliability of observation of primitive reflexes. Illingworth writes of the asymmetrical tonic neck reflex (ATNR) that "in normal babies passive rotation of the head causes some increase of tone of the upper limb on the side to which the rotation occurs, but one rarely sees full extension of the limb."[2] He mentions that it is difficult to produce a TNR unless it persists beyond an appropriate age or increases, as in cerebral palsy, and he cites at length the Bobaths' descriptions of primitive reflexes in this context. The latter descriptions have appeared frequently in literature familiar to physical therapists, but the Bobaths have cautioned that although

> postural reflexes . . . can be observed in patients with lesions of the (central nervous system), where their release has led to their appearance in an exaggerated form . . . even then it is difficult to isolate the various postural reactions, as the picture is usually complicated by the simultaneous action of a number of reflexes, and by the patient's volitional efforts.[33]

We do not infer from this any reduction in the importance to treatment of observing and recording the presence of primitive reflexes, but we do not feel that the "Inventory" format lends itself to that type of recording. For example, if a reflex persists in an exaggerated form, it is not accurate to say that the child in whom it persists is functioning like a normal child, who is younger than the average age for disappearance of the reflex. Individual narrative recording is much more informative than fitting an individual pattern into a description designed to be representative of a primitive reflex.

2. Controversy over the mechanisms that are responsible for primitive reflexes. The tonic neck reflexes are the ones most often mentioned in general infant examinations. Ausubel labors over differentiation between nonreflex behavior and reflex behavior (including tonic neck reflexes in the latter) and comes up with much overlapping of their distinguishing qualities.[34] Illingworth speaks of the tonic neck reflexes as postural determinants in the neonate with firmer stimulus—response connections in the child with cerebral palsy.[2] Gesell refers to the tonic neck reflex as a postural attitude which "almost literally paves the way for prehension."[35]

Milani-Comparetti, in his (gross motor) Developmental Examination includes primitive reflexes among "evoked responses" and cites the normal age of disappearance for each.[7] His terminology is acceptable in the light of the above studies of normal children since he has set out to identify diagnostically significant dominance of motor patterns of behavior. Presumably, in order to dominate behavior, persistent primitive patterns would be exaggerated and more strongly connected to a specific stimulus than transient primitive patterns in the normal subject. If primitive patterns do not persist or cannot be evoked beyond the stated age, progress in the form of neurological maturation is assumed, but in order to equate their absence with progress in behavioral development one must show that their disappearance coincides with achievement of more advanced activities as Gesell theorizes from observing normal children.[35] But Bobath has found that inhibition of the reflexes does not ensure their replacement by purposive movements. "Reflex-inhibiting postures create only the pre-condition for the use of facilitation techniques" and "a permanent carry over of treatment into activities of daily life . . . will depend on the extent to which active normal sequences of movement can be facilitated, and their patterns firmly established."[36] It is the utilization of these "normal sequences of movement" which are listed on the Inventory.

3. Our clinical experience and reports of others indicate that where primitive reflexes persist they are sometimes modified for purposive movements.[37] We have observed a patient whose posture is dominated by the asymmetrical tonic neck reflex using it to lift her spoon from her plate. She uses an adapted spoon and requires stabilizing assistance, but she insists upon feeding herself. She is unable to walk, speak, or care for herself in any other way. In her case, loss or inhibition of the reflex could not be equated with progress.

Bobath describes a "pattern . . . in reaching for an object with the jaw arm (of the ATNR) and then for grasping purposes making it the skull arm by turning the head away to the opposite side,"[33] and, speaking more generally, alleges that "the combination of tonic reflex activity and compensatory activity pro-

---

man beings, *see:* Hellebrandt, F. A., M. Schade, M. L. Carns, Methods of evoking tonic neck reflexes in normal human subjects. Amer. J. Phys. Med., 41:90, 1962.

duces patterns of standing and walking which are fairly characteristic for every type of (cerebral palsied) patient."[37] It is desirable, if possible, to avoid deformities which result from consistent use of reflex patterns by replacing them with normal patterns. In severe cases, better patterns may not be possible,[36] and in those cases any motion may be better than none. Brunnstrom has written, "While no unrealistic hope should be aroused . . ., no method of training which might produce desirable results should be left untried. It may well be that a subcortical motion synergy which can be elicited on a reflex basis may serve as a wedge by means of which a limited amount of willed movement may be learned."[38]

The "Inventory" should suggest goals of treatment and not method.

Although the progression of item placement in the "Inventory" is from simple to complex, and some more difficult items obviously build upon the simpler ones, no single item is considered absolutely indispensable to a child's development.

Adjustment for prematurity need not be made except in the examiner's expectations for the very young premature infant and interpretation of test results to his parents. It has been shown that the premature infant "catches up" in his development, and this will be indicated on serial testing.[39]

Allowances can be made for adaptations within the criterion that a child performs the activity with as much ease and precision as the average child at the average chronological age of achievement. For example, "walking alone" at fourteen months is unsteady, with frequent falls; it is limited to level surfaces, and a child at that age may pull up to standing in order to walk. If a patient wearing braces and using crutches can perform comparably, he is credited with achievement. By the same token, if a patient wears braces most of the time (for support or control during the waking period when he is most active), he must be able to perform any item on the inventory while wearing the braces. Credit for items related to dressing must include appropriate areas of brace management (Table 4).

Scoring

In the Cerebral Palsy Activity Record[21] the zone (chronological age group of items) with a score of more than 50 per cent indicates the "maturity level." The Dallas Motor Test,[17] which is used by West Haverstraw,[18] and the Edith Hartwell Clinic Motor Age Examination[19] are scored in month values; the calculations are already done, and the examiner need only refer to the printed chart, which is a part of the score sheet, to determine the value in months of each item. The method for calculating the month value for each item is described as follows:

"The amount of months given to each individual item has been determined by the number of items at each age group divided by the number of months between age groups."[18]

There is no accompanying explanation of the reason for choosing this valuation. To the best of my knowledge, there is no study that shows that each of several skills, usually attained in the same three-month period, takes an equal part of that period for attainment. This is what is suggested, but consider an example:

Age Level: 3 months

Items: Hand Use:

1. Holds toy (½" peg) actively.
2. Arms activate on sight of toy.
3. Symmetrical head and arm posture (supine).

Number of items in this group=3.

Number of months between age groups (0–3 mos.)=3.

3/3=1 month value each.

The three items are neither interdependent, nor are they arranged in time order of appearance. Yet, if a child achieves only the first item, he is credited with one month of development for his ability to do something which is usually achieved at or about the third month of life.

The method could be compared to that used in standard psychometric tests, although the number and interrelationship of items are not comparable. One could not say, on the basis of the above example, that a child who achieves only item number one is only doing one-third of the things the average three-month child does.

On the "Inventory of Development," the area score is the highest level at which a child can perform at least half of the items in that area. The therapist can then assess the importance of any items missed to the individual child and decide the need to try to perfect them.

The raw score of a developmental scale is usually expressed in units of months or years or both: It is an indication of the developmental level, *i.e.*, a child who achieves a score of eighteen months is able to perform activities which the average child can do at eighteen months chronological age.

The Developmental Quotient (D.Q.) is more informative because it compares a child's chronological age with his developmental age (raw score): "It indicates how far the child has developed in relation to the average level of development at that age; and no implication is made that it will not alter as future years go by."[2]

The author believes that results of developmental testing are most useful as a chart of progress if they are presented in graphic form providing a comparison of developmental quotients achieved on serial testings spaced six months apart (Fig. 1). From the standpoint of the behavioral sciences the most important comparison presented on the graph is a child's performance in relation to his own past performance. Restated in terms of pure science: This is a measure of the velocity of development, which is much more valuable to know than the distance it has gone at any given point.[40]

Administration of the Test

The entire Inventory can be administered in one hour, although it is seldom necessary to run through the entire test with one child: successful completion of all of the items means obviously the test need not be repeated unless one wants to document regression of a child with a progressive disease. Test administration need not be completed in a single sitting. It can be included in one or more treatment periods, or achievements can be recorded as they occur and summarized on the graph at six-month intervals.

Who shall administer the test? Ideally for the child who has multiple disabilities, the physical therapist will administer the gross motor section (dealing with posture and locomotion), the occupational therapist will administer the fine motor (eyes and hands) and personal-social (self-care, play, and social interaction) section, and the speech pathologist or audiologist will administer the communication (hearing, language, and speech production) section, and all will have the benefit of a composite result. However, the physical therapist working without co-workers in the allied therapies still needs a complete assess-

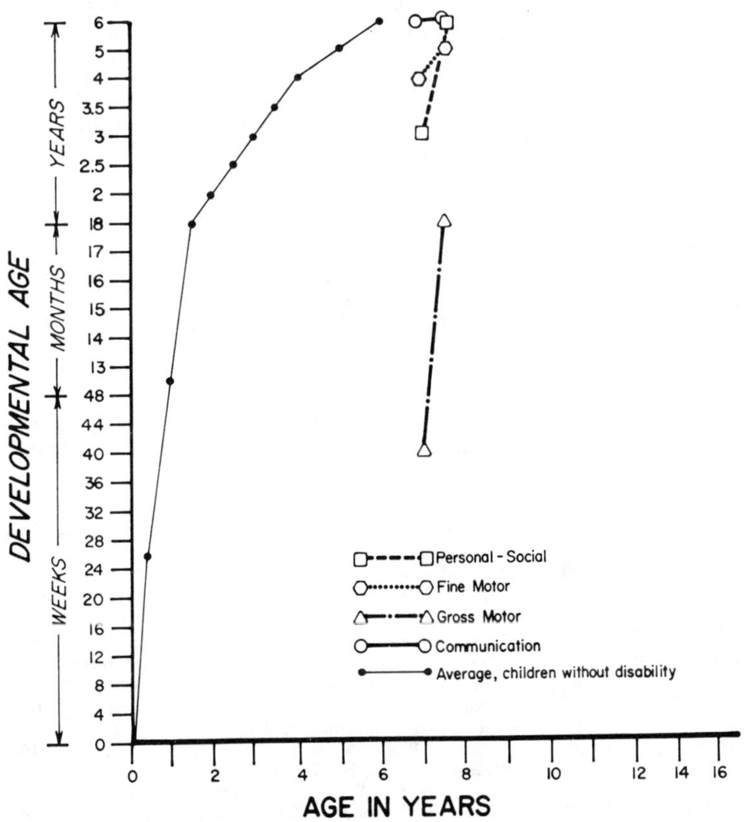

Fig. 1. Graphic representation of child's development as assessed on inventory.

ment of each child's development in order to avoid unnecessary frustrations and to set practical goals and gear treatment to the appropriate level of complexity.

It has been questioned whether physical therapists are prepared to administer and evaluate performance in all areas of a Gesell-modelled test.[16] The directors of forty-three curricula in physical therapy were queried (by mail) regarding the amount of normal human growth and development included in preparation of their physical therapy students. Thirty-eight responses were received. The results as summarized in Table 6 indicate that the subject is most often incorporated into a variety of courses of the basic physical therapy curriculum, and this seldom includes observation of normal human infants.

TABLE 6
RESUME OF COURSE CONTENT RELATED TO HUMAN GROWTH AND DEVELOPMENT IN THIRTY-EIGHT BASIC CURRICULA IN PHYSICAL THERAPY

Presentation of Human Growth and Development in Basic Physical Therapy Curriculum	Lecture	Lab or Observation
Separate course	9	2
Included in other courses	29	6
Other courses in which the subject is included:		
Therapeutic exercise	24[a]	..
Psychology	7	..
Medicine	7	..
Pediatrics	5	..
Kinesiology	3	..
Neurology	2	..
Evaluation procedures	2	..
Neurophysiology	2	..
Orthopedics	1	..

[a] Four of the curricula that had separate courses also mentioned applications in therapeutic exercise.

Summary

Increased knowledge and improved techniques are making possible earlier diagnosis, and physical therapists are asking to see patients as soon as possible to try to avoid defective patterns of motor behavior, contractures, and other deformities.[41] It is, therefore, necessary for physical therapists to have a working knowledge of patterns of development, care, and handling of children from the time of birth. "The Inventory of Development" can offer guidelines and documentation of progress made during the course of physical therapy.

All of the items in the "Inventory of Development" have been cross-checked with the Gesell Schedules [26] so that descriptive material is available from the original reference.[1] In addition, an attempt is made to describe stimuli and behavioral responses on the checklist itself in such a way that no specialized knowledge is required of the physical therapist to administer the "Inventory"; rather, the physical therapist needs to be able to interpret the results of the testing in order to utilize the specialized knowledge he possesses to plan and carry out treatment.

"The Inventory of Development" is recommended as a chart of progress. Each administration gives information about the current developmental status of a patient. The graphic representation compares present with past developmental status and illustrates progress or the lack of it. It is not intended as an instrument for prognostication. Studies of the prognostic value of more detailed tests modeled after the Gesell Schedules are controversial.[32, 42] The results of the "Inventory" cannot be construed as a direct measure of effectiveness of treatment because it does not separate out the influence of physiological maturation. It can indicate ineffectiveness of treatment, *i.e.,* no progress is made despite whatever therapeutic measures are tried. Hopefully, retrospective comparison of test results, degree of disability, and amount and type of therapy received among a large population of patients will yield an indication of the effectiveness of treatment.

REFERENCES

1. Gesell, A., H. M. Halverson, H. Thompson, F. L. Ilg, B. M. Castner, L. B. Ames, and C. S. Armatruda, The First Five Years of Life. Harper, New York, 1940.
2. Illingworth, R. S., The Development of the Infant and Young Child. Williams and Wilkins, Baltimore, 1966.
3. Knobloch, H., Developmental Screening Instrument. Child Development Service, The Children's Hospital, Columbus, 1963. (Mimeographed)
4. Haynes, Una, A Developmental Approach to Casefinding with Special Reference to Cerebral Palsy, Mental Retardation, and Related Disorders, Children's Bureau Publication #449–1967, Washington, D. C., reprinted, 1967.
5. Gentry, E., and L. M. Paris, Tools to evaluate child development. Amer. J. Nurs., 67, 1967.
6. Frankenburg, W. K., and J. B. Dobbs, The Denver Developmental Screening Test. J. Pediat., 71:181–191, 1967.
7. Milani-Comparetti, A., and E. A. Gidoni, Routine developmental examination in normal and retarded children. Develop. Med. Child Neurol., 9:631, 1967.
8. Anderson, R. M., M. Miles, P. A. Matheny, Communicative Evaluation Chart from Infancy to Five Years. Business Forms, Inc., Golden, Colorado, 1964.
9. Anderson, R., E. Bargowski, W. H. Blodgett, A Code Method for Evaluating Function in Cerebral Palsy. Detroit Orthopedic Clinic, Detroit, Michigan, 1966.

——Developmental Inventory as a Chart of Progress——

10. Charney, E., Examination of the preschool child. New Eng. J. Med., 270:1408, 1964.
11. Kendall, H. O., and F. P. Kendall, Normal flexibility according to age groups. J. Bone Joint Surg., 30-A: 690, 1948.
12. Bobath, K., The long-term results of treatment. Develop. Med. Child Neurol., 1962.
13. Fiorentino, M., Reflex Testing Methods for Evaluating Central Nervous System Development. Springfield, Illinois, Charles C Thomas, 1963.
14. Semans, S. R., R. A. Phillips, M. Romanoli, R. Miller, and M. Skillen, A cerebral palsy assessment chart: Instructions for administration of the test. J. Amer. Phys. Ther. Ass., 45:463–468, May 1965.
15. Keats, S., Cerebral Palsy. Charles C Thomas, Springfield, Illinois, 1965, pp. 141–142.
16. Semans, S. R., Specific tests and evaluation tools for the child with central nervous system deficit. The Child with Central Nervous System Deficit. Children's Bureau, U. S. Department of Health, Education, and Welfare, Washington, D.C., 1965, pp. 129–134.
17. Dallas Society for Crippled Children, The Dallas Motor Development Test. 1963. (Mimeographed)
18. Miller, A. S., M. D. Stewart, M. A. Murphy, and A. C. Jantzen, An evaluation method for cerebral palsy. Amer. J. Occup. Ther., 9, May–June 1955.
19. Johnson, M. K., F. N. Zuck, and K. Wingate, Measurement of motor handicap in children with neuromuscular disorders such as cerebral palsy. J. Bone Joint Surg., 33A:698–707, 1951.
20. Da Costa, M. I. L., In Doll, Edgar A., editor, The Oseretsky Tests of Motor Proficiency. Educational Publishers, Inc., Chicago, 1946.
21. Ingram, A., J. Withers, and E. Speltz, Role of physical and occupational therapy in the treatment of cerebral palsy: testing and results. Arch. Phys. Med., 40:429–438, 1959.
22. Footh, W. K., and K. L. Kogan, Measuring effectiveness of physical therapy in the treatment of cerebral palsy. J. Amer. Phys. Ther. Ass., 43:867–873, 1963.
23. Hazel, Sylvia, Chief Physical Therapist, Cerebral Palsy Treatment Center, Dallas Society for Crippled Children, Dallas, Texas. Personal communication.
24. Wingate, Kathleen, R.N., retired, University of Rochester Medical Center, Rochester, New York. Personal communication.
25. Tyler, Nancy, O.T.R., Spastic Children's Clinic and Preschool, Seattle, Washington. Personal communication.
26. Gesell Developmental Schedules, The Psychological Corporation, New York.
27. Kephart, N. C., Perceptual-motor aspects of learning disabilities. Exceptional Children, 201–206, December 1964.
28. Tuddenham, R. D., Jean Piaget and the world of the child. Amer. Psychol., 21:207–217, October 1967.
29. Ayres, A. J., Southern California Test Battery for Assessment of Dysfunction. Western Psychological Services, Los Angeles, California.
30. Frostig, M., W. Leferver, and J. R. B. Whettlesey, Developmental Test of Visual Perception, Consulting Psychologist Press, Palo Alto, California.
31. Tueber, H. L., and R. G. Rudel, Behavior after cerebral lesions in children and adults. Develop. Med. Child Neurol., 4:3–20, 1962.
32. Bayley, N., Value and limitations of infant testing. Children, 5:129, 1958.
33. Bobath, B., A study of abnormal postural reflex activity in patients with lesions of the central nervous system—I. Physiotherapy, 40:259, 1954.
34. Ausubel, D. P., Theory and Problems of Child Development. Grune and Stratton, New York, 1958, pp. 205–211.
35. Gesell, A., and C. S. Amatruda, Developmental Diagnosis, Second Edition, Hoeber, New York, 1960, pp. 32–33.
36. Bobath, K., and B. Bobath, The facilitation of normal postural reactions and movement in the treatment of cerebral palsy. Physiotherapy, 50:246–262, 1964.
37. Bobath, K., and B. Bobath, An analysis of the development of standing and walking patterns in patients with cerebral palsy. Physiotherapy, 48:144–153, 1962.
38. Brunnstrom, S., Associated reactions of the upper extremity in adult patients with hemiplegia—an approach to training. Phys. Ther. Rev., 36:4, 1957.
39. Shirley, M. M., Development of immature babies during their first two years. Child Develop., 9:347–360, 1938.
40. Falkner, Frank, Physical growth and development of the preschool age child. Institute on Growth and Development, Kentucky State Department of Health, Louisville, May 1958.
41. Bobath, B., The very early treatment of cerebral palsy. Develop. Med. Child Neurol., 9:373–390, 1967.
42. Knobloch, H., and B. Pasamanick, Predicting intellectual potential in infancy, some variables affecting the validity of developmental diagnosis. Amer. J. Dis. Child, 106:77–85, 1963.

SELECTED BIBLIOGRAPHY

1. Illingworth, R. S., An Introduction to Developmental Assessment, Little Club Clinics in Developmental Medicine, No. 3, National Spastics Society, London, 1962.
2. Caldwell, Bettye M., and R. H. Drachman, Comparability of three methods of assessing the development of young infants. Pediatrics, 34:51, 1964.
3. Illingworth, R. S., Difficulties in Developmental Prediction. National Spastics Society, London, 1960.
4. Gesell, A., and L. B. Ames, The development of directionality in drawing. J. Genet. Psychol., 68:45–61, 1946.
5. Abercrombie, M. J. L., R. L. Lindon, M. C. Tyson, Direction of drawing movements. Develop. Med. Child. Neurol., 10:93–97, 1968.

what's the answer?

queries and replies of concern to therapists

What are some of the problems in the evaluation and treatment of the child with cerebral palsy?

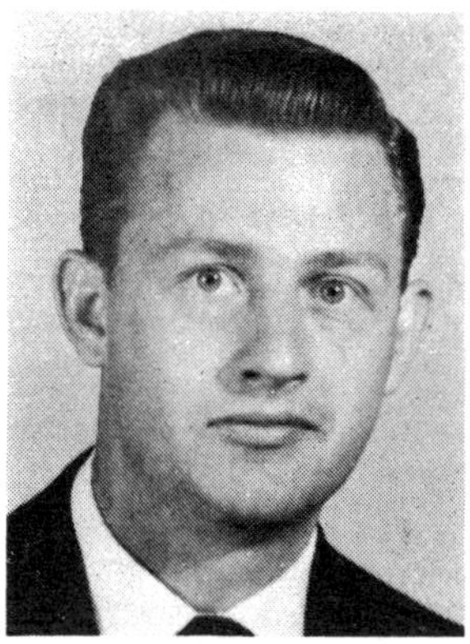

Stanley G. Daily

The rise and decline in popularity during the past twenty years of numerous treatment philosophies and techniques reflect physical therapists' continual search for something better for the child with palsy. This is as it should be; however, therapists persist in flitting from one technique to another as if they expect eventually to find the magic combination. Some therapists believe that the technique per se, rather than the perceptiveness of the therapist, determines the effectiveness of a treatment program.

This search for the magic answer can be a major cause of the frustration which many therapists, both experienced and inexperienced, exhibit. Hasn't every therapist met parents who, in the therapist's opinion, are unable to accept their child's handicap? Yet aren't some therapists equally guilty of being unable to accept their patients' abnormal movement patterns, and of dwelling too long on their deficits rather than determining their assets and building upon them? Although therapists must strive for normalcy of movement in their patients, the possibility of completely achieving that goal is extremely limited; therefore, both therapists and physicians, are obligated to determine when the emphasis of treatment should focus primarily on function, with the pattern of movement of secondary importance. The concept that abnormal movement is preferable to no movement should be kept in mind when planning the patient's activities.

A serious problem of some therapists who work with children with cerebral palsy is the attitude that they are fulfilling their obligations to their patients merely by performing the prescribed treatment. They seem to feel that their professional responsibilities are limited to working with the child in the clinic for thirty to sixty minutes two to five times per week, plus an occasional conference with his parents. They are presumptuous in thinking that such a relatively insignificant period of time spent with the patient will significantly alter his motor patterns or will even begin to achieve the maximum potential. If the therapist does not extend his services outside the therapy unit, he is offering little more than a token service, regardless of his skill, technique, or educational background.

Another problem which sometimes thwarts optimal care of the child with cerebral palsy is the relationship between the prescribing physician, who is usually an orthopedist, and the physical therapist.

Mutual understanding and respect between physician and therapist is basic to an effective treatment regime. Although therapists readily acknowledge the physician's leadership role, many of them resent and disagree with the orthopedist's use of bracing and surgery. Fortunately, most therapists are sufficiently dedicated to medical ethics not to transfer their reservations about the physician's medical direction to the patient or his family. Under no circumstances can failure to conform to medical ethics be tolerated; however, this does not mean the therapist need always accept the physician's judgment unequivocally. If the therapist finds his concept of treatment differing from the referring physician's, a logical first step would be to examine carefully his own treatment philosophy in an attempt to evaluate objectively the reasons for his own attitudes. The therapist may be unduly influenced by some of the currently popular concepts of treatment which minimize the orthopedic approach to the treatment of the child with cerebral palsy. The frequently heard expression that cerebral palsy is a neurological rather than orthopedic problem and should be treated "neurologically" is responsible for many problems. To deny orthopedic treatment to patients who have developed secondary orthopedic problems is as ludicrous as to refuse orthopedic measures to a patient who has had an amputation as the result of diabetes simply because the problem is not of orthopedic origin.

If, after honest soul-searching, the therapist cannot reconcile his views with those of the prescribing physician, he should attempt to discuss those differences with the physician in an unobtrusive, tactful manner. The professionally secure physician is usually most receptive to such discussions. In addition, he realizes that the therapist frequently knows the patient much better than he does, and is therefore in a position to offer significant information pertinent to the total management of the child.

Another problem concerns the inflexibility in the scheduling of patients. The therapist's willingness to alter his schedule in order to provide intensive treatment to postoperative patients can mean the difference between a successful and an unsuccessful surgical procedure. Such scheduling may involve temporarily discontinuing treatment for some patients in order to provide maximal therapy for other children at a crucial postoperative period. Incidentally, institution of a postoperative therapy program should not be postponed until the casts are removed. The child with cerebral palsy is especially vulnerable both psychologically and physically to prolonged immobilization; therefore, the therapist must work closely with the surgeon to encourage resumption of therapy as soon as possible after surgery.

Another equally important aspect of scheduling is to provide time for the involvement of fathers in their children's treatment programs. Too often, fathers are not included because they are unable to take time from their jobs during regular working hours. When this is the case, the therapist should arrange special appointments so that the father's contribution to the treatment program can be fully utilized.

The final problem to be discussed here is related to the widely recognized need for objective measuring instruments for the evaluation and treatment of children with cerebral palsy. The question arises as to whether therapists are fully utilizing their present means of measurement, as limited as those measurements might be. One device which could be used to a much greater extent is movies, using established key developmental milestones as standards by which the child's motor performance is recorded, evaluated, and graded from infancy to adolescence. Taking sixteen-millimeter black-and-white movies every two years, using fifty feet of film per take, would cost about $50.00 per child—a rather insignificant figure when compared with the total amount expended on the average patient with cerebral palsy during the first twenty-one years of his life.

Many therapists do not record joint range of motion; instead, they enter some comment in the progress note about the existence of "much tension" or "moderate tightness"—statements which are practically worthless. The therapist's range-of-motion measurements should be especially helpful to the orthopedist who understandably does not usually have sufficient rapport with a child to obtain an accurate range of motion. Often the therapist who objects so vigorously to surgery is the same therapist who has not recorded range-of-motion measurements which could have influenced the orthopedist in his surgical decision.

The greater utilization of graphs and charts in quantitatively recording various activities of daily living and basic motor skills can also be a motivating force to both patient and therapist.

A key factor in providing physical therapy to the child with cerebral palsy is the therapist's attitude and personal feeling toward his patient. The therapist's sincerity, enthusiasm, and confidence will contribute much toward eliminating his problems and toward providing a therapeutic spark to patient, parents, and fellow workers.

Stanley G. Daily
Physical Therapy Consultant
Bureau of Crippled Children's Services
Department of Public Health
Berkeley, California

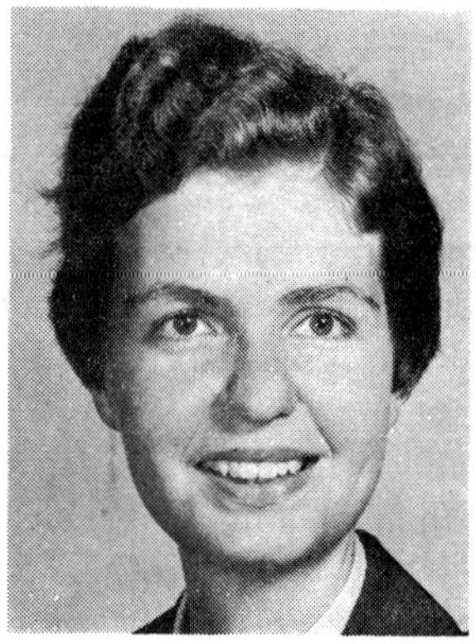

Jolene K. Tomlan

The question, what are some of the problems in the evaluation and treatment of the child with cerebral palsy?, was submitted by Jolene K. Tomlan, CPT, USA, a physical therapist at Fitzsimons General Hospital, Denver, Colorado.

Neonatal Assessment: An Overview

BARBARA H. CONNOLLY

The purpose of this paper is to provide an overview of assessment techniques used by physical therapists in the assessment of the neonate. An additional purpose is to provide a review of prenatal and postnatal development in the areas of muscle tone, range of motion, somatosensory skills, and reflex development. The role of the physical therapist on the neonatal team is discussed relating to the types of assessments physical therapists might use in evaluating the neonate. General considerations for assessment are provided, and specific areas including physical examination, behavioral assessment, evaluation of muscle tone, reflex assessment, oral motor evaluation, and sensory systems assessment are discussed. Physical therapy for the neonate has been considered as a specialty area of pediatrics. Physical therapists, however, are being asked to function in neonatal units in hospitals as a part of their practice in the general hospital setting. This article provides information for the inexperienced clinician who is interested in working with the neonate and for the experienced clinician.

Key Words: *Neonatology, Physical therapy.*

Physical therapists have become more involved in assessments of the neonate over the last decade. As the number of neonatal intensive care units increases, more physical therapists are receiving referrals from physicians (neonatologists, pediatricians, and geneticists) to assess newborns during their stay in and after their discharge from these units or after the infant's transfer to less specialized units. Although growth and development courses are required in physical therapy curricula, emphasis is usually placed on the development that occurs after the neonatal period. Most physical therapists may know what occurs during the neonatal period but do not know the specifics of the development of somatosensory systems, tone, oral mechanisms, or reflex functioning during this period. In addition to knowledge of expected developmental abilities during the neonatal period, many therapists (especially those treating neonates in intensive care nurseries) require knowledge of the physiological state, postural attitudes, muscle tone, and motor behavior of the developing neonate who is between the gestational age of 28 and 42 weeks.

This article presents information that is needed by those physical therapists who assess the preterm as well as the full term infant. Information on various types of assessments (eg, motor, behavioral, muscle tone, postural attitudes, organizational behavior, sensory states, and family status) will be included.

DEFINITIONS

The neonatal period typically refers to the first four weeks of life.[1] For the preterm infant, this period refers to the period of time that lapses until the infant reaches an adjusted age of four weeks. Preterm infants, however, are not on a timetable and, thus, at an adjusted age of 10 days, may not be comparable to full term infants in size, tone, movement, or reflex development.[2]

The following definitions are used in describing classifications of newborn infants either by gestational age or birth weight: Full term—Infant born between 38 to 42 weeks of gestational age; Preterm—Infant born before the end of the 37th week of gestation; Postterm—Infant born at the onset of the 42nd week of gestation or anytime thereafter; Appropriately grown for gestational age (AGA)—Infants whose rate of intrauterine growth was normal prior to the time of birth; Small for gestational age (SGA)—Infants whose rate of intrauterine growth was slower than expected prior to the time of birth; and Large for gestational age (LGA)—Infants whose weight at the time of birth falls above the 90th percentile on the intrauterine growth curve.

Infants are usually classified according to their gestational age and their birth weight (eg, a full term infant who is large for gestational age or a full term infant who is small for gestational age).

HIGH RISK INFANTS

Preterm and low birth weight infants make up a large proportion of infants who are classified as high risk. The incidence of severe central nervous system dysfunction seems to be greater in preterm infants who are small for gestational age than in any other group.[3]

Numerous neonatal conditions may be associated with high risk births. In addition to prematurity and low birth weight, factors such as hemorrhaging, cardiorespiratory distress, and placental anomalies may contribute to problems during the neonatal period and later in life. Of those infants who have either periventricular hemorrhage or intraventricular hemorrhage, poor neurologic outcome may be associated with the more severe hemorrhages.[4] Cardiopulmonary problems may include asphyxia at the time of delivery, apnea, meconium aspiration, or respiratory distress syndrome (RDS). Although most infants do survive RDS, neuromuscular development of these infants may be influenced by factors associated with the

Dr. Connolly is Associate Professor, Department of Rehabilitation Sciences, Program in Physical Therapy, The University of Tennessee Center for the Health Sciences, 800 Madison Ave, Memphis, TN 38163 (USA).

This invited paper was submitted December 26, 1984, and was accepted April 30, 1985.

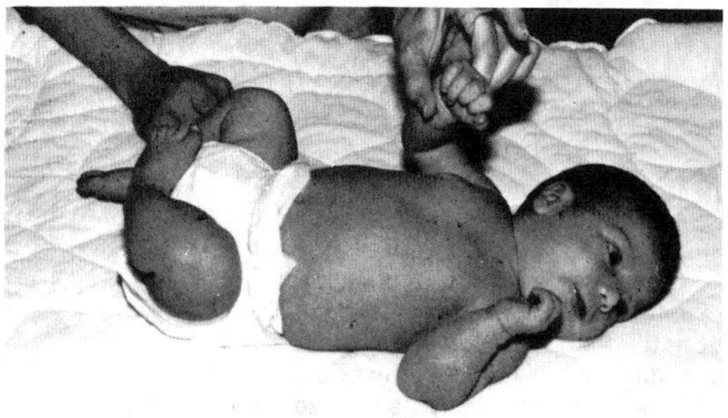

Fig. 1. Normal physiological flexion of the arms and legs in the neonate in the supine position.

treatment of RDS. According to Kraybill, immobilization of the extremities, confinement under oxygen hoods, prolonged endotracheal intubation, delayed oral feedings, inappropriate sensory stimulation, and separation from the parents may adversely influence early neuromuscular development.[5]

ROLE OF PHYSICAL THERAPY

The role of the physical therapist on the neonatal team varies not only with the status of the neonate but also with the philosophy of the medical facility. In general, however, the role encompasses assessment of behavioral status, muscle tone, reflex development, oral assessment, developmental skills, sensory system development, and parent-child interactions. Physical therapists may also be involved in the care of the child's cardiopulmonary system.

Physical therapists assess and treat neonates in a variety of settings, including neonatal units in hospitals, developmental centers, and children's hospitals. In any situation, assessments are necessary before a treatment program is initiated.

Not every infant in the neonatal unit will be referred to physical therapy for evaluation, but usually those infants who have a birth history that indicates neurologic problems may exist will be referred. Initially, some of these infants may be observed by the physical therapist without actual handling until that infant is medically stable. Infants showing abnormal tone or posture are often referred to the physical therapist while the infant is in the neonatal unit. The physical therapist is requested to advise the staff on the proper positioning of the infant or on oral stimulation. Infants who sustain injuries to the peripheral nervous system or to the spinal cord and infants who have soft tissue injuries, such as sternocleidomastoid trauma, may also be referred for physical therapy.

A role of the physical therapist may be to help establish bonding between the infant and the parents. Many parents may feel awkward in handling their infant or in interacting with the infant through the incubator. Proper instruction from the physical therapist and other staff in the intensive care unit in the use of appropriate handling techniques, such as touching the baby through the portholes of the incubator, may help the parents relate to the infant.

PHYSICAL THERAPY ASSESSMENTS

General Considerations

The sequence of the portions of the assessment is usually a matter of personal preference. Most therapists, however, proceed in a manner that relates to the amount of disturbance they cause the infants. Observation without contact is probably the least disturbing portion of the examination and provides a tremendous amount of information.

The infant's posture is informative about his muscle tone and reflex state. Normal flexion (physiological flexion) in the extremities indicates good muscle tone, but increased flexion may indicate hypertonicity (Fig. 1). A lack of flexion may be indicative of hypotonicity. A preterm infant should be expected to have a less flexed posture than the full term infant even though his age is equivalent to the age of the full term infant.[6] Predominance of the asymmetrical tonic neck reflex or tonic labyrinthine reflex might also be noted during the observation of the infant.

Spontaneous movement of the infant may be observed if the infant is not disturbed. Infants with normal development have sporadic, well-coordinated movements. A lack of spontaneous movements or decreased movements may indicate significant depression (lethargy) or hypotonia in the infant.

The therapist should be aware of the types of any seizures during the neonatal period. Subtle seizures account for approximately 50% of seizure activity in newborns.[7] The signs of subtle seizure activity include tonic horizontal or vertical deviations of the eyes; repetitive blinking or fluttering of the eyes; oral and buccal movements such as drooling, sucking, or yawning; tonic posturing of the limbs; apnea; cycling or swimming movements; hyperpnea; and vasomotor changes. Infants of less than 34-weeks gestational age can have multifocal clonic seizures consisting of clonic movements of the limbs in a nonordered fashion. Tonic seizures in the neonate may consist of movements that resemble decorticate posturing in older children. Eye deviations and apnea may be present with tonic seizure. Focal clonic seizures are uncommon in neonates unless the infant has a focal traumatic injury.

Neonates are frequently tremulous, which should not be confused with seizure activity. Tremulous infants do not exhibit abnormalities of gaze or eye movements. Stimulation of the infants usually causes them to be tremulous, which is expressed as a movement tremor, not a clonic jerk. The tremor usually ceases with passive flexion of the child. The tremulous condition is often associated with hypocalcemia, hypoglycemia, hypoxic ischemia, encephalopathy, and drug withdrawal.

Observation of respiratory patterns may yield information about the cardiopulmonary status of the infant. Retractions may be seen if cardiopulmonary distress is present. An increase in the anteroposterior diameter of the chest may indicate overexpanded lungs resulting from RDS. If the left side of the chest is larger than the right, cardiomegaly may be present.

Once observations are made, handling may be the next step in the assessment. With newborns, the physical therapist must be careful not to chill the infant. Ideally, the infant should not be uncovered for periods longer than one to two minutes at a time unless the baby is in a warming device. Temperature regulation is extremely crucial in the care of the low birth weight infant. Neonates usually have almost no shivering responses and must produce most of their heat metabolically. A highly specialized brown fat, which has a rich supply of blood vessels, is present in newborns and is their primary source of thermogenesis. When the infant is chilled, sensors in the skin cause an increase in the production of norepinephrine that causes metabolic reactions in the brown fat. These reactions involve the splitting of triglycerides into glycerine and fatty acids. In turn, the fatty acids are released into the infant's bloodstream and oxidized or reesterized with a production of heat. In preterm babies, problems with heat production occur because of the large amount of skin area in juxtaposition to the small weight of the infant, a decreased amount of subcutaneous fat and brown fat, and a decreased ability to mobilize norepinephrine and brown fat. Additionally, most preterm infants are unable to take in enough calories to provide nutrients for thermogenesis. Therefore, the calories the body needs for growth may be used to keep the chilled infant warm.

Physical Examination

Infants who sustain birth trauma involving injuries to the peripheral nervous system or spinal cord may be treated by the physical therapist in the neonatal unit. Assessment of facial nerve injury should include observation of spontaneous facial movements and feeding sessions. If central nerve damage is present, the infant will have asymmetry of the face during crying with a smoothness to the damaged side of the face. The nasolabial fold will be missing, and the corner of the mouth will droop. If the peripheral nerve is damaged, only asymmetrical posturing of the face during crying will be noted. If a peripheral branch injury is present, asymmetric crying facies will be noted, but the paralysis will be limited to the forehead, eye, and mouth.[8]

Brachial plexus injuries are often related to traumatic deliveries. In vertex deliveries, brachial plexus injuries result from a stretch injury when the head is laterally flexed excessively toward one of the shoulders with damage occurring to the brachial plexus on the opposite side. Brachial plexus injuries may also occur in breech deliveries when the body of the infant is flexed laterally just before the delivery of the head. Three types of brachial plexus injuries may be seen. In Erb's palsy, the most common type, the spinal roots of C5 and C6 are involved. The affected arm is adducted and internally rotated at the shoulder with the elbow extended. The forearm is pronated and the wrist is flexed. Moro, biceps, and radial reflexes are absent on the affected side, but the grasp reflex is intact. The affected arm is held passively at the infant's side.

Klumpke's paralysis involves the nerve trunks that originate from the lower spinal roots of C7, C8, and T1. The intrinsic muscles of the hand are involved, but the grasp is intact. Biceps and radial reflexes continue to be present. The upper extremity extends and abducts normally when the Moro reflex is tested, but the wrist and fingers remain flaccid. The third type of brachial plexus injury, the Erb-Duchenne-Klumpke type, involves an injury to the entire brachial plexus, resulting in an entirely flaccid arm with all reflexes absent.[9] Usual management of these infants includes proper positioning of the upper extremity to prevent injury and range of motion activities. Facilitation activities and splinting may also be used.

Spinal cord injuries in newborns are rare complications of vaginal breech deliveries. As with other spinal cord injuries, the complications of the injury vary with the site of involvement.

The most common soft tissue injury in the neonate treated by physical therapists is sternocleidomastoid muscle injury. The injury may result from birth trauma with a hematoma forming inside the muscle. Limitations in range of motion of the neck may occur as the hematoma mass enlarges. Assessment of range of motion and initiation of passive movement are often performed by the therapist during the neonatal period.

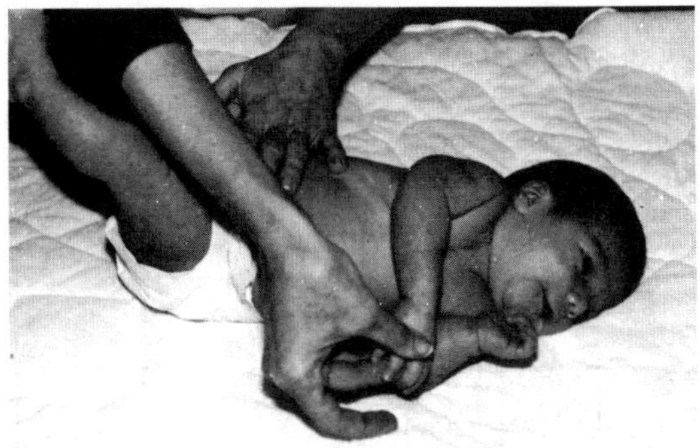

Fig. 2. The scarf test for extensibility at the shoulder in the neonate.

Assessment of musculoskeletal status can be performed when the infant is undressed. Mild degrees of tibial bowing or torsion are considered a normal result of fetal positioning during the last trimester. Many infants will also have forefoot adduction because of their fetal position. Full term infants' feet are compressed in utero and may take several days to unfold. Often, when the foot is put in dorsiflexion, it is possible to have the dorsum of the foot touch the lateral border of the lower leg. Plantar flexion is limited in newborns because of the extreme dorsiflexion that is present. Greater than normal range of motion in the neck and shoulder will also be seen in the preterm infant. The preterm infant shows greater range of motion in the scarf sign (movement of the arm across the chest) than the full term infant (Fig. 2). Additionally, hyperextensibility of the joints will be noted in infants who are hypotonic.

Clinical signs of congenital hip dislocation should be known by physical therapists who assess neonates. Although hip dislocation is generally diagnosed by the infant's physician, occasionally the physical therapist may be the first to suspect a dislocation. Clinical findings in congenital dislocation of the hip include shortening of the thigh with bunching of the soft tissue and larger skinfolds, limitations of abduction caused by shortening of the adductor muscles, lowered knee on the affected side when the knees and hips are flexed, and telescoping or pistoning of the thigh when the hip is flexed.[9]

Behavioral Assessments

The behavioral states have been defined as "distinct conditions each having its specific properties and reflecting a particular mode of nervous system functioning."[10] The state of arousal of the infant may influence all aspects of the neurologic examination of the newborn. Therefore, a description of the infant's behavioral states is an essential part of the interpretation of the examination.

Prechtl has presented the five states commonly used in describing infants[11]:

State I—Eyes closed, regular respiration, no movement.

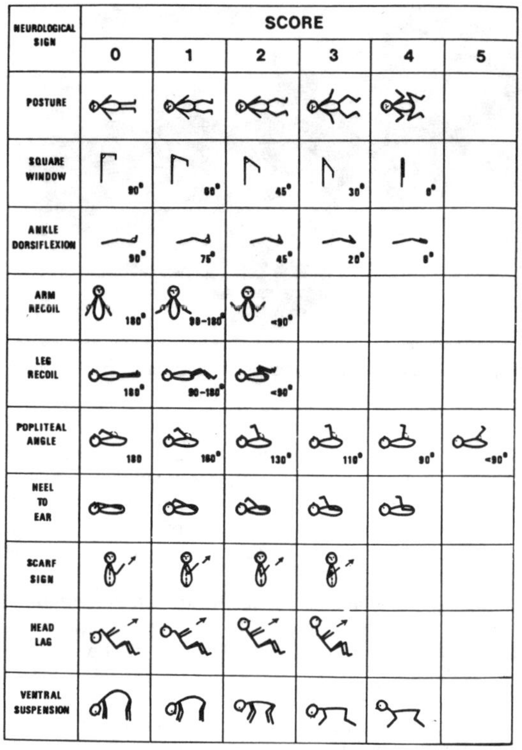

Fig. 3. Dubowitz scoring system for neurologic criteria for assessment of gestational age.[16]

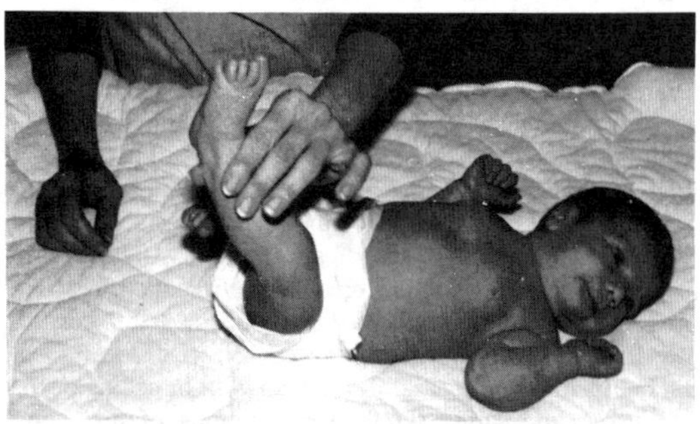

Fig. 4. Foot flapping. A test for passivity in the neonate. Tightening of the foot musculature should occur after several excursions.

State II—Eyes closed, regular respiration, small movements; gross body movements may occur.
State III—Eyes open, quiet, no gross movements.
State IV—Eyes open, gross movements, no crying.
State V—Eyes open or closed, crying.
The ideal states for assessment of the infant are States III and IV. Other variables may affect the arousal state of the infant and should be considered. Hunger or sleepiness will inhibit some spontaneous activities and reflex reactions. If the infant is not in the optimal state for assessment, the therapist must either awaken or calm the infant or reschedule the examination.

The Neonatal Behavioral Assessment Scale (NBAS), a behavioral analysis instrument that is often used by the Neonatal Intensive Care Unit personnel other than the physical therapist, allows for evaluation of the infant's behavioral responses as they are integrated into the overall functioning of the child.[12] The NBAS includes biobehavioral items that assess the infant's capacity to organize states of consciousness, habituate reactions to disturbing events, attend to and process simple and complex environmental events, control motor activity and postural tone, and perform integrated motor acts.[13] The NBAS also includes 20 reflex items but is not considered a comprehensive neurological examination. The Assessment of Preterm Infants' Behavior may also be used by therapists to assess the behavioral capabilities of the preterm infant.[14] Specialized training, however, is required for the administration of both tests.

Muscle Tone

Assessment of muscle tone in the neonate includes evaluation of passive and active tone. Passive tone may be defined as the amount of resistance given by a muscle to passive movement by the therapist.[15] Active tone is directly related to static postures and the strength and coordination of elicited reflexes, automatic reactions, and spontaneous movements.

A review of selected activities illustrating the development of tone is shown in Figure 3.[16] This scoring system, developed in 1970, allows for an estimation of gestational age through examination of certain neurological signs. A full explanation of the use of this tool is described in detail by Dubowitz et al.[16] An excellent review of the development of muscle tone prenatally has also been done by Campbell.[17]

During assessment of muscle tone, the preterm infant may appear to have better extensor muscle tone in the prone position than the full term infant because of the progression of development of tone in utero and because of extrauterine experience in antigravity movement.[6] Extension develops in the seventh month, rotation in the eighth month, and flexion in the ninth month. Therefore, the preterm infant has a greater range of movement than the full term infant because of decreased flexor muscle hypertonicity. Additionally, infants with intrauterine hypoxia may appear hypotonic and may not flex at rest. Straightening of the arms or legs will not be followed by a return to flexion.

In assessing neuromuscular maturation, clinicians should have a good understanding of tone in the neonate. Passive tone is usually determined by the extensibility and passivity of the muscles. Extensibility is measured by the amount of elongation that a muscle allows when its points of origin and insertion are separated. Tests for extensibility include evaluation of adductor angle, heel to ear maneuver, popliteal angle, and scarf sign. Tests for passivity include evaluation of amplitude of movement in foot flapping and hand flapping (Fig. 4). Passive tone in the spinal axis is assessed through ventral flexion of the head and trunk, extension of the trunk, and lateral flexion of the trunk. Evaluation of tone in more detail is described by Amiel-Tison and Grenier.[15]

Evaluation of active tone is accomplished by moving the infant and examining coordinated movements of muscle groups. Lifting the infant from a supporting surface provides information on the infant's ability to adjust to a new position. The full term infant has some degree of overall muscle tone and will attempt to right his head when held in an upright position. The infant with too much tone will feel stiff and may hyperextend the neck, fist his hands, or extend the legs when held. Good cuddling responses are not seen. In contrast, the infant with too little tone may appear limp and be difficult to cuddle because of his lack of postural adjustments.

The pull-to-sit activity is used for assessing head control and the traction response of the arms in infants. When pulled to sit, normal, full term infants contract the shoulder and arm muscles and flex the neck (Fig. 5). When sitting is accomplished, the infant controls the head with his neck muscles to keep the head from falling forward or backward. The baby will right his head with minimal difficulty if it falls forward. Hypotonic infants do not elicit the traction response when pulled to sit. In sitting, the neck muscles appear lax and the head bobbles. In infants with hypertonicity of the neck muscles, the increased tone prevents the head from being mobilized forward, and the head does not fall forward at the end of the maneuver.

In addition to pull-to-sit activities, global straightening of the trunk should also be examined. The infant should be placed in a standing position with the examiner's hand around the infant's chest, the middle finger holding the infant at the axilla, and the index finger providing support under the infant's chin. By straightening the legs, the normal neonate should be able to support himself in this position without any additional assistance.

When the infant is in the supine position, the neck should be normally flexed with little or no space between the cervical spine and the supporting surface. Spontaneous rotation of the head should be present. Abnormal posturing of the head in the supine position includes hyperextension of the neck and head in an arched position or in the opisthotonic posture. Asymmetric tonic neck reflex activity is observed often in newborns with extension of the arm and leg on the chin side and flexion on the occipital side (Fig. 6).

The infant should be able to rotate the head spontaneously in the prone position and lift the head high enough to clear the nose from the supporting surface. In the prone position, the arms should be relatively inactive in contrast to the activity of the legs. Alternate volleys of flexion and extension, however, may be noted in the arms and legs in both the prone and supine positions. When the head is aligned with the axis of the trunk, movements should be symmetrical in all extremities. Asymmetries in posture should alert the examiner to potential abnormalities in the infant.

Generally, the newborn's hands are closed both in the prone and supine positions. Spontaneous opening and closing of the hands may be noted when the infant is sleeping or resting. Special attention should be paid to the infant whose thumb is adducted and flexed across the palm in a clenched position, particularly if this is the only position of the infant's hand noted.[15] This position may be seen in young infants but only as one of a variety of positions of the thumb.

Reflex Development

Neonatal reflex assessment is a critical area of evaluation but is also somewhat subjective in nature. In addition to noting the presence or absence of certain reflexes, the therapist must observe if the reflex is obligatory or if it interferes with the function of the infant.

The primary reflexes present during the first month of life are as follows[11,18]:

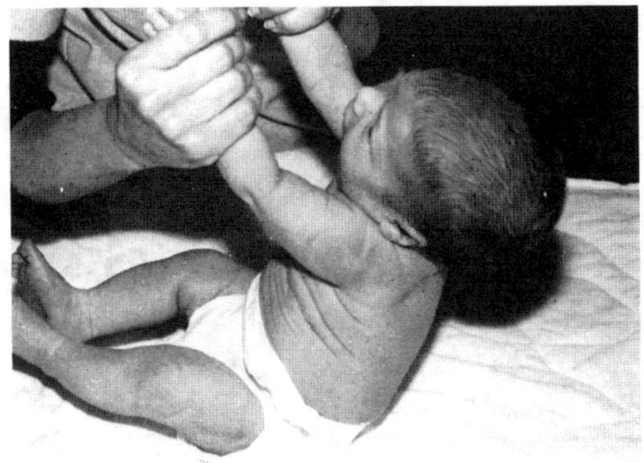

Fig. 5. Pull-to-sit responses in the normal neonate. Contraction of the shoulder and arm muscles is followed by flexion of the neck.

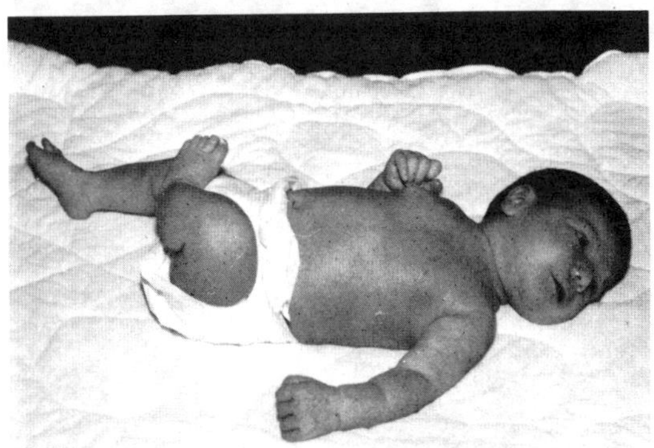

Fig. 6. Spontaneously occurring asymmetrical tonic neck reflex responses in the neonate with flexion of the arm and extension of the leg on the occipital side of the head and extension of the arm with flexion of the leg on the chin side.

1. Galant—Stimulation of the skin on the back from the 12th rib to the iliac crest should produce brisk incurving to the side stimulated. This reflex is present from approximately 20 to 24 weeks gestational age and should be a consistent reflex response in the normal newborn.
2. Palmar grasp—The palmar grasp reflex is normally strong in newborns and appears between 28 to 30 weeks gestational age (Fig. 7). The palmar grasp reflex may be weak in premature or depressed infants. The response may be asymmetrical in cases of hemiplegia, brachial plexus injuries, or in fractures of the clavicle or humerus.
3. Automatic walking—Automatic walking is seen in infants from 32 to 36 weeks gestational age (Fig. 8).
4. Moro—This reflex is present in all normal neonates and begins at about 28 weeks gestational age (Fig. 9). If an extremity does not respond, one should suspect a localized neurologic defect such as a brachial plexus injury or a fracture of the clavicle or humerus. Suboptimal vigor of the overall response may be seen in depressed infants or in hypotonic infants. In preterm infants, the response may be disorganized and incomplete to varying degrees

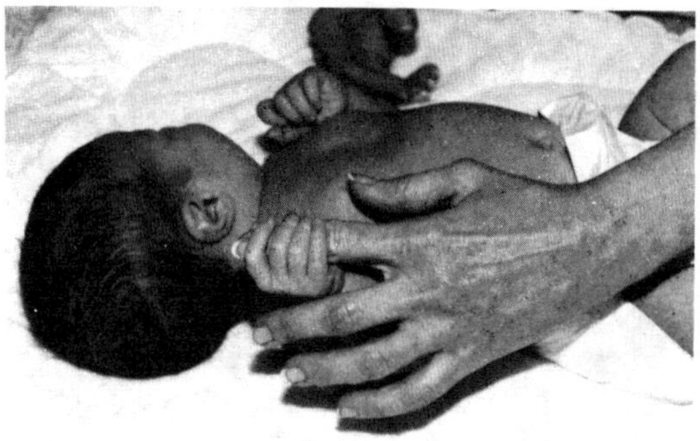

Fig. 7. Grasp response in the neonate elicited by pressure to the palmar surface of the hand.

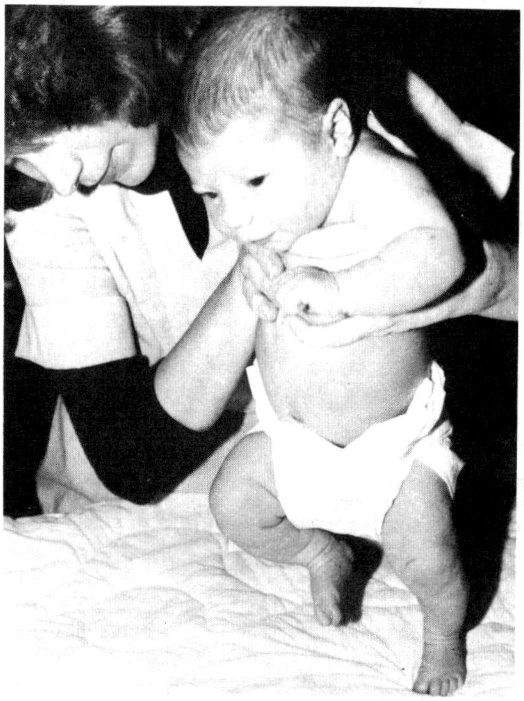

Fig. 8. Primitive walking occurring in response to the neonate held standing and tilted forward.

as a result of the randomness of movements and the predominance of extensor muscle tone in these infants.[3]

5. Crossed extension—The crossed extension response is present from 32 to 36 weeks gestational age and should be strong in the full term infant. Decreased responses may be seen in the infant with low muscle tone. Additionally, decreased flexion responses may be seen in the preterm infant.
6. Flexor withdrawal—This response should be brisk in the full term infant with a short latent period. Preterm infants will have a decreased response from the lack of flexor muscle tonicity.
7. Asymmetrical tonic neck reflex (ATNR)—The ATNR is found in infants who are approximately 34 to 36 weeks gestational age. The upper extremities usually show more tone changes than the lower extremities. The normal infant should be able to move in and out of the reflex position spontaneously and should be able to bring the thumb to the mouth with minimal difficulty.
8. Plantar grasp—Pressure under the toes of the infant should elicit flexion of the toes (Fig. 10). This reflex should be strong and consistent in the neonate.
9. Traction—The traction response should be strong enough in the infant so that while being lifted by the hand or wrist, he can support all or a portion of his own weight.
10. Righting of the head—When held in ventral suspension, the infant should have a predominance of tone in the neck extensor muscles. The infant should hold the head in line with the trunk while he is suspended.

Oral Assessment

Feeding is a developmental skill that is a major component of neonatal behavior. Referrals may be made to physical therapists on infants who demonstrate difficulties with sucking or other oral functions.

Reflexes to be assessed in the newborn include sucking and rooting reactions. In normal infants, the sucking response should be immediate, forceful, and coordinated. Preterm infants may have the sucking reflex because this response is present from about 28 weeks gestational age; however, the effort of sucking may fatigue the infant. Rooting reactions, turning the head toward a tactile stimulus to the cheek, should be present from 24 weeks gestational age. Those infants, however, who have been fed recently or those infants who are lethargic or depressed may only purse their lips or not respond at all to the stimulus. Infants who draw away from the stimulus or who become irritable during feeding may have facial hypersensitivity that may interfere with normal sucking activity.

Determination of breathing patterns is also necessary when evaluating feeding problems in neonates. Normal infants are obligatory nose breathers to allow sucking with the lips sealed. If the infant has difficulty breathing while nursing, he may be a mouth breather and may have an oral facial muscle imbalance.[19]

The normal infant should exhibit rhythmical suck-swallow responses. The neonate under 33 to 34 weeks gestational age may not have a coordinated suck-swallow response; these infants are usually not good candidates for total oral feedings.[19]

Assessment of the Sensory Systems

Sensory systems can be used effectively in the treatment of neonates because many of these systems are fully developed even in the preterm infant. Assessment of each system should be done separately because infants generally do better with one task at a time. Care should be taken in testing the preterm infant because these babies are vulnerable to sensory overload.[2] The organization of sensory input is a major task for all neonates. Therefore, intense stimuli may cause an acute decompensation of behavior with a change in the infant's color or instability of vital signs. Fast movements and sudden noises may be stressful to the neonate and should be avoided.

Overstimulation of the infant should be avoided before feedings because this may produce poor sucking, decreased gastrointestinal mobility, and vomiting or spitting in some infants.[2] The following sensory systems should be assessed.

Tactile. Neonates have been found to look at the body part that is being touched by the examiner.[20,21] Therefore, the examiner should touch the infant in a variety of places. Hypersensitivity or hyposensitivity to touch should be noted.

Proprioception. Proprioception is assessed in infants by evaluating their ability to contour into the arms of the holder. The proprioceptive system is also indirectly evaluated by assessing the infant's posture, muscle tone, and reflexes.

Visual. In newborns, pupil changes should be seen in response to light, but blinking usually occurs only in response to tactile stimuli. Acuity in neonates is thought to be approximately 20/150, although by 6 to 12 months of age, the infant's acuity is similar to that of adults.[20]

Fixation responses first occur in neonates when in a face-to-face position (Fig. 11).[20] Fixed focus occurs at a distance of about 19 cm, which is approximately the distance from the breast-fed neonate to the mother's face.[20]

Tracking in neonates is usually brief and may occur when an object interferes with an ongoing activity such as sucking. Neonates tend to attend to colored rather than grey objects and seem to prefer high contrast figures such as the human face.[21-23]

Auditory responses. Neonates will respond to loud noises, perhaps because of the vibration but not from the pure auditory stimulus.[24] Neonates seem to have a higher threshold for sounds, particularly in response to high frequencies, than older infants.

Responses to sounds in neonates include changes in muscle tone, blinking of eyes, disruptions in breathing, changes in heart rate, and alterations of activity with startle reactions.

Vestibular. Vestibular assessments in neonates should include observation of the infant's response to slow linear movements. A fast rotary movement assessment is not recommended for young infants because they do not naturally make these movements. As with proprioception, vestibular functioning is also assessed through observation of the infant's posture, muscle tone, and reflex reactions.

Parent-Infant Interactions

Assessment of parent-infant interaction is a very important part of the total evaluation of the neonate. Parents may feel uncomfortable in dealing with the infant and need guidance in the proper handling of their child.

In the assessment of parent-infant interactions, the therapist must note the amount of handling by the parents in activities other than routine care-giving activities. Unfortunately, the routine handling of the infant is usually related to medical procedures or high stimulus activities if the child is in a neonatal unit. Parents need to be aware that activities such as stroking and cradling the infant are needed in addition to those activities that stimulate the child.

Parents must also be cautioned against overhandling, particularly if their child is an infant of low birth weight. Long et al, in a study of 30 infants with a low birth weight, found that 75% of the hypoxemia suffered by the infants was associated with handling by personnel in the NICU.[25] They recommended that 1) unnecessary handling be decreased in infants who experienced hypoxemic episodes and 2) infants receive continuous, transcutaneous oxygen monitoring if handling was necessary.

Signs of overhandling of the infant include changes in the infant's color, which might be seen as circumoral cyanosis or mottling of the skin, a marked increase or decrease in respiratory rate, an increase or decrease in heart rate, abrupt

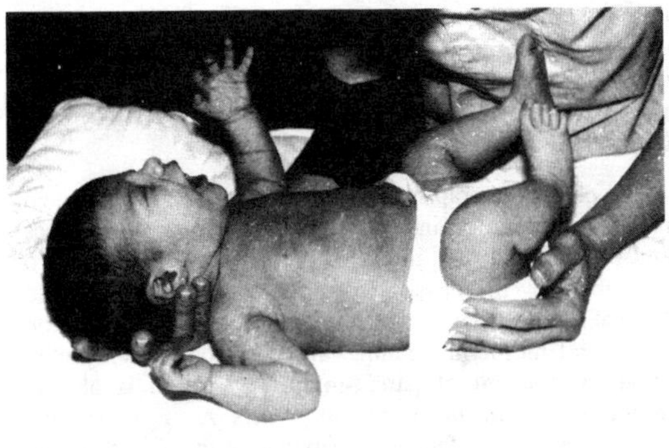

Fig. 9. The initial stage of Moro reflex with abduction and flexion of the arms.

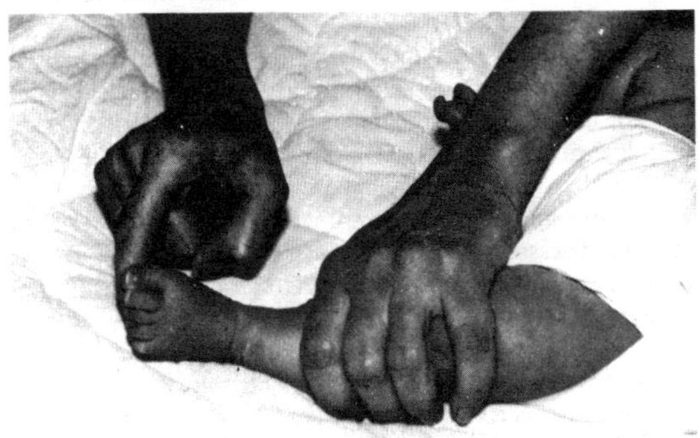

Fig. 10. Plantar grasp or curling of the toes occurring in response to pressure under the neonate's toes.

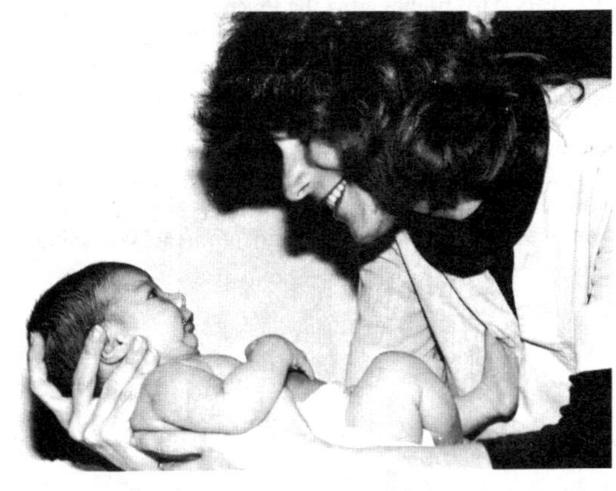

Fig. 11. Initial fixation responses in the neonate occur in the face-to-face position.

limpness, or sudden fussiness. When the infant experiences one or more of these signs, handling should be ceased and the infant allowed to rest.

DISCUSSION

The physical therapist should include a review of pertinent medical information including medical history and physical and neurological data in assessments of neonates. Areas of assessment by the physical therapist may include musculoskeletal status, behavioral states, muscle tone, reflex development, oral motor functioning, and somatosensory development. Assessment of parent-infant interaction is also an important part of the evaluation process. A single examination of the infant offers only a small amount of information regarding the infant's clinical state. Repeated assessments of the infant give more information about the status of the infant and, therefore, allow the therapist to make more realistic plans for the infant.

Numerous assessment tools have been developed for use by physical therapists and others who deal with neonates. Three types of neonatal assessments are available to the therapist: neurological assessments, gestational age assessments, and behavioral assessments. Each type contains evaluations of muscle tone and motor functioning. The prognostic value of neonatal assessments, particularly the neurological and behavioral assessments, are of concern to professionals who use these tools. Minkowski and Saint-Anne Dargassies, in a longitudinal study of 74 newborns, found that none of the newborns who had normal results of neurological examinations at birth received abnormal results of assessments at 2 years of age.[26] One half of the neonates suspected of being abnormal at birth, however, were classified as normal at 2 years, and one half of the neonates who were assessed as abnormal initially were considered suspect for abnormalities at 2 years. Two studies using the Prechtl neurological assessment further raised questions regarding the validity of neonatal assessments. In a four-year study of 252 neonates, Prechtl found that 88 of the 102 infants classified as normal continued to be classified normal at 2 and 4 years of age.[27] Of the 150 infants with abnormal results of evaluations at birth, 110 infants continued to be rated abnormal. In a later study, however, researchers using the Prechtl neurological assessment reported that the vast majority of infants who initially had abnormal examinations did not display neurological deficits at 18 months of age.[28]

The predictive value of behavioral assessments has also been questioned. In a study of 18 normal, full term infants who were 10 weeks of age, Sostek and Anders found that the NBAS could be used as a predictor of mental scores on the Bayley Scales of Infant Development but not on the psychomotor developmental quotient.[29] In a comparison study of the MBAS and the Prechtl neurological assessment, the NBAS was found to be similar to the Prechtl neurological assessment in identifying abnormal infants.[30] When the infants were reexamined at 7 years of age, the Prechtl neurological assessment had identified 13 of the 15 abnormal children, and the NBAS had identified 12 of the same 15 abnormal children. The Prechtl neurological assessment had classified 43 infants as suspect-abnormal, however, and only 13 turned out to be abnormal, but the NBAS had identified only 21 newborns in the suspect-abnormal rating with 12 children classified as abnormal at 7 years of age.

Even with the availability of these formal neonatal assessment instruments, the physical therapist must be aware that supplemental information may be needed, particularly in the area of sensorimotor development, in addition to the information from the assessment tool. Additionally, the therapist should 1) become familiar with the nature of each of the assessments available, 2) understand the purpose of each assessment, and 3) be cautious in interpreting the prognostic abilities of the assessment. Palisano and Short additionally cautioned that "parts of assessments should not be combined because conclusion based on testing of selected items, in a manner other than the standardized procedure, may not be valid."[31]

SUMMARY

This article has presented an overview of the information necessary for the assessment of the neonate, both preterm and full term. This information should be useful both to the therapist who is beginning to deal with the neonate and to the therapist whose practice is primarily devoted to assessment and treatment of the neonate. More information is needed in the area of neonatal care, and physical therapists have the opportunity and challenge to participate in increasing this knowledge base.

PRACTICE

REFERENCES

1. Thomas A, Chesni CY, Saint-Anne Dargassies S: Neurological Examination of the Infant. Little Club Clinics in Developmental Medicine. No. 1, London, England, National Spastics Society with Heinemann Medical Books, 1960, p 10
2. Sammons William AH: Premature behavior and the neonatal intensive care unit environment. In Cloherty JP, et al (eds): Manual of Neonatal Care. Boston, MA, Little, Brown & Co Inc, 1980, pp 359–363
3. Korones SB: High Risk Newborn Infants: The Basis for Intensive Nursing Care, ed 3. St. Louis, MO, C V Mosby Co, 1981, p 133
4. Williamson WD: Early neurodevelopmental outcome of low birth weight infants surviving neonatal intraventricular hemorrhage. J Perinat Med 10:34–41, 1982
5. Kraybill EN: Medical problems of special babies. In Slaton DS, et al (eds): Caring for Special Babies. Chapel Hill, NC, University of North Carolina, 1983, pp 14–24
6. Carter RE, Campbell SK: Early neuromuscular development of the premature infant. Phys Ther 55:1332–1341, 1975
7. Volpe JJ: Neonatal intracranial hemorrhage: Pathophysiology, neuropathology and clinical features. Clin Perinatol 4:77–102, 1977
8. Coulter DM: Birth trauma. In Cloherty JP, et al (eds): Manual of Neonatal Care. Boston, MA, Little, Brown & Co Inc, 1980, pp 251–255
9. Hensinger RN, Jones ET: Neonatal Orthopaedics. Orlando, FL, Grune & Stratton Inc, 1981
10. Prechtl HFR: The behavioral states of the newborn infant: A review. Brain Res 76:185–212, 1974
11. Prechtl HFR, Beintema D: Neurological Examination of the Full Term Newborn Infant, ed 2. Philadelphia, PA, J B Lippincott Co, 1977
12. Brazelton TB: Neonatal Behavioral Assessment Scale. Philadelphia, PA, J B Lippincott, 1973
13. Stengel TJ: The Neonatal Behavioral Assessment Scale: Description, clinical uses and research implications. Physical and Occupational Therapy in Pediatrics 1:39–57, 1980
14. Als H, Lester BM, Tronick E: Assessment of preterm infant's behavior (APIB). In Fitzgerald H, et al (eds): Theory and Research in Behavioral Pediatrics, Vol 1. New York, NY, Plenum Publishing Corp, 1982
15. Amiel-Tison C, Grenier A: Neurological Evaluation of the Newborn and the Infant. New York, NY, Masson Publishing USA Inc, 1983, pp 15–38
16. Dubowitz LMS, Dubowitz V, Goldberg C: Clinical assessment of gestational age in the newborn infant. J Pediatr 77:1–10, 1970
17. Campbell SK: The developing infant: Neuromuscular maturation. In Wilson JM (ed): Infants at Risk: Medical and Therapeutic Management. Chapel Hill, NC, University of North Carolina, 1981, pp 63–68
18. Illingworth RS: The Development of the Infant and the Young Child: Normal and Abnormal, ed 6. Edinburgh, Scotland, Churchill Livingstone, 1975, pp 80–95
19. Garliner D: Myofunctional Therapy. Philadelphia, PA, W B Saunders Co, 1976, pp 7–13
20. Bower TGR: A Primer of Infant Development. New York, NY, W H Freeman & Co Publishers, 1977
21. Bower TGR: Human Development. New York, NY, W H Freeman & Co Publishers, 1979
22. Cohen LB, DeLoache JS, Strauss MS: Infant visual perception. In Osofsky O (ed): Handbook of Infancy. New York, NY, John Wiley & Sons Inc, 1978
23. Haaf RA, Bell RQ: A facial dimension in visual discrimination by human infants. Child Dev 38:893–899, 1967
24. Eisenberg RB: Development of hearing in man: An assessment of current status. Journal of the American Speech and Hearing Association 12:199–223, 1970
25. Long JG, Alistair GSP, Lucey JF: Excessive handling as a cause of hypoxemia. Pediatrics 65:203–207, 1980
26. Minkowski A, Saint-Anne Dargassies S: Le retentissement de l'anoxic toetale sur le systeme nerveux control. Rev franc et clin biol 1:531, 1956. Cited in Parmelee AH: European studies of the newborn. Child Dev 33:169–180, 1962
27. Prechtl HFR: Prognostic value of neurological signs in the newborn infant. Proceeding of the Royal Society of Medicine 58:3–4, 1965
28. Bierman-van Eenderburg MEC, Jurgens van der Zee AD, Olina AA, et al: Predictive value of neonatal neurological examination: A follow up study at 18 mos. Dev Med Child Neurol 23:296–305, 1981
29. Sostek A, Anders TF: Relationships among the Brazelton neonatal scale, Bayley infant scales, and early temperament. Child Dev 48:320–323, 1977
30. Tronick E, Brazelton TB: Clinical uses of the Brazelton Neonatal Behavioral Assessment. In Friedlander BZ, et al (eds): Exceptional Infant: Assessment and Intervention, Vol 3. New York, NY, Brunner/Mazel Inc, 1975
31. Palisano RJ, Short MA: Methods for assessing muscle tone and motor functions in the neonate: A review. Physical and Occupational Therapy in Pediatrics 4:43–54, 1984

Scoring Sheet for the Infant Neurological International Battery (INFANIB)

Suggestion from the Field

PATRICIA H. ELLISON

The scoring sheet for the Infant Neurological International Battery (INFANIB) was not published in the September 1985 issue (Phys Ther 65:1326–1331, 1985) with the research article by Ellison et al entitled "Construction of an Infant Neurological International Battery (INFANIB) for the Assessment of Neurological Integrity in Infancy." The sheet is printed here to permit clinicians working with infants to use this method for a quantified evaluation of tone and posture. Further details that describe each item and more information about the use of the method are available from the author.

Dr. Ellison is Research Professor, Department of Psychology, University of Denver, 2030 S York St, Denver, CO 80208 (USA).

PRACTICE

INFANIB

Date of Exam ______

Corrected Gestational Age ______

ITEM	START SCORE	MAJOR CHANGE	NAME	CIRCLE ONE							
1	Birth		**SUPINE** Hands closed/open	Closed	Sometimes Closed	Open					
2	Birth		Scarf sign	Less Than #1	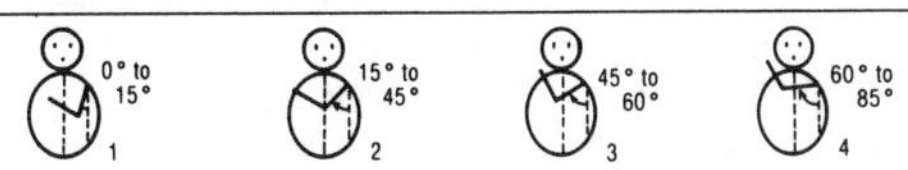 0° to 15° (1)	15° to 45° (2)	45° to 60° (3)	60° to 85° (4)	Past #4		
3	Birth		Heel to ear	Over 100°	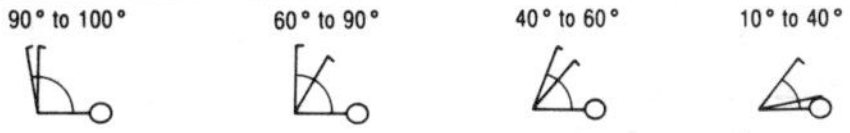 90° to 100°	60° to 90°	40° to 60°	10° to 40°	Under 10°		
4	Birth		Popliteal angle	Under 80°	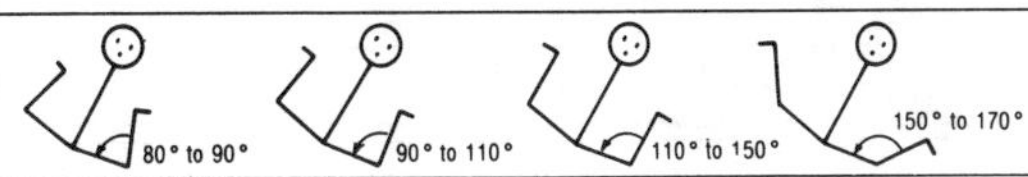 80° to 90°	90° to 110°	110° to 150°	150° to 170°	Over 170°		
5	Birth		Leg abduction	Under 40°	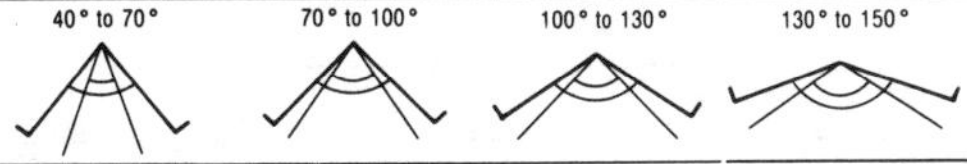 40° to 70°	70° to 100°	100° to 130°	130° to 150°	Over 150°		
6	Birth		Dorsiflexion of foot	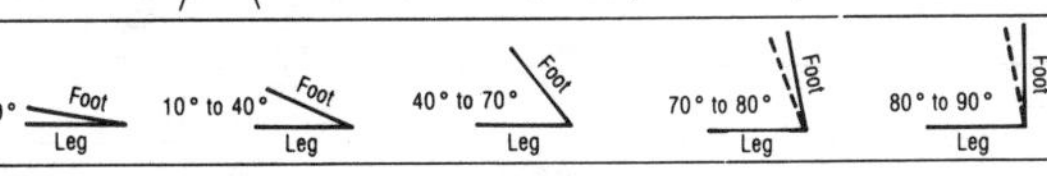 0° to 10° (Foot / Leg)	10° to 40° (Foot / Leg)	40° to 70° (Foot / Leg)	70° to 80° (Foot / Leg)	80° to 90° (Foot / Leg)			
7	Birth	9 mos.	Foot grasp	No Grasp	Barely Grasp	Grasp					
8	Birth	6 mos.	Tonic labyrinthine supine	Absent	Shoulder retraction or some extension of trunk or legs	Shoulder retraction and full leg extension					
9	Birth	6 mos.	Asymmetric tonic neck reflex	Absent	Postures in, can move out	Persistent					
10	Birth		Pull to sitting	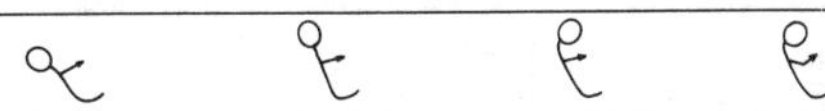 Head extended Arms extended	Head up Arms ext.	Head flexed Arms ext.	Head flexed Arms flexed				
11	4 mos.		Body derotative	Present to both sides	Slow or mildly asymmetrical	Absent or markedly asymmetrical					
12	9 mos		Body rotative	Present	Poor	Absent					
13	Birth		**PRONE** All fours	Lifts Head	Head up 45°	Forearms only	Head up 90°	Bears weight on extended arms	Assumes all fours unsteadily	Assumes all fours well	Stands up through Plantigrade
14	Birth	9 mos.	Tonic labyrinthine prone	Absent	With Head Flexion: Shoulder protraction or some flexion of legs	With Head Flexion: Shoulder protraction and arms, hips, or legs under trunk					
15	Birth		**SITTING** Sitting position	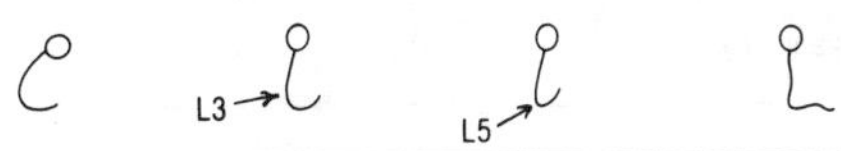	L3	L5					
16	6 mos.		Sideways parachute	Present in both arms	Slow or mildly asymmetrical	Absent or markedly asymmetrical					
17	9 mos.		Backwards parachute	Present in both arms	Slow or mildly asymmetrical	Absent or markedly asymmetrical					
18	Birth		**STANDING** Weight bearing	Primitive reflex	No weight bearing	Poor weight bearing Breaks at knees	Unequal weight bearing	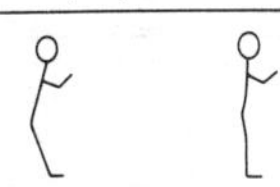			
19	3 mos.		Positive support reaction	Feet flat	5 to 30 sec. on toes then drop to feet flat	>30 sec. on toes					
20	7 mos.		**SUSPENDED** Forward parachute	Present	Slow or mildly asymmetrical	Absent or markedly asymmetrical					

FACTOR SCORES

TOTAL SCORE

↓ Corrected gestational age

SCORING

Overall: Normal = 5, Mildly abnormal = 3, Markedly abnormal = 1

ITEM	0-.9	1-1.9	2-2.9	3-3.9	4-4.9	5-5.9	6-6.9	7-7.9	8-8.9	9-18 months	Comments
1.	Closed		Sometimes closed	Open						Matches age = 5	One stage delay = 3 Two stage delay = 1 One closed, one open = 1
2.	 0 - 15° 1			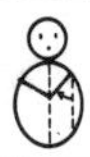 15 - 45° 2			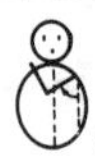 45 - 60° 3			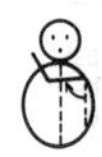 60 - 85° 4	5 = Picture matches age 3 = One stage away ← or → 1 = Two stages away ← or →
3.	100 - 90°			90 - 60°			60 - 40°			40 - 10°	
4.	80 - 90°			90 - 110°			110 - 150°			150 - 170°	As above except definite asymmetry = 1
5.	40 - 70°			70 - 100°			100 - 130°			130 - 150°	As for # 2 & 3
6.	0 - 10° = 1			10 - 40° = 3			40 - 70° = 5			70 - 80° = 3 80 - 90° = 1	
7.	Exaggerated Grasp = 1, Other = 5									Absent = 5 Barely Grasp = 3 Grasp = 1	
8.	Exaggerated TLS = 1, Other = 5									Absent = 5 Some = 3 Full = 1	
9.	Exaggerated ATNR = 1, Other = 5						Absent = 5		Postures in Can move out = 3	Persistent = 1	
10.	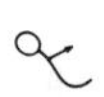			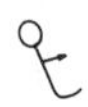	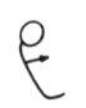	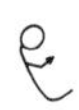	Full = 5 Partial head lag or not using arms = 3 Complete head lag and not using arms = 1				Picture matches age = 5 One stage delay = 3 Two stage delay = 1
11.					Present to both sides = 5		Slow or mildly asymmetrical = 3			Absent or markedly asymmetrical = 1	
12.										Present = 5 Poor = 3 Absent = 1	
13.	Lifts Head		Head up 45°	Forearms only	Head up 90°	Bears weight on extended forearms		All fours unsteadily	All fours well	Plantigrade	Picture matches age = 5 One stage delay = 3 Two stage delay = 1
14.	Exaggerated TLP = 1, Other = 5									Absent = 5 Some = 3 Full = 1	
15.	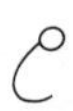			L3 → 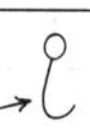		L5 → 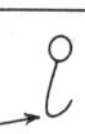		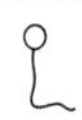			Picture matches age = 5 One stage delay = 3 Two stage delay = 1
16.							Present in both arms = 5		Slow or mildly asymmetrical = 3	Absent or markedly asymmetrical = 1	
17.										As Above	
18.	Primitive Reflex	No Weight-bearing	Poor weight bearing Breaks at knee			Unequal weight bearing		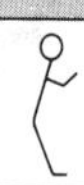		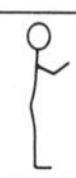	Picture matches age = 5 One stage delay = 3 Two stage delay = 1 Persistent weight-bearing (> 60 sec) at 2.5 - 5 months = 1
19.				Maintains weight feet flat = 5		5 - 30 sec. on toes then drop to feet flat = 3				> 30 sec on toes = 1	
20.								Present = 5	Slow or mildly asymmetrical = 3	Absent or markedly asym. = 1	

Degree of normality/abnormality based on total score

Less than 4 months	4 to 8 months	8 months or more
Abnormal ≤ 48	Abnormal ≤ 54	Abnormal ≤ 68
Transient 49 - 65	Transient 55-71	Transient 69-82
Normal ≥ 66	Normal ≥ 72	Normal ≥ 83

Category of abnormality

If abnormal, choose a category

☐ Spastic Tetraparesis/Dyskinesia ☐ Spastic Hemiparesis ☐ Spastic Diplegia ☐ Hypotonia

1/85

Norm-Referenced and Criterion-Referenced Tests

Use in Pediatrics and Application to Task Analysis of Motor Skill

PATRICIA C. MONTGOMERY
and BARBARA H. CONNOLLY

The purposes of this article are 1) to compare the similarities and differences between norm-referenced and criterion-referenced tests and 2) to summarize how each should be used in the assessment of developmental performance in children. Specific developmental assessments, the populations they address, and the information they provide are described briefly. The need for additional criterion-referenced tests in physical therapy is discussed, and an example of how task analysis can be applied to movement or motor skills in the development of a criterion-referenced test is provided. Physical therapists can enhance the credibility of their assessments by appropriate use of norm-referenced and criterion-referenced tests.

Key Words: *Pediatrics, evaluation; Physical therapy.*

Physical therapists use various tests to document children's motor behavior and sensory-perceptual, cognitive-language, and social-emotional functioning. The purposes of this article are 1) to define norm-referenced and criterion-referenced tests and 2) to describe their use in pediatrics. In addition, the need for criterion-referenced tests that are related to physical therapy intervention is discussed, and an example of how task analysis can be applied to movement and used in the development of a criterion-referenced test is included.

NORM-REFERENCED AND CRITERION-REFERENCED TESTS

Physical therapists often use published developmental tests to ensure credibility in the assessment of children. The purpose of testing must be determined by the therapist if the appropriate test is to be selected. If the purpose of a test is to identify children with motor handicaps in a school system or to establish a specific age level for an individual child, a norm-referenced test would be used. If a physical therapist wants to plan an intervention program or determine its effectiveness by examining an individual child's performance, however, a criterion-referenced test would be appropriate.

Norm-referenced tests are designed to examine individual performance in relation to the performance of a representative group. Criterion-referenced tests document individual performance in relation to a domain of information or specific set of skills.[1]

A standardized test is inferred usually to be a norm-referenced test, but criterion-referenced tests also may be standardized. *Standardization* is the process of administering a test under uniform conditions to each child who is to be tested. A normative test is a test that has been administered in a standardized manner to large numbers of children at various ages. A test, therefore, may be standardized in its administration, but not normed, as in some criterion-referenced tests. In addition to purpose, factors such as how the test was developed and how the test scores are interpreted help to distinguish between norm-referenced and criterion-referenced tests.[2] According to Swezey, a test is criterion-referenced if the scoring is based on absolute rather than relative standards, its primary use is to measure mastery of specific skills or tasks, and the test items are based on known performance objectives associated with the tasks of interest.[2]

Glaser introduced the term *criterion-referenced measures.*[3] He stated that the concept of proficiency measurement was a continuum of skill ranging from no proficiency at all to a perfect performance. Knowledge of an individual's performance on a criterion-referenced measure provides explicit information as to what he can and cannot do, thereby providing an index of competence that is independent of the performance of others. The child's performance on criterion-referenced tests is compared with an external criterion or standard of performance without regard to the distribution of scores achieved by other individuals of the same age.[2] Unless the criterion-referenced test is normed and administered in a standardized manner, it cannot be used to assign age levels as a normative test. Tests that are domain referenced, competency based, and objectives referenced can be subsumed under the category of criterion-referenced tests.

Criterion-referenced tests are related directly to instructional objectives, are based on task analysis, and are designed to measure changes in successive performances of an individual. Criterion-referenced tests, therefore, are sensitive to and can be used to measure the effects of instruction. Conversely, norm-referenced tests generally are not related to instructional objectives, do not use task analysis, and are designed to delineate differences among individuals. Norm-referenced tests, therefore, are not sensitive to and should not be used to evaluate the effects of instruction.[1–3]

Although some uncertainty has existed about appropriate measures for determining reliability and validity of criterion-referenced instruments,[4] models of test theory can be applied to criterion-referenced tests.[2,5] Criterion-referenced tests should demonstrate the same interrater and test-retest reliability as norm-referenced tests, and issues of validity (particularly content, concurrence, and predictive value) also are applicable, depending on the purpose of the test. Similarities and differences between norm-referenced and criterion-referenced tests are summarized in Table 1.

Dr. Montgomery is in private practice with Therapeutic Intervention Programs, Inc, 2217 Glenhurst Rd, St. Louis Park, MN 55416 (USA).
Dr. Connolly is Associate Professor, Program in Physical Therapy, University of Tennessee, 800 Madison Ave, Memphis, TN 38163.

TABLE 1
Similarities and Differences Between Norm-Referenced and Criterion-Referenced Tests

Norm-Referenced Tests	Criterion-Referenced Tests
Purposes: to examine individual performance in relation to a representative group; can be used to establish age levels; used for diagnosis and placement.	Purposes: to examine individual performance in relation to a criterion or external standard; cannot be used to establish age levels unless normed; used for program planning and evaluation because items are sensitive to effects of instruction (intervention).
Test construction: items usually not developed from task analysis; test items may or may not be related to the objectives of instruction (intervention).	Test construction: items developed from task analysis; test items are related to the objectives of instruction (intervention).
Administration: must be administered in a standard manner.	Administration: may or may not be administered in a standard manner.
Scoring: based on standards relative to a group; variability of scores (ie, means and standard deviations) is desired with normal distribution.	Scoring: based on absolute standards; variability of scores is not obtained because perfect or near-perfect scores are desired.
Psychometric properties: test should demonstrate reliability and validity.	Psychometric properties: test should demonstrate reliability and validity.

NORM-REFERENCED TESTS IN PEDIATRICS

Two examples of norm-referenced tests for young children are the Bayley Scales of Infant Development[6] and the Gesell developmental scales.[7] The Bayley scales were standardized on 1,400 children between 1 and 15 months of age and 160 children between 18 and 30 months of age. The main purpose of the Bayley scales is to establish current developmental status (motor and mental scales) to identify problems and the need for intervention. The Gesell scales were administered to groups of children between 4 weeks and 36 months of age with the purpose of identifying even minor deviations in the areas of adaptive, gross and fine motor, language, and personal and social development. The motor performance of older children can be evaluated using the Bruininks-Oseretsky Test of Motor Proficiency (ages 4.5-14.5 years)[8] or the Stott-Moyes-Henderson Test of Motor Impairment (ages 5-12 years).[9] Both tests have normative data and are designed to be used in making decisions about appropriate educational and therapeutic placement.

CRITERION-REFERENCED TESTS IN PEDIATRICS

The Brigance Diagnostic Inventory of Early Development can be used with children whose developmental ages range from birth to 7 years.[10] This criterion-referenced test is based on items from norm-referenced tests, and its purpose is to assess general development as a guide to subsequent instruction. Developed as a response to Public Law 94-142 for children with developmental handicaps, it is used appropriately for programming, but not as a diagnostic or placement test. A second criterion-referenced test is the Milani-Comparetti Motor Development Screening Test.[11] This test is a neurodevelopmental examination of children from 0 to 2 years of age with tasks designed to measure developmental reflexes and motor skill development. Although its purpose is to determine "whether one child's motor development corresponds to that of a normal child,"[11] normative data are unavailable.

Another criterion-referenced test is the Movement Assessment of Infants (MAI), which was designed to provide measures of muscle tone, reflex development, automatic movement, and volitional movement in the first year of life and to provide an assessment of risk for motor dysfunction at 4 months of age.[12] The MAI is a good example of a criterion-referenced test that currently is being subjected to reliability and validity testing and to the process of standardization and normative data collection so that its use as a norm-referenced test eventually may be appropriate. The Peabody Developmental Motor Scales (ages 0-7 years) is an example of a norm-referenced test that also can be used as a criterion-referenced test, depending on the purpose of its use and the interpretation of the child's performance.[13]

USING TEST RESULTS

Although formal testing is only a part of the overall assessment of children, quantifiable data are essential for communicating information regarding motor and other types of performance and developmental levels. Norm-referenced tests, however, are not particularly helpful to the physical therapist in planning qualitative intervention and may be used inappropriately to develop intervention objectives or to teach the next developmental skill. As motor development tests are developed, items often are chosen from previously published normative tests, resulting in similar test items that are reflective of major motor milestones, rather than documenting qualitative factors that may exist. Tests measuring sensory-based functions are more innovative and often more qualitative in nature than tests of motor development. These tests may have more questionable construct validity, however, because they are more theoretical in nature. Sensory-based tests such as the Miller Assessment for Preschoolers (ages 2 years 9 months to 5 years 8 months)[14] and the Sensory Integration and Praxis Tests (ages 5-10 years)[15] complement tests of motor skills and can be psychometrically sound.

Physical therapists use clinical observations and expertise in assessing motor development to determine why a child has motor delays or dysfunction, and intervention usually is aimed at underlying problems. Criterion-referenced motor development tests consisting of task analyses, therefore, are usually more helpful in planning intervention programs and measuring change than are norm-referenced tests.

CONSTRUCTING CRITERION-REFERENCED TESTS

Physical therapists need more criterion-referenced tests to evaluate the sensory and motor abilities of children and adults. The characteristics of well-constructed criterion-referenced tests have been established,[16] and physical therapists should consider constructing tests that meet their specific program planning and evaluation needs. Criterion-referenced tests can be designed for a particular group or subgroup of patients or to assess specific functional abilities.

In developing criterion-referenced tests, several models can be used. According to Swezey, in criterion-referenced measurement test items are developed directly from an analysis of tasks to be performed.[2] For physical therapists working with children, these tasks often would be related to normal motor development. Current criterion-referenced tests often provide a standard of performance for motor skills, but may not use external criteria of interest to physical therapists. For example, rolling is a developmental motor skill often assessed as either present or absent. Table 2 illustrates some performance components related to physical therapy intervention that could be observed during rolling, such as the ability to roll in both directions, motor planning, the influence of postural reactions and primitive reflexes, and the vestibular response to self-induced movement.[17] Specific standards of performance by which to judge the child's performance are listed in the Appendix. Such a task analysis would be appropriate for use as a pretest and posttest device to identify problem areas underlying poor performance. This information would be helpful to the therapist in treatment planning and in subsequent reevaluations of performance as one way to measure change. Performance on such a test could be used as a screening technique, but unless criterion-referenced tests are administered to a large number of children at different ages, they could not be used as diagnostic tools for assigning specific age (or normative) levels or for determining program placement.

CONCLUSIONS

Physical therapists include norm-referenced and criterion-referenced tests in the assessment process. One essential element in determining the appropriateness of the test selected is how it is to be used. Norm-referenced tests, in which the child's performance is compared with that of a normative group, are used for diagnostic and placement purposes. Criterion-referenced tests compare a child's performance against his own performance or an external standard, rather than against the performance of others. Criterion-referenced tests

TABLE 2
Analysis of Rolling

Task	Performance Level[a]		
	Poor	Fair	Optimal
Rolls both directions	1	3	5
	Lt —	Lt —	Lt —
	Rt —	Rt —	Rt —
Motor planning	1	3	5
Body righting	1	3	5
Head righting			
Prone	1	3	5
Supine	1	3	5
Lateral	1	3	5
Asymmetrical tonic neck response			
Right	1	3	5
Left	1	3	5
Antigravity flexion	1	3	5
Antigravity extension	1	3	5
Hips flexed			
Knees flexed			
Arms flexed			
Becomes dizzy (vestibular)	1	3	5
			TOTAL ____

[a] No score given if subject unable to perform task. (See Appendix for criteria.)

APPENDIX
Analysis of Rolling

Instructions: Child rolls about 12 ft[a] in a straight line (place masking tape line on carpet or mat). Ask child to roll from one end to the other and back. Demonstrate, if necessary.
Criteria (Score: 1 = Poor, 3 = Fair, 5 = Optimal)

Rolls both directions. Poor: Child rolls to one direction only. Fair: Child tends to roll to one direction, but will roll both directions when encouraged (check side to which child does not roll spontaneously). Optimal: Child rolls both directions easily and spontaneously.

Motor planning. Poor: Child cannot roll from one point to another; may roll in circular pattern. Fair: Child has some difficulty rolling in a straight line, but can correct direction to arrive at designated point. Optimal: Child rolls easily in a straight line in both directions. If response is asymmetric, check side to which child has more difficulty motor planning.

Body righting. Poor: Child log rolls; no segmentation of hip, trunk, or shoulders. Fair: Child log rolls, but occasionally uses segmental movement. Optimal: Child performs smooth segmental roll in both directions with hip or shoulder leading. If response is asymmetric, check side to which child does not use body righting.

Head righting. Poor: As child rolls, head touches floor occasionally, or child cannot lift head off surface. Fair: Child lifts head up, but occasionally drops it without touching floor. Optimal: Child's head "rights" in all positions and does not touch floor. Evaluate when child is in prone, supine, and side-lying positions during rolling.

Asymmetrical tonic neck response (ATNR). Poor: Child uses ATNR to roll by turning face to elicit arm extension and increase momentum for rolling (check direction face is turned if ATNR response occurs). Fair: Child occasionally uses ATNR to roll. Optimal: Child rotates left shoulder before right shoulder when rolling to right side (if child uses ATNR, right arm will lead). Evaluate when child is rolling in both directions.

Antigravity flexion. Poor: Child routinely assumes hyperextended position of neck or trunk when positioned supine. Fair: Child occasionally assumes hyperextended position when positioned supine. Optimal: Child assumes extended position of trunk momentarily when positioned supine.

Antigravity extension. Poor: Child assumes flexed posture when in prone position (note whether hips, knees, and arms are flexed). Fair: Mild flexion is evident when in prone position. Optimal: Child does not flex when in prone position.

Becomes dizzy (vestibular). Poor: Child reports or displays dizziness or nausea or becomes disoriented and cannot complete task. Fair: Child reports dizziness or nausea or becomes disoriented, but can complete task with some difficulty. Optimal: Child may report mild dizziness, but does not become disoriented and completes task easily.

[a] 1 ft = 0.3048 m.

are used for program planning and evaluation, and task analyses used in the development of criterion-referenced tests can be applied to movements or motor skills of interest to physical therapists. In addition, external standards of performance can be chosen that relate directly to physical therapy intervention. Although physical therapists use their observational skills to evaluate the qualitative aspects of movement, norm-referenced and criterion-referenced tests are essential for ensuring credibility in the assessment process and for communicating information regarding the need for intervention, the type of intervention necessary, and changes in the child's function. Such data are essential not only to the physical therapist, but also to the child's family, other health care professionals, and third-party payers.

REFERENCES

1. Swanson HL, Watson BL: Educational and Psychological Assessment of Exceptional Children: Theories, Strategies, and Applications. St Louis, MO, C V Mosby Co, 1982, pp 38–61
2. Swezey RW: Individual Performance Assessment: An Approach to Criterion-Referenced Test Development. Reston, VA, Reston Publishing Co Inc, 1981, pp 3–19, 141–158
3. Glaser R: Instructional technology and the measurement of learning outcomes: Some questions. Am Psychol 18:519–521, 1963
4. Boehm A: Criterion-referenced assessment for the teacher. Teachers College Record 78:117–126, 1973
5. Shaycoft MF: Handbook of Criterion-Referenced Testing: Development, Evaluation and Use. New York, NY, Garland Publishing Inc, 1979
6. Bayley N: The Bayley Scales of Infant Development. New York, NY, The Psychological Corporation, 1969
7. Knobloch H, Stevens F, Malone AF: Manual of Developmental Diagnosis: The Administration and Interpretation of the Revised Gesell and Amtruda Developmental and Neurologic Examination. Hagerstown, MD, Harper & Row, Publishers Inc, 1980
8. Bruininks RH: Bruininks-Oseretsky Test of Motor Proficiency: Examiner's Manual. Circle Pines, MN, American Guidance Service, 1978
9. Stott DH, Moyes FA, Henderson SE: Test of Motor Impairment. Guelph, Ontario, Canada, Brook Educational Publishing Limited, 1984
10. Brigance AH: Brigance Diagnostic Inventory of Early Development. Woburn, MA, Curriculum Associates Inc, 1978
11. Milani-Comparetti A: The Milani-Comparetti Motor Development Screening Test. Omaha, NE, Meyer Children's Rehabilitation Institute, University of Nebraska Medical Center, 1977
12. Chandler LS, Andrews MS, Swanson MW: Movement Assessment of Infants: A Manual. Rolling Bay, WA, Chandler, Andrews, and Swanson, 1980
13. Folio MR, Fewell RR: Peabody Developmental Motor Scales and Activity Cards. Allen, TX, DLM Teaching Resources, 1983
14. Miller L: Miller Assessment for Preschoolers. Littleton, CO, The Foundation for Knowledge in Development, 1982
15. Ayres AJ: Sensory Integration and Praxis Tests. Pasadena, CA, Western Psychological Services, to be published
16. Popham WJ: Criterion-Referenced Measurements. Englewood Cliffs, NJ, Prentice-Hall Inc, 1978, pp 89–141
17. Richter EW, Montgomery PC: The Sensorimotor Performance Analysis. Laurel, MD, RAMSCO Publications, to be published

Measuring Infant Movement

Clinical and Technological Assessment Techniques

SUSAN R. HARRIS
and CAROLYN B. HERIZA

Assessment of infant movement patterns is an important evaluation component in the early identification and management of high-risk and handicapped infants. Differences in infant movement patterns may provide early clues to the diagnosis of cerebral palsy and other developmental disabilities. The ultimate goal of early identification of movement disorders is the provision of early intervention services, such as developmental physical therapy. Qualitative analysis of infant movement differences can assist the clinician in developing treatment strategies aimed at facilitating normal movement patterns during the critical period of early central nervous system plasticity. This article presents four measurement strategies for quantifying such qualitative differences. Three clinical assessment tools—the Movement Assessment of Infants, the Bayley Motor Scale, and the Peabody Developmental Motor Scales—are described. Finally, new technological advances for kinematic analysis of infant movement are presented.

Key Words: *Child development disorders; Infant; Pediatrics, evaluation; Physical therapy.*

Traditionally, physical therapists in pediatrics have relied on norm-referenced, developmental motor assessment tools in the evaluation of motor-risk infants. Although such tools assess the attainment of developmental motor milestones, they fail to provide information on qualitative aspects of infant movement patterns that are important elements in early diagnosis and early therapeutic programming efforts. An infant may achieve a developmental motor milestone "on schedule," but the movement patterns used to achieve the milestone may be atypical. Infants with Down syndrome, for example, frequently roll from a prone to a supine position in advance of their nonhandicapped peers (ie, at 1-2 months vs 4-5 months). A qualitative evaluation of this "precocious" milestone, however, reveals that this early rolling pattern is actually a brisk "flip over" into a supine position, which is accomplished because of a lack of co-contraction of trunk muscles and an inability to grade the movement adequately.[1]

Although the use of norm-referenced developmental assessment tools is an important component of infant movement evaluation, a need exists for standardized qualitative assessment tools as well. Following are examples of a qualitative movement assessment tool (the Movement Assessment of Infants[2]) and two norm-referenced developmental motor assessment scales (the Bayley Motor Scale[3] and the Peabody Developmental Motor Scales[4]).

MOVEMENT ASSESSMENT OF INFANTS

Developed by three physical therapists in pediatrics, the Movement Assessment of Infants (MAI)[2] assesses four different components of movement: 1) muscle tone (readiness of muscles to respond to gravity), 2) primitive reflexes, 3) automatic reactions, and 4) volitional movement. Included across these four components are 65 items, each with individual, objective scoring criteria. Whereas most instruments that assess attainment of developmental motor milestones use nominal scoring criteria such as "pass-fail" or "present-absent," the MAI uses either a four-point or a six-point ordinal scale in measuring the infant's behavior on each of the 65 items. Thus, qualitative assessment of the infant's movement is incorporated into a quantitative scoring system for each item.

Although the MAI is intended for clinical use with infants up to the age of 12 months, its use as a research tool has been limited to infants who range in age from 3.5 to 4.5 months. Included in the MAI manual is a 4-month profile that suggests age-appropriate scores for 48 of the 65 items. If an infant receives an item score that is not considered to be age-appropriate or typical for a 4-month-old infant, the score is circled and becomes a risk score. Circled item scores then are summed to attain a total risk score. Currently, the 4-month profile is based on limited normative data. Nonetheless, the use of the total risk score has been validated empirically in a retrospective analysis of its ability to detect early signs of cerebral palsy.[5]

Early studies examining the overall reliability and validity of the MAI suggest that it has acceptable levels of interrater and test-retest reliability,[6] in addition to some measure of concurrent and predictive validity.[5] Recent item analysis studies have shown that certain items have much greater reliability and predictive ability than do other items.[7,8] Future research should be directed at developing a refined version of this tool. It would use only the most reliable and predictive items and would be strengthened further by the collection of normative data. Despite these shortcomings, the MAI represents an important first step toward the clinical measurement of qualitative aspects of infant movement.

Dr. Harris is Associate Professor and Program Coordinator of Physical Therapy, School of Allied Health Professions, University of Wisconsin, 1300 University Ave, Madison, WI 53706 (USA). She was Physical Therapy Department Head, Clinical Training Unit, Child Development and Mental Retardation Center, and Research Assistant Professor of Pediatrics, School of Medicine, University of Washington, Seattle, WA 98195, when this article was written.

Dr. Heriza is Associate Professor, Department of Physical Therapy, School of Allied Health Professions, St. Louis University Medical Center, St. Louis, MO 63104.

BAYLEY MOTOR SCALE

The Bayley Motor Scale is one of three scales of the Bayley Scales of Infant Development (BSID), a norm-referenced, standardized developmental assessment tool developed by a psychologist and published in 1969.[3] Normalized on 1,262 infants in the mid-1960s, the BSID is one of the most widely used developmental assessment tools both in clinical practice and in research. The other two components of the BSID are the Mental Scale and the Infant Behavior Record.

The Bayley Motor Scale consists of 81 developmental motor milestones covering an age span of 2 to 30 months. Each item is scored as either "pass" or "fail" based on standardized administration and scoring guidelines included in the instruction manual. Items that are omitted or that are based only on parent report are scored as failures. The majority of items are in the gross motor area, although some fine motor items (ie, prehension, combining, ball throwing) are included as well.

The reliability of the BSID is high.[9] The instruction manual advises, however, that scores attained during infancy are not valid predictors of later performance.[3] Both the Bayley Mental Scale and the Bayley Motor Scale have been used in numerous research studies with both high-risk and handicapped infants, including studies conducted by physical therapists.[6,10-12] Recent research has suggested, however, that the 1969 BSID normative data are out-of-date and should be renormed.[13]

The Bayley Motor Scale assesses the attainment of developmental motor milestones without judging the qualitative performance used to achieve those milestones, whereas the MAI both qualitatively and quantitatively assesses infant movement. An item on the Bayley Motor Scale entitled "unilateral reaching," for example, would be passed easily by an infant with early signs of spastic hemiplegia. The infant's motor deficit actually would enhance his ability to pass this item in that he would be unable to reach bimanually.

Based on its shortcoming in measuring qualitative movement differences, we could hypothesize that the Bayley Motor Scale would be less sensitive than the MAI in identifying early signs of cerebral palsy. A recent retrospective study supports this hypothesis.[14] The MAI was shown to be more than twice as sensitive as the Bayley Motor Scale in identifying low birthweight infants who were diagnosed later as having cerebral palsy.

PEABODY DEVELOPMENTAL MOTOR SCALES

Published in 1983, the Peabody Developmental Motor Scales (PDMS) are standardized, norm-referenced gross and fine motor scales that were developed by a physical educator and a special educator.[4] Normative data were collected in 1981-1982 on a stratified sample of 617 children ranging in age from 1 to 83 months.[15] Because the PDMS consists of both gross and fine motor scales and spans an age range of birth to 7 years, it has broad appeal for use by physical therapists in pediatrics.

The Peabody Gross Motor Scale and the Peabody Fine Motor Scale consist of 170 and 112 items, respectively. Each item is scored on a three-point scale (0 = unsuccessful; 1 = clear resemblance to item criterion, but criterion not fully met; 2 = successful performance, criterion met). Standardized administration procedures, materials, position of the child, and scoring criteria are included in the PDMS manual.[4,15]

Both interrater and test-retest reliability are high ($r \geq .80$) for the PDMS. As reported in the PDMS manual, the correlation coefficient for concurrent validity of the Peabody Gross Motor Scale with the Bayley Motor Scale was .37 ($p = .02$); the Peabody Fine Motor Scale scores were correlated significantly with the Bayley Mental Scale scores ($r = .78$, $p = .001$).

A recent study by Palisano examined concurrent and predictive validities of the Bayley Motor Scale and the PDMS in a sample of 44 infants (23 full-term and 21 healthy premature) aged 12, 15, and 18 months.[16] Correlation coefficients for current validity ranged from .63 to .93 between scores on the Bayley Motor Scale and scores on the Peabody Gross Motor Scale and between .17 and .59 for scores on the Bayley Motor Scale and scores on the Peabody Fine Motor Scale. Predictive abilities of 12-month scores to 18-month scores generally were poor ($r \leq .60$) with the exception of the scores of the Peabody Fine Motor Scale for the premature group ($r = .75$).[16]

The PDMS demonstrates some obvious advantages when compared with the Bayley Motor Scale. The scoring criteria of the PDMS are broader in that it uses a three-point ordinal scale, whereas the Bayley Motor Scale uses a nominal scale of pass or fail. Normative data for the PDMS were collected more recently than those for the Bayley Motor Scale (early 1980s vs mid-1960s); however, the normative sample for the PDMS is only half as large as that for the Bayley Motor Scale, despite its expanded age range. The PDMS also has the added advantage of including both gross motor and fine motor scales.

Nonetheless, numerous drawbacks have been outlined recently for the PDMS (K. Kinderer, P. Richardson, S. Atwater; unpublished manuscript; April 1987). Some age levels are loaded heavily with items from certain skill categories. Seventy percent of the items at 36 to 41 months on the Peabody Gross Motor Scale, for example, are locomotor activities, whereas 50% of the items at the next age level (42-47 months) are ball skills. Although the PDMS has five different skill categories, these categories are not represented equally at each age level. Other concerns noted about the PDMS in this manuscript are the failure to place items in correct developmental sequence, such as skipping preceding galloping; poor quality of many of the test materials; failure to include several test materials in the site, thus threatening standardization; failure of the test manual to include specific criteria for a score of 1; and discrepancies in correspondence between age equivalents and z scores.

Despite the deficiencies noted in both the Bayley Motor Scale and the PDMS, pediatric physical therapists must continue to rely on norm-referenced, developmental assessment tools as well as qualitative movement assessment instruments such as the MAI. Both types of clinical tools may be useful in the early identification and treatment of infants with movement differences. Finally, data from norm-referenced tools often are required to qualify an infant to receive state-funded developmental intervention services. We advocate that both types of tools be used concurrently to measure reliably infant movement and motor development.

KINEMATIC ANALYSIS

Kinematic analysis is a detailed descriptive analysis of a movement pattern.[17-20] Such analysis delineates temporal and spatial qualities of movement. It reveals how the segments of the body are coordinated with one another and the structure of the movement. Kinematic variables used to describe and analyze movement are joint position and angle, time, linear and angular displacements, limb velocities, and accelerations.[18-20]

Although physical therapists traditionally have used visual observations to conduct kinematic assessment of movements,

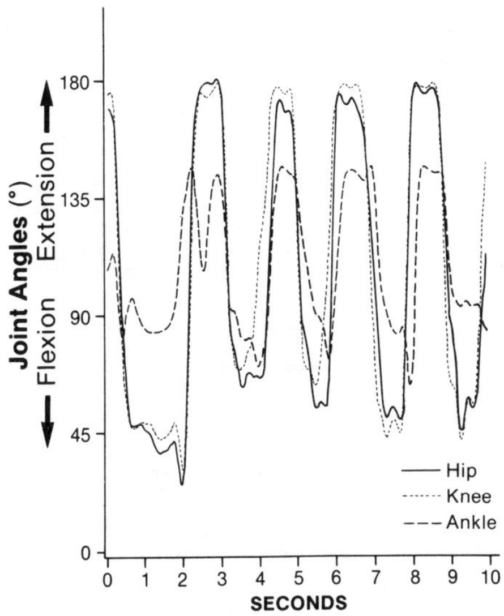

Fig. 1. Angle-time diagram of joint angle rotations of typical kicking movements of a 34-week gestational age infant. Decreasing angles indicate flexion.

such description is subjective relying on the clinical experience and knowledge of the therapist.[17,19–21] Imaging techniques (television, cinematography, and optoelectric systems) have been used in laboratory settings to provide objective kinematic analysis of movement. With recent advances in technology, these techniques are being incorporated into clinical settings. The various imaging techniques differ in cost and sophistication. For detailed descriptions of imaging techniques and of their advantages and limitations, the reader is referred to Craik and Oatis,[17] Yack,[20] Gronley and Perry,[22] Medeiros,[23] and Winter and associates.[19,24] The advantages of imaging measurement techniques, especially the automated systems, indicate that they will become the preferred method of describing, analyzing, and assessing movement.[17] Such objective measurements of movement will provide a quantitative source of information that will complement the qualitative descriptions based on visual observation.[23]

Kinematic analysis of infant movements using imaging techniques provides a permanent record of movement from which the therapist objectively can 1) describe the movement pattern, 2) identify infants early who may have a movement dysfunction, 3) classify movement dysfunction, and 4) determine the effectiveness of treatment. In addition, kinematic analysis can provide data that may help to answer the following questions: How do motor coordination and control develop? What fundamental processes drive developmental change? What mechanisms are responsible for producing abnormal movement? What precisely happens when an infant practices a movement?

Numerous studies have used kinematic analysis to analyze infant movement.[25–37] Kicking and stepping movements have been described in premature and full-term infants.[26–30] Changes in motor coordination during the transition from prelocomotion to crawling have been documented.[25] Studies have delineated the spatial and temporal characteristics of first independent walking and walking over the second year.[31–34] The kinematic characteristics of reaching movements have been described in full-term infants and in infants ranging in age from 3 to 9 months.[35,36] The relationships between speech events and arm movements also has been studied.[37] Recently, kinematic analysis of leg movements in premature infants has demonstrated that dynamic movement analysis may be a sensitive instrument for the identification of neuromuscular dysfunction at early ages.[26,27]

Kinematic data conventionally have been displayed graphically resulting in a visual permanent record of movement. These diagrams can be reviewed for evaluation purposes, compared with other movement sequences of the same infant, or compared with movement patterns of other infants. Kinematic descriptors can be either time-dependent representations in which the patterns of joint displacement are plotted as a function of time (Fig. 1) or time-independent representations such as angle-angle diagrams (Fig. 2) and amplitude-velocity phase-plane trajectories (Fig. 3). These typical plots can provide useful interpretative data about the movement path of a body segment with respect to time or the movement path of one body segment versus another, as well as the movement path's velocity, direction, and magnitude.

Kinematic analysis is a sensitive quantitative measurement system that 1) captures the dynamic quality of movement; 2) objectifies movement by describing it according to the kinematic variables of time, displacement, velocity, and acceleration; and 3) provides a permanent record from which questions can be asked as to how and why movement was produced. This analysis is essential for conducting advanced motion analysis of the underlying kinetics or distribution of forces that provides information on the underlying cause of a movement disorder.[19,20] In addition, kinematic analysis can be coupled with electromyography for insights into the neural control of movement.[17,20,38]

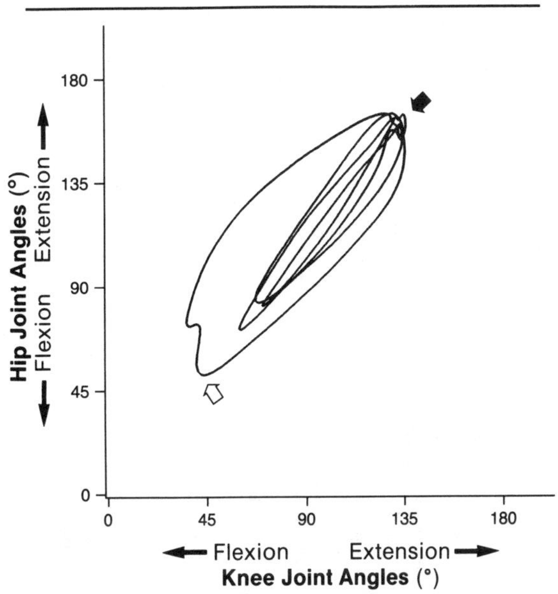

Fig. 2. Typical angle-angle diagram of the rotation of the hip versus the angular rotation about the knee during spontaneous kicking in a 35-week gestational age infant. Note that as the hip flexes, the knee flexes, and as the hip extends, the knee extends. The filled arrow indicates the beginning of a kick flexion movement; the open arrow indicates peak flexion.

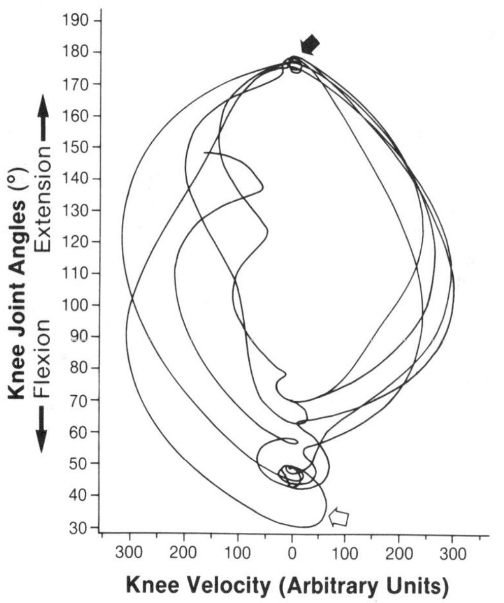

Fig. 3. Typical phase-plane trajectory of the amplitude of movement and peak velocity of the knee joint during spontaneous kicking of a 34-week gestational age infant. The filled arrow indicates the beginning of a kick flexion movement; the open arrow indicates peak flexion.

CONCLUSIONS

We are gratified to note that physical therapists are contributing to both clinical and technological advances in measuring infant movement. As trained observers of human movement, we must continue to make contributions that will assist in the early identification of infant movement disorders and in the therapeutic management of such disorders. As we further refine these clinical and technological measurement tools, we should do so with the goal of measuring change as a result of intervention. Our failure to document successfully the efficacy of our early intervention strategies, in part, is due to the lack of sensitivity of our dependent measures. We hope that the emergence of new methods for quantifying infant movement, as described in this article, will assist physical therapists in documenting change as a result of treatment and in identifying movement disorders during infancy.

REFERENCES

1. Harris SR: Down syndrome. In Campbell SK (ed): Pediatric Neurologic Physical Therapy. New York, NY, Churchill Livingstone Inc, 1984, pp 169–204
2. Chandler LS, Andrews MS, Swanson MW: Movement Assessment of Infants: A Manual. Rolling Bay, WA, Chandler, Andrews, and Swanson, 1980
3. Bayley N: The Bayley Scales of Infant Development. New York, NY, The Psychological Corporation, 1969
4. Folio MR, Fewell RR: Peabody Developmental Motor Scales and Activity Cards. Allen, TX, DLM Teaching Resources, 1983
5. Harris SR, Swanson MW, Andrews MS, et al: Predictive validity of the Movement Assessment of Infants. J Dev Behav Pediatr 5:336–342, 1984
6. Harris SR, Haley SM, Tada WL, et al: Reliability of observational measures of the *Movement Assessment of Infants.* Phys Ther 64:471–475, 1984
7. Haley SM, Harris SR, Tada WL, et al: Item reliability of the Movement Assessment of Infants. Physical & Occupational Therapy in Pediatrics 6(1):21–38, 1986
8. Harris SR: Early neuromotor predictors of cerebral palsy in low birthweight infants. Dev Med Child Neurol 29:508–519, 1987
9. Werner E, Bayley N: The reliability of Bayley's revised scale of mental and motor development during the first year of life. Child Dev 37:39–50, 1966
10. Harris SR: Effects of neurodevelopmental therapy on motor performance of infants with Down syndrome. Dev Med Child Neurol 23:477–483, 1981
11. Haley SM: Postural reactions in infants with Down syndrome: Relationship to motor milestone development and age. Phys Ther 66:17–22, 1986
12. Campbell SK, Wilhelm IJ: Development from birth to 3 years of age of 15 children at high risk for central nervous system dysfunction: Interim report. Phys Ther 65:463–469, 1985
13. Campbell SK, Siegel E, Parr CA, et al: Evidence of the need to renorm the Bayley Scales of Infant Development based on the performance of a population-based sample of 12-month-old infants. Topics in Early Childhood Special Education 6(2):83–96, 1986
14. Harris SR: Early detection of cerebral palsy: Sensitivity and specificity of two motor assessment tools. Journal of Perinatology 7(1):11–15, 1987
15. Palisano RJ, Lydic JS: The Peabody Developmental Motor Scales: An analysis. Physical & Occupational Therapy in Pediatrics 4(1):69–75, 1984
16. Palisano RJ: Concurrent and predictive validities of the Bayley Motor Scale and the Peabody Developmental Motor Scales. Phys Ther 66:1714–1719, 1986
17. Craik RL, Oatis CA: Gait assessment in the clinic: Issues and approaches. In Rothstein JM (ed): Measurement in Physical Therapy: Clinics in Physical Therapy. New York, NY, Churchill Livingston Inc, 1985, vol 7, pp 169–205
18. Smidt GL: Biomechanics and physical therapy: A perspective. Phys Ther 64:1807–1808, 1984
19. Winter DA: Biomechanics of Human Movement. New York, NY, John Wiley & Sons Inc, 1979, pp 16–25
20. Yack HJ: Techniques for clinical assessment of human movement. Phys Ther 64:1821–1830, 1984
21. Krebs DE, Edelstein JE, Fishman S: Reliability of observational kinematic gait analysis. Phys Ther 65:1027–1033, 1985
22. Gronley JK, Perry J: Gait analysis techniques: Rancho Los Amigos Hospital gait laboratory. Phys Ther 64:1831–1838, 1984
23. Medeiros J: Automated measurement systems for clinical motion analysis. Phys Ther 64:1846–1850, 1984
24. Winter DA, Greenlavo RK, Hobson DA: Television computer analysis of kinematics of human gait. Comput Biomed Res 5:498–504, 1972
25. Benson JB, Welch L, Campos JJ, et al: The Development of Crawling in Infancy. Read at the Eighth Bienniel Meeting of the International Society for the Study of Behavioral Development, Tours, France, July 6–10, 1985
26. Heriza CB: Kinematic analysis of leg movements in premature and full-term infants: Research in progress. Physical & Occupational Therapy in Pediatrics 6(3/4):320–321, 1986
27. Heriza CB: A Kinematic Analysis of Leg Movements in Premature and Full-term Infants. Doctoral Dissertation. Edwardsville, IL, Southern Illinois University at Edwardsville, 1986
28. Thelen E, Bradshaw G, Ward JA: Spontaneous kicking in month-old infants: Manifestations of a human central locomotor program. Behav Neural Biol 32:45–53, 1981
29. Thelen E, Fisher DM: Newborn stepping: An explanation for a "disappearing reflex." Developmental Psychology 18:760–775, 1982
30. Thelen E, Fisher DM: The organization of spontaneous leg movements in newborn infants. Journal of Motor Behavior 15:353–377, 1983
31. Clark JE, Phillips SJ: The Organization of Upright Locomotion. Read at the Bienniel Meeting of the Society for Research in Child Development, Toronto, Ontario, Canada, April 25–28, 1985
32. Forssberg H: Ontogeny of human locomotor control: I. Infant stepping, supported locomotion, and transition to independent locomotion. Exp Brain Res 57:480–493, 1985
33. Thelen E, Cooke DW: The relationship between newborn stepping and later locomotion: A new interpretation. Dev Med Child Neurol 29:380–393, 1987
34. Sutherland DH, Olshen R, Cooper L, et al: The development of mature gait. J Bone Joint Surg [Am] 62:336–353, 1980
35. von Hofsten C: Catching skills in infancy. J Exp Psychol [Hum Percept] 9:75–85, 1983
36. von Hofsten C, Lindhagen K: Observations of the development of reaching for moving objects. J Exp Child Psychol 28:158–173, 1979
37. Dowd JM, Tronick EZ: Temporal coordination of arm movements in early infancy: Do infants move in synchrony with adult speech? Child Dev 57:762–776, 1986
38. Craik RL: Biomechanics: A neural control perspective. Phys Ther 64:1810–1811, 1984

Movement Science Series

Movement Analysis—An Aid to Early Diagnosis of Cerebral Palsy

Susan R Harris

The purpose of this article is to review research related to the use of clinical analysis of movement as an aid to the early diagnosis of cerebral palsy. A historical perspective of clinical techniques used by physicians and physical therapists in the early diagnosis of cerebral palsy will be presented first, including recent research findings on clinical signs that were most predictive of this movement disorder. Predictive neuromotor behaviors common across several recent studies will be highlighted. Future trends in the use of movement analysis, including digitized kinematic analysis of term and preterm infants and fetal ultrasound techniques, will be discussed as well. [Harris SR. Movement analysis—an aid to early diagnosis of cerebral palsy. Phys Ther. 1991;71:215–221.]

Key Words: *Cerebral palsy; Kinesiology/biomechanics, general; Movement; Pediatrics, development; Pediatrics, evaluation.*

The purpose of this article is to review research related to the use of clinical analysis of movement as an aid to the early diagnosis of cerebral palsy (CP). A historical perspective of clinical techniques used by physicians and physical therapists in the early diagnosis of CP will be presented first, including recent research findings on clinical signs predictive of this movement disorder. Future trends in the use of movement analysis as an aid to the detection of CP will be discussed as well.

Historical Perspective on Early Diagnosis of Cerebral Palsy

The most universally accepted definition of CP was provided by Bax in 1964: "A disorder of movement and posture due to a defect or lesion of the immature brain."[1(p295)] Bennett[2] has further defined CP as a nonprogressive disability resulting from damage or defect in the brain that occurs during the period of rapid brain growth—either prenatally, perinatally, or up to 3 to 5 years following birth. Classification of the different types of CP has been based historically on predominant neurological signs, including abnormalities in muscle tone and extrapyramidal functions.[3] Barabas and Taft[3] have listed six different types of CP using this form of classification system: spastic, choreathetoid, ataxic, dystonic, hypotonic/atonic, and mixed; spastic CP has been further classified by the limb involvement as either quadriplegia, hemiplegia, or diplegia. The value to physical therapists of such a medically oriented classification system has been questioned by Sahrmann, who has suggested that physical therapists themselves must

> classify or categorize, by specific assessments, the components of the movement dysfunction that will provide definitive guidelines for treatment and for a prognosis.[4(p1705)]

For example, physical therapists are beginning to use kinematic data to quantitatively describe movement in children with CP with the goal of developing specific guidelines for treatment.[5]

Descriptive Literature on Early Diagnosis of Cerebral Palsy

Until the late 1970s, most of the literature on the early diagnosis of CP was based on clinical impressions of neurologists, pediatricians, and physical therapists who had acquired extensive experience in evaluating children with this developmental disorder. Emphasis was placed on the assessment of muscle tone, absence or persistence of primitive or postural re-

SR Harris, PhD, PT, FAPTA, is Associate Professor, School of Rehabilitation Medicine, University of British Columbia, T325-2211 Wesbrook Mall, Vancouver, British Columbia, Canada V6T 2B5, and a Mary E Switzer Distinguished Fellow of the National Institute on Disability and Rehabilitation Research, US Department of Education.

flexes, attainment of righting reactions, and asymmetries in motor development.[6–9] *Muscle tone* has been defined traditionally as resistance to passive elongation or stretch[10]; in the assessment of infants at risk for CP, tone has been differentiated further as active tone or passive tone. As Wilson has noted,

> Active tone is defined as the power and adaptability of the muscles during spontaneous movement, and passive tone refers to resistance of the muscle when movements are imposed by the examiner.[11(p362)]

The historical emphasis on primitive reflexes as diagnostic markers for early CP raises interesting questions about the role of infant reflexes in development. Oppenheim, in citing the work of McGraw,[12] Peiper,[13] and Touwen,[14] has commented that infantile or primary reflexes "typically disappear within the first year or so of life."[15(p87)] Easton,[16(p591)] however, has suggested that reflexes "form the basic language of the motor program" and underlie most, if not all, volitional movements. In attempting to diagnose CP during infancy, child neurologists and developmental pediatricians have concerned themselves primarily with the persistence or exaggeration of primitive reflexes.[17]

Contradictory views on the prognostic importance of the various primitive reflexes among experts in the field of neuromotor assessment prompted the following comments from Scherzer, a leading developmental pediatrician:

> The literature is replete with differing views of the significance of early reflex behaviors. For example, St.-Anne Dargassies . . . places little importance on the Galant reflex, but considers crossed extension to be critical in maturation. Taft . . . stresses the predictive significance only of the asymmetric tonic neck and crossed extension reflexes. Our own clinical experience of predictability has led to the use of the following reflexes: Moro, palmar grasp, rooting, sucking, and asymmetric tonic neck. The postural reflexes we emphasize include neck and body righting, parachute (protective extension), and Landau. . . . Delineation of which reflex behaviors have the most reliable predictive value would be a major contribution, worthy of extensive study by any research group.[18(p126)]

As Scherzer[18] noted in his concluding comment, it is only through systematic research efforts, both retrospective and prospective, that real clues to the early diagnosis of this disorder can be uncovered. Fortunately, data-based studies conducted during the past two decades have begun to identify important clinical signs that can be used in the early identification of CP. Unfortunately, there has been little attempt to summarize or consolidate these findings in order to identify commonalities across these studies. As a result, those movement behaviors that are most predictive of CP are just beginning to be identified.[19] The goal of the following section is to provide a summary of those findings.

Research Findings on Early Diagnostic Signs of Cerebral Palsy

In a descriptive study of 1,743 term newborn infants, Amiel-Tison and colleagues[20] examined the importance of neck extensor hypertonia as a clinical sign of insult to the central nervous system. This study was based on the clinical impressions of the authors that there was an association between increased neck extensor muscle tone and perinatal insult to the central nervous system.

Six procedures were used to examine active and passive tone of the neck. Initially, the infant's neck position was observed with the infant positioned supine in order to evaluate the presence of spontaneous hyperextension. The infant's head was passively flexed four times to determine whether there was increasing resistance to passive flexion. With the infant still lying supine, the examiner then attempted to provoke opisthotonus by lifting the infant slightly between the neck and scapulae. Active flexor and extensor tone of the neck were assessed by pulling the infant into a sitting position from the supine position and by then pushing the infant smoothly back into a supine position. The examiners observed the infant's ability to co-contract flexor and extensor muscles. By rocking the infant backward and forward in supported sitting, the examiner assessed the "equality of tone" of the flexor and extensor muscles. Normal and abnormal reactions were described for each of the procedures; infants were considered to show neck extensor hypertonia if they demonstrated abnormalities in both active and passive tone.

There were 57 infants who showed neurologic abnormalities beyond the first 3 days of life. For example, disturbances such as tone or reflex disturbances, irritability, and seizures were noted. Of those 57 infants, 47% had neck extensor hypertonia. Of 31 infants with transient neurological signs (less than 3 days), 6% showed neck extensor hypertonia, whereas only 0.7% of the remaining 1,655 neurologically normal infants showed neck extensor hypertonia (for 1 day).

The prognostic significance of neonatal extensor hypertonia among this sample of term infants was questionable because only 5 of the 43 infants followed to the age of 1 year showed persistent neurological abnormalities. The authors stressed the need, however, to conduct future studies with follow-up at least until school age. They also emphasized the danger of examining individual neurological signs in isolation.[20]

This was a descriptive study with limited prognostic value; however, it represents one of the earliest attempts to systematically document the presence of specific neurological signs by using a standardized assessment procedure. Later studies have corroborated the importance of neck extensor hypertonia as an important diagnostic sign for the early identification of CP.

In 1981, Ellenberg and Nelson[21] published the results of a retrospective study that examined the relative value of certain physical findings and behavioral responses of 4-month-old infants in predicting CP at early school age.

Because the study was part of the Collaborative Perinatal Project of the National Institute of Neurological and Communicative Disorders and Stroke, the sample consisted of approximately 32,300 infants who were examined at 4 months of age and then again at 7 years of age. Diagnoses of CP were made, as appropriate, at the examination at age 7 years. The predictive value of physical and behavioral measurements at 4 months of age was analyzed by using corrected chi-square statistics to demonstrate the incidence of children who showed each behavior versus children without the behavior. Predictive behaviors were examined for "low birth-weight" infants (≤2,500 g) as well as for "term birth-weight" infants (>2,500 g). *Relative risk* was defined as

> the number of times more frequently CP occurred among children with a given characteristic compared with those without that characteristic.[21(p707)]

Movement behaviors found at 4 months of age that were associated with an increased risk for CP among the low birth-weight infants in the sample included tremulous or jittery patterns of movement. In the term birth-weight infants, writhing movements were associated with later CP. Asymmetrical movements were not predictive of CP in general or of hemiplegic CP in either birth-weight group.

Specific developmental milestones were associated with an increased relative risk for CP. These developmental milestones included the infant's failure to maintain hands open, to support weight on the forearms in the prone position, to hold the head erect in supported sitting, or to engage interest in her or his mirror image. These behaviors were associated with relative risks of 4, 12, 15, and 17, respectively. Muscle tone abnormalities at age 4 months were strongly related to later CP, with neck and trunk hypertonia being of even greater relative risk (74 and 71, respectively) than hypertonia in the limbs (55 in the arms and 52 in the legs). Hypertonia was associated consistently with greater relative risks than hypotonia, particularly in the low birth-weight infants.[21] The finding that neck extensor hypertonia at age 4 months was associated with a 74-fold increase in later CP supported the contention of Amiel-Tison and colleagues[20] that this is an important diagnostic marker for central nervous system insult.

Because Nelson and Ellenberg[22] previously studied prognostic indicators of CP among newborn infants in this same sample, they concluded that neck extensor hypertonia at 4 months of age was an even greater cause for concern than neck extensor hypertonia during the neonatal period. Whereas the presence of this sign was followed by later CP in 4% of the term birth-weight neonates but in none of the low birth-weight neonates, 15% of term 4-month-olds and 42% of low birth-weight 4-month-olds who demonstrated this sign received later diagnoses of CP.[21] This sign was absent in 99.9% of infants who did not develop later CP.

In 1983, Touwen and Hadders-Algra[23] published a prognostic study of the effects of neck and trunk hyperextension and shoulder retraction in infancy on neurological outcome at 18 months of age. Their sample consisted of 105 infants, all of whom showed hyperextension of the neck and trunk with shoulder retraction at an initial examination conducted during the first few months postnatally and subsequently at home (according to the mothers). Forty-two were full-term infants, and 63 were preterm. The investigators assessed the infants two or three times during the first few months postnatally using Touwen's[24] standardized neurological examination. Based on neurological findings from this examination, the infants were classified as

> *marked,* when evident signs of hypertonia, hypotonia, hemisyndrome or deviant reactions and responses were found; *mild,* when comparable signs were present with, however, less intensity; and *none,* if no neurological deviations were found besides the target symptoms.[23(p202)]

The final follow-up visit in Touwen and Hadders-Algra's[23] study was conducted at approximately age 18 months or when the infant could walk independently. Of the 38 infants with no additional neurological signs, 37 were neurologically normal at the last follow-up visit, and 1 was classified as "suspect," which indicated the presence of "mild neurological signs, such as mild hypotonia or slight hypotonia."[23(p203)] For the 45 infants labeled initially as mild, 23 developed normally, 21 were deemed suspect, and 1 was severely impaired. Of the remaining 22 infants, who had been classified as marked during the early months postnatally, 20 were severely impaired and 2 were identified as suspect at the final follow-up visit.

Based on these findings, the authors concluded:

> Hyperextension and shoulder retraction in neonatally neurologically normal infants appeared to be without much clinical significance, even when some slight additional neurological abnormality is present.[23(p204)]

Nonetheless, the fact that 42.8% of infants identified initially *because* of this sign were subsequently labeled as either suspect or abnormal at about 18 months of age suggests that this sign is an important diagnostic predictor of neurological dysfunction, especially if found in combination with other neurological signs. The authors did not statistically analyze the relative risk for having this sign or any of the other neurological findings during the first few postnatal months; thus, comparison of their results with those of Ellenberg and Nelson[21] or with those of subsequent studies[25] is not really possible. Although most researchers agree that no single neurological sign is predictive of later CP, statistical analyses can at least measure the relative effectiveness of different signs, with the goal of improving prediction in subsequent prospective studies. The focus by Touwen and Hadders-Algra[23] on an isolated neurological

Table. *Comparison of Positive and Negative Signs During Infancy for Later Cerebral Palsy*[a]

Study	Neck Hyperextension/ Shoulder Retraction	Abnormal Trunk Tone	Abnormal Extremity Tone	Asymmetrical Movements	Tremulousness	Positive Support Reflex	Inability to Keep Hands Open	Inability to Bear Weight on Forearms	Head Balance in Supported Sitting
Ellenberg and Nelson[21]	+	+	+	−	+	−	+	+	+
Touwen and Hadders-Algra[23]	+	NA	NA	NA	NA	NA	NA	NA	NA
Harris[25]	+	+	+	−	−	−	+	+	+

[a] + = predictive sign of later cerebral palsy, − = sign that failed to discriminate later cerebral palsy, NA = behavior not assessed.

sign provides limited prognostic information for the practicing clinician.

In a retrospective study, Harris[25] statistically analyzed the predictive power of selected items from the Movement Assessment of Infants (MAI)[26] in identifying CP in a sample of low birth-weight infants who were examined initially at 4 months' corrected age. The MAI is a 65-item neuromotor assessment tool developed by physical therapists to examine motor behaviors in four areas: muscle tone, primitive reflexes, automatic reactions, and volitional movement. Based on a "4-month-profile" developed by Chandler and colleagues,[26] 48 of the 65 items of the MAI can be scored as either "risk" or "no-risk."

The 229 infants in this sample were followed until 3 to 8 years of age. A variety of standardized and nonstandardized tests were administered at the follow-up visits. Medical diagnoses of different types of CP were made for 36 of the children. Using chi-square tests, Harris analyzed the presence or absence of risk scores for each of the 48 risk items for the group of children with CP and a group who were deemed "normal," or nonhandicapped, at the final follow-up visit (n=118). Data for a third group of children with developmental delay were not analyzed at this time.[25]

There were 32 MAI items that discriminated between the group of children with CP and the nonhandicapped children. In addition, the group of children with CP was subdivided into three diagnostic categories: spastic diplegia, spastic hemiplegia, and quadriplegia. Each diagnostic category contained 7 items that were significantly different for the children with spastic diplegia and spastic hemiplegia versus the nonhandicapped group. For the subgroup with quadriplegia, many of whom were moderately to severely involved, 35 items were significant predictors. Similarities between Harris's[25] findings and those of the previous studies by Amiel-Tison et al,[20] Ellenberg and Nelson,[21] and Touwen and Hadders-Algra[23] will be highlighted in an effort to examine commonalities across the four studies.

Although the MAI does not have a specific item labeled as "neck hyperextension," the item that most closely measures this behavior is a primitive reflex item—tonic labyrinthine reflex in the supine position. Using procedures similar to those described by Amiel-Tison and colleagues[20] and Touwen and Hadders-Algra,[23] this behavior is assessed through both visually observing the child's neck and shoulder girdle and passively moving the child's head, shoulders, and hips against gravity.[26] A risk score is attained if there is only "occasional arching of the neck and/or some retraction at the shoulder girdle."[26(p31)] These criteria suggest a milder degree of neck hyperextension and shoulder retraction than was used to determine risk in the studies by Amiel-Tison and colleagues[20] and Touwen and Hadders-Algra.[23] This MAI item was significantly discriminative of later CP, both in the CP group as a whole and in the quadriplegic subgroup. Fifty-four percent of the children in the CP group and 90% of the children in the quadriplegic subgroup received a risk score for this item versus approximately 18% of the nonhandicapped group. Thus, all four studies reviewed suggest that this is an extremely important movement behavior to assess as an aid to the early diagnosis of CP (Table).

Another diagnostic predictor common to findings in the studies by Ellenberg and Nelson[21] and Harris[25] was the infant's ability to support weight on the forearms. This behavior is measured in part by several different MAI items: the infant's antigravity muscle tone when placed in the prone position, the tonic labyrinthine reflex in the prone position, and active weight bearing through the shoulders in the prone position. The first two behaviors were significantly different for the CP group as a whole. The volitional movement item—active weight bearing through the shoulders—was scored as a risk behavior for 34.3% of the children who developed CP versus 12.8% of the children who were labeled nonhandicapped at the final follow-up visit. A child's inability to support weight on the forearms at 4 months of age had a relative risk of 12 in Ellenberg and Nelson's study; 4.8% of low birth-weight infants and 2.1% of term birth-weight infants who showed this sign had CP at the age of

7 years. The similarities in these findings across two studies conducted on 4-month-old infants suggest that the inability to assume and maintain a prone-on-elbows posture is an important diagnostic risk behavior (Table). One difference between the two studies, however, is that Harris assessed infants at 4 months' corrected age, whereas Ellenberg and Nelson used the infants' chronological age. Another difference between the two studies concerns their respective samples. Harris's sample consisted primarily of premature infants; Ellenberg and Nelson's much larger sample consisted of both term and preterm infants.

A common finding across these two studies[21,25] was the lack of predictive significance of asymmetries (Table). Ellenberg and Nelson concluded:

> Asymmetrical movements were not a statistically significant predictor of CP in general, nor of hemiparesis in particular, in either birthweight group or in the total.[21(p707)]

The MAI provides for assessment of asymmetry in each of the four sections of the tool. Harris concluded:

> For the overall CP group, asymmetry was a predictive finding *only* in the section on muscle tone (p=0.021). For the subgroups, asymmetry of tone was predictive only for the quadriplegia group. In the sections on automatic reactions and volitional movement, there were higher proportions of asymmetry risk scores among the group of children who were subsequently non-handicapped than for the CP group as a whole.[25(p516)]

These findings suggest that asymmetries, except perhaps in the area of muscle tone, are normal movement behaviors at 4 months of age and probably earlier. Whether asymmetrical movement behaviors are predictive of CP at 5 or 6 months of age or even later remains open to study.

The inability to sit with support with head erect was 15 times more common among infants who later developed CP than among infants with subsequent normal development in Ellenberg and Nelson's[21] study. The most analogous MAI item is a volitional movement item that assesses the child's ability to maintain a stable head position in supported or independent sitting. A risk score is attained if the infant's head bobs, even if there is "some ability to hold head upright."[26(p47)] Risk scores for this item were obtained by 33.3% of children in the CP group as a whole and by 60% of children in the quadriplegia subgroup versus 11.3% of the normally developing children, making this behavior a significant discriminator of later CP. This dual finding suggests the importance of assessing head control in supported sitting as a diagnostic marker of later CP, at least for 4-month-old infants (Table).

Common to both studies by Ellenberg and Nelson[21] and Harris[25] was the importance of abnormal muscle tone as a predictor of CP. Whereas the earlier study by Ellenberg and Nelson demonstrated that hypertonia was a more ominous sign than hypotonia, the data analysis by Harris did not differentiate these two types of tone, despite the fact that the MAI does allow for scoring of both hypotonia and hypertonia. Whereas Ellenberg and Nelson's study showed that abnormal truncal tone had a greater relative risk than abnormal tone of the extremities, Harris's study using the MAI demonstrated that risk scores for *both* behaviors occurred in a significantly higher proportion of children in the CP group than in the nonhandicapped group (42.9% versus 16.1% for trunk tone; 60% versus 26.5% for extremity tone).

Another somewhat contradictory finding between Ellenberg and Nelson's[21] study and Harris's[25] study was related to the presence of tremulousness. Whereas tremulousness in the low birth-weight children was associated with a sixfold increase in the rate of CP by Ellenberg and Nelson, the MAI item measuring tremulousness did not significantly predict later handicap for the CP group as a whole or for any of the subgroups. Nonetheless, the proportion of children in the CP group who demonstrated a risk score on tremulousness was more than twice as great as the proportion of nonhandicapped children with a risk score in Harris's MAI study (17.1% versus 6.8%).

Neither Ellenberg and Nelson's[21] study nor Harris's[25] study demonstrated predictive significance of the positive support reflex among low birth-weight infants, except for the subgroup of children with quadriplegia in Harris's study.

Clinical Implications of Recent Research Findings

Although it is difficult to draw perfect comparisons among studies that used different assessment tools and different samples of infants assessed at somewhat different ages, it is nonetheless helpful to try to assess similarities and differences among these studies with the aim of identifying movement behaviors that could be the most predictive of CP in both clinical and research settings. Attempts should also be made to behaviorally define these movements for consistency in visual analysis rather than to infer their underlying cause. An example is the MAI item "tonic labyrinthine reflex in supine." The movement behaviors that are actually being measured are neck hyperextension and shoulder retraction. Whether these deviant behaviors are caused by abnormal primitive reflex patterns, abnormal muscle tone, or a combination of these factors is of less concern to the physical therapy diagnostician than is a reliable means of assessing their presence or absence or their relative strength or frequency. The fact that the incidence of these behaviors ranged from 42% to 90% of the infants who later developed CP or other neurological handicap across the three prognostic studies[21,23,25] suggests that assessment of these behaviors is extremely important.

Other movement behaviors that appear to be of diagnostic value in the 4-month-old infant are the ability to bear weight on the forearms in the prone position and the ability to maintain a stable head position in supported or independent sitting.[21,25] Similar prognostic "milestone" behaviors need to be developed for other age levels based on prospective longitudinal studies. The lack of predictive significance of asymmetrical movements at 4 months of age is another important commonality across the studies by Ellenberg and Nelson[21] and Harris.[25] Pediatric physical therapists traditionally have placed great import on the presence of asymmetrical movements; although such movements may be important in the older infant with early CP, they are probably of little prognostic significance in infants up to at least 4 months of age unless they are extreme and obviously interfere with normal movement patterns.

Muscle tone abnormalities also appear to be important predictors of CP in 4-month-old infants. It is probably more important to operationally define movement differences as seen in antigravity postures, for example, than to infer that these differences are due to underlying tone disorders. Of the six individual muscle tone items on the MAI, three are active tone items that involve a visual analysis of the infant's ability to move against gravity in the prone, supine, and prone suspension positions.[26] All three of these "tone" items were highly significant predictors of later CP. In contrast, of the three passive tone items—which involve handling and passive manipulation rather than visual analysis of movement patterns—only one (extensibility) was as significant a predictor. These findings support Milani-Comparetti's[27] clinical assertion that watching how the infant moves against gravity is of greater diagnostic value than trying to stimulate responses through passive manipulation or handling.

The ultimate goal of early diagnosis of CP is the provision of early therapeutic intervention, often in the form of developmentally based physical therapy or occupational therapy. Recent research[28] examining the relative efficacy of early physical therapy intervention, in the form of neurodevelopmental treatment (NDT), as compared with a more global infant stimulation program, suggested that the latter approach effected more positive developmental motor outcomes than did the NDT approach. Criticism has been directed at this study because of apparent inequities between the two groups in terms of severity of neurological impairment and because of the researchers' use of outcome measures that were not sensitive to the goals of NDT.[29,30] Future efficacy research in CP should include outcome measures that are congruent with the aims of treatment. For example, Kluzik and colleagues[5] studied the effects of NDT on qualitative aspects of reaching in children with spastic quadriplegia via quantitative kinematic analysis of the "smoothness" of the reach.

Earlier diagnosis of CP (ie, within the first postnatal year) will enhance our abilities to examine further the efficacy of early treatment. Although the study by Palmer and colleagues[28] included infants with spastic diplegia, ranging in age initially from 12 to 19 months, no study has been published attempting to examine the effectiveness of early physical therapy intervention for infants with CP who are *less* than 1 year of age.

Future Trends in Movement Analysis for the Early Diagnosis of Cerebral Palsy

As we expand our role to become diagnosticians, we must rely increasingly on reliable and standardized techniques for assessing movement differences as an aid to diagnosis. Assessment tools such as the MAI have been shown to be both reliable and valid in the assessment of high-risk infants,[31–33] but additional research is needed to increase the sensitivity and specificity of such tools in the early diagnosis of CP.

The traditional medical emphasis on the passive assessment of muscle tone and primitive reflexes must be replaced by a new focus on systematic analysis of movement differences through visual observation, videotapes, and kinematic recordings. The assessment of primitive reflexes has perhaps been overemphasized to the exclusion of more important and more functional movement behaviors such as early motor patterns required for feeding, visual tracking, eye-hand coordination, and parent-infant interaction. Research[31,33] on the reliability and predictive validity of the MAI has shown that primitive reflexes, as a group, "are the least reliable and valid predictors of later motor handicap."[33(p339)]

Through movement analysis of videotapes of neurologically normal and high-risk infants, physical therapists could begin to operationally define movement differences between these two groups. Longitudinal follow-up of such infants could assist in determining which movement behaviors were most predictive of later neurological handicap. Attempts must be made to quantify the frequency and variety of movement patterns through standardized observational protocols. Exciting progress is being made in the area of kinematic analysis of infant movements by physical therapist researchers using digitized data from videotapes to examine organization of infant movements[34,35] and possible differences in movement between preterm and full-term infants.[36] Longitudinal follow-up of the developmental outcome of these infants would allow for evaluation of the prognostic significance of movement differences.

Another exciting avenue for future research is the diagnosis of movement differences in utero through the use of fetal ultrasound. Milani-Comparetti[37] has proposed that perinatally acquired CP could perhaps be prevented or minimized by obstetrical modifications for infants identified in utero as having impaired movements. As physical therapists become increasingly involved in fetal analysis of movement differences,[38] it is hoped that we can assist in prenatal diagnosis of CP.

As specialists in movement analysis, physical therapists must continue to conduct research that will aid in the diagnosis and treatment planning for movement disorders such as CP. As Rose concluded in his description of the roles and functions of physical therapy diagnosis, "Excellence in practice, now and in the future, requires physical therapists to be skillful diagnosticians."[39(p537)]

It is hoped that this review of recent research on diagnostic movement predictors of CP will assist physical therapists in their ability to identify children with CP and physical therapist researchers in developing hypotheses for prospective studies aimed at further defining and classifying this important movement disorder during early infancy.

References

1 Bax MCO. Terminology and classification of cerebral palsy. *Dev Med Child Neurol.* 1964;6:295–297.

2 Bennett FC. Cerebral palsy: the how and why of early diagnosis. *Consultant.* 1984;24:151–173.

3 Barabas G, Taft LT. The early signs and differential diagnosis of cerebral palsy. *Pediatr Ann.* 1986;15:203–214.

4 Sahrmann SA. Diagnosis by the physical therapist—a prerequisite for treatment: a special communication. *Phys Ther.* 1988;68: 1703–1706.

5 Kluzik JA, Fetters L, Coryell J. Quantification of control: a preliminary study of effects of neurodevelopmental treatment on reaching in children with cerebral palsy. *Phys Ther.* 1990;70:65–76.

6 Paine RS. The early diagnosis of cerebral palsy. *RI Med J.* 1961;44:522–527.

7 Illingworth RS. The diagnosis of cerebral palsy in the first year of life. *Dev Med Child Neurol.* 1966;8:178–194.

8 Milani-Comparetti A, Gidoni EA. Routine developmental examination in normal and retarded children. *Dev Med Child Neurol.* 1967;9:631–636.

9 Bobath B, Bobath K. *Motor Development in the Different Types of Cerebral Palsy.* London, England: William Heinemann Medical Books Ltd; 1975:2–19.

10 *Dorland's Illustrated Medical Dictionary.* 27th ed. Philadelphia, Pa: WB Saunders Co; 1988.

11 Wilson JM. Cerebral palsy. In: Campbell SK, ed. *Pediatric Neurologic Physical Therapy.* New York, NY: Churchill Livingstone Inc; 1985:353–408.

12 McGraw MB. Cited by: Oppenheim RW. Ontogenic adaptations and retrogressive processes in the development of the nervous system and behaviour: a neuroembryological perspective. In: Connolly KJ, Prechtl HFR, eds. *Maturation and Development: Biological and Psychological Perspectives.* Philadelphia, Pa: JB Lippincott Co; 1981:73–109.

13 Peiper A. Cited by: Oppenheim RW. Ontogenic adaptations and retrogressive processes in the development of the nervous system and behaviour: a neuroembryological perspective. In: Connolly KJ, Prechtl HFR, eds. *Maturation and Development: Biological and Psychological Perspectives.* Philadelphia, Pa: JB Lippincott Co; 1981:73–109.

14 Touwen BCL. Cited by: Oppenheim RW. Ontogenic adaptations and retrogressive processes in the development of the nervous system and behaviour: a neuroembryological perspective. In: Connolly KJ, Prechtl HFR, eds. *Maturation and Development: Biological and Psychological Perspectives.* Philadelphia, Pa: JB Lippincott Co; 1981:73–109.

15 Oppenheim RW. Ontogenetic adaptations and retrogressive processes in the development of the nervous system and behaviour: a neuroembryological perspective. In: Connolly KJ, Prechtl HFR, eds. *Maturation and Development: Biological and Psychological Perspectives.* Philadelphia, Pa: JB Lippincott Co; 1981:73–109.

16 Easton TA. On the normal use of reflexes. *American Scientist.* 1972;60:591–599.

17 Capute AJ. Early neuromotor reflexes in infancy. *Pediatr Ann.* 1986;15:217–226.

18 Scherzer AL. Primitive reflex profile. *Dev Med Child Neurol.* 1985;27:126–127. Letters to the Editor.

19 Harris SR. Early identification of cerebral palsy. In: Gottlieb M, Williams J, eds. *Developmental-Behavioral Disorders: Selected Topics (vol 4).* New York, NY: Plenum Publishing Corp. In press.

20 Amiel-Tison C, Korobkin R, Esquevaucouloux M. Neck extensor hypertonia: a clinical sign of insult to the central nervous system of the newborn. *Early Hum Dev.* 1977;1/2: 188–190.

21 Ellenberg JH, Nelson KB. Early recognition of infants at high risk for cerebral palsy: examination at age four months. *Dev Med Child Neurol.* 1981;23:705–716.

22 Nelson KB, Ellenberg JH. Neonatal signs as predictors of cerebral palsy. *Pediatrics.* 1979;64:225–232.

23 Touwen BCL, Hadders-Algra M. Hyperextension of neck and trunk and shoulder retraction in infancy: a prognostic study. *Neuropediatrics.* 1983;14:202–205.

24 Touwen BCL. *Neurological Development in Infancy.* Philadelphia, Pa: JB Lippincott Co; 1976.

25 Harris SR. Early neuromotor predictors of cerebral palsy in low-birthweight infants. *Dev Med Child Neurol.* 1987;29:508–519.

26 Chandler LS, Andrews MS, Swanson MW. *The Movement Assessment of Infants: A Manual.* Rolling Bay, Wash: Chandler, Andrews, & Swanson; 1980:1–53.

27 Milani-Comparetti AM. Developmental diagnosis. Read at the 10th Annual Sensorimotor Integration Symposium; July 9–11, 1982; San Diego, Calif.

28 Palmer FB, Shapiro BK, Wachtel RC, et al. The effects of physical therapy on cerebral palsy: a controlled trial in infants with spastic diplegia. *N Engl J Med.* 1988;318:803–808.

29 Mettler JL. Commentary. *Physical & Occupational Therapy in Pediatrics.* 1989;9(2):5–7.

30 Harris SR. Commentary on "The effects of physical therapy on cerebral palsy: a controlled trial in infants with spastic diplegia." *Physical & Occupational Therapy in Pediatrics.* 1989;9(3):1–4.

31 Harris SR, Haley SM, Tada WL, Swanson MW. Reliability of observational measures of the Movement Assessment of Infants. *Phys Ther.* 1984;64:471–475.

32 Haley SM, Harris SR, Tada WL, Swanson MW. Item reliability of the Movement Assessment of Infants. *Physical & Occupational Therapy in Pediatrics.* 1986;6(1):21–39.

33 Harris SR, Swanson MW, Andrews MS, et al. Predictive validity of the Movement Assessment of Infants. *J Dev Behav Pediatr.* 1984;5:336–342.

34 Heriza CB. Organization of leg movements in preterm infants. *Phys Ther.* 1988;68: 1340–1346.

35 Gross MT, Cochrane CG. A method for quantifying the activity and rest periods of spontaneous kicking. *Physical & Occupational Therapy in Pediatrics.* 1988;3(2):59–70.

36 Heriza CB. Comparison of leg movements in preterm infants at term with healthy full-term infants. *Phys Ther.* 1988;68:1687–1693.

37 Milani-Comparetti A. The neurophysiologic and clinical implications of studies on fetal motor behavior. *Semin Perinatol.* 1981;5: 183–189.

38 Sparling JW. *A Study of the Use of Prenatal Ultrasound and Its Relationship to Parental Adaptation and Infant Behavior.* Chapel Hill, NC: University of North Carolina at Chapel Hill; 1987. Doctoral dissertation.

39 Rose SJ. Physical therapy diagnosis: role and function. *Phys Ther.* 1989;69:535–537.

Pediatric Orthopedics Series

Assessment of Lower-Extremity Alignment in the Transverse Plane: Implications for Management of Children with Neuromotor Dysfunction

The authors present nine clinical assessment procedures designed to detect factors contributing to transverse-plane structural and joint alignment abnormality in children with neuromotor dysfunction. Where applicable, each assessment is accompanied by a discussion of the normal features of pediatric lower-extremity torsional and rotational alignment; limitations of the assessment procedures as regards reliability, specificity, and age-related normative findings; and clinical management suggestions. The authors urge clinical evaluators to expand the existing knowledge base. [Cusick BD, Stuberg WA. Assessment of lower-extremity alignment in the transverse plane: implications for management of children with neuromotor dysfunction. Phys Ther. 1992;72:3–15.]

Beverly D Cusick
Wayne A Stuberg

Key Words: *Lower extremity, general; Neuromotor disorders, general; Orthopedics, general; Pediatrics, evaluation.*

Children with chronic neuromotor dysfunction commonly exhibit deviations in transverse-plane (torsional and rotational) alignment of the pelvis and lower extremities (Fig. 1). Abnormal weight bearing and muscle action and shortened soft tissues impose forces that combine to impede and impair normal maturation of torsional and rotational features of skeletal structure and joint alignment. Unlike children with normal neuromotor status, most children who lack normal neuromuscular function do not develop efficient mechanisms to compensate for these structural abnormalities.[1] Alignment problems generally worsen with increasing age.[2–19]

The clinician should base management decisions on findings gained through a combination of gait analysis, posture evaluation, and a thorough biomechanical assessment.[3,17,20,21] To determine whether a clinical biomechanical finding indicates the presence of pathology, a clinician must identify and acknowledge normal maturational changes in skeletal architecture and joint configuration as they are currently understood.[1] We believe that research is needed to establish adequate norms and to evaluate the efficacy of interventions.

The purpose of this article is to raise the therapist's awareness of certain biomechanical components that can influence lower-extremity transverse-plane alignment and function and of the need to expand the existing body of research pertaining to the significance of clinical findings. Following a brief review of terminology, we present nine clinical biomechanical assessment procedures. The discussion pertaining to these assessments covers normative data, normal maturational changes in structural and joint configuration, limitations of the procedures as regards reliability and validity issues, and clinical management implications of assessment results.

Terminology

Rotation—a movement of one or both joint segments in a plane that is perpendicular to the axis of the motion.[22,23] Medial rotation and lateral rotation occur when a joint segment is rotated toward and away from midline, respectively, around a vertical axis.

BD Cusick, MS-CCT, PT, is Clinical Specialist, Lucille Packard Children's Hospital at Stanford, 725 Welch Rd, Palo Alto, CA 94304. She also teaches, consults, and is involved in private practice. Address all correspondence to Ms Cusick at 415 Velarde St, Mountain View, CA 94041 (USA).

WA Stuberg, PhD, PT, is Director of Physical Therapy, Meyer Rehabilitation Institute, Associate Professor, Division of Physical Therapy Education, and Assistant Professor, Department of Anatomy, University of Nebraska Medical Center, 600 S 42nd St, Omaha, NE 68198-5450.

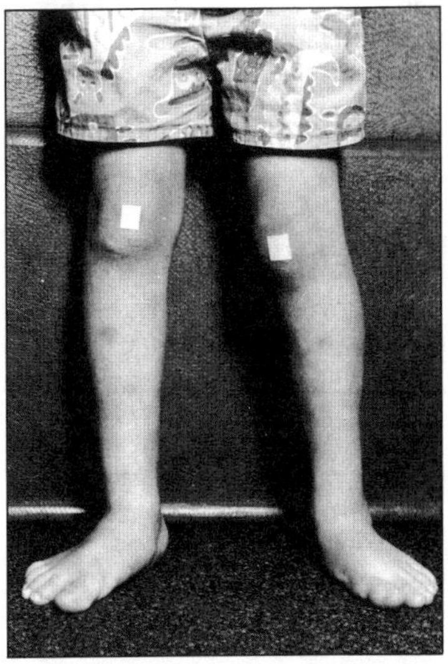

Figure 1. *Malalignment, characterized by medially rotated patellae (left more than right), positive foot progression angle, and bilateral foot pronation.*

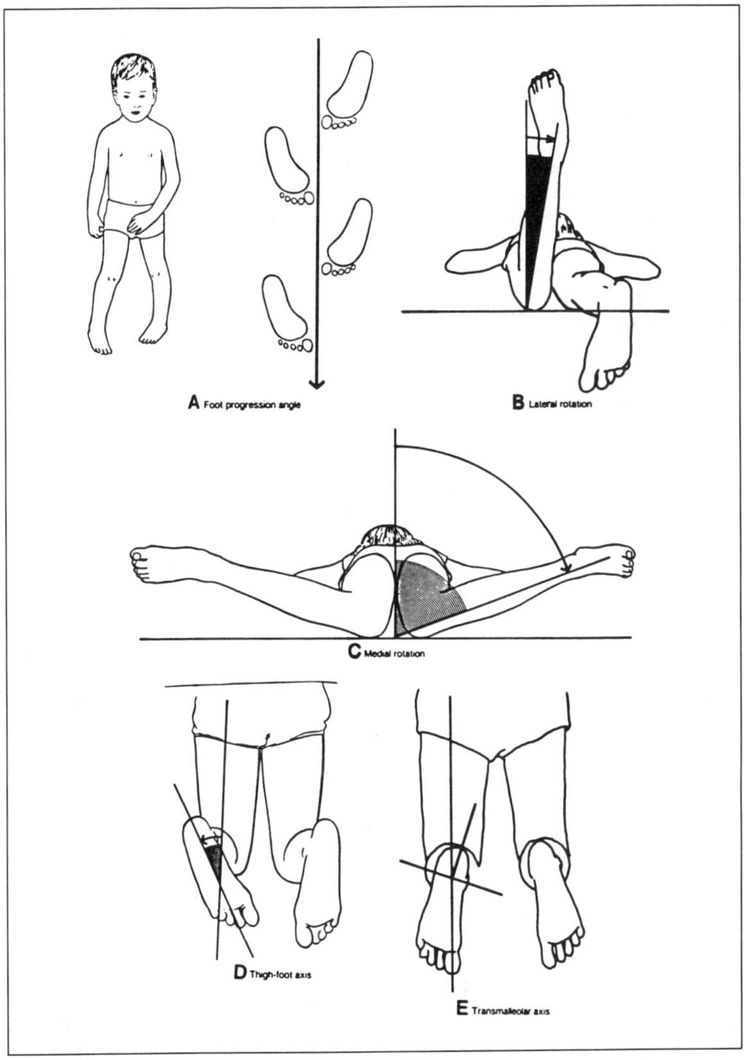

Figure 2. *Staheli's "Rotational Profile": (A) foot progression angle; (B) hip lateral rotation; (C) hip medial rotation; (D) thigh-foot angle; (E) transmalleolar axis-thigh angle.*

Torsion—a structural, osseous state of twist in a bone along its longitudinal axis.[24] "Femoral antetorsion" and "medial femoral torsion" are synonymous terms describing a femur that bears a medial twist of the distal-on-proximal ends.[3,25,26] "Femoral retrotorsion" and "lateral femoral torsion" are also synonymous terms that describe a deformity ranging from a lack of normal medial torsion to a true lateral twist of the distal-on-proximal ends of the femur.[3,25,26] Clinical tibiofibular torsion describes a state of twist, either medial or lateral, in the long axis of the tibiofibular unit.

Version—"The act or process of turning something or changing direction."[24(p1830)] For example, the femoral head and neck are described as anteverted when the head lies anterior to the frontal plane and retroverted when the head lies posterior to the frontal plane. Version and torsion are not identical, although they may occur together. Version describes a position in space relative to a plane. Torsion describes a twist in structure.

Genicular position—an abnormality in the relative ranges of medial or lateral axial tibiofibular rotation with the knee joint flexed 90 degrees.[25]

Clinical Biomechanical Assessment Procedures

At least 13 biomechanical factors can be cited as contributing to lower-extremity malalignment in the transverse plane: (1) pelvic rotation in the transverse plane[7]; (2) immature acetabular anteversion[19,27–32]; (3) soft tissue restriction of hip joint medial or lateral rotation mobility[19,25,33–35]; (4) abnormal magnitude of femoral torsion*; (5) abnormal activity of the

*References 4, 7, 19, 21, 25, 26, 33, 36–45.

medial hamstring muscles[3,4,21,36,39,46]; (6) medial or lateral genicular position[23,25,43,47]; (7) abnormal magnitude of tibiofibular torsion[†]; (8) abnormal transverse-plane alignment of the talar body within the ankle mortise[49,50]; (9) persistent talar neck adduction relative to the talar body[38]; (10) abnormal foot pronation, resulting in midtarsal joint abduction[36,45,51–53]; (11) abnormal foot supination, resulting in midtarsal joint adduction[21,52,53]; (12) metatarsus adductus[37,44,45]; and (13) overpull of the abductor hallucis muscle ("searching toe").[54,55] We refer the reader to the cited references for information that is beyond the scope of this article.

We present a battery of nine assessment procedures that constitute a general screening. The battery features elements of Staheli's "Rotational Profile," which includes foot progression angle (FPA), medial and lateral hip rotation mobility with the hips extended, thigh-foot angle, transmalleolar axis (TMA)-thigh angle, and foot configuration (Fig. 2).[9,44,45,55–58] We have expanded Staheli's profile by adding pelvic rotation in the transverse plane, Ryder's test for femoral torsion, axial tibiofibular rotation mobility, and tibiofibular torsional status with the knee joint extended.

The assessment process is begun by observing the foot progression angle (FPA) to provide a basis for investigating specific components of limb structure and joint mobility. The remaining eight tests proceed from proximal to distal body segments.

General Alignment

Test 1—foot progression angle. This test helps determine the angle formed by the foot and the line of forward progression. Abnormal FPA is commonly described as a gait deviation characterized by toeing-in or toeing-out beyond the normal mean.

Procedure. The therapist dusts the soles of the child's feet with chalk and obtains a series of footprints. We measure FPA as the angle formed by the longitudinal bisection of the foot and the line of progression (Fig. 2). The longitudinal bisection of the foot normally falls between the center of the plantar heel and the second and third metatarsals.[59] We obtain at least six measurements for each foot and calculate the average FPA. Toeing-in is indicated by a negative value, and toeing-out is indicated by a positive value.

Norms. Normative studies[60,61] have shown a mean FPA of 4 to 10 degrees in infants, children, and adults. The variability is greatest in children younger than 2 years of age.[60,61]

Limitations. Replicability of findings is hindered by the problem of establishing a precise reference for the line of progression, as few children walk in a purely straight line. Pronation and supination foot deformities induce compensatory lateral and medial deviations, respectively, of the axis of the forefoot relative to that of the hindfoot. We use the longitudinal bisection of the hindfoot to measure FPA in children with neuromotor dysfunction. The orientation of the hindfoot bisection to the sagittal plane offers a closer manifestation of proximal rotary and torsional influences on foot alignment than does that of the bisection of the compensating forefoot. The longitudinal forefoot bisection divides the second and third metatarsals.

Clinical implications. Toeing-in, which typically occurs in fewer than 30% of infants without neuromotor dysfunction, usually resolves by the age of 4 years.[40,47,48] An FPA of −1 to −10 indicates a mild abnormality, an FPA of −10 to −15 degrees indicates a moderate abnormality, and an FPA beyond −15 degrees indicates a severe abnormality. Adults rarely exhibit a negative FPA.[40,43,47,48,62] Children without neuromotor dysfunction who show persistent toe-in gait typically show no evidence of functional deficit.[63] A positive FPA exceeding 15 degrees imposes abnormal pronatory forces on the foot structures, as weight is borne abnormally on the medial aspect of the midfoot.[53]

Motion analysis reveals the occurrence of lateral rotation of the femur and, to a greater degree, the tibia during the mid-stance and propulsion phases of gait in all children, including early walkers.[40,64] As the ligaments of the knee joint and foot gain integrity, these stance-phase lateral torque forces descending on the foot evidently induce spontaneous correction of toeing-in.[1,51]

Children with abnormal muscle activity or myelomeningocele often demonstrate an abnormal magnitude of FPA.[4,7,36,39,40,65] Abnormal FPA in children with cerebral palsy depletes stability in the early stance phase of gait; necessitates that double-support stance begin prematurely; and reduces normal acceleration, velocity, and step length.[36] The components that contribute to abnormal FPA are discussed in the context of the remaining tests.

Proximal Alignment Features

We urge therapists to observe the postural alignment of each knee joint and patella relative to the sagittal plane of the limb. If the knee axis and patella align medially in quiet stance, we look for pelvic rotation, soft tissue restriction on lateral hip rotation, and evidence of abnormally increased medial femoral torsion (see tests 2–4). If medial deviation increases in gait, we assess hamstring muscle length[4,39] using the popliteal angle test as described by Jones and Knapp[21] and Rang et al.[16] If the patella and knee axis align laterally, we look for restriction on medial hip rotation mobility and femoral retrotorsion (see tests 3 and 4).

†References 7, 9, 19, 23, 25, 36, 44, 47, 48.

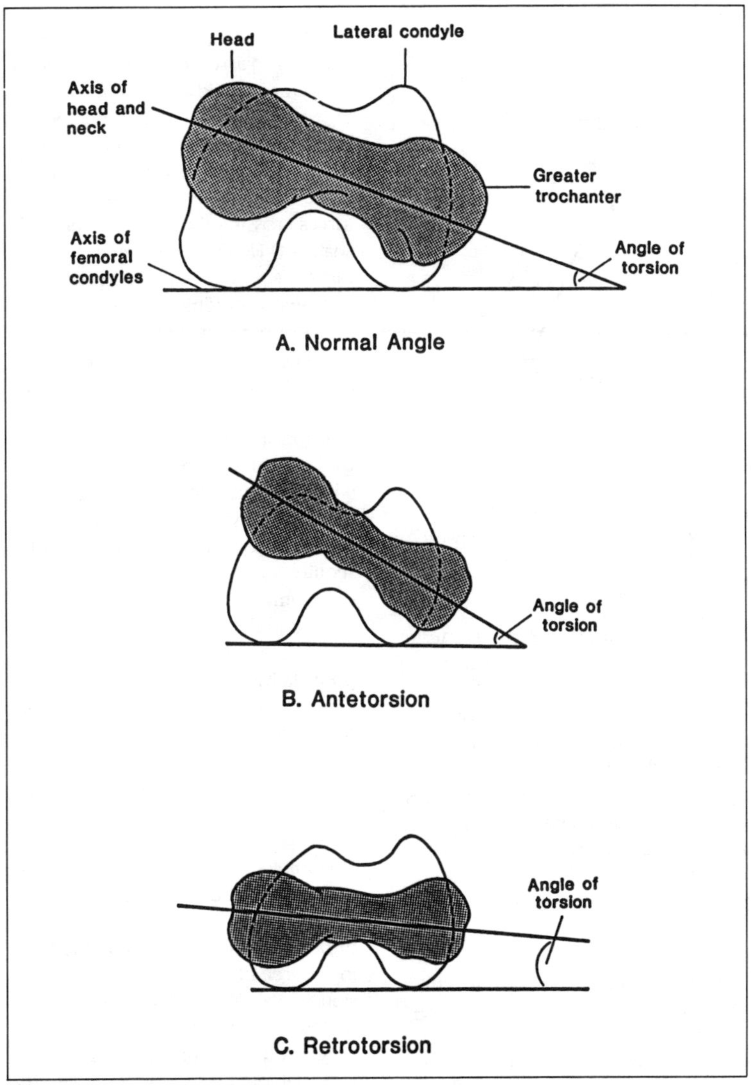

Figure 3. *Proximal and distal reference axes for femur of an adolescent (unshaded) and an adult (shaded): (A) normal mean antetorsion (12°–20°); (B) abnormal or immature antetorsion (>20°); (C) femoral retrotorsion (<12° antetorsion).*

Test 2—pelvic rotation. As the child stands and walks, we observe pelvic rotation in the transverse plane and note whether the right or left anterior superior iliac spine is anterior to a frontal-plane reference line.

Norms. The pelvis ideally aligns on the frontal plane.[66(p144)]

Clinical implications. If abnormal rotation is evident, the acetabulum on the anterior side may consequently be more anteverted than the acetabulum on the posterior side. Thus, the femur on the anterior side might falsely appear to be medially rotated.[19,30] Acetabular anteversion normally diminishes with skeletal maturation.[30,32,67,68] Persistence of structurally increased acetabular anteversion can cause toeing-in when femoral torsion is normal, or it can occur in conjunction with increased femoral antetorsion.[19,30] We know of no clinical test to determine acetabular orientation. Radiographic confirmation is needed.

Test 3—Ryder's test. The magnitude of femoral torsion is measured as the angle formed by the transverse-plane intersection of the femur's proximal reference axis (PRA) and distal reference axis (DRA). The PRA bisects the femoral head and greater trochanter, and the DRA lies parallel to the posterior aspects of the femoral condyles and is known as the transcondylar axis (TCA).

Femoral antetorsion is evident when the TCA is placed on the frontal plane and the femoral head lies anterior to the frontal plane (Fig. 3). Femoral retrotorsion is evident when the TCA is placed on the frontal plane and the femoral head lies less than 10 to 12 degrees anterior to the frontal plane (Fig. 3).[25,26,43] The orientation of these axes to each other can only be estimated on clinical examination using Ryder's test, which features palpation of the position of the greater trochanter while rotating the femur.[4,19,25]

Procedure. Position the child prone, supine, or sitting with the knee flexed to 90 degrees. The findings should be consistent in all positions, as they should represent the bony configuration. The examiner holds the leg proximal to the ankle and rotates the hip while palpating the anterior and posterior borders of the greater trochanter. When the trochanter reaches the most lateral position in the arc, we presume that the femoral neck and head are aligned on or near the frontal plane (Figs. 4, 5). We then measure the resulting position of hip rotation.

We use a straight line connecting the mid-patella and the mid-ankle as the DRA.[69] If measuring with a goniometer, we use the table surface as the PRA (frontal plane) and subtract the resulting value from 90. We prefer to use a 7.62-cm-diameter (3-in-diameter), gravity-driven angle

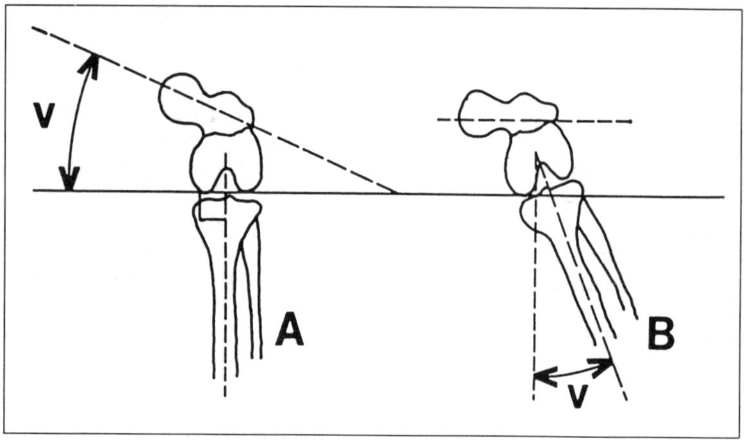

Figure 4. *Skeletal representation of Ryder's test in context of increased left medial femoral torsion: (A) When the distal reference axis (DRA) of the tibia is aligned on the sagittal plane, the greater trochanter lies posterior to the frontal plane; (B) when the proximal reference axis of the greater trochanter and the femoral neck is aligned on the frontal plane, the distal DRA of the tibia deviates laterally to represent a position of hip medial rotation. (V-angle of femoral torsion.)*

finder,[‡§] adapted by holding an extended straightedge against the shorter side of the angle finder (Fig. 5). The angle finder offers a vertical-plane reference, which is a gravitational constant.

Norms. The magnitude of medial femoral torsion at birth approaches a mean of 40 degrees. Thereafter, the mean torsion angle reduces to 31 degrees at age 2 years, decreases to 25 degrees by age 8 years, and drops rapidly to the adult mean of 16 degrees between ages 14 and 16 years.[5,70] Stuberg and colleagues[71] reported mean medial rotation values of 10 to 13.5 degrees (SD=3.3°=3.9°) obtained by three testers on a group of 17 subjects, aged 3 to 22 years.

Limitations. Age-related reliability coefficients and normative data for Ryder's test results have not been established. Stuberg et al[71] used a different goniometric technique from the one we suggest and showed a mean intertester difference of approximately 3 degrees. Reliability improved with the testers' clinical experience. Thickness of soft tissues overlying the greater trochanter can affect the precision of palpation. Age-related torsional normative values for computed tomography (CT) or magnetic resonance imaging (MRI) findings have not been established or validated against measurements on anatomic specimens.

Clinical implications. Given the current available data comparing CT results with both Ryder's test results and measurements taken on an anatomic femur specimen, one can presume that the femur is twisted medially approximately 20 degrees more than the measured hip rotation value indicates.[7,71,72] For example, 5 degrees of lateral rotation (the distal leg deviates medially) represents a femur with approximately 15 degrees of medial torsion, whereas 5 degrees of medial rotation (the distal leg deviates laterally) suggests the presence of approximately 25 degrees of medial torsion.

Children with spastic cerebral palsy exhibit increased femoral antetorsion,[‖] as do many children with myelomeningocele.[19,73] These children typically show persistent hip flexion contractures, with a concurrent lack of adequate extension and lateral rotation forces crossing the proximal femoral shaft.[1,3,38] Habitual sleep and play postures, such as W sitting, correlate with persistence of femoral antetorsion.[19,41,43,74,75] Staheli[45] has described a malalignment syndrome that causes awkward gait and chondromalacia in children with normal neuromotor function. This syndrome is characterized by increased femoral antetorsion, which persists into adolescence with compensatory, excessive lateral tibiofibular torsion. Correction would require femoral and tibial derotational osteotomy. Because the most rapid decline in femoral antetorsion normally occurs during the first 4 years postnatally,[70] we advise the pediatric clinician to intervene early to gain biomechanically efficient limb alignment before this malalignment syndrome evolves in children with neuromotor deficits.

No radiologic or anatomic studies have documented the effects of twister cables, antirotation braces, exercises, orthoses, splints, or shoes on the existing degree of femoral or tibial torsion.[5,25,38,41,47,57,74,76] Twister cables are not recommended for femoral antetorsion, as they may promote excessive lateral tibiofibular torsion or rotation.[38] Until research proves that exercise, positioning, and orthoses offer no benefit, we base our management recommendations on the principle that the application of correct forces is required for optimum skeletal modeling before the skeleton ossifies[6,11,12] and on findings relating habitual limb positioning to torsional abnormality. For children with adequate innervation, from birth to 8 years of age, we recommend multiple daily repetitions of resisted hip extension and lateral rotation, the reduction of hip and knee flexion and femoral medial rotation postures in stance and gait, the im-

‡Macklanburg Duncan Inc, Oklahoma City, OK 73118.

§Model AF100, Dasco Pro Inc, 2215 Kishawaukee St, Rockford, IL 61101.

‖References 2, 5, 7, 9, 10, 13, 14, 18, 41, 70.

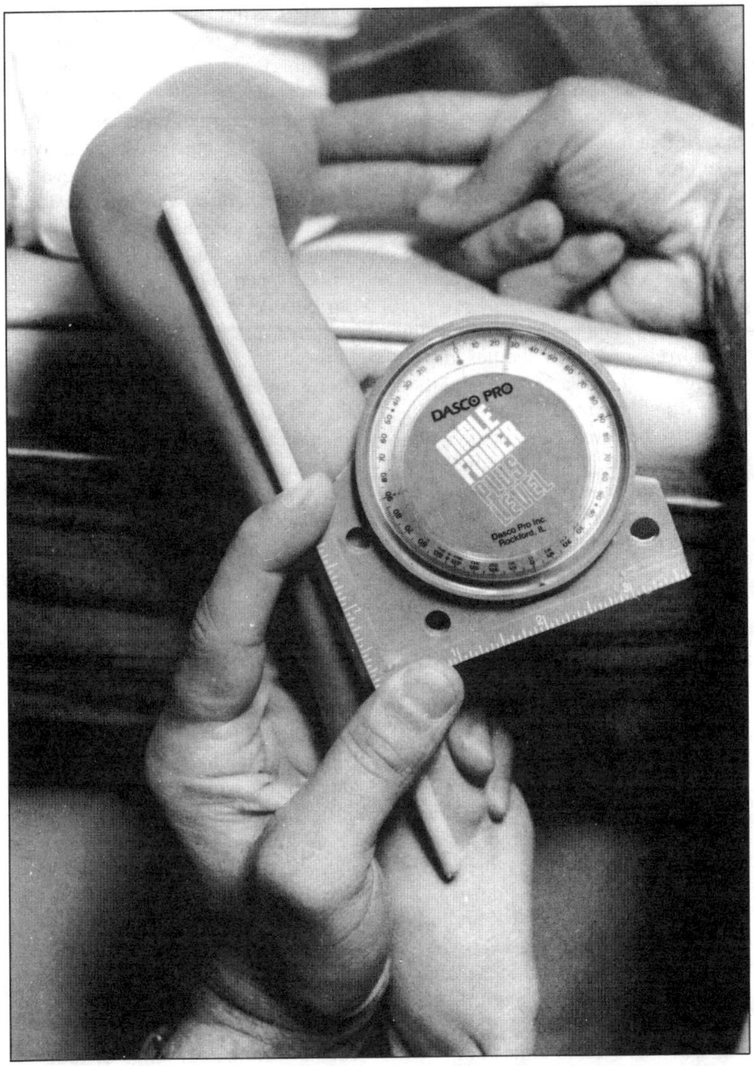

Figure 5. *Ryder's test for femoral torsion. Palpate the greater trochanter and align it in its most lateral position. Use the adapted angle finder to measure hip rotation. Landmarks: mid-patella and mid-ankle.*

provement of lateral and posterior weight transfer skills over the feet, and the institution of a consistent positioning program. Because abnormal foot pronation deformity is believed to promote medial rotation of the proximal limb structures,[52,53] we protect the foot from pronating abnormally by serial casting to gain full ankle dorsiflexion mobility (minimum of 10°) and by combining the consistent use of appropriate splints or orthoses with weight transfer training.

The general opinion among orthopedists is that femoral derotation osteotomy is the only effective treatment for antetorsion for children aged 7 years and older.[5,7,19,39,63] Tachdjian[19] and Staheli[45] discuss criteria for osteotomy for the neurologically normal child. Hoffer et al[7] report good results and minimal complications following supracondylar femoral derotational osteotomy, undertaken for 11 children with spastic cerebral palsy, aged 7 to 15 years ($\bar{X}$=9.5).

Test 4—hip rotation mobility test. Another way to assess femoral torsional status and to evaluate soft tissue extensibility is to measure passive hip medial rotation and lateral rotation (Fig. 2).

Procedure. The therapist positions the child prone with knees flexed 90 degrees and tibias vertical. Keeping the pelvis level, the therapist allows the feet to fall apart from each other until gravity stops the motion. Range of motion (ROM) is measured using the same DRA landmarks as described for the Ryder's test (see test 3 and Fig. 5). To measure lateral rotation mobility, the pelvis is gently kept level, and the therapist laterally rotates each hip 10 to 20 times to reduce any influence of soft tissue restriction.[19]

The therapist identifies soft tissue effects on rotation by noting whether the magnitude of ROM changes with the hip and knee flexed 90 degrees (sitting).[19,25] Evidence of abnormal femoral torsion is supported when the same findings are obtained with the hip flexed and extended.[25]

Norms. Lateral rotation contracture normally limits medial rotation mobility in infancy.[35,77] As the contracture reduces, medial rotation increases. At age 24 months, medial rotation exceeds lateral rotation by an average of 7 degrees.[77] A normative study of medial rotation findings for school-aged children showed a mean approximating 40 to 50 degrees (range=15°–65°), whereas the mean lateral rotation value approached 70 degrees before age 1 year and decreased to approximately 45 degrees (range=25°-65°) from age 5 years through mid-adulthood. This study examined between 11 and 28 children in age groups of 1 year each greater than 1 year.[61]

Limitations. Reliability studies for measurements obtained from medial rotation/lateral rotation tests on children have not been published, nor have medial rotation/lateral rotation findings been validated using CT or MRI analysis of torsion. This test cannot be used to identify abnormal femoral torsion in children less than age 2 years because of persistence of normal intrauterine lateral rotation contracture of the hip joint.[35,40,77] If lax ligaments allow abnormally increased medial rotation and lateral rotation mobility, the findings cannot be used to discern torsional status. We believe the medial rotation/lateral rotation test cannot be used to distinguish femoral torsion from abnormal acetabular anteversion or retroversion. We use Ryder's test as an adjunct to the medial rotation/lateral rotation test, and we repeat the medial rotation/lateral rotation test in the sitting position.

Clinical implications. Clinically significant medial femoral torsion is evident when medial rotation is greater than 60 degrees and lateral rotation is less than 25 degrees.[38,44,45] Limitation of lateral rotation range is the principal finding.[19] If medial rotation/lateral rotation findings corroborate those obtained with the Ryder's test, we try to manage torsional deformity as suggested for the Ryder's test (see test 3). If soft tissue limitation becomes evident, we use positioning, soft tissue mobilization techniques, and exercises to gain mobility.

Distal Limb Features

If the hindfoot FPA is negative and the patella aligns on the sagittal plane, we look for a medial genicular position, excessive activity or shortening of the medial hamstring and popliteus muscles, medial tibiofibular torsion, or a combination of these factors (see tests 5–8).[25,42,50,54,78] If the forefoot FPA is negative, we look for evidence of increased talar torsion,[38] foot supination, or forefoot adductus (see tests 5, 6, and 9). If the patella aligns either medially or normally and the hindfoot FPA is abnormally positive, we look for a lateral genicular position or excessive lateral tibiofibular torsion, or both (see tests 5–8). If a line bisecting the forefoot deviates laterally on the hindfoot, we evaluate for foot pronation, which is characterized by midtarsal joint dorsiflexion and abduction (see test 9).

Test 5—thigh-foot angle test. Staheli[44,45,57] uses this test to assess tibiofibular torsional status. We suggest instead that it is a composite test of axial tibiofibular rotation position, tibiofibular torsion, subtalar joint alignment, and foot configuration (ie, adduction, supination, pronation, and so forth).

Procedure. The therapist positions the child prone with the knee flexed 90 degrees, the tibia vertical, and the ankle dorsiflexed to 0 degrees. As this test is used to evaluate structures distal to the femur, we believe the position of proximal femoral rotation or hip abduction is not relevant. We hold the foot in the subtalar joint neutral position (neither supinated nor pronated) and use the bisection of the plantar surface of the hindfoot only as the DRA to eliminate forefoot deviations as a factor in measurement. We measure the angle formed by the bisecting line of the thigh (PRA) and the longitudinal axis of the hindfoot (DRA) (Fig. 2). Medial deviation (adduction) of the foot results in a negative value; lateral deviation (abduction) produces a positive value.

Norms. The range of normal findings is wide, especially during infancy.[61] Through age 2 years, the mean angle lies between 0 and −10 degrees (range=−25°–20° at birth). The angle gradually increases to a mean of 10 degrees (range=−5°–30°) from middle childhood on.[61]

Limitations. Normative clinical data represent small age-specific study groups of 11 to 28 children.[61] Reliability data are not available for this test, nor are validity data available for comparisons of thigh-foot angles and tibiofibular torsion CT or MRI findings for children of more than 9 months' gestational age.[49] Age-related normative data for CT and MRI findings are also not available. The thigh-foot angle results might reveal factors that falsely indicate the presence of medial tibiofibular torsion, such as normal infantile hyperextensibility of the knee joint ligaments and capsule, which interferes with stabilizing and identifying the rotary position of the proximal tibia[42]; normal neonatal medial rotation bias of the knee joint ligaments and capsule[79]; medial hamstring and popliteus muscle activity or shortening[25]; release of the screw-home mechanism with knee flexion, which allows medial axial tibiofibular rotation to occur[25,66,80,81]; or persistence of medial genicular position attributable to habitual sleep or play postures. Talar torsion or medial rotation of the talar body in the ankle mortise might position the well-aligned foot in medial rotation under the tibia and fibula.[49,50] We believe this factor accounts primarily for the failure of Badelon et al[49] to find a correlation between the thigh-foot angle test and the status of anatomic tibiofibular torsion in fetal cadaver specimens.

Clinical implications. Staheli[57] states that, if the thigh-foot angle is greater than −5 degrees (child's age unspecified), medial tibial torsion is present. We use the thigh-foot angle as a global indicator of change rather than as a reliable or valid indicator of tibiofibular torsion. We supplement this test with the axial tibiofibular rotation test (see test 8), the TMA-thigh angle test (see test 6), and examination of tibiofibular torsion status with the knee joint extended (see test 7) before proposing a management program.

Test 6—the transmalleolar axis-thigh angle test. The TMA-thigh angle moves the scope of assessment to the segment proximal to the subtalar joint.[9,19,45,55,61]

Procedure. The therapist positions the child prone with the knee and ankle flexed 90 degrees and the tibia vertical. We locate the anterior-posterior (AP) malleolar bisections and mark a line joining them on the plantar surface of the foot, representing the TMA. We also mark a perpendicular line from the TMA posteriorly on the heel. This perpendicular line is the DRA. The PRA is the long bisection of the posterior thigh. We measure the

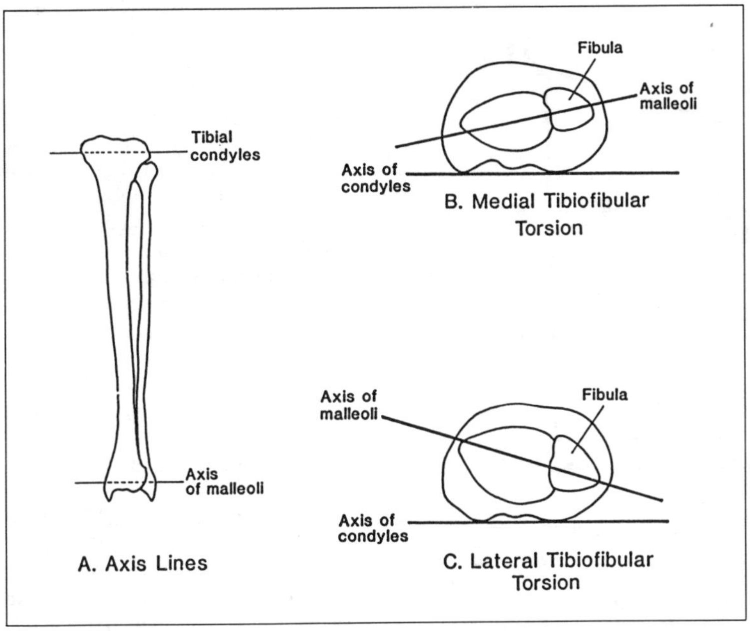

Figure 6. *(A) Proximal and distal reference axes for tibiofibular (TF) torsion; (B) medial TF torsion; (C) lateral TF torsion.*

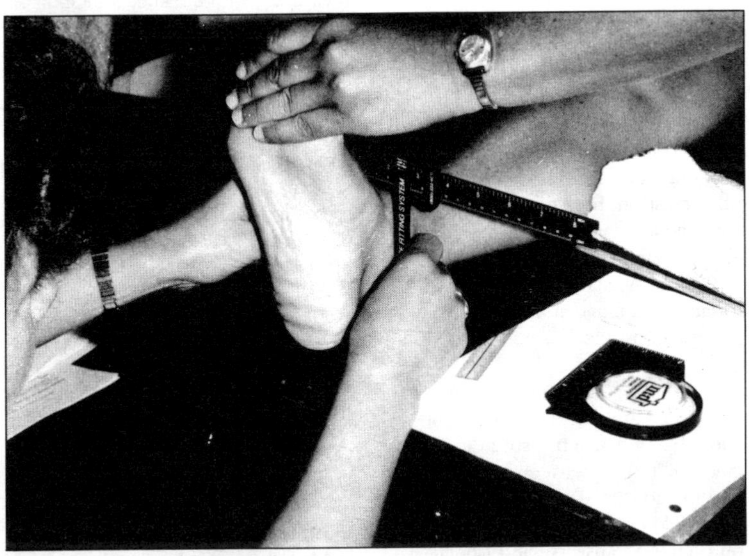

Figure 7. *Measure the width between the malleolar bisections by carefully aligning the measuring device (photo shows a medial-lateral caliper) on both the transverse and frontal planes. Do not take a diagonal width measurement.*

angle formed by the PRA and DRA (Fig. 2).

Norms. The normative values for TMA-thigh angle are higher than those for thigh-foot angle by approximately 10 degrees.[61] The mean TMA-thigh angle at birth is about 0 degrees (range=−30°–20°), gradually increasing to approximately 20 degrees (range=0°–45°) during and after middle childhood.[61] In our opinion, these normative values, when compared with those for thigh-foot angle, reveal evidence of a normal medial rotation of the foot under the malleoli.

Limitations. The same reliability and validity issues discussed in reference to the thigh-foot angle test pertain to the TMA-thigh angle test. "Pseudolack of malleolar torsion" describes a low orientation of the TMA to the frontal plane that might falsely suggest medial tibiofibular torsion.[#] Although a rather high incidence (30%) of toe-in gait has been reported for infants without neuromotor dysfunction,[48] Rosen and Sandick found "a surprising lack of true [internal] TF torsion"[23(p854)] among 2-year-old children who exhibit a toe-in gait.

Clinical implications. We advise using the TMA-thigh angle to measure change, rather than to indicate tibiofibular torsion in children with neuromotor deficits. We evaluate axial tibiofibular rotation and torsion with the knee extended before intervening. Computed tomography provides the most accurate impression of torsional status, but age-related normative data are not yet available.

Test 7—tibiofibular torsion test in knee extension. Tibiofibular torsion is measured clinically as the angle (DRA) formed by the intersection of a frontal-plane bisection of the knee joint (PRA) and a line bisecting the medial and lateral malleoli (TMA). On CT scans, the frontal-plane bisection of the proximal tibial condyles forms the PRA (Fig. 6). After aligning the PRA on the frontal plane, medial tibiofibular torsion is evident when the medial malleolus lies posterior to the frontal plane. Lateral tibiofibular tor-

[#]References 23, 25(p103), 34(p326), 62(p311), 82(p308).

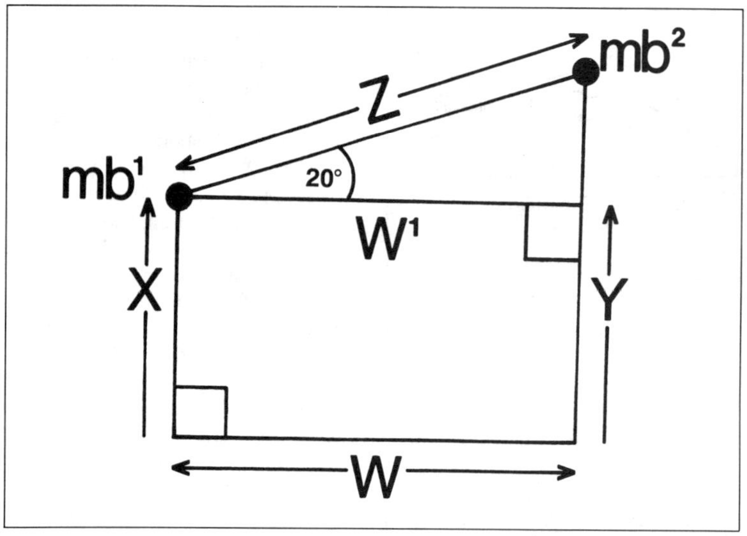

Figure 8. *Calibrating tibiofemoral torsion. (X=distance between malleolar bisection (mb¹) and surface. Y=distance between malleolar bisection (mb²) and surface. W=width between malleolar bisections, measured parallel with the transverse and frontal planes. W¹ represents the frontal plane, connects mb¹ and Y, and lies parallel to line W. Z=transmalleolar axis (TMA), connecting mb¹ and mb². The angle formed by the intersection of lines W¹ and Z indicates that the TMA is oriented 20° to the frontal plane.)*

sion is evident when the lateral malleolus lies posterior to the frontal plane.

The collateral and cruciate ligaments and the popliteus muscle become taut with the knee extended, locking the fully extended mature knee joint against transverse- and frontal-plane motions.[42,83,84] Given that the knee joint ligaments are intact and not hyperextensible, and that the extensibility of the knee joint capsule allows full knee extension to occur, we believe that extending the knee joint to measure tibiofibular torsional status secures the proximal tibia against rotating and reduces measurement error.

Procedure. The therapist positions the child sitting or supine on a firm table surface with the knee fully extended and the ankle and foot hanging off the table edge. The table surface represents the frontal plane of the limb and serves as the PRA for this test. The therapist then places the knee joint axis on the frontal plane by flexing the knee a few times in the pure sagittal plane. An assistant supports the knee at 0 degrees of extension, stabilizing it against rotating.

We rotate the tibiofibular unit medially and laterally under the stabilized distal femur. If the joint allows more than 10 degrees of rotation, we carefully align the tibial tuberosity and tibial crest on the sagittal plane and have the assistant stabilize the tibia. The assistant then dorsiflexes the ankle on the sagittal plane to the comfortable end-range and holds the ankle in that position.

We mark a dot on the AP bisection of the medial and lateral malleoli (mb^1 and mb^2). We also measure the distance (X and Y) between each malleolar bisection (mb) and the table surface. Holding a medial-lateral caliper on both the transverse and frontal planes, we measure the width (W) between the malleoli (Fig. 7). All three measurements are transferred onto graph paper, using W as the baseline and setting X and Y at each end of the baseline (Fig. 8). We draw a horizontal line (W^1) from the top of the shorter mb line to the longer mb line, parallel to the baseline. Another line (Z), connecting the dots at mb^1 and mb^2 and representing the TMA, is drawn. A goniometer is used to measure the angle formed by Z and W^1. We believe lateral tibiofibular torsion is evident when the medial mb line is longer than the lateral mb line and is recorded as a positive value. Medial tibiofibular torsion occurs when the lateral mb line is longer than the medial mb line and is recorded as a negative value.

Norms. Existing normative values vary in magnitude, having been obtained using a variety of anatomical landmarks and knee joint positions.[23,48,49,85–89] We refer the reader to cited references for details. Because McCrea[25] measures tibiofibular torsional status with the knee joint extended, we report his stated normative values, as follows: −5 to 10 degrees in infancy, 10 to 15 degrees by age 2 years, and 20 to 30 degrees by age 5 to 7 years through adulthood. Jakob et al[89] found a mean tibiofibular torsion of 30 degrees in adult cadavers, measuring with the knee joint extended. Badelon et al[47] assessed fetal cadavers and found a mean anatomical angle of 20 degrees (range=10°–32°) at 9 months' gestational age, suggesting that the tibiofibular unit might achieve a mature magnitude of lateral torsion at birth. If so, the reported normative values for infants and very young children may be affected by medial genicular position.

Limitations. Reliability coefficients and age-related, normative values for the tibiofibular torsion assessment procedure described are not established. Age-related normative values do not exist for CT or MRI measurements of tibiofibular torsion.

If the knee joint cannot be fully extended, the screw-home mechanism cannot operate to secure the proximal tibia. If the lateral malleolus is abnormally enlarged, as often occurs with supination deformity, the width of the ankle might be misrepresented.

Clinical implications. If true medial tibiofibular torsion is present in young children, it usually improves spontaneously, whereas lateral tibiofibular torsion often worsens.[45] Valmassey (RL Valmassey; personal communication; June 28, 1991) and various authors[25,40,43,90] suggest intervening early to reduce a significant, negative FPA, using serial casting, night splinting bars, and counterrotation devices. The criteria for using such interventions, however, are not specified. Radiologic studies are needed to ascertain the efficacy of these interventions. It is likely that these interventions actually impose lateral rotation on soft tissues within the knee joint, as they do not secure the proximal tibia.[43,47] The immediate and long-term biomechanical influences of these interventions on tibiofibular torsion and knee joint status have not been investigated.[45,47]

Staheli[45,58] has reported suggested guidelines for surgical osteotomy for children with normal neuromotor status. For children with cerebral palsy, abnormal lateral tibiofibular torsion may be a greater biomechanical problem than medial tibiofibular torsion. Õunpuu et al[65] recommend supramalleolar derotational osteotomy for children with cerebral palsy who show evidence of increased tibiofibular lateral torsion. They claim results that show improved sagittal-plane gait features at the knee and ankle after reducing the mean FPA from 31.8 to 11.5 degrees.

Test 8—axial tibiofibular rotation test. We believe this test helps to distinguish axial rotation mobility and alignment from tibiofibular torsional status. Maximum axial rotation occurs with the knee joint flexed between 60 and 90 degrees.[91] Infants normally exhibit 20 to 30 degrees of rotary mobility with the knee joint extended.[42,92]

Procedure. The therapist positions the child prone with the knee flexed 90 degrees, the tibia vertical, and the ankle flexed to 0 degrees. Refer to the illustration for thigh-foot angle in Figure 2 for landmarks of measurement. Holding the foot and malleoli as a stable unit, we rotate the leg, ankle, and foot medially to the maximum comfortable end-range. We align the arms of a small goniometer on the longitudinal heel bisection and parallel to the longitudinal axis of the thigh, with the axis posterior to the heel border. We measure the resulting angle, rotate the leg and foot laterally, and repeat the measurement. We suggest repeating the measurement with the hips flexed over the edge of the mat table and the knees flexed on a bench. McCrea[25] describes a similar measurement procedure in which the child is positioned sitting and supine; however, we believe the reference axes are more difficult to ascertain with this procedure, thus impeding potential measurement replicability.

Norms. McCrea's[25] clinical experience suggests that children without neuromotor dysfunction under age 3 years, positioned sitting with hips and knees flexed 90 degrees, show a normal medial rotation-to-lateral rotation ratio of between 1:1 and 1:2, with normal findings of 45 to 65 degrees for medial rotation and 45 to 95 degrees for lateral rotation.[25] By age 3 to 4 years, the knee joint typically gains integrity, and rotation range decreases.[42,92] An unpublished study, lacking specification of reference axes, revealed that the mean total range of axial tibiofibular rotation in women without neuromotor dysfunction approached 40 degrees (SD=8°), with a lateral rotation-to-medial rotation ratio of approximately 2:1. Axial tibial rotation with the knee extended was 0 degrees.[93] Other authors report unsubstantiated values ranging from 10 degrees of medial and lateral rotation[80,81] to 30 degrees of medial rotation and 45 degrees of lateral rotation.[79,94]

Limitations. Reliability studies and studies to determine age-specific pediatric normative values have not been undertaken for this test. Clinical judgment must rest on the merits of reported clinical experience. Correlation has not been established between axial tibiofibular rotation mobility and FPA or between axial tibiofibular rotation and foot deformity.

Clinical implications. A medial genicular position is evident when medial rotation exceeds lateral rotation. The medial rotation bias can be caused by soft tissues or medial tibiofibular torsion, or both.[25] If lateral rotation mobility diminishes in hip flexion, then consider shortened medial hamstring muscles to be a limiting factor. Clinical findings often reveal a medial genicular position in preschool-aged children with spastic diplegia, particularly when the medial hamstring muscles are overactive and shortened and the child habitually kneel-sits with legs rotated medially. The same problem often occurs in children with meningomyelocele who can voluntarily control only the medial (and not the lateral) hamstring muscles. We believe early positioning and night splinting to maintain full medial hamstring muscle ROM and to gently rotate the leg laterally under the flexed knee may reduce the functional problems relating to this medial rotational bias. Gait studies and radiographic assessments are needed to evaluate the structural and functional effects of these interventions.

Medial hamstring muscle lengthening has been shown to produce a significant and perhaps pathological increase in FPA in children with spastic cerebral palsy over age 4 years.[3,44] The resulting stability of the tibiofemoral articulation was not evaluated.

We find that children with hemiparesis who exhibit equinovarus deformity at the foot and ankle often reveal increased lateral axial tibiofibular mobility. The rigid, supinating foot imposes lateral rotation forces on the tibiofibular unit during the stance phase of gait. We suggest reducing this deforming strain by gaining dorsiflexion and pronation mobility through progressive casting, use of night splints and orthoses, or, if casting yields no gain of mobility, surgical intervention.[1,95]

Test 9—foot configuration. Consider the shape of the foot as a factor affecting FPA when proximal factors are normal.

Procedure. The therapist positions the child prone to allow a view of the plantar surface of the foot. We stabilize the foot in the subtalar neutral position of maximum congruity (ie, neither supinated nor pronated) and view the plantar surface. We align the arms of a small goniometer on the longitudinal bisection of the heel and parallel with a line bisecting the second and third metatarsals.

Norms. The ideal hindfoot/forefoot angle is 0 degrees.[53,59,88,96]

Limitations. Reliability and validity tests are needed for this procedure. Age-related normative values have not been established.

Clinical implications. Metatarsus adductus and supination or pronation deformities affect the FPA.[45] A straight foot positioned in adduction (medial rotation) under a normally aligned femur and TMA suggests the presence of increased talar torsion or medial rotation of the talar body within the ankle mortise.[38,49,50]

In young children with spastic diplegia who bear excessive weight on the medial forefoot, we often see foot pronation deformity, characterized by an abducted forefoot on an adducted hindfoot. The lateral forefoot deviation masks a negative hindfoot FPA. In this case, we believe that when the foot is supported in proper alignment with an orthosis, toeing-in appears or worsens. Clinicians should alert caretakers to this possibility prior to intervening to protect the foot pronation deformity from progressing, as caretakers usually perceive toeing-in as a more serious problem than progressive foot pronation.

As children with spastic diplegia grow beyond preschool age, some develop lateral tibiofibular rotation and torsion as well as foot pronation, which increases the hindfoot FPA.[27] The medial knee joint ligaments and capsule become overstretched by abnormal loading forces.[19,27,38,53,54,78] Having identified the presence of shortened triceps surae muscles, we work to reduce foot pronation and strain on the knee joint and tibiofibular unit by (1) gaining ankle dorsiflexion mobility with serial casting or stretch splinting, or surgery if these measures fail; (2) applying appropriate orthoses or splints to maintain ideal foot alignment; and (3) facilitating lateral/posterior weight transfers over the foot.[1,95,97]

Because the forefoot adducts on the hindfoot in individuals with foot supination deformity, the hindfoot FPA might be more positive than that of the forefoot. We reduce the supination deformity with serial casting and the use of orthoses as needed to achieve a more normal FPA.[1,95,97]

Summary

The field of biomechanical analysis as it applies to children with neuromotor deficits is clearly in its infancy. The clinical assessment procedures presented in this article require further research to establish their validity and reliability for children with and without neuromotor dysfunction. Large-scale normative studies should follow, recording coincidental measures of the FPA. Sophisticated radiographic techniques should be used to determine the efficacy of commonly prescribed splinting apparatuses and therapeutic exercise programs. Such studies would contribute greatly to our understanding of the functional significance and management of transverse-plane biomechanical factors for children with neuromotor dysfunction.

References

1 Cusick BD. *Progressive Casting and Splinting for Lower Extremity Deformities in Children with Neuromotor Dysfunction.* Tucson, Ariz: Therapy Skill Builders; 1990.

2 Beals RK. Developmental changes in the femur and acetabulum in spastic paraplegia and diplegia. *Dev Med Child Neurol.* 1969;11:303–313.

3 Bleck EE. *Orthopedic Management of Cerebral Palsy.* Philadelphia, Pa: JB Lippincott Co; 1987.

4 Chong KC, Vojnic CD, Quanburg AO, Letts RM. The assessment of internal rotation gait in cerebral palsy: an electromyographic gait analysis. *Clin Orthop.* 1978;132:145–149.

5 Fabry G, MacEwen GD, Shands AR. Torsion of the femur. *J Bone Joint Surg [Am].* 1973;55:1726–1738.

6 Frost HM. *Intermediary Organization of the Skeleton.* Boca Raton, Fla: CRC Press; 1986.

7 Hoffer MM, Prietto C, Koffman M. Supracondylar derotational osteotomy of the femur for internal rotation of the thigh in the cerebral palsied child. *J Bone Joint Surg [Am].* 1981;63:389–393.

8 Kasser JR, MacEwen GD. Examination of the cerebral palsy patient with foot and ankle problems. *Foot Ankle.* 1983;4:135–144.

9 King HA, Staheli LT. Torsional problems in cerebral palsy. *Foot Ankle.* 1984;4:180–184.

10 Laplaza FJ, Root L, Tassanawipas A, Burke S. Femoral torsion and neck-shaft angles in patients with cerebral palsy. *Dev Med Child Neurol.* 1989;31:27. Abstract.

11 LeVeau BF. Developmental biomechanics and the principles of growth. In: Wilson JM, Davis LA, eds. *Orthopedic Aspects of Developmental Disabilities.* Chapel Hill, NC; University of North Carolina Press; 1980:1–27.

12 LeVeau BF, Bernhardt DB. Developmental biomechanics: effect of forces on the growth, development, and maintenance of the human body. *Phys Ther.* 1984;64:1874–1882.

13 Lewis FR, Samilson RR, Lucas DB. Femoral torsion and coxa valga in cerebral palsy. *Dev Med Child Neurol.* 1964;6:591–597.

14 Majestro TC, Frost HM. Cerebral palsy: spastic internal femoral torsion. *Clin Orthop.* 1971;79:44–56.

15 Mann R. Biomechanics in cerebral palsy. *Foot Ankle.* 1983;4:114–119.

16 Rang M, Silver R, de la Garza J. Cerebral palsy. In: Lovell WW, Winters RB, eds. *Pediatric Orthopaedics.* 2nd ed. Philadelphia, Pa: JB Lippincott Co; 1986:345–396.

17 Samilson RL, Dillin L. Postural impositions on the foot and ankle from trunk, pelvis, hip, and knee in cerebral palsy. *Foot Ankle.* 1983;4:120–127.

18 Staheli LT, Duncan WR, Schaefer E. Growth alterations in the hemiplegic child. *Clin Orthop.* 1968;60:205–212.

19 Tachdjian MO. *Pediatric Orthopedics.* 2nd ed. Philadelphia, Pa: WB Saunders Co; 1990.

20 Hoffer MM, Perry J. Pathodynamics of gait alterations in cerebral palsy and the significance of kinetic electromyography in evaluating foot and ankle problems. *Foot Ankle.* 1983;4:128–134.

21 Jones ET, Knapp DR. Assessment and management of the lower extremity in cerebral palsy. *Orthop Clin North Am.* 1987;18:725–738.

22 Cole TM, Tobis JS. Measurement of musculoskeletal function. In: Kottke FJ, Lehmann JF, eds. *Krusen's Handbook of Physical Medicine and Rehabilitation.* 4th ed. Philadelphia, Pa: WB Saunders Co; 1990;20–71.

23 Rosen H, Sandick H. The management of tibiofibular torsion. *J Bone Joint Surg [Am].* 1955;37:847–855.

24 *Dorland's Illustrated Medical Dictionary.* 27th ed. Philadelphia, Pa: WB Saunders Co; 1988:1830.

25 McCrea JD. *Pediatric Orthopedics of the Lower Extremity: An Instructional Handbook.* Mount Kisco, NY: Futura Press; 1985.

26 Smith C, Fuller E. *Biomechanics III—Syllabus.* San Francisco, Calif: California College of Podiatric Medicine.

27 Feltz WL. The prenatal development of the human femur. *Am J Anat.* 1954;94:1–44.

28 Lloyd-Roberts GC, Harris NH, Chrispin AR. Anteversion of the acetabulum in congenital dislocation of the hip: a preliminary report. *Orthop Clin North Am.* 1978;9:89–95.

29 McKibbin B. Anatomical factors in the stability of the hip joint in the newborn. *J Bone Joint Surg [Br].* 1970;52:148–159.

30 McSweeney A. A study of femoral torsion in children. *J Bone Joint Surg [Br].* 1971;53: 90–95.

31 Stanisavljevic S. Congenital dysplasia, subluxation, and dislocation of the hip in stillborn and newborn infants. *J Bone Joint Surg [Am].* 1963;45:1147–1158.

32 Watanabe RS. Embryology of the human hip. *Clin Orthop.* 1974;98:1–26.

33 Engel GM, Staheli LT. Natural history of torsion and other factors influencing gait in childhood. *Clin Orthop.* 1974;99:12–17.

34 Hlavac HF. Major considerations in the clinical evaluation of the lower extremity. In: Sgarlato T, ed. *A Compendium of Podiatric Biomechanics.* San Francisco, Calif: California College of Podiatric Medicine; 1971:321–344.

35 Pitkow RB. External rotation contracture of the extended hip. *Clin Orthop.* 1975;110: 139–145.

36 Gage JR. An overview of normal and cerebral palsy gait. *Neurosurgery: State of the Art Reviews.* 1989;4:379–401.

37 Alexander I. Evaluation of in-toeing in children. In: *The Foot: Examination and Diagnosis.* New York, NY: Churchill Livingstone Inc; 1990:149–160.

38 Bleck EE. Developmental orthopaedics, III: toddlers. *Dev Med Child Neurol.* 1982;24: 533–555.

39 Sutherland DH, Schottstaedt ER, Larsen LJ, et al. Clinical and electromyographic study of seven spastic children with internal rotation gait. *J Bone Joint Surg [Am].* 1969;51: 1070–1082.

40 Sutherland DH. *Gait Disorders in Childhood and Adolescence.* Baltimore, Md: Williams & Wilkins; 1984.

41 Swanson AB, Greene PW, Allis HD. Rotational deformities of the lower extremity in children and their clinical significance. *Clin Orthop.* 1963;27:157–174.

42 Valmassy RL. Biomechanical evaluation of the child. In: Ganley JV, ed. *Symposium on Podopediatrics.* Philadelphia, Pa: WB Saunders Co; 1984;563–579.

43 McDonough MW. Angular and axial deformities of the legs of children. In: Ganley JV, ed. *Symposium on Podopediatrics.* Philadelphia, Pa: WB Saunders Co; 1984:601–620.

44 Staheli LT. Torsional deformity. *Pediatr Clin North Am.* 1977;24:799–811.

45 Staheli LT. The lower limb. In: Morrissy RT, ed. *Lovell and Winter's Pediatric Orthopaedics.* 3rd ed. Philadelphia, Pa: JB Lippincott Co; 1990;1:741–766.

46 Sullivan RC, Krzyzanowski JA, Harris GF. Rotational changes in the lower limbs following distal medial hamstrings surgery for cerebral-palsied children. *Dev Med Child Neurol.* 1986;28:107. Abstract.

47 Scoles PV. Lower extremity development. In: Scoles PV. *Pediatric Orthopedics in Clinical Practice.* 2nd ed. Chicago, Ill: Year Book Medical Publishers; 1988:82–121.

48 Hutter CG, Scott W. Tibial torsion. *J Bone Joint Surg [Am].* 1949;31:511–518.

49 Badelon O, Bensahel H, Folinais D, Lassale B. Tibiofibular torsion from the fetal period until birth. *J Pediatr Orthop.* 1989;9:169–173.

50 Ritter MA, DeRosa GP, Babcock JL. Tibial torsion? *Clin Orthop.* 1976;120:159–163.

51 Jordan RP, Cusack J, Resseque B. Foot function and its relationship to posture in the pediatric patient with cerebral palsy and other neuromotor disorders: course materials and lecture notes. Symposium, presented by Langer Biomedical Group, sponsored by the Neurodevelopmental Treatment Association; May 20–22, 1983; New York, NY.

52 Oatis CA. Biomechanics of the foot and ankle under static conditions. *Phys Ther.* 1988;68:1815–1821.

53 Root ML, Orien WP, Weed JH. *Normal and Abnormal Biomechanics of the Foot: Clinical Biomechanics.* Los Angeles, Calif: Clinical Biomechanics Corp; 1977: vol 2.

54 Kumar SJ, MacEwen GD. Torsional abnormalities in children's lower extremities. *Orthop Clin North Am.* 1982;13:629–639.

55 Staheli LT. Torsional deformity. *Pediatr Clin North Am.* 1986;33:1373–1381.

56 Staheli LT, Engel GM. Tibial torsion. *Clin Orthop.* 1972;86:183–186.

57 Staheli LT. Rotational problems of the lower extremities. *Orthop Clin North Am.* 1987;18:503–512.

58 Staheli LT. Torsion: treatment indications. *Clin Orthop.* 1989;247:61–66.

59 Aharonson Z, Voloshin A, Steinbach TV, et al. Normal foot-ground pressure pattern in children. *Clin Orthop.* 1980;150:220–223.

60 Scrutton D. Footprint sequences of normal children under five years. *Dev Med Child Neurol.* 1969;11:44–53.

61 Staheli LT, Corbett M, Wyss C, King H. Lower extremity rotational problems in children. *J Bone Joint Surg [Am].* 1985;67:39–44.

62 Sgarlato T. *A Compendium of Podiatric Biomechanics.* San Francisco, Calif: California College of Podiatric Medicine; 1971:311.

63 Staheli LT, Clawson DK, Hubbard DD. Medial femoral torsion: experience with operative treatment. *Clin Orthop.* 1980;146:222–225.

64 Sutherland DH, Olshen R, Cooper A, Dale D. The development of mature gait. *J Bone Joint Surg [Am].* 1980;62:336–353.

65 Õunpuu S, Andrews M, Gage JR. The effects of internal tibial derotation osteotomy on the gait of children with cerebral palsy. *Dev Med Child Neurol.* 1989;31(suppl 59):8. Abstract.

66 Hoppenfeld S. *Physical Examination of the Spine and Extremities.* East Norwalk, Conn: Appleton-Century-Crofts; 1976:144, 186–189.

67 Dega W. Richerche anatomiche e meccaniche sull'anca fetale rivolte a chiarire l'etiologia e la patogenisi della lussazione congenita. *Chir Organi di Movimento.* 1933;18:425–505.

68 Ogden JA. *Skeletal Injury in the Child.* Philadelphia, Pa: Lea & Febiger; 1982:16–40.

69 Forero N, Okamura LA, Larson MA. Normal ranges of hip motion in neonates. *J Pediatr Orthop.* 1989;9:391–395.

70 Shands AR, Steele MK. Torsion of the femur: a follow-up report of the use of the Dunlap method for its determination. *J Bone Joint Surg [Am].* 1958;40:803–816.

71 Stuberg WA, Koehler A, Wichita M, et al. Comparison of femoral torsion assessment using goniometry and computerized tomography. *Pediatric Physical Therapy.* 1989;1(3): 115–118.

72 Murphy SB, Simon SR, Kijewski PK, et al. Femoral anteversion. *J Bone Joint Surg [Am].* 1987;69:1169–1176.

73 Carroll NC. Assessment and management of the lower extremity in myelodysplasia. *Orthop Clin North Am.* 1987;18:709–724.

74 Crane L. Femoral torsion and its relation to toeing-in and toeing-out. *J Bone Joint Surg [Am].* 1959;41:421–428.

75 Knight RA. Developmental deformities of the lower extremities. *J Bone Joint Surg [Am].* 1954;36:521–526.

76 Knittel G, Staheli LT. The effectiveness of shoe modifications for intoeing. *Orthop Clin North Am.* 1976;7:1019–1025.

77 Phelps E, Smith LJ, Hallum A. Normal ranges of hip motion of infants between nine and 24 months of age. *Dev Med Child Neurol.* 1985;27:785–792.

78 Kling TF. Toe in, toe out. *Emer Med.* March 1986:32–46.

79 Wilkins KE. Bowlegs. *Pediatr Clin North Am.* 1986;33:1429–1438.

80 Grimsby O. *Fundamentals of Manual Therapy: A Course Workbook.* 2nd ed. Vagsbygd, Norway: Sorlandets Fysikalske Institutt A/S; 1980.

81 Schafer RC. *Clinical Biomechanics: Musculoskeletal Actions and Reactions.* 2nd ed. New York, NY: Marcel Dekker Inc; 1987.

82 Tax HR. *Podopediatrics,* 2nd ed. Baltimore, Md: Williams & Wilkins; 1985.

83 Kisner C, Colby LA. The knee. In: Kisner C, Colby LA. *Therapeutic Exercise Foundations and Techniques.* 2nd ed. Philadelphia, Pa: FA Davis Co; 1990:345–356.

84 Warren R, Arnoczky SP, Wickiewicz TL. Anatomy of the knee. In: Nicholas JA, Hershman EB, eds. *The Lower Extremity and Spine in Sports Medicine.* St Louis, Mo: CV Mosby Co; 1986:657–694.

85 Le Damany P. La torsion des tibias, normale, pathologique, experimentale. *J de l'Anat Phys.* 1909;45:598–615.

86 Wynne-Davies R. Talipes equinovarus: a review of eighty-four cases after completion of treatment. *J Bone Joint Surg [Br].* 1964;46: 464–476.

87 Dupius PV. La torsion tibiale. In: *Son Interet Clinique: Radiologique et Chirurgical.* Paris, France: Masson et Cie; 1951:3–68.

88 Root ML, Orien WP, Weed JH, Hughes RJ. *Biomechanical Examination of the Foot.* Los Angeles, Calif: Clinical Biomechanics Corp; 1971: vol 1.

89 Jakob RP, Haertel M, Stussi E. Tibial torsion calculated by computerized tomography and compared to other methods of measurement. *J Bone Joint Surg [Br].* 1980;62:238–242.

90 McCollough NC. Orthotic management. In: Lovell WW, Winter RB, eds. *Pediatric Orthopaedics.* 2nd ed. Philadelphia, Pa: JB Lippincott Co; 1986:1038–1039.

91 Larson RL. Physical examination in the diagnosis of rotary instability. *Clin Orthop.* 1983;172:38–44.

92 Valmassy RL. *Normal and Abnormal Development of the Lower Extremity in the Infant: Treatment of Common Pediatric Musculoskeletal Disorders—Course Syllabus.* San Francisco,

Calif: California College of Podiatric Medicine; 1990.

93 Mossberg K, Smith LK. Axial rotation of the knee in adult females. Cited in: Lehmkuhl LD, Smith LK. *Brunnström's Clinical Kinesiology,* 4th ed. Philadelphia, Pa: FA Davis Co; 1983:292.

94 Weber D, Agro M, eds. *Clinical Aspects of Lower Extremity Orthotics.* Oakville, Ontario, Canada: Elgan Enterprises; 1990.

95 Cusick BD. *Serial Casts: Their Use in the Management of Spasticity-Induced Foot Deformity.* Rev ed. Tucson, Ariz: Therapy Skill Builders; 1990.

96 Seibel MO. *Foot Function: A Programmed Text.* Baltimore, Md: Williams & Wilkins; 1988.

97 Rang M, Wright M. What have 30 years of medical progress done for cerebral palsy? *Clin Orthop.* 1989;247:55–60.

Part IV: Schools and Education

The Chicago Public Schools' Experiment in the Education of the "Spastic Child"

By Mabel C. Smart

A professional woman in one of her books relates the following incident and draws from it an interesting analogy concerning the learning processes. To those who know the "spastic" child it presents a perfect picture of his social discomfort—a discomfort that amounts to suffering. The author says:

"The last bi-monthly tea of the X. Y. Z. Club was the setting for one of life's little dramas. I was reluctant to leave my home that evening for the weather was severely cold. I braved the storm, however, and set out through the drifting snow and the cutting wind toward the shelter of the clubhouse. As I entered the reception room, whose color and warmth in contrast to the cold and darkness without made it unusually attractive, and saw the many groups of guests scattered about, a sense of well-being came over me. I settled myself in a comfortable nook to indulge in my favorite pastime, namely, to philosophize over the scene before me. That evening I learned a lesson in psychology in a new and forceful way. As each newcomer entered the room, he hesitated a moment at the threshold and looked about him. I observed that the first arrival, after this moment of hesitation, was at once appropriatead by a group which eagerly listened whenever he expressed an opinion. The next guest was welcomed into another group but not quite so spontaneously. The third one seemed a bit different from the average person and wandered about from group to group before he found his niche. Then a fourth came. He hesitated quite a long time at the door, then walked about the room wih his hands in his pockets. He looked wistfully at the gayety about him, but no one noticed him, nor extended a hand, nor gave him a friendly nod. Then other interests attracted me and I forgot him for awhile. When I remembered him a half hour later, I noticed that he had his hat and coat and was leaving, passing from the frigid, social atmosphere within to the cold and darkness without." In the social isolation of the fourth man we see the untrained spastic child today, tomorrow, and throughout his life.

Twice in my early experience I had recognized his type. I had seen him in the person of a pupil in a school I attended as a child. He was most repulsive in appearance. His gait was a drunken stagger and his speech was the bane of my life because he was an unsolvable by facial contortions. He was born of drunken parents and the current opinion was that he had been "marked." Naturally, the children avoided him. I know now that he was palsied or "spastic." Years later I became a second grade teacher and again I saw this "fourth man." Again he was in the person of a misfit boy. This boy was the bane of my life because he was an unsolvable problem that was ever before me. When the class marched, his feet were out of step and out of line; when it sang, his coarse monotone ruined the purity of the group tone; when it played ball, he crashed into the home base; in fact, there was no such thing as team work because his personality stuck out like a sore thumb. Nobody wanted him. He was shunted from room to room as the semesters rolled by. He was a drag in every class and an irritation to every teacher. Yet it never occurred to one of us to find out whether she irritated him. Had we done so, he might have paraphrased Shylock, saying, "Has not a 'spastic' hands, organs, dimensions, senses, affections, passions, fed by the same food, warmed and cooled by the same winter and summer, as a non-spastic is?" I never forgot these boys even though years passed before I met their type again. Then the contact came in a school for crippled children.

It is as a teacher in the Spalding School that the social discomfort of these particularly misfit children has been forced upon my attention. It has been forced upon my attention first, because of the prevalence of the type. At Spalding School, out of a membership of eight hundred fifty, one hundred fifteen are "spastic cases." One of the foremost surgeons of Baltimore, while holding clinics in Maryland, was amazed to find the following percentages of "spastics": 14%—10%—8%—12½%—23%—4%—19½%. Dr. Bronson Crothers of Boston says that he can select from any every-day-clinic group enough palsied cases to demonstrate for hours without making a special effort to bring them in. He thinks the number is larger than in the poliomyelitis group because the latter is usually epidemic while the former is continuous.

It has been forced upon my attention secondly, because of the great needs of the group. One of these needs is that of psychological research. Children whose lack of speech, facial contortions, and drooling would classify them as feeble-minded have an untrained native intelligence that cannot express itself. There are cases who, by the present standardized tests rate low, yet, who show unmistakable signs of good thinking ability. Dr. Arnold Gesell of Yale and Miss Elizabeth Lord, formerly of Yale, have standardized the reactions of normal infants at different month levels. It may be just to compare a month old palsied baby with a month old normal baby, but we wonder whether it is fair to measure an older, palsied child by the same measure that is used for a physically normal child of the same age. Their developmental opportunities certainly have not been equal. Dr. Gessell, in his book, *Infancy and Human Growth,* gives over an entire chapter to a plea for the better understanding of the cerebral palsied child. Dr. Abraham A. Low of the Illinois Research Hospital of Chicago is doing at present a fine piece of research among children. Only a careful, scientific study of each individual "spastic" child will make it possible to determine his physical and mental potentialities.

Another great need is a recognition of the urgency for adjusting the environment to the physical condition. The child with "lesion in the central nervous system" (after Lord, a term more inclusive than the term "spastic") is over stimulated by regular class room procedures because his inhibition is low. Competing with his classmates, both as to quantity and to quality of achievement, irritates him. If he remains in the class room, he is in a continual state of tension; if he is excluded from school room environment, he is deprived not only of motor and academic training, but also, usually, of medical study. He goes out of the ill-adapted school situation into a bleaker outside world.

The third and fourth necessities are medical and vocational study. These unmet needs cause the social discomfort and the suffering of this "fourth man," and the resultant cry among all workers with the handicapped, "What shall we do with the 'spastic'?"

While Miss Jane A. Neil was principal of the Spalding School for Crippled Children in Chicago, she was constantly seeking the answer to this question. As she travelled about the country, she followed every lead that presented itself, one of which was a visit to Dr. Ivory Shepherd Franz, formerly of St. Elizabeth's Hospital, Washington, D. C., who gave her her first great inspiration to "carry on." When she returned, she opened to us visions of what might be done. After years of persistent and constructive building toward a plan, Miss Neil has developed a scheme which affords an opportunity at least to study this problem. The objective of the plan is to attempt to determine whether segregation and special technique in teaching methods will reduce the tension and the irritation that are incident to regular class room procedures. To that end a department was opened, known as "The Experimental Unit."

The personnel of the unit consists of fifty cases having intelligence quotients not lower than seventy, in so far as that can be determined. The selections were made on the basis of intelligence and motor handicap. The organization of the unit is as follows: There are two main divisions, the Home-Room Group and the Motor-Academic Group. The former reside in their own segregated class rooms, while the latter are scattered throughout the school from kindergarten through the high school. The Home-Room Group is subdivided into the Primary Room and the Nursery School. A third group, an Infant Clinic, will complete the unit.

Authorities in this field regard infant clinics as indispensable. Dr. Crothers says:

"It is indefensible to leave palsied babies without training until they reach school age. Their training is a matter of education rather than of medication. Parents need to understand that this education must be better than that of other children; that it must be begun in infancy and carried on in pre-school days; hat it is a matter of years as is all the rest of the child's education."

Miss Neil had long felt the need for the earliest possible training. Results obtained from education begun after the sixth year were not the best; mental and muscle habits were too strongly fixed; home attitudes toward the individual were too set to be easily changed. Her conception of the remedial work under existing conditions is to work down to the lower age levels as fast as circumstances and the ripening of public opinion will permit. It may be that some day preparatory training for the Nursery School in the form of an infant clinic will be, not a dream, but a reality, as it is already under consideration.

The Nursery School, opened in February, 1930, affords fine opportunities to the palsied child of ages two to four years. These age limits are flexible. The Board of Education provides the room, heated and lighted. The Sunbeam League and a patroness of the school provide the teacher and the splendid equipment we now have. The Nursery has its own playground and an activity room. A teacher, trained at National Kindergarten College, with nursery school technique as a background and an ever growing knowledge of the physical side, is in charge. The little ones, twelve in number, are transported by the school bus service. Rest and nutrition are carefully arranged for in each day's program. Speech training, muscle training, (including swimming), and regular nursery school curricula are given. The children enter having had little or no training in habits of sleep and rest, behavior, toilet needs, food reactions, etc. In the year's time they have learned to sleep and rest at regular intervals; tantrums, weeping, and enuresis have been practically cured; food is accepted as served. They are being taught to feed themselves, to swallow, to balance themselves, to walk, etc. The physiotherapist teaches them through games to use the large muscle co-ordinations. This group affords a wealth of material for research. We find that they enter the Primary room showing a higher level of physical and behavior adjustment than do those who have not had this training.

The Primary Group is made up of about twelve children of varying ages of the first, second, and third grade levels. They reside in the home room and are in charge of a regular teacher of primary academic subjects. They go to the occupational therapist for corrective handwork, to the physiotherapist for muscle training and swimming, and to the teacher of speech correction, if necessary. The curriculum is two-fold:

(a) Individualized. The tool subjects are taught, as far as possible, through individualized material. Thus each child progresses at his own rate, independent of the group.

(b) Socialized. This includes all the training that makes a child socially desirable. Games, music, rhythm, stories, and social situations are used to develop cooperation both physical and physic. Training in toilet habits, self-feeding, cleanliness, etc., create self respect. Correction of speech defects, though slow, develops a feeling of social security. At the end of each semester those cases who continue to need this intensive training are retained in the group but the rest are placed in the regular class rooms and become members of the Motor-academic Group.

Inasmuch as the grammar grade teachers find it difficult to determine just how to adjust the palsied students because there is no way to determine what they really know, the Motor-academic study is incorporated into the plan. The grade distribution is from the third grade through the high school. The basis of selection is serious disturbance of motor expression, either oral or written, or both. The children reside in the regular grade rooms and go to the unit teacher for help in academic subjects that require motor expression. In some cases a helper is employed by the hour to be "hands" for the individual. Thus far facilities permit this part of the plan to be carried out only meagerly. Another angle of the problem is to develop a sort of course of study that will be suited to these individuals and yet be so standardized as to be acceptable to educators.

The activities of the unit are three-fold: The academic, already partially alluded to, the physical and the social. The academic features have been discussed in the previous paragraphs, except as to expression. The type of expression to be used depends upon the purpose it is to accomplish. When a mental outlet is in view (for Spalding holds that, while the motor abilities must be developed to the last degree possible, nevertheless, such training should not be given at the expense of mental efficiency) then the least resisted pathway to expression must be sought. Typewriting is being experimented with as a medium for such an outlet. To that end some fourth, fifth, and sixth grade cases are being trained by a competent teacher of commercial subjects to use the typewriter. The hope is that by the time the seventh and eighth grades are reached, these children will have obtained a sufficiently serviceable amount of skill to enable them to express themselves with a fair degree of ease. When therapeutic or vocational results are in view, then the school shops afford about fourteen different means of activity; namely, printing, manual training, brace repairing, basketry, pottery, weaving, novelty making, personal hygiene, sewing, cooking, dining room management, and child care (practice in which is received by assisting in the Nursery School and the Primary Room). In these shop activities the academic and the physical merge more or less.

Dr. Crothers in the following remarks to physiotherapists strikes the keynote in physical care. He says:

"The diagnosis of cerebral palsy, as far as physiotherapists are concerned, should be physiological rather than anatomic. They must train residual cells to make new patterns. First search for the assets. The functional disability is usually greater than the organic one. Encourage the child to use more activity than he is accustomed to use. Build up a morale and a sense of sufficiency." Our physical therapy program seeks to develop the residual cells through swimming, muscle training, occupational therapy, the use of appliances, when necessary, and speech correction.

The Nursery School children are taken into the water twice a week; the Primary Group are taught swimming three times a week; the Motor-academic Group, once a week. Special cases are given additional treatments as far as possible. The objectives in swimming developed in the order named, are: courage, breathing, walking, floating, swimming, and diving.

Children above the Nursery School age have occupational therapy every day. The physiotherapist makes the recommendations as to what movements are desired and the occupational therapist applies the exercise in terms of hand work. The work done is strictly curative.

In the Nursery School speech is very informal; in the Primary Room it is carried on largely through plays and games; but in the older group it is more precise. For all ages a certain amount of definite muscle training in the speech organs is indicated.

The use of appliances is limited largely to wheelchairs. The adjustment of wheelchairs and tables to patients is carefully watched. As rapidly as possible wheelchair cases are urged to sit at regular desks and to walk. Part of the technique is to analyze the physical steps that go to make the co-ordination desired; to teach the child what these steps are after having first made clear to him what it is that he is being asked to do.

Such a physical and academic program cannot function efficiently in the school unless it is vigorously supported by the home. Therefore a program of social activities must be carried on concurrently. It includes parent education and vocational guidance. A visiting nurse or teacher is the link (at present a missing link) between the school on the one hand and the home and economic world on the other. Parents need education in regard to the child's emotional needs, to the right attitude toward behavior problems, to a proper health program, to his treatments, to operative work, to the use of appliances, to his training, and to planning his future.

Vocational guidance, training, and placement are the crux of the whole matter. To accomplish these steps we endeavor: to link psychological testing with all training; to link the child's aptitudes with industries and professions; to link the school with industries and professions; and to educate the public to employ the paralyzed. In the effort to direct the child, conferences have been held in which have sat the parents, the psychologist, the physiotherapist, the occupational therapist, the teacher of speech correction, the grade teacher, the shop and art teachers, the vocational guidance worker, the principal, and, where possible, the superintendent of special schools. The object of the conferences has been to get the composite of the individual's assets through the slants contributed by each worker who has contact with him. By ruling out his liabilities an attempt is made to map out his future. Some of the recommendations of these conferences have been as follows: home-keeping, child care, training for certain kinds of factory work, and a course of training that will lead into Scout work. How practical these recommendations are remains to be seen.

The whole matter may be epitomized:

In our creed: That all previous care, cure and education find their consummation in final placement of the palsied in their own homes, in industry, or in the professions.

In our hope: For the co-operation of education, medicine, and industry; for the time when these palsied will

For the time when these palsied will not be like the fourth man at the tea, but will have been trained and helped until they have become integrated into some niche suited to their abilities.

In our aim: To give to every child with lesion in the central nervous system

"1. The best physical condition it is possible for him to attain.

"2. The best education he can assimilate.

"3. To help him find his place for service in the world's work."

CHILD CRIPPLES GET FULL COURSE AT MORTON HIGH*

ONLY SUCH GROUP IN STATE HOUSED WITH NORMAL KIDS

By Ruth De Young

Mary Jane, 12 years old, is walking this year for the first time in her life—slowly and falteringly, but her little legs are working just like other boys' and girls'.

"Oh," she exclaimed the other day, "It's so nice to be high up like other folks!"

It was her answer to the question of Miss Leona H. Fette, director of the orthopedic school at J. Sterling Morton High School, Cicero, who was making inquiry about the result of her recent treatment. This little girl is one of 81 children at the school who are learning to use their arms and their legs at the same time that they are acquiring their readin' and writin' and 'rithmetic. Mary Jane's case is typical of many another that has come under Miss Fette's care during the seven years of the school.

It has been proved repeatedly that it is unnecessary for handicapped children to remain prisoners in wheel chairs, but it takes years of scientific care to make it possible for them to walk with crutches and years more for them to make the transition to braces alone.

ONLY SCHOOL OF KIND IN STATE

There are well known schools in Chicago and elsewhere that care only for these handicapped children, but the orthopedic school at Morton is the only orthopedic school in Illinois that is housed under the same roof and directed by the same officials as a city or township high school. Miss Fette said this close association with the secondary school provides a complete curriculum for the little cripples, courses that a school run solely for handicapped children might be unable to offer because of the small demand. Another advantage is in the service that the high school students give for the asking in serving meals and assisting generally their less fortunate neighbors.

*Reprinted from the Re-Aides Post.

From kindergarten through the last year of high school these 81 boys and girls in the Morton orthopedic school receive treatment and care during school hours, each one under the direction of a private or a clinic physician. They are called for and taken home daily in busses furnished by the board of education with the exception of those children living at the greatest distances. In these cases two private cars call for and return the children.

Corrective Exercises Given

During the day exercise and corrective therapy are administered to each child as the physician in charge of his case prescribes. Alpine rays and massage, rest hours for those who need it—all of these items come first on the program. Studies are pursued according to each child's ability to handle them.

The school is housed on the first floor of the Morton High School building. It was in 1924 that Harry Victor Church, superintendent of the J. Sterling Morton schools, took advantage of the state appropriation through action of the board of education to establish the orthopedic school. Miss Fette was called immediately to take charge. Her experience had been varied, for she had served as an instructor in the Columbia University Teachers' College, the Oregon Agricultural College, and during the war had been a reconstruction aide after an intensive training course in the Harvard Medical School.

In September, 1924, five pupils enrolled and one teacher assisted Miss Fette—this in contrast to 81 pupils today and a teaching staff of five. These instructors are Mrs. Olive Parkhurst, Miss Marion Muir, Miss Ann Dolezal, and Miss Stella Uehren.

Few Clinics at School

Children are admitted to the school only upon recommendation of their own orthopedic surgeon or after examination at any one of the large hospitals of the city. This is a change from the plan on which the school was first run when Dr. Henry Bascom Thomas of the department of orthopedic surgery at the University of Illinois Medical School conducted clinics at Morton.

"It is only occasionally that we have a clinic in Cicero now," Miss Fette explained. "The first in many months is to be held Oct. 26 under the auspices of the Cicero Rotary Club, which has assisted generously in the work of the school. Dr. Thomas is coming to conduct this clinic, when 14 pupils now in school will be examined and when any other crippled children in the township may be brought for examination."

The Morton Orthopedic School is grateful not only to the Rotary Club, but also to the Berwyn Kiwanis Club and the board of education, groups which have aided materially in making the little cripples happy. There's nothing that these boys and girls anticipate more than their annual Christmas party and their annual trip to the circus, both provided by the Berwyn Kiwanians.

Clubs Arrange Hospital Care

Through their efforts a number of the children have been given medical attention gratis by Dr. B. H. Moore at the Shriners' Hospital. The Rotarians, through their crippled children's committee, headed in recent years by John Carlander and Ben Braun, have obtained care for some of the boys and girls at the Illinois Research Hospital.

Each member of the high school board of education has given personal attention to the orthopedic school and the handicapped children enrolled, Miss Fete said. George G. Tucker is president of this board and Oscar E. Rox, Henry Langner, John J. Sherlock, and Frank A. Svoboda are all members.

Infantile paralysis is responsible for the condition of most of the children in the school. Tuberculosis of the bone, which is not contagious, cardiac and the spastic cases constitute the bulk of the others.

It is the grouping of handicapped children in a school or a department of their own that has solved many of their difficulties, Miss Fette believes.

"In their social life, in their work, and in their play," she said, "they are competing with their equals; their handicaps are forgotten to a certain extent because all have them. We put the emphasis here on their strength, not their weakness."—Chicago Tribune.

The Spastic Child in the Classroom

Eleanor V. Givins

From the viewpoint of the teacher, the spastic child probably presents the greatest problem in the schoolroom. He has greater difficulty in conforming to the usual classroom procedure. However, because of the large number of spastics in the schools, they bear special consideration.

Mrs. Hazel C. McIntire, Director of Special Schools in Ohio, reported that in the school year 1935-1936, there were 205 spastic children in public special schools, 16.5 per cent of the total enrollment of 1241.[1] She remarked that the large number (next to infantile paralysis) was due, not to a great increase in such cases, but because there is more interest in this group and they now are receiving a fair chance. Last year, 1936-1937, Charles Feilbach School of Toledo reported

Teacher, Charles Feilbach School, Toledo, Ohio.

28 spastic children, over 14 per cent of our total enrollment.

Doctor Carlson states that there is a wide range of difference in the mental resources of the birth injured—from idiocy to purely motor handicaps with little or no mental disturbance.[2] Tremulous rigidity, violent irrelevant movements, delayed or difficult speech, and drooling have no validity as evidences of mental defect. There is a difference between a feeble mind and a good mind that has been damaged. He contends that we cannot rely too much on intelligence tests as criteria of their mentality, as the majority of tests require the use of muscles over which the child may have little or no control. However, he does believe that the intelligence tests may serve as a starting point and if subsequent tests show higher rating, we know that the child is making progress.[3]

Records of 628 crippled children in Ohio schools for the school year 1936-1937 showed that the median Intelligence Quotient was 89, just one point below the normal I.Q., but the median Intelligence Quotient of spastics only was 82. Last year, the spastic children at Feilbach School had a median Intelligence quotient of 81 as compared with an Intelligence Quotient of 94 for other crippled children, exclusive of spastics. The Intelligence Quotient of a considerable number of these children is such as to justify serious effort at their education.

The methods in the schoolroom must be adapted to help the spastic child. There may be disabilities of speech or hearing or vision which interfere with his schooling and which should receive special consideration. The question of handedness should be investigated.[4] Anxiety, fear and self-consciousness should be reduced as much as possible. He should be comfortable and feel secure in a chair which permits him to put his feet firmly on the floor. His paper could be held in place by thumb tacks. Let him use large arm movements in writing, using paper with lines of more than the usual width. It may be necessary for the teacher or another pupil to write his work for him. He should have time to express himself without being conscious of impatience on the part of the teacher. Whenever possible he should be permitted to perform the same activities as the other children but at a slower rate. Competition with others should be avoided. School work in which the element of time enters tends to overstimulate him and he cannot do his best work.

Behavior and psychiatric problems are present in almost every case, according to Doctor Carlson. The spastic child may use his handicap as a defense mechanism. Inability to cope with nervous overflow reaction may drive him to despair.[5] Unfavorable comparisons tend to deepen a feeling of incompetence and arouse jealousy, resentment, diffidence, or sullenness. Attitudes of pity or contempt towards him are disastrous. Morale can be built up by making requirements simple and thus permitting some degree of success. The level of expected performance should be set at a level challenging his ability but not so high that failure is likely.

Thomas and Rogers claim that the spastic child should be given more rather than less education than the average child because he will need more strength of mind, more courage, and a stronger philosophy of life to be able to hold his own.[6] Spastic children should be considered a group of interesting, soluble problems in education, rather than a dull, pitiful group of dependent cripples.[7]

Bibliography

1. McIntire, Hazel C.: An Analysis of Crippling Conditions and the Age-Grade Distribution in Orthopedic Classes in Ohio.
2. Carlson, Earl R.: Neurological Aspects and Treatment of Birth Injuries. New York State Jour. of Med., Vol. 34, Oct. 1, 1934, No. 19; p. 831-836.
3. Ibid. p. 831.
4. Ibid. pp. 831-832.
5. Carlson, Earl A.: The Problem of the Spastic Child. The Crippled Child Magazine, August 1935, Vol. XIII, No. 2, p. 58.
6. Thomas, Leah C. and Rogers, G. Gage: The Spastic as a Child. Physiotherapy Review, May-June 1934, p. 60.
7. Crothers, Bronson: Physiological Management of Children Handicapped by Cerebral Palsy." Lecture, June 11, 1929. Published by Visiting Nurse Association of Chicago, 1929.

Value of Nursery School Training for Cerebral Palsy Patients

Eleanor H. Farrell

When people first became interested in the cerebral palsy patients the physician worked out operative procedures and the teacher devised new educational methods. But the problem today has become far more complicated. If the child with cerebral palsy is to receive maximum benefits, all problems arising out of his physical disability must be considered. These problems center around abnormal physical growth, interferences in mental development, difficulties in social adjustments, the questions arising out of emotional disturbances and the introduction of personality complications. All of these profoundly affect normal development. As our task is to help the cerebral palsy patient become as nearly normal as he is capable of becoming, we are concerned with all problems which arise and interfere with this normal development. If we wait until the child is 6 or 7 years of age the problems have become too complicated and the child a product of them. Attempts to solve the problems should be made as they arise. Most of the difficulties first present themselves in babyhood and during the nursery school years. That is the time to start treatment.

There are three main classifications of cerebral palsy: the true spastic, the athetoid and ataxic types; and although there is a difference in treatment, basically it is relaxation and muscle reeducation. In the first group, the true spastic, treatment consists in relaxing the spastic or tense group and strengthening the flaccid group through muscle reeducation. We know that all his life the spastic has flexed, inward rotated and adducted, and consequently has developed strong tensions in these muscles. Conversely he has rarely experienced outward rotation, abduction and extension. These are the stretched and weak muscles. The aim is to balance these two groups of muscles and so coordinate their work that improvement in the mobility of the joint results. As the stretch reflex interferes in improvement, the movement, therefore, should be slow and easy and the muscles never forcibly stretched. The arc of motion is limited by the first sign of tension but is increased as the spastic group relaxes and the flaccid group strengthens.

The second group are the athetoids, and their chief treatment is relaxation, increased muscle power through muscle reeducation, and gradual buildup of control over involuntary movements. Work from the passive exercise, through active

Physical therapist, Spalding School for Crippled Children, Chicago, Ill.

assistive, to active exercise in back lying, then sitting and last standing. Persistently urging control of involuntary movements causes a rigidity akin to spasticity. This is to be avoided. It is far better to progress slowly and make the transition by easy steps to more difficult actions.

The third group of cerebral palsy are the ataxic type. There is no involuntary motion and no spasticity. Their difficulty is to give the direction to the movement that is intended. The treatment is training in coordination. They are told to walk directly toward an object. Physical activities are introduced which encourage direction to a specific object. Exercises which help to stabilize balance are of most help to them.

Next it is well to introduce progression in sitting, standing and walking. Fear accompanies every step of progress, so stress security all along the way. From learning to sit on a child's chair, with head rest, back rest, side supports and with thigh straps and a broad band to hold the child securely, progress to greater independence by removing first the head rest, then the band, then thigh straps and the side supports. The child then learns to sit at his table in an ordinary chair and finally sits without back support.

The progress in standing alone is equally slow. He first learns to stand on his feet with a worker taking the major part of the support. Gradually he takes more and more of his own weight. The next step is to get him to stand without the aid of human support. Place him in a corner where he learns that by leaning against the walls he can stand securely and without fear of falling, with only the aid of the walls for outside support. Later let him learn that one wall gives him the same aid and the same security. The next step is to return him to the corner. Sit facing him. He has the two walls in the rear and you in front for security. Let his body sway away from the walls and then fall backward to them. Count to five as he stands away from the wall. Then let him fall back to the walls for support, increase the count until he can stand alone for a minute or more. Now he is ready to learn to walk, for he has learned he can stand alone for a moment, which gives him a sense of security.

The cerebral palsy patient passes through many stages before he learns to walk. On the bicycle he learns the rhythmical flexion and extension of the legs. After learning to stand on his feet, he is taught to use a walker with the horse shoe top, which gives him upper body support. He progresses to the push walker, to the walking bars, to walking around furniture, and then to independent walking. This last, because of fear, is difficult to obtain. It is secured in two ways. Standing with his back to the wall, he stands away from it and takes one step toward the worker. This is gradually increased until he takes several steps. After this the child is encouraged to walk forward with the worker in the rear, giving the minimum amount of support. His tendency is to fall back toward that support, but more and more he can be encouraged to become independent of it. He is now taught to walk between two pieces of furniture. Thus the human aid is eliminated. He is now on his own.

The child with cerebral palsy is deprived of many of the concepts of touch, kinesthetic sensations, large mucle group coordinations and physical contacts with his world. He is deprived of all their accompanying emotional reactions which give meaning to the normal child's world. These children need help in finding out about their world. But there are many parents, over-anxious, over-protective who stand in the way of their child's development. Children enter the nursery whose parents have foreseen all the child's needs and then done everything for the child. Some of these children have rarely initiated a movement. These children have just looked and listened, that is all. They have never entered into any activity. They do not know that they can. How much meaning can the world have for them? To them it is truly only a vision. Little of it is of their own making. Their world can come to have real meaning only when they take part in it.

One of the first things the nursery school does is to try to get the child to initiate physical activity. Stimulating the child to initiate activity comes only after the child is adjusted to his new environment. With the increase in initiative comes increased physical improvement. But more than that comes the awakening of the mind. From a child who casually views his environment there emerges one who is actively interested in his world and wants to participate in it. Improvement is evident and comes rapidly after that.

There is a mechanical device which gives pleasure and also helps start initiation of physical activity. It is the bicycle. It was mainly for this reason that it was introduced. Its values consist in the following: (1) Children are the initiators of the activity. (2) Pleasure in the activity supplants attention to spastic and athetoid seizures. Consequently we find the spastic has less spasm and the athetoid less athetosis. (3) Peddling is easy to do. It gives the necessary momentum for movement that some of the children need and starts them on the road to improvement. (4) It develops power in the muscles. (5) Peddling makes an excellent preliminary exercise for walking. It is particularly satisfactory for the athetoid, who needs to find a transition for control in an activity between sitting and standing. (6) Children unable to carry head erect over a sustained period of time have an incentive for doing so. Such cases markedly improve. The doodle bug proves an excellent and pleasant way to develop the upper body.

Physical disability affects the speech. There is many a cerebral palsy patient with delayed speech who is handicapped for years through lack of oral expression. Acquisition of new facts, knowledge of environment, social adjustments, emotional outlets, reflective thinking find no expression in words. The child loses opportunties for mental growth and expansion. His thoughts die in him. Time and again there comes into the nursery school a child who finds no expression except in crying and laughing. Mostly it is crying. What chance has such a child for mental development? How can he make adjustments so necessary to his development?

Many mothers who are patient and interested will help the child build a series of signs which take the place of speech. Many frown upon this. It interferes in speech development. I know this is contrary to the accepted idea in speech training. If the child's speech development is swallowed up in sign language the need for speech is not there. Teachers of speech insist he make an effort to give verbal expression to his wants. But he cannot do this. In the meantime are we to allow all means of expression to lay dormant? If we do we stand in the way of the child's mental growth. We must seek another way to teach the child to express his thoughts and his wants. That way lays through pantomine. I wonder what this would mean in helping him to understand his environment. What chances it gives for self expression and what opportunities it might give him for contact with others. One mother I know has a flare for expressing a thought by an effective movement which she teaches her child. There is little need for the spoken word between these two.

Physical disability affects emotional development. The cerebral palsy child is deprived of the emotions which come through contact with the outside world. The trend away from the normal pattern is further increased by emotional maladjustments, conditioned by parental fears, overindulgence, neglect. These in turn are intensified by physical fears and inability to make his wants known.

The irritability that arises from his inability to make his wants known fade away when adults learn to read the signs and interpret the sounds that express his thoughts. Questioning and watching for a change of expression, an utterance of a sound, a movement of the body that expresses his thought, makes it possible for the adult to understand the child and the child's needs. Irritability recedes.

Fear plays an important part in the picture of most cerebral palsy patients. Our first efforts are directed toward giving the child a sense of physical security in all situations. This is done by conducting all activities on or near the floor, adjusting seats to give him a sense of security and giving additional support at every evidence of fear.

Because the environment and experiences of the cerebral palsy patient are limited, fear is too often expressed at new faces and new places. Their introduction into his life is made gradually and quietly. Preparation by way of talks explaining new experiences make their acceptance easier. Thus more and more new experiences and people are injected into his life, until he comes to accept most new people and new experiences without fear.

Bound up into the emotional life of the child are emotionally disturbed parents. Parents of a child with cerebral palsy often are a greater problem than the child. A child with cerebral palsy is born into the family. Parents are frustrated and unable to cope with the problem. Many are so emotionally disturbed at the inability to adjust that the whole family suffers. The child reflects these disturbances and the combination of emotionally disturbed parents and the child creates many behaviour problems.

One of our first tasks, therefore, is parental education. This would be most difficult, but it is made possible by two effective arguments. One is that the detrimental effect of the emotional instability of the parents interferes with the progress of the child. The contact between a mother and a child with cerebral palsy is close, so much closer than that between a mother and a normal child. This is true because the child with cerebral palsy is much more dependent on the mother than the normal child. She is practically his world. Much of the emotional instability of the mother is readily reflected in the cerebral palsy patient. This is very evident to workers in the nursery. When once a mother realizes her emotional life prevents improvement in her child, she makes desperate efforts to adjust to more normal balance.

Another forceful argument is that the child receives no treatments from the physical therapist until he is adjusted. Emotion in a child has a way of possessing the attention of the child to the exclusion of everything else. A child, emotionally disturbed, cannot give his attention wholly to the treatments of the physical therapist. It is difficult enough to gain and hold the attention of the nursery school child without having him diverted by emotion. The child receives no physical therapy. The mother knows this, consequently she seeks to remedy the trouble and helps in her child's adjustments. Besides, the physical therapist does not wish to have her treatments associated with unpleasant experiences and emotions. She knows there is grave danger the child might acquire a dislike of exercise. Above all, she does not want this to occur.

It is important that children like to do their exercise. At the first sign of resistence, stop work or change to some other form of exercise. Return to the exercise at another more favorable time. If a child resists an exercise day after day, either because he does not like it, is physically uncomfortable, or unable to do it with a fair degree of success, we are only strengthening the will of that child against his own physical improvement. The best way to develop a strong will in a child against any activity is to persist in doing it against that child's will, when he continues to resist the exercise day after day. More and more exercise becomes bound up with emotional disturbances. There are exceptions when the physical therapy technician should assert her will over the child. But you can impose those exceptions only when the child accepts you and most of your work.

It is excellent training for a parent to come and stay in the nursery school through the morning. She learns many things which help her and her child to adjust. If she stays, she stays on three conditions: One is that she bows to the routine of the nursery. The second is that she care for and start her child in the morning routine. Then she is to pay no attention to him until lunch time, after which time she takes him home. The third condition is that she perform certain duties and care for one or two children other than her own. The impersonal attitude she assumes and the success she invariably has under the direction of the nursery school director in handling a child other than her own gives her confidence in more successfully caring for her own child.

Physical disability interferes with social development. Lack of child companions is one of the greatest handicaps suffered by the child with cerebral palsy. He has few opportunities to learn to know others, to form social habits and to make social adjustments. Contact with others helps him to form habits of behaviour. So we see the cerebral palsy patient loses much in character building. Children stimulate each other to new activities. They like to do what they see other children do. Imitation stimulates children to initiate activities which the efforts of adults could not arouse. Pitting one child against another is one of the greatest stimulations for physical as well as mental progress. What possible chance has a child of nursery school age to develop a well balanced personality when he has no playmates to condition his anger, fears, jealousies; no companions to increase his powers of independence and initiative.

The nursery school for cerebral palsy patients offers the child a social life with children of his own age. Many children are for the first time introduced to child companions. They participate for the first time in group activity, in rhythms, games, singing, dramatics and stories. Active children assist and play with inactive children. Children, in their behaviour, are conditioned by the group and by each other. Many of the benefits which normal children derive from the nursery school experiences are given to the cerebral palsy patient in their nursery school.

Cerebral injury is responsible for part of the handicap of these patients. But as the years pass, habit plays an increasingly prominent role. If at the very start the baby could use conscious control, probably athetosis and spasticity in later years would not be so pronounced. In addition, emotion is a powerful aid in greatly increasing the habit of spasticity and athetosis. The more intelligent a child is, the more fearful he is, for he knows he has not the controls that allow him to sit securely and stand safely. He frequently gives physical expression to his fears. Just as often as he is seized with fear, just as frequently does he give expression to his fear in seizures of spasticity and athetosis. These repeated seizures induced by emotion, together with seizures eminating from stimulation of the brain centers that produce spasticity and athetosis, over which he has no control, build deep seated habits.

The value of the nursery school for the cerebral palsy patient becomes evident. The nursery is primarily interested in habit formation. The mind and body of the child are pliable and flexible at this age. This is the time to start conscious control. With every added year the habits become more deeply fixed and difficulty in establishing controls increases. This is the time, too, to break down fears and gradually substitute physical security. Every opportunity is given the child for physical and oral expression and for social adjustments. The nursery school offers the handicapped child all phases of development, much of which he might not otherwise have had if left at home.

Handicapped with a physical defect that no amount of education and training will completely eradicate, the child with cerebral palsy should be encouraged to foster and develop those powers which remain intact. The nursery school starts the training and lays the foundation in the child. The child's informal activities in the nursery are the foundations of the formal work in school and college. The gross coordinations of the child evolve into the finer coordinations of the adult. His early speech patterns become the tools of oral and written expression. The nursery is concerned with elementary problem solving. Out of it grows increasing interest, persistence, concentration, accuracy and initiative. The child is constantly adjusting to new people and new situations, and his increasing ability to adjust makes his future life in society more secure. The first five years form the foundation. From this foundation spring the urges, stimulations, the patterns for future habits, attitudes and action. The firmer the foundation is laid, the surer is the chance for a successful adult life. For on the whole as the nursery school child, so is the boy, and later that boy is the man.

The average child is given the opportunity to develop normally, whether he is in the home or in the nursery school, but the cerebral palsy patient, too often, has not that opportunity. If education is to reclaim more of these unfortunate children, more opportunities should be given them to lay the foundation early. Kindergarten is too late, for by that time wrong habits are too firmly established. The child with cerebral palsy needs training early and he needs it more urgently than the normal child, because he starts with such a tremendous handicap. The time to obtain the best results is when the mind is plastic and the body pliable. That time is at the nursery school age.

The Physical Therapist Looks at the School Child

Esther Hutchinson

A glance at your morning newspaper reveals headlines bearing testimony of the topsy-turvy condition of the world. Even the flavor of your breakfast coffee does nothing to add a note of normality to the picture. It is interesting in these abnormal times to find one healthy, normal note. Picture some of the headlines you have seen—"The Handicapped Help Defense," "Crippled Employed in War Industries," "Hundreds of Handicapped Find Jobs." People are discovering what normal things the handicapped can do. This is healthy, hopeful news.

Why does the story of handicapped people working make feature material for the *Saturday Evening Post?* Chiefly for the reason that while the crippled child makes an emotional appeal to the general public, the crippled adult has been considered just an unfortunate. Perhaps in the past we who have worked with the crippled child have unwittingly promoted such an attitude through segregation which, unless handled carefully, tends to place a premium on being crippled. The child has grown to expect favors and the general public has not learned that the cripple can work at the side of the normal. Throughout the years we have placed too much emphasis on the fact that these people are crippled and not enough emphasis on what they can do.

If the child is to take his place in society as a well-adjusted, self-respecting and economically independent adult, the school must share in a coordinated program with other individuals and agencies interested in the welfare of children. Recognizing this, special education, as conducted today, is no longer so highly "special." It is regular education geared to meet the individual needs of certain children, physically as well as academically. The child with a paralyzed arm or a scoliosis has more in common with the so-called normal child than he has differences. He carries the same academic work, has the same desires and interests as other children and spends his out-of-school time with parents, brothers, sisters and friends. Although normal in most respects there are times when the child's physical disability prevents him from carrying the regular school routine. It is then that we in the schools must help him to secure maximum physical improvement and assure him the same educational opportunities as other children through an enriched program which will round out his field of experience.

Since crippled children vary widely in the extent of their handicaps and in their needs, the special education program is made flexible enough to serve all types of crippled children. Protective care and curative treatment are included when indicated, but are gradually withdrawn as the child gains strength and confidence in his own ability. The educational program may be either in the form of individual instruction given at home or in the hospital, or group instruction in special class, combination special and regular class, or in regular school on a modified program. The end of each year shows a comparatively large turnover in each group, for children are advanced just as rapidly as it is thought advisable by the attending physician. The measure of success of the special program is not how many children are kept under protective care, but how many are prepared for normal living.

In Ohio the crippled child needing special school placement may enter a centralized school housing only crippled children or a special unit in a regular school building. Of the 25 special schools in the state, 20 are located in regular school buildings with normal children.

The centralized schools housing only crippled children are in the larger cities and from the administrative angle have certain advantages, particularly from the point of building arrangement, transportation and attendant care. They also offer greater opportunities for fitting the school to the child. But in fitting the school to the child, one must always keep in mind the fact

Supervisor, Physical Therapy, Dept. of Education, Division of Special Education, Columbus, Ohio.

Read before Pre-Convention meeting of the Orthopedic Section of the American Physiotherapy Association with the Therapeutic Section of the American Association for Health, Physical Education and Recreation, Cincinnati, Ohio, April 12, 1943.

that our main objective is fitting the child for normal life. He must receive normal treatment along with his special treatment. This is more difficult to do in a centralized school serving only crippled children, but it can and is being done successfully.

It is believed by many, and this belief is shared by the Division of Special Education, that it is easier for the crippled child to grow normally when he is in association with regular school children. The normal majority group tends to raise the standards of achievement. In orthopedic units, housed in regular school buildings, the child who needs transportation, rest or physical therapy will receive these services the same as in a centralized school, but in addition he has an opportunity to attend regular classes and participate in a program with normal children. His schoolmates of today will be his working companions of tomorrow.

Advocates for the centralized orthopedic school may object on the grounds that the crippled child will not be accepted completely in the regular school. Their point is well taken, for, unless the special and regular teachers share in the responsibility for educating these children, the child may become more isolated than if he were in a special class full time. One superintendent has said, "The regular teacher's attitude should be one not of mere tolerance, but rather of keen interest in guiding his educational and social development. It is her privilege and obligation to do for the child that which the special teachers cannot do, namely, make him feel that though he has a physical disability he is not inferior to normal children in other respects. She is in a position to do much to help him build up confidence in himself by explaining to the regular children the purpose of the special class, striving to develop among regular children a wholesome attitude toward the crippled child, encouraging the crippled child to participate in group activities of the normal grade children, and insisting that he grow in responsibility to himself."

As many orthopedic disabilities in children respond well to treatment, physical therapy has been included as part of the special school program. Although children in the class are given first consideration, in the more rural areas this service has been extended to a limited number of preschool, high school, home instruction, and regular school children. In planning the school day, rest and physical therapy are woven into the program in such a way that the child has the advantage of treatment with a minimum loss of time from his academic work.

The first duty of the physical therapist is to give the massage, light or muscle training which has been prescribed by the child's physician. This may be either to improve function or to prepare for further surgery. Many of the school children are seen by the orthopedist only once in every three or four months. As they outgrow braces and crutches and during their period of growth tend to develop further deformity, it is important that they be watched during these intervals. The physical therapist keeps in close contact with the orthopedists and frequently attends clinic with the children in order to discuss changes in treatment. In a few centers the orthopedists examine children at school.

Another step in rehabilitating the child is to teach him to use what power he has to the best advantage. We are preparing him to go on from the protected class into normal society, and he will need skills and self-reliance. It may be necessary to teach him to feed and dress himself, get in and out of chairs and climb stairs, and this can best be accomplished with practice in actual situations. Most children want to do what other children are doing, and school provides the necessary incentive. He learns to climb stairs so he can go out to class and he feeds himself because other children are doing this. One year a little boy with cerebral palsy entered school, and, although not too badly handicapped, had never learned to dress himself nor was he anxious to start at that time. However, he did love to go in the pool and when he realized that he must at least help with the dressing if he continued, it was no time until he could care for himself.

During the period the child is under close supervision every effort is made to improve his physical condition and general appearance, increase his endurance and instill in him a desire to improve. Of course, the amount of improvement which can be expected will vary with each individual. Most of the children will return to regular school, but some few will never reach a point where they are self-sustaining individuals. For these we also have certain responsibilities. If they can be taught to entertain themselves and care for at least a few of their personal needs, they will be much happier and less of a burden to other members of the family.

This year a class was opened for some of the more handicapped children with cerebral palsy. Badly handicapped children are usually overprotected and Martha was one of these. The whole family life had been built around her and for seven years the parents had watched and worried over every movement. Martha was unable to attend the local special class, so it was decided to place her in the cerebral palsy unit where she might live in the convalescent home in which the unit operates. You can imagine what it meant to sell the family on the idea of placing her in a school 150 miles from home, and as the family physician was to be consulted, the plan must be presented to him. At first the physician was a bit dubious about the whole thing, but in the end he replied, "I'll do all in my power to help. I don't know how much you can do with Martha, but I believe such a plan might save the married life of a fine young couple. The mother is now on the verge of a nervous breakdown just from worry over the child." Through the efforts of various people in the community Martha entered school in September. The family is now delighted with her school progress, slight physical improvement, and the opportunity she is having to enter into the social life of the group. She will return to a much more stable home in June. The special class is helping to build a more normal life for badly handicapped children and their parents.

Parents are likely to help crippled children too much. Nurses and physical therapists sometimes help parents too much. It is usually easier for the nurse or physical therapist to take the child to clinic and care for brace adjustments than it is to persuade parents to assume these duties. We often hear the nurse or physical therapist say, "But I can get these things done in half the time and I know they're done right." True, but in doing this are we preparing the child and the parents to take over responsibility which may be theirs for many years to come?

We wish to emphasize here, how the physical therapist and special teacher can help in laying a foundation which will aid the child, the parents and the regular teacher in their future planning for care, treatment and education. Many children have had little contact with physicians and hospitals before entering school, and a question familiar to any physical therapist is: "What are they going to do to me?" As some children will need a series of operations and long periods of aftercare, she can help in getting the child's cooperation by explaining briefly what to expect in the hospital and what the aftercare will be. Parents, too, at times are confused. They come to the physical therapist with some such statement as this: "The physician explained what he was going to do, but I didn't understand and was afraid to ask him again." Both parents and children must have a general understanding of what is to be done, and why, if maximum improvement is to be achieved.

It is only within the last few years that children with cardiac disabilities have been included in the special education program and there still is much to be done in this field. From studies made, it is estimated that one to two per cent of all school children have some type of heart disease. Congenital heart disease is more or less stationary, but rheumatic heart disease, which is responsible for 95 per cent of the cardiac disabilities in children, presents quite a different picture. During the active stage, when acute symptoms are present, complete bed rest is indicated, but during the inactive stage, functional ability fluctuates. At times the child may need a greatly restricted program, and then again, his condition may permit only slight limitation or allow him to participate in normal activity.

Most cardiologists and pediatricians are opposed to long periods of school segregation, believing that the child should learn to "live with his heart" and receive protective care only so long as the actual need exists. Parents and physicians frequently differ on the amount of restriction required by the child in school. For a better program parents must be informed on the needs of a child with rheumatic heart disease, and facilities for the examination and care of these children must be placed within the geographical and financial reach of the parents. Children with cardiac as well as orthopedic disabilities should have adequate medical care, a wholesome understanding of their handicap, and be encouraged to participate in physical activity within the limits of their functional capacity.

In regular school, there will be found certain children who would benefit by, but, for various reasons, have never received remedial care. Some of these are discovered by the physician and nurse, and some by the physical education instructors. In a number of cities, the physical therapist and physical education teachers work together in examining and planning activity programs for crippled children. The physical therapist follows those needing intensive individual work, and the physical education teacher, the others—most of whom are able to participate in a modified program. A majority of the school physical therapists have had physical education background. We believe this is desirable, for the girls seem to fit more easily into school routine and, too, they usually are better prepared for carrying on a recreational program.

Sometimes we are asked why there are special classes for crippled children at elementary level and not at high school level. It has been found that most corrective surgery has been completed by the time the child finishes the elementary grades, and he has then gained self-reliance which will permit him to compete with regular high school pupils even though some adjustment may need to be made in the physical program. The regular high school, with its extensive curriculum, provides more normal educational and social opportunities than could be offered in a special school. If a pupil is too badly handicapped to attend high school, he may continue his education under home instruction.

During his years of schooling, the child is accumulating occupational information. He is learning what people do, first, in relation to the home, then the community, and later to society as a whole. Good educational and vocational counseling will help him to evaluate his abilities and limitations and become interested in those vocations for which he is best suited. When the crippled youth makes more intelligent selections in the field of vocations, there will be fewer employers identifying failure with a physical handicap.

The physical therapist looks at the crippled child. She sees his need for protection and treatment. In looking at the crippled child and his crippled condition, we must always remember his normalities and make his school and life situations as full of normal experiences as possible.

Cerebral Palsy as an Educational Problem

Martin F. Palmer, Sc.D.

The present day growing enthusiasm for the solution of the problems of individuals handicapped by cerebral palsy is gratifying and yet dangerous. It is gratifying because these children have been too long neglected and it is dangerous because clinics are being started here, there, and elsewhere in this country without proper planning and without proper staffing. Inadequately trained personnel, no matter whether it be in medicine, surgery, or in any of the educative and nursing fields, can only militate eventually against this whole movement.

I. As Educational Problem

The presentation contained in this paper is aimed at the essential core of the cerebral palsy problem, which is, after all, an educational as much as a medical matter. All clinics which have accepted the heavy responsibility of dealing with cerebral palsy have been started by some individual trained in one or another specialty. Thus we have a picture of a clinic run primarily from the logopedic point of view, etc. No clinic in this field can be completely successful unless the very highest skills are available in the various specialties which are involved in the solution of this distressing problem. Thus, the best clinic, achieving the best results, will be that clinic which has the most highly skilled physical therapist, the most highly skilled vocational therapist, the most highly skilled logopedist, and, perhaps not least of all, the most highly skilled public school teacher.

In the historical development of the prominent clinics of this country in this field, each of these specialists, in turn, has realized the necessity gradually of bringing into the picture the knowledge available only in other specialties of science. Thus, the pediatrician has had to rely on the physical therapist, on the neurologist, on the logopedist, on the educator for knowledge which cannot be obtained in the one specialty of pediatrics. The logopedist, on the other hand, has had to reply on the other specialties more and more as his clinical development gained momentum. It is safe to say, in these introductory remarks, that no single specialist and no single specialty can possibly know all there is to know about cerebral palsy. In the mind of the pediatrician, cerebral palsy is a medical problem primarily pediatric in nature because it begins in childhood and many of the distressing complications are childhood phenomena which must be taken care of before adulthood is reached. In the eyes of the neurologist many of the distressing phenomena are neurological resulting from injuries to the nervous system of one sort or another which must be taken care of from a neurological point of view and thus cerebral palsy becomes a neurological problem. From the standpoint of the physical therapist, the problem is one of poor coordination of muscles which must be corrected insofar as possible by the application of the most highly skilled physical therapy technics. In the eyes of the logopedist, the problem is primarily one of speech because it is, in effect, a speech disorder as well as a general motor disorder.

Director, Institute of Logopedics, Wichita, Kansas
Reprinted in part from The Spastic Review, Vol. 8, No. 9, September 1947.

Physical Therapy in Schools for Crippled Children

Ruth E. Pratt

An important aspect of physical therapy is its use in schools for crippled children (usually those who have chronic orthopedic disabilities, such as cerebral palsy, poliomyelitis, tuberculosis of bone and joint, birth anomalies, and other long-term disorders). In providing such schools, the communities grant these children the same educational opportunities which their friends enjoy, with the added assistance of treatments. Specific portions of the daily program are set aside for the treatment prescribed by the child's physician, and these treatments are scheduled with the classroom teacher. Because of this training the child is better equipped to fit into his educational and social program.

The physical therapist, working with a staff of educators and nurses, has the privilege of seeing the whole child. He contacts many of the community physicians through conferences and clinics, and his knowledge and training grows because of their varied approaches to the problems. Often he has the responsibility for organizing clinic services and assisting parents in learning of the community facilities available to help their child. Whereas the hospital or private-office physical therapist sees the patient only during treatment period, the school physical therapist has more opportunity to follow the child in his peer groups.

In most large cities the special school is a unit in itself, providing specific treatment as well as guidance in play and vocational activities. Many small communities provide special rooms in regular schools for similar programs.

While some physical therapists are civil service appointees, many have appointments as special teachers, with the same privileges and responsibilities as teachers. These privileges may include continuing contracts, regular increments, sick leave, and retirement benefits. The requirements for appointment are much the same as for teachers, including training in methods of education and psychology and certificates or degrees, depending upon the standards of the school system in question. Besides the basic education, the candidate must have completed a course in physical therapy at an approved school. The administrations of many school systems expect and encourage further study and attendance at conferences, and provide the necessary time for these activities.

It is felt by some that work in the field of chronic ailments is depressing, but this is a misconception. Although there are cases in the school physical therapy program which do not fall in this classification, the larger group is composed of chronic poliomyelitis and cerebral palsy cases. Many of these enter at the kindergarten level and continue throughout high school. There is great satisfaction in having an active part in the physical and social adjustments which are accomplished over a long period. A child may enter school unable to walk, with severe speech involvement, and with anti-social attitudes. Through the combined efforts of the entire staff, and through contacts in his own social group, he is helped to develop his latent abilities so that he may find a satisfactory place in society, rather than be dependent upon the community.

This is a rich and happy field if one enjoys and appreciates children. Opportunities are constantly presenting themselves as the educational systems expand and the handicapped child is encouraged to take his rightful place.

Physical Therapist, Randall Condon School, Cincinnati, O.

Vol. 30, No. 10 THE PHYSICAL THERAPY REVIEW 415

Daily Activity Inventories of Cerebral Palsied Children in Experimental Classes*

Mary Eleanor Brown

Forty-seven children with cerebral palsy in four classes in three public schools were checked on their daily activity status as part of the Cerebral Palsy Program of the New York State Department of Health. The work was done under the direction of Morton L. Levin, M.D., Assistant Commissioner of Health, and his successor, I. Jay Brightman, M.D., and with the assistance of the staff of the Division of Medical Services. The forty-seven inventories are being used as a baseline of activity against which to check progress, and will be taken again at specified times as a continuation of the state's program. The inventories were taken by the

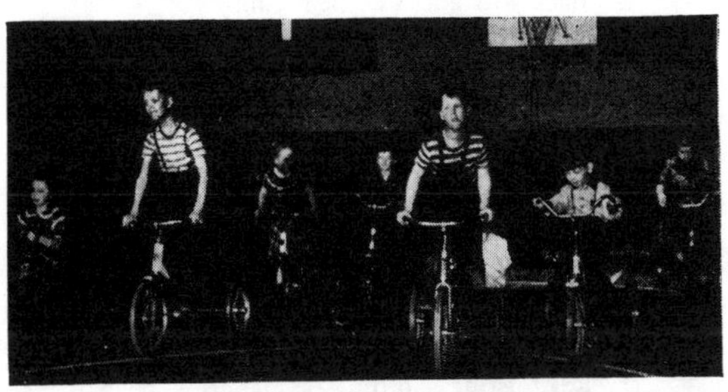

Courtesy Tri-Village Cerebral Palsy Association, New York (Canajoharie, Fort Plain, St. Johnsville).

Figure 1. The children in the Special Class for Cerebral Palsied at the Fifth Ward Public School, Amsterdam, New York, are fortunate in having their classroom next to the regular school gymnasium where they spend many of their recreational and therapy periods as well as mingle and play with the other school children.

Director, Cerebral Palsy and Rehabilitation Services, Eastern New York Orthopedic Hospital-School, Inc., Schenectady, New York.

*Read at the 27th Annual Conference of the American Physical Therapy Association, Cleveland, June 1950.

author who was loaned by the Eastern New York Orthopedic Hospital-School, Inc., Schenectady, to the Department of Health as Physical Therapy Consultant in Cerebral Palsy.

The three schools were the Day School for Crippled Children in Buffalo, the Pleasant Valley School in Schenectady, and the Fifth Ward School in Amsterdam. The inventories were taken between December 8, 1949, and March 28, 1950. The ages of the children were from five years and two months to sixteen years and four months. Twenty-seven of the children were boys, and twenty, girls. The records are in graphic form, convenient for purposes of study and comparison, and bring out points which may be of value in improving cerebral palsy facilities.

Record Forms and Procedure

The record forms and procedure were prepared by this author. The Daily Activity Inventory and Progress Record for Those with Atypical Movement is designed to check disabled persons, who have movement difficulties, on their ability to perform one hundred activities of daily life. It is for use by workers who undertake daily activity teaching of those with atypical movement, that is, persons who have or have had congenital defects, disease or trauma affecting the bones, ligaments, joints, muscles, nerves, or blood vessels, which produce disabilities influencing movement by muscular weakness, limitation, and/or disturbed coordination. The inventory's one hundred activities are arranged in twelve groups with time allowances for their performance. They are listed below:

Daily Activities

I. Speech
1. Speech

II. Bed
2. Back to right side, bed-lying
3. Right side to abdomen, bed-lying
4. Abdomen to right side, bed-lying
5. Right side to back, bed-lying
6. Back to left side, bed-lying
7. Left side to abdomen, bed-lying
8. Abdomen to left side, bed-lying
9. Left side to back, bed-lying
10. Edge to edge, bed
11. Lying to sitting, bed
12. Sitting to lying (not falling), bed
13. Urinal, bed (motions)
14. Adjusting clothing as if for bedpan use
15. Readjusting clothing as if after bedpan use
16. On bedpan
17. Off bedpan
18. Cleansing after bedpan activities (motions)

III. Bathing and Grooming
19. Combing hair (motions)
20. Brushing teeth (motions)
21. Washing body (motions)
22. Shaving or applying cosmetics (motions)

IV. Dressing and Undressing
23. Dressing, except for fastening shoes or tying shoestrings and putting on and adjusting necktie
24. Fastening shoes or tying shoestrings
25. Putting on and adjusting necktie
26. Undressing

V. Eating
27. Cutting meat-substitute
28. Spoon to mouth with food-substitute
29. Fork to mouth with food-substitute
30. Drinking from cup with handle
31. Drinking from glass

VI. Desk
32. Writing or printing
33. Opening envelope, removing, unfolding paper
34. Folding new paper, placing in new envelope, sealing envelope
35. Drawing straight line with pencil, using ruler
36. Cutting along line with scissors
37. Telephone

VII. Wheelchair
38. Bed to wheelchair
39. Wheelchair to bed
40. Forward 30 ft.
41. Backward 10 ft.
42. Revolution to right
43. Revolution to left
44. Pushing door open, clearing doorsill, closing door
45. Pulling door open, clearing doorsill, closing door
46. Up ramp
47. Down ramp
48. Wheelchair to chair
49. Chair to wheelchair
50. Wheelchair (chair or stool) to toilet
51. Toilet to wheelchair (chair or stool)
52. Adjusting clothing as if for bowel evacuation
53. Readjusting clothing as if after bowel evacuation
54. Cleansing after bowel evacuation (motions)
55. Wheelchair to automobile
56. Automobile to wheelchair
57. Wheelchair to floor
58. Floor to wheelchair
59. On floor 30 ft., lying, sitting, or crawling

VIII. Bathtub
60. Into bathtub
61. Out of bathtub

IX. Appliance
62. Putting on appliances
63. Removing appliances
64. Locking appliances
65. Unlocking appliances

X. Locomotion, Upright
66. Forward 30 ft.
67. Backward 10 ft.
68. Sideward to right 10 ft.
69. Sideward to left 10 ft.
70. Pushing door open, clearing doorsill, closing door
71. Pulling door open, clearing doorsill, closing door
72. Up ramp
73. Down ramp
74. Up 3 steps, right handrail

75. Down 3 steps, right handrail
76. Up 3 steps, left handrail
77. Down 3 steps, left handrail
78. Up 3 steps, no handrail
79. Down 3 steps, no handrail
80. Up curb
81. Down curb
82. Into bus
83. Out of bus

XI. STANDING-TO-SITTING AND SITTING-TO-STANDING

84. Standing to bed
85. Bed to standing
86. Standing to wheelchair
87. Wheelchair to standing
88. Standing to chair
89. Chair to standing
90. Standing to toilet
91. Toilet to standing
92. Adjusting clothing as if for bowel evacuation
93. Readjusting clothing as if after bowel evacuation
94. Cleansing after bowel evacuation (motions)
95. Standing to automobile
96. Automobile to standing
97. Standing to floor
98. Floor to standing

XII. TRAVELING, UPRIGHT

99. Crossing dummy street on green light
100. Public vehicles

The aim of the daily activity inventory is to gauge the extent to which a disabled person is independent, with regard to his daily personal needs of locomotion, self-care, and the use of the hands. Daily work inventories are needed to gauge ability in job activities. Since every human being is a prospective vocational problem, it is appropriate to give him an independence index, no matter what his age or the cause of his condition may be. Such a record may follow him through his medical and educational period and serve as an inventory, progress record, and guide to those who help him to find a place for himself in his own home, industry, business, or the professions.

Each daily activity is analyzed under the following headings: Explanation to Examiner, Starting Position, Instructions to Subject, Need, Satisfactory Performance, Equipment. The daily activity inventory, with its instructions for use, has been prepared for flexible use by groups and individuals. Equipment is specified as "standard," and the exact measurements are not given. There is great variation among standard pieces of furniture and equipment. In order to use this inventory for comparative purposes, it would have been ideal to have checked all the children with identical supplies, equipment, furniture, vehicles, and under identical conditions. This not being possible, it was attempted to make the checking conditions as similar as possible. Measurements were made of all equipment used, in order to sort out the comparable items. Furthermore, the inventory is not a scientifically standardized test at the present time, although such a possibility is undergoing consideration as a research project. Some items are objective, some are not. The number of items, both objective in character and for which the equipment was essentially similar, were thirty-five. They are Nos. 2-12, 16-17, 32-37, 60-61, 84-85, 88-91, 97-98. However, since one checker took all the inventories, there is a greater chance for the nonobjective items to approach significance. In any case, gross conclusions of a practical nature can be drawn.

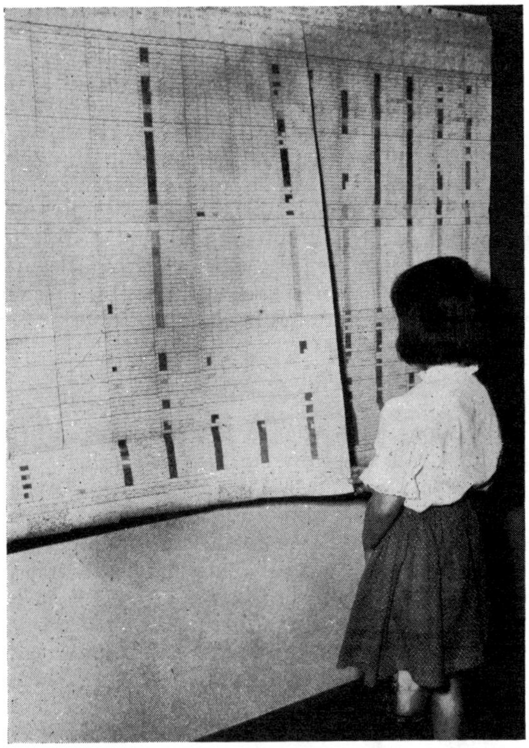

Courtesy Eastern New York Orthopedic Hospital-School, Inc., Schenectady, New York.

Figure 2. These daily activity inventories are those of the children in the Special Class for Cerebral Palsied at the Pleasant Valley Public School, Schenectady, New York. The overlapping feature of the eleven-inch wide record forms focuses attention upon the individual graphs at the righthand side of each. Thus space is saved, and yet each record has its own classification, key and list of activities, is a complete unit by itself, and as such may be examined, filed, or transmitted at any time.

EXPENDITURE OF TIME

The number of hours spent taking the inventories was approximately seventy; the average length of time spent per child was one hour and a half. It is likely that such a period of time can be incorporated in the routine of handling cerebral palsied children, and it is recommended that centers consider organizing to allow for such inventory-checking.

It required a total of nineteen working days for preparation and eighteen for taking the inventories. The preparation involved, mainly: (1) choosing and collecting the supplies, equipment, furniture, and vehicles; (2) describing to carpenters the pieces of equipment which needed to be constructed; and (3) arranging space and setting up supplies, equipment, furniture, and vehicles for each item, including provision for the use of automobiles, buses, bathtubs, and suitable toilets when not on the premises.

EQUIPMENT

The long preparation period is significant. The daily activity inventory aims to show achievement of everyday acts, involving commonly-found supplies, equipment, furniture, and vehicles, yet the classes were neither set up for daily activities, nor were they readily adaptable to a daily activity program. A few outstanding missing items, of an ordinary, standard character, which required time to locate and acquire, were: beds, bathtubs, bedpans, steps, cups and saucers, glasses, scissors, wheelchairs, doors with doorsills, space for distance-walking (thirty feet for locomotion forward and sixty feet for street-crossing), autos, and buses. Two eight-inch wooden platforms to serve as curbs, and one wooden ramp to be attached to one platform are the only special pieces needed.

SCORES

The scores are the number of activities satisfactorily performed. They range from 0 to 90. Eleven scores are 15½ and below. Nine are below 10. There are three scores of 3 and two of 0. There are fourteen below 50. These are very severely disabled children requiring custodial care all day and all night. The thought occurs that, even if educable, perhaps they should not be in public school classes on the basis of their severe physical disability, alone. If they are kept in school, or wherever they may go, they need floor space for exploration of the floor and learning to move from place to place on it, with and without the use of overhead pulley devices, parachute and other walkers, creepers, and the like. Sufficient floor space with suitable floor covering is almost always lacking.

DISCUSSION OF GROUPS OF ACTIVITIES

The following figures suggest comments which are given:

Fifteen satisfied the speech item. This is a very grossly and crudely checked item. These fifteen were understood but do not necessarily lack speech defects. The other thirty-two were not understood or had no speech. Speech training is obviously greatly needed.

Seven performed all seventeen bed activities; ten, less than one-half; two, none; fifteen did not get from edge to edge of the bed. With forty unable to perform all the bed activities, the need for a bed for checking and teaching these activities becomes evident. With fifteen unable to satisfy the conditions for getting from edge to edge of the bed, the conclusion is that someone in the households of these children is moving them on the bed the first thing every morning, and possibly at other times during the day and night, too.

Twenty-five performed no bathing and grooming activities; twenty-one did not get in and out of the bathtub. A bathroom of ordinary proportions, containing standard fixtures, connected and functioning, should be the center of activities in a cerebral palsy facility of any kind. If it is possible to have various sizes of fixtures, this is all the better for teaching purposes, but it is most important of all to have the ones usually found in ordinary homes. There is no better exercise than washing hands and face, taking care of toilet needs, using faucets and plugs, getting into a bathtub, handling soap, sponges, brushes, water, washcloths, and towels, and getting out of a bathtub safely. The cerebral palsied need to learn hygienic habits young. They must be all the more immaculate to help to offset their motion difficulties. It is desirable to check these activities at first hand, and teach them early, and with concentration, rather than to rely on the motions used, as has been necessary in the case of some of the inventory items.

Thirty performed no dressing and undressing; fourteen, undressing, but not dressing; none accomplished all dressing and undressing (the necktie item was disregarded in this statement); nineteen in the upright position did not readjust clothing after toilet activities. Dressing and undressing have been outstandingly difficult. These activities require considerable coordination. A very great difficulty, however, is the unsatisfactory clothing—fastenings which do not fasten; shoestrings that are too short and often untipped, tearing at the least force; overalls and suspenders that are too tight and do not hook or stay hooked; buttons on trousers which are so small as to defy buttoning, or which have buttonholes which do not permit the entrance of the buttons; long underwear, buttoning in the back with tiny ineffectual buttons; dresses with minute buttons at the top of a tight neckband; slip-over sweaters, often too small, in layers. . . . Inability to adjust and re-adjust clothing before and after toilet activities reinforces further the need for more care with children's clothes, as well as a better selection. The minutes per day spent on such activities by parents and therapists add up to hours that might be turned to better account for all concerned.

Why not capes, instead of layers of tight turtle-neck sweaters? Why not sturdy, diaper-like pants with snaps, instead of flimsy ones which get torn being pulled off and on over braces? Why not wrap-around skirts, or culottes, instead of tight overalls or slacks? Why not ski pants that zip up the sides? Why not dresses and blouses with zippers or large buttons and buttonholes in the front, rather than unreachable ties and microscopic buttons in the back? Why not narrow bands with buckles on braces, instead of wide bands with laces? And why not shorter hair on those who cannot manage their own, instead of long curls which get tangled up in the sweaters, bibs, slings and back braces?

Ten wear braces which contain a total of twenty-five slip locks (ten hip, fifteen knee); only one child managed his locks; none did all the brace activities; one removed his braces; four wear long, double, lower-extremity braces with pelvic band and back brace attached and cannot put them on or take them off, cannot lock or unlock them. The four children are among the low-scoring (3, 10, 3, 3) discussed earlier. These are essentially helpless children, and an investigation would indicate many minutes per day being spent in putting on and taking off braces which it may not ever be possible for them to manage independently. The question becomes, should these children not be taught to use some variation of a wheelchair or walker or even learn to creep as means of locomotion? It should also be noted that the braces themselves are sometimes too small, have locks which do not work, or function with great difficulty, and present problems in the bathroom because underwear is worn underneath.

Nine performed no eating activities; none did all. The motions of eating are often not sufficient in the case of cerebral palsied for checking or teaching. This is another group of activities needing more detailed analysis and concentrated teaching, with the coordination of all therapies.

Twenty-seven did not accomplish any of the desk activities; none did all; eleven performed the telephone item (which requires knowledge of numbers for dialing); two drew straight lines. The desk activity results reveal a need for increasing acquaintance with these skills. The use of paper, envelopes, pencils, rulers, scissors, telephones, writing, and printing is essential and basic to many vocations and should be learned early, through schoolwork, occupational therapy, and recreation. Paper-folding books, valentines, Christmas tree ornaments, and puppet-making are a few of the many possible activities. Trades have proved impossible to learn and jobs have been lost by disabled adults who were not exposed to such activities when young.

Six sat in wheelchairs, but did not use them; only one used a wheelchair, and he to the extent of performing half of the twenty-two activities; four do not sit in wheelchairs, but require special chairs; thirty-six are in the upright position not needing wheelchairs. Wheelchair manipulation requires skill, and is, too, an excellent exercise for strength and coordination. Here is evidence that such exercise is not being taught sufficiently. It is advisable that wheelchair technics be taught by graduated activities, early, when this mode of locomotion can improve independence. It is interesting to note that, whereas thirty-six children are independent of wheelchairs, dressing, undressing, eating, and desk activities are not accomplished. This reinforces the too-little-emphasized idea that teaching a child to "walk" is not the sole aim.

Thirteen of the thirty-six in the upright position did not satisfy the items of moving forward and backward; twenty-three did not do all the step, curb, and bus activities; twelve did not cross the dummy street. These figures show the following needs, mentioned before: space is required for distance-walking; steps, curbs, and bus practice are indicated. A valuable recommendation for groups laying plans for rehabilitation centers is to urge that standard, daily-activity supplies, equipment, furniture, and vehicles be included in their building, equipment, and organization plans, so as to give the disabled sufficient acquaintance and practice with materials they will find elsewhere and thus facilitate their absorption into normal life. It has been found unwise to build facilities for crippled children with an over-abundance of special features to the exclusion of standard and usual conditions. Attention is called to the lack of the usual staircases in some centers and the over-use of ramps. Inability to climb stairs has stood in the way of many a disabled person's getting and holding a job. A similar comment may be made with regard to school buses. The children who can be taught to climb in satisfactorily should not only be taught, but should be allowed to do so daily. In one school, where school buses were plentiful, no child was seen to enter a bus by its front door. Rather, they all entered the rear ends of the buses, which were backed up to specially-built platforms. It is possible that therapists could arrange with the school staff to alleviate this condition, to the advantage of all the children, without decreasing the efficiency of the school's program. In many centers the children are carried in and out of autos and buses. Everyday equipment of many varieties is needed in all facilities handling people with conditions impairing movement. This is particularly true in the case of the cerebral palsied. Even though some of these items are not customarily found in schools, they need to be acquired, retained, and used for cerebral palsied, as well as for other children with motion handicaps.

USE OF THE DAILY ACTIVITY INVENTORIES

The daily activity inventory is a guide to teaching. A physical therapist may wish to re-check the inventory if she has not been the one to take it originally. Then, from among the activities which were not performed, a selection of those most needed by the subject, after a survey of home, school, and working conditions has been made, is marked for teaching. In studying further the daily activity needs of the subject, some not appearing on the basic list may prove to be more valuable to the subject. In the case of the cerebral palsied, a few of these would be: blowing noses, cleaning teeth with tongue, learning not to drool, cutting finger and toe nails, learning to wash and care for hair, and others relating to personal hygiene and good grooming. Detailed supplementary check-lists, to cover eating, speech, and any others appearing only grossly on the inventory, are suggested. The inventory can serve to indicate when further examination into details of a particular group of skills is necessary. Each activity should be broken down into its elemental components and taught by means of graduated equipment. Once the methods are selected and perfected, then the activity should be practiced over and over again for speed and endurance. The questions to ask oneself are: Which of the activities on the daily activity inventory are accomplished? Are there any not on the list which should be checked? Are the activities done every day by the subject? Is there sufficient endurance? Is there enough speed? Can variations of the activities be done? Are they done customarily? Do all people handling the subjects have access to and use the above information?

CONCLUSIONS

Thus, the inventory results show that the daily activity phase of the cerebral palsied child's needs is not being adequately covered.

The Crowded School Day

Many speeches and articles begin: "Cerebral palsied children are, first, children. They need everything the normal child needs, but more of it." To this should be added, "and often many special services, physical, occupational, and speech therapy, hearing and vision correction and instruction, special surgery, etc." The school week is five days, the school hours are nine to three with an hour and a half to two hours, and even more, for lunch and rest. How can a child receive all that the normal child is exposed to, and more of it, as well as the specialized therapies and other services he may need, within these hours? It is a common complaint of the school teacher that she barely gets started with a child when he is whisked away for nursing care, physical therapy, speech therapy, or occupational therapy. Then there are library hours, field trips, movies, parties, holiday celebrations. These are very valuable to the cerebral palsied child, but how is everything to be fitted in? A solution might be to stagger the therapy and school days by having the therapists functioning earlier and later and some children come earlier and others stay later. A therapy week of Tuesday through Saturday would allow Monday free for school work exclusively, but transportation difficulties would often interfere with a Saturday program.

More Exercise Needed

It was noticed anew that the cerebral palsied children are often not given vigorous exercise, are treated relatively gently, are given considerable light, formal exercise, often of a passive nature, on a table, and are scheduled for extensive rest periods. One physical therapist was heard to say, "I see the importance of daily activities, but how I do love my table work!" The children as a whole need more exercise of the vigorous, resistive kind, more daily activity work on many kinds of everyday equipment, group exercises, and games of a type to build strength, skill, and endurance in whatever motor powers they may have, and, especially, more floor exercise, involving moving from place to place by varying methods, and playing active games. Pulley and other exercises for improving joint range and strength should be worked out along recreational lines for center and home use. Lack of physical activity is very evident.

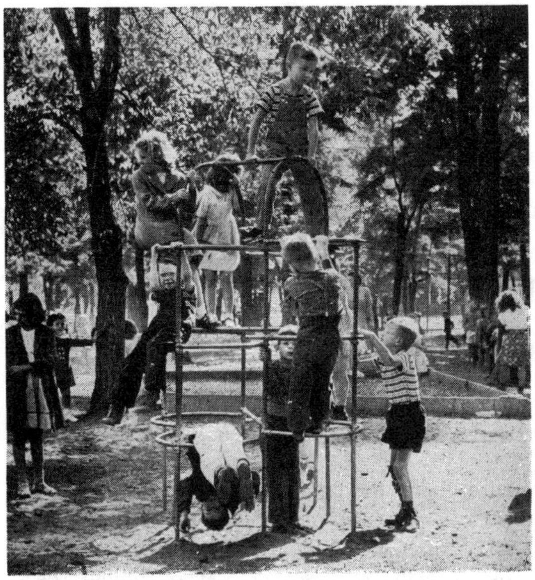

Courtesy Schenectady Gazette.

Figure 3. Cerebral palsied children play with the other children on the playground, attend school assemblies and movies with the other children, have fire drills at the same time as the other children, at Pleasant Valley Public School, Schenectady, New York.

Attitudes

Cerebral palsied children are not sick from cerebral palsy. What they are sick from, often, is the constant reference to them as any or all of the following: "weakly," "tired," "fearful of falling," "nervous," "shy," "hating doctors," "lacking in concentration," "afraid of being alone," "frightened of new places and people," and "needing rest." It is advisable to keep reiterating that overprotective attitudes on the part of therapists and parents prevent the child from developing initiative, concentration, strength, and endurance. Over-praise of activities which should be taken for granted gives him the wrong perspective of himself. Positive suggestions, plenty of forceful exercise in the center and at home, and expecting a lot from the child, yield results in vim, vigor, and accomplishment. Often the cerebral palsied person does not know what work means because he never really tried it.

Screening

It is possible that the daily activity inventory may serve as a supportive screening device for admission and discharge. It might be worked out on a score basis. That is, those with scores of less than thirty-five or forty should not be admitted, but, rather, given some outpatient and home therapy until the designated score is reached; those who do not progress ten points within a certain period should step out of school, either temporarily or permanently. Such decisions, of course, should be made in staff conferences with the benefit and agreement of all specialists. Perhaps a composite score could be evolved to aid in solving the difficult problems of admission and discharge.

Further Studies

A study is now in process at the Pleasant Valley Public School's Classes for Cerebral Palsied Children, the medical services for which are provided by the above Hospital-School. The study is in the form of a daily time schedule kept by each staff member, containing twenty-five activities, including time spent with children in bathroom, giving nourishment and medication, undressing and dressing, taking braces off and putting them on, teaching, testing and therapy, minor repairs to shoes and braces, records, meetings, home visits, telephone, transportation from room to room, taking off outside clothes and putting them on in the morning, for playground at lunchtime, and to go home, lunch and rest, visits of physicians, publicity, and visitors. It is believed that the results may spotlight items for further study toward a better regulation of the crowded days of cerebral palsied school children.

BIBLIOGRAPHY

1. Report of the New York State Joint Legislative Committee to Study the Problem of Cerebral Palsy. Legislative Document (1949) No. 55.
2. Levin, Morton L., M.D., Brightman, I. Jay, M.D., and Burtt, Edith J.: The Problem of Cerebral Palsy. New York State Journal of Medicine, Volume 49, No. 23, December 1, 1949.
3. Brown, Mary Eleanor: "Daily Activity Inventory and Progress Record for Those with Atypical Movement." Published serially in American Journal of Occupational Therapy, beginning Vol. IV, No. 5, September-October 1950. Daily Activity Record Blanks are supplied by Eastern New York Orthopedic Hospital-School, Inc., 124 Rosa Road, Schenectady 8, New York.

clinical reports

Integrating Physical Therapy into a Cerebral Palsy Early Education Program

MARION MARX, M.A.

Just as early infant movement comes as the natural response to frequent physical handling by the mother and to multisensory stimulation, so the young child uses his body most vigorously in play with other children and in response to toys and activities that he enjoys. This is true for handicapped as well as for normal children; therefore, therapy takes place more naturally in the schoolroom or playground, rather than in a separate therapy room.

Based on this premise, a program has been started at United Cerebral Palsy of Manhattan that integrates therapy and early education. The program is geared toward three- to six-year-old children, most of them having a diagnosis of cerebral palsy in all degrees of severity. The children are grouped according to age and intelligence, with eight children and two teachers in each class. The program includes the services of a psychiatrist, psychologist, social worker, physical therapist, occupational therapist, and speech therapist. Except for the purposes of evaluation, all of the ancillary staff try to provide services to the children within the context of the classroom, either by direct participation in classroom (or playroom) activities, or by instruction to the teachers. Parent instruction and conferences take place frequently and involve any or all of the staff members. For the purpose of this article, the role of physical therapy in this integrated program will be described, even though the other disciplines play an equally active part.

POSITIONING CHILDREN AND STIMULATING MOVEMENT

The physical therapist helps the teacher in positioning the children, either in chairs or on the floor, depending on where an activity is taking place. When children move from one spot to another in the classroom, the physical therapist advises the teacher on how she can assist the children if they cannot move independently, or how she can carry or position them if they are totally dependent.[1] Keeping in mind the developmental motor sequence[2] as well as the need for proper postural alignment, the physical therapist can recommend more advanced movement patterns and demonstrate how the teacher can encourage these in her children. This may run the gamut from stimulating emerging righting reflexes as a child wants to rise from the floor, to adjusting a child's standing alignment at the sand or water table, to teaching tricycle riding and advanced climbing activities.

With the severely physically involved children, we have found the use of neurodevelopmental treatment methods most effective, and have used them as fully as staff knowledge has permitted.[3,4]

Mrs. Marx is a physical therapist and Assistant Director, Early Education Program, United Cerebral Palsy of New York City, 339 E. 44th Street, New York, NY 10017.

In our program, we have found that a large playroom can be used satisfactorily as the main arena where teacher and therapist can work together on the children's gross motor development. In the smaller classrooms, one must keep in mind that no young child should remain in one position for more than fifteen to twenty minutes, and, in this situation, the physical therapist helps the teacher place the children in alternate positions.

The physical therapist also advises the teacher on the use of braces and crutches for those children who come to school with them, on how and when to lock and unlock braces, and on techniques of putting them on and taking them off. Medical instructions from doctors at the children's hospital affiliations are followed whenever given.

SELF-CARE

The instruction in self-care skills also falls naturally into the school setting and represents another area of teacher-therapist cooperation. These skills involve the taking off and putting on of outer clothing, as well as braces, shoes, and socks which are frequently removed during playroom time. They include toileting and the related necessary adjusting of clothes.

Independent eating and drinking during snack and lunch time is another goal of the school program. Teachers and the therapy staff (occupational therapy, physical therapy, and speech therapy) work together to place children in the optimal position for self-feeding. They stabilize plates and cups (with tape) whenever necessary or provide children with special adaptive eating devices. The social worker advises parents to send the types of food that permit optimal eating independence as well as good nutrition. This makes the preparation of "school food" a learning experience for parents. Most popular are finger foods, such as frankfurters, cheese, or sandwiches with adherent fillings, and sticky spoon foods, such as cottage cheese, apple sauce, or puddings.

PERCEPTUAL TRAINING

An important part of early education for brain-damaged children is the use of gross motor activities for perceptual training.[5,6] Our teachers and therapists jointly plan activities that will enhance learning in perceptual areas.

Figure-ground perception is reinforced by games that involve stepping on rubber flagstones; crawling between two ropes, or straddling one rope; or hide and seek, using people or objects to hide.

Body awareness is reinforced, for example, by follow-the-leader games that involve touching body parts, by wrapping body parts with colored wool, by imitation of movement activities, by numerous mirror games, and by using a box with different-sized holes to insert body parts of appropriate size.

Position in space (such as the concepts of up, down, over, under, in front of, in back of, in, out, through) can be reinforced by the use of obstacle courses, by play on slides and seesaws, and by games that utilize boxes, tunnels, inflatables, and large balls and rolls.

Motor planning skills can be taught logically in a playroom setting when children have to move certain objects out of the way to get to a desired toy. Sometimes objects need to be placed together to provide the setting for dramatic play, such as a train, bridge, boat, and dock. When children ride tricycles, rules of the road have to be established, all of which involve motor planning by the children. All games with balls and bean bags are excellent ways of training in perceptual skills. Perceptual skills developed in gross motor activities are later carried on in increasingly finer activities in the classroom.

Most of the above mentioned activities (and others) are carried out with small or large groups of children. The same activity does not provide the same learning experience for each child. For example, a game of "imitate my movements" may improve one child's successful hand grasp on the plastic pointer that is being used to touch body parts; it may increase another child's awareness of the parts of his body; it may stimulate language in another child; and it may provide a fourth child with his first social experience of being a group leader. For all the children, the group stimulation reinforces learning, and the joint teacher-therapist activity planning widens the learning horizon. In making activity analyses (such as the one just described), the staff focuses on developing activities appropriate for and consistent with the objectives established for each child at staff conferences.

Acknowledgment. The program described in this article was developed under the leadership of Berta Rafael, Director, Early Education and Day Care, United Cerebral Palsy of New York City, Inc.

REFERENCES

1. Finnie N: Handling the Young Cerebral Palsied Child at Home. New York, E. P. Dutton & Co., 1970
2. Frankenburg WK, Dodds JB: The Denver developmental screening test. J Pediatr 71:181–191, 1967
3. Bobath B: The very early treatment of cerebral palsy. Dev Med Child Neurol 9:4:373–390, 1967
4. Bobath B: Motor development, its effect on general development, and applications to the treatment of cerebral palsy. Physiotherapy 57:526–532, 1971
5. Kephardt N: The Slow Learner in the Classroom. Columbus, OH, Merrill, 1960
6. Getman GN: How to Develop your Child's Intelligence. Wayne, PA, Research Publications, 1962

Severely Handicapped Children in the Public Schools

A New Frontier for the Physical Therapist

BARBARA H. CONNOLLY, MEd,
and ROBERT M. ANDERSON, EdD

Recent court decisions are currently generating the need for the development of a more humane, school-based system of educational options for severely and profoundly handicapped children. This natural commitment, which includes provisions for various ancillary services, has major implications for the profession of physical therapy. This paper includes the problems, issues, and trends related to the development of public school physical therapy programs and presents some guidelines and suggestions which might be helpful in the implementation of such programs.

Right-to-education laws are being passed in virtually every state of the Union. These laws mandate public school services for all handicapped children regardless of their level of mental functioning or physical disability. Although such laws vary with respect to specific provisions, they all share a common major focus on the development of programs for severely and profoundly handicapped children. The right-to-education laws were generated by a series of court decisions, two of which are generally considered to be landmark cases. The first suit, filed by the Pennsylvania Association for Retarded Children (1973), resulted in the decision that all mentally retarded children should receive free public education.[1] The second suit, Mills vs. Board of Education of the District of Columbia (1972), was even more significant inasmuch as it expanded the implications of the Pennsylvania case to *all* handicapped children, not just those labeled mentally retarded.[2]

The fact that the new legislation now includes provisions for physically and multiply handicapped children obviously has major implications for the utilization of physical therapists in public school systems.

For example, in Tennessee, the Policies Governing the Development of Programs and Services for the Handicapped (1974) states that "Physical and/or occupational therapy shall be provided for handicapped students whose physical impairments require appropriate therapeutic attention if the students are to receive full benefit from the instructional program provided them."[3] Unfortunately, many school systems in the state did not have a physical therapist at the time this law was passed. In addition, the few physical therapists who were already employed were not adequately prepared to handle the severely and profoundly retarded children who began attending the public schools following transferral from the state institutions. Many states have experienced or are experiencing the same difficulties as Tennessee in complying with their educational laws. This paper will focus on some of the major trends, issues, and problems associated with the development of physical therapy programs designed to meet the needs of the severely and profoundly handicapped now being included in the public schools. Some tentative guidelines and suggestions that might be helpful in program development are included.

DEFINITION OF SEVERE AND PROFOUND RETARDATION

The American Association on Mental Deficiency (AAMD) has published six manuals on terminology and classifications of retardation. The latest manual published by Grossman in 1973 defines mental retardation as "significant subaverage general intellectual functioning existing concurrently with deficits in adaptive behavior and manifested during the developmental period."[4] The level of retardation is determined by comparing the developmental age of the child with his chronological age. If the developmental age is the same as the chronological age, the

Ms. Connolly is Chief of Physical Therapy, Child Development Center, University of Tennessee, 711 Jefferson Ave, Memphis, TN 38105.

Dr. Anderson is Professor in the Department of Special Education and Rehabilitation, College of Education, Memphis State University, Memphis, TN 38152.

child is said to have an intelligence quotient (IQ) of 100 which is termed average. In severe mental retardation, the child would have an IQ somewhere in the range of from 20 to 35 and in profound retardation the IQ would be 19 or below. These scores denoting the level of retardation are based on the Stanford-Binet and the Cattell Intelligence Scales.[4] In looking at scores from intelligence tests, the viewer should realize that the test is interpreting the child's level of functioning only at the time the test was administered. Only with further testing can a prognosis for future functioning be determined. Of importance also is what treatment and programs are provided for the child after he has been identified as retarded.

Adaptive levels of behavior can be used in predicting motor behavior in the severely and profoundly retarded. Heber states that the severely retarded child from birth to 5 years of age will have poor motor development and the profoundly retarded child may have minimal capacity for sensorimotor functioning.[5] From age 6 to 21 years, the severely retarded child will probably learn to walk but continue to develop very slowly. The profoundly retarded child from age 2 to 21 years may never learn to walk but some motor development will occur.

THE CHANGING ROLE OF THE PHYSICAL THERAPIST

With the passage of the new legislation concerning education of the severely handicapped child, physical therapists in the public school are being faced with the treatment of many children who previously would have been institutionalized. In the past, the majority of the children treated by therapists in the public schools have functioned at the levels of normal intelligence or mild to moderate retardation. Various articles have been published regarding programs for children functioning at these levels.[6–8] Physical therapists have also participated in screening programs as described by Cronis[9] but very little has been written about their role with the severely handicapped in the schools.

In 1966, Ethun wrote that most severely and profoundly retarded persons with associated physical handicaps resided in state or private institutions.[10] At that time, Ethun found that of 468 residential facilities for the mentally retarded, only 50 actually employed registered physical therapists. A need for qualified physical therapists in these institutions was clearly evident but was not being met. This need for qualified therapists has been further dramatized by the inception of the philosophy of normalization and the subsequent deinstitutionalization of handicapped children. Whereas one physical therapist would typically work with a large number of children in an institutional setting, more physical therapists will be needed as these currently institutionalized children are dispersed to a number of public schools.

DeHaven, in 1974, questioned the assumptions set forth by the provisions for physical therapy services in special education legislation.[11] The primary assumption questioned was that all physical therapists have an extensive background of academic training and professional experience in working with severely handicapped children. Another assumption that caused concern was the knowledge of most therapists about the educational model and how easily they can adapt to this model. Probably the least accurate of the assumptions set forth in the provisions for services is that unlimited numbers of physical therapists are prepared to work with severely handicapped children in the schools.

In dealing with severely handicapped children in the public schools, physical therapists must be aware of limitations in their ability to provide optimal treatment for the total child unless adequate ancillary services are available. Many therapists are finding the interdisciplinary approach to be a major asset. Delays in all areas of development of severely handicapped children necessitates the utilization of the skills of other professionals such as occupational therapists, speech therapists, and educators. One must be aware of treatment provided by other disciplines so that he can reinforce target behaviors in physical therapy. For example, if certain words or sounds are being stressed in speech therapy, these words should be used during physical therapy. Likewise, if a behavior modification program is being used to decrease or increase selected target behaviors in a child, there should be consistency in using the same reinforcers for those behaviors in physical therapy.

The physical therapist must learn to rely upon the skills of the classroom teacher in the total management of the child. In many cases, severely handicapped children are not seen daily in therapy, and teachers must become responsible for daily activities for the children. At the same time the teacher must be taught special positioning of the child, simple stimulation techniques, and methods of promoting the child's independence in activities of daily living. If teachers are not aware of the activities that are being used in therapy, they may unknowingly be reinforcing behaviors and postures that are inconsistent with the physical therapy program. Lectures and workshops for the classroom teachers and teachers aides are necessary if the physical therapy program is to be successful.

The physical therapist in the school must also be willing to act as a consultant for children who are no longer in need of active treatment in physical therapy. The physical therapist is often requested to work with the physical education teacher in providing developmental play activities for retarded children. In these cases, even though the children are not in need of specialized treatment, therapists must be willing to suggest activities or references that would be beneficial in physical education programs.

Physical therapists in the school program must also realize that the parents of the child are important members of the treatment team. Programs conducted only in the school environment are generally not as effective as those programs which extend beyond the school. The parents, like the teachers, must learn how to handle the child and understand the goals of treatment. One must be able to make a judgment concerning the extent of the abilities of the parents who will be asked to carry out an exercise program at home. Problems must be recognized that the parents and the family of the child are experiencing that would limit or deter their being involved in programming. If possible, the family should be referred to proper agencies to help alleviate these problems. In many instances, physical therapists have more contact with the family than other professionals and become the family's liaison with the school. To fully understand the families of the retarded and their relationships with the retarded child, physical therapists should become familiar with research done with families of retarded children. Odle and co-workers have provided an overview of research conducted with families of retarded persons and a summary of needs of these families.[12] In addition, several books which focus on working with families of the retarded are now available to physical therapists.[13–15]

TECHNIQUES

Physical therapists employed to work with the severely and profoundly handicapped in a school system are often faced with a child who is noncooperative, nonverbal, and inactive. Techniques used previously with adult patients or mildly retarded children will rarely work. Frequently the child being seen is functioning at a developmental level far below that of walking or crawling. Many therapists who work with children at this level for the first time are frustrated before even starting their exercise regimens.

A systematic program to evaluate the child fully should be implemented before any treatment is started. The Bayley Scales are frequently used to evaluate the level of a child's development[16]; however, the Bayley Scales are not organized into as discrete sequential levels as the Gesell Scales and may not be as useful when used for children with very delayed development.[17] Each child should also be evaluated in terms of his postural reflex development. Fiorentino and Bobath have described in detail the testing of these reflexes.[18, 19] Good results from treatment may not be achieved if an exercise program is initiated with a child without consideration of the presence of abnormal postural reflexes (ie, an asymmetrical tonic labyrinthine reflex or Moro's reflex). In 1973, Hoskins and Squires developed an evaluation form that encompassed developmental levels as well as reflex development.[20] This form may be used without difficulty in the classroom for rapid testing of children.

Traditional range-of-motion, muscle tone, and muscle strength evaluations may be included in the full evaluation of some children. Muscle testing on uncooperative or very young children presents a major problem. How can one determine if the child can use a muscle against gravity or with resistance if the child does not understand directions? One method used is to place the child in positions that elicit normal postural reflexes and then note the muscular responses. Another method is to observe the child's use of muscles during play or gross motor activities. Evaluation of body alignment is also important in the evaluation. Physical therapists often may be the first to notice problems such as scoliosis, hip subluxation or dislocation, and leg length discrepancies which need to be evaluated further. In addition, body alignment problems must be evaluated in order for therapists to recommend specialized seating for the child if necessary.

Specific Approaches

Once a child is assessed, a treatment program should be initiated. Goals for the program should include such items as stimulation of postural reflexes, inhibition of abnormal postural reflexes, stimulation of gross motor development, reduction of increased muscle tone and prevention of faulty body alignment. Specific goals should be set for each child.

Various books have been published regarding techniques used most frequently with children with developmental disabilities.[21–23] The four approaches that appear to be most widely accepted are Bobath, Rood, Brunnstrom, and proprioceptive neuromuscular facilitation (PNF).

Each of these treatment approaches contain certain similarities. Each approach stresses that movement develops in an orderly, sequential manner and that voluntary movement is superimposed on a reflex foundation. All four approaches also provide for facilitation of normal reflexes in the treatment programs. Only the Bobath and the Rood approaches, however, place importance on the inhibition of abnormal reflexes. Proprioceptive input or exteroceptive input are common to all approaches. In the PNF approach, specific sensory input is required, whereas in the other approaches the input is a component of the total activity program.

Each approach has its own merit in the treatment of the severely handicapped child. The Bobath approach, which relies on the stimulation and inhibition of postural reflexes, can be used well with the child who is unable to cooperate because of his chronological or developmental age. Likewise, the Rood approach, utilizing specific sensory stimulation such as vibration and stroking, allows for response even in the noncooperative or severely involved child. The Brunnstrom approach has been used primarily in the rehabilitation of hemiplegic children. This approach depends on the cooperation of the child; use of the approach will be difficult if the child is uncooperative or if the child does not actively use the uninvolved side. The PNF approach can be used with the child who is unable to cooperate or who does not wish to cooperate, through the use of positioning, manual contacts by handling, stretch, traction, approximation, and graded or careful resistance. For therapists interested in further study of these approaches, *Physical Therapy Services in the Developmental Disabilities,* edited by Pearson and Williams, provides a comprehensive and current interpretation of each approach.[21] Many other sources are also available to inquiring therapists.[24–31]

Perceptual Training

Perceptual training should also be included in treatment planned for the severely handicapped. This training is more applicable to ambulatory children who present problems with coordination and balance. Therapists should be familiar with gross motor activities that can be incorporated with a child's physical education program that would enhance perceptual development. Cratty has divided the learning of perceptual skills into six phases: 1) impulse control, 2) body image training, 3) perceptual motor competencies, 4) seriation, 5) pattern recognition, and 6) decision making and problem solving.[32] The first three phases are ones in which a physical therapist would play a major role. The first phase, impulse control, encompasses relaxation training, controlling movements, and prolonging tasks. The second phase, body image training, includes the learning of body planes, body parts, and structuring in space. The third phase (and probably the most well known by therapists) focuses on perceptual motor competencies which include the learning of balance, agility, locomotor skills, manual skills, and ball throwing and catching. These perceptual skills often develop very slowly in severely and profoundly handicapped children. To develop the desired skills in a child, therapists must recognize the importance of starting at the child's level of mental development rather than chronological development. Therapists must also utilize skills of teaching that will enhance a child's learning. For example, therapists must present tasks which are broken down into sequential steps that are achievable, use repetition of materials, and use concrete examples in addition to oral instructions. Activities suggested by Kephart[33] and Ayres[34] for perceptual motor development would be useful to the therapist involved in such programs.

Behavior Modification

Operant conditioning or behavior modification is the technique which is usually most effective but often the least understood by physical therapists in the treatment of severely involved children. Many times these youngsters are often unable to cooperate or to respond to the instructions. To involve a child in his program, the child's attention first must be gained by establishing eye contact. Next, the therapist must find a method of motivating the child to respond to his program. Nawas and Braun divide the task of conditioning into two areas: 1) increasing the frequency of the desired behavior and 2) decreasing the frequency of undesired behavior.[35] Positive reinforcers are stimuli which are given immediately after a behavior which will increase the frequency of that behavior. Consumables such as food and drink are used as well as other positive reinforcers and have been used successfully to teach the profoundly retarded child to walk, dress, and feed himself.[36–38] Experiments using food reinforcers have also shown that children can be taught to cooperate when no prior cooperation had been elicited. Visual, auditory, and social stimuli such as praise and affection have also proved effective as positive reinforcers.

Tokens can be used as a positive reinforcer with some children. The tokens are given to the children for desirable behaviors and, at the end of a set period, the tokens are exchanged for primary reinforcers such as food; however, this technique is usually more successful with higher functioning children. Behaviors may be increased in frequency by avoidance or escape procedures. For example, a child will perform an activity if the activity prevents him from receiving an aversive or noxious stimuli.[36]

Techniques to decrease the frequency of undesired behaviors are *extinction* and *punishment*. In *extinction*, a positive reinforcer following a behavior is taken away. Food may be removed, for example, if an undesirable behavior occurs.[38, 39] In *punishment*, an aversive stimulus such as a slap or physical restraint is used following the undesired behavior. In recent years, many arguments have arisen against the use of aversive conditioning.[40, 41] In particular, the qualifications of the person applying the aversive procedures are most often questioned. Most advocates of behavior modification believe that other means, such as positive reinforcement, should be tried before using aversive conditioning.

In view of the increasing arguments against some of the methods used in behavior modification, physical therapists wishing to use behavior modification should ideally attend an education course on the use and abuse of behavior modification. An alternative to a special course would be a team effort between a physical therapist and a school psychologist.

Implementation of Techniques

In the treatment of severely involved children, therapists must be able to integrate techniques from all the approaches that provide optimal improvement of the child. No single approach is effective for all children. New graduates have developed what Griffin terms "integrating behavior" which allows them to integrate the approaches based on their knowledge of neurophysiologic principles.[42] For those persons already working in the field, integrating behavior which includes the following skills is also important:

1. Ability to make decisions and to evaluate the outcomes of the decisions made
2. Ability to construct new learning relationships which provide for change
3. Ability to be flexible in new situations
4. Ability to derive one's own meaning and conclusions
5. Ability to question tradition.

ASSOCIATED PROBLEMS

With the compliance of the mandatory education laws concerning physical therapy services, many states like Tennessee will find that a variety of problems are associated with the development of services.

Such problems as too few therapists to serve the population, too little money to finance all necessary services (occupational therapy and speech therapy as well as physical therapy), and limited space available in pre-existing schools have been encountered in all parts of the state. The issue of whether a prescriptive referral is necessary for all children seen by a therapist presents a real problem, especially for proposed screening programs. There have been difficulties in Tennessee in the past with the certification of therapists as teachers. Recently, however, therapists have been hired in Tennessee without certification being required. Many other states are still requiring their therapists to become certified as teachers even though the competencies needed to work with handicapped children have already been acquired by therapists.

The ability to evaluate children accurately and then to plan appropriate programs that can be implemented by classroom teachers is a must for school therapists. They must be able to determine what program must be done by therapists and what program can be adequately handled by teachers. Therapists must undergo a process called "role release" in many cases.[21] They will be unable to provide all services and must allow others to aid in carrying out the program for the child. Most teachers with instruction, prove to be invaluable assets to the overall physical therapy program.

SUMMARY

The treatment of severely and profoundly retarded children in the classroom presents a challenge to physical therapists. New laws regarding public education demand that children receive physical therapy that will facilitate their optimal growth and development. Physical therapists in a school program must become aware of the interdisciplinary approach to handling severely and profoundly retarded children in addition to becoming more adept in providing optimal physical therapy services.

Physical therapists who work with severely handicapped children must be prepared to continue their education through workshops and lectures as well as through formal education in graduate school if they are to provide optimal treatment for children.

Fortunately, an increasing number of articles have been written during the past five years designed to educate practicing therapists in more effectively treating these children. Campbell has provided much information in the education and treatment of the young child.[43, 44] Marx and Connolly have also written about the use of physical therapy in early intervention programs.[45, 46] Gilbert and Wilbur have contributed suggestions for special equipment for use with severely handicapped children.[47, 48] In the future, even more information from experienced therapists working the severely handicapped must be shared. This field is indeed a new frontier for most therapists.

REFERENCES

1. Pennsylvania Association for Retarded Children v. Commonwealth of Pennsylvania, Civil Action No. 71-42 (3 Judge Court, E.D. Pennsylvania), January 1971
2. Mills v. Board of Education, Civil Action No. 1939-71 (District of Columbia), August 1972
3. Policies Governing the Development of Programs and Services for the Handicapped. Nashville, Tennessee Department of Education, 1974
4. Grossman HJ (ed): Manual on Terminology and Classification in Mental Retardation. Washington, American Association on Mental Deficiency, 1973
5. Heber R (ed): A Manual on Terminology and Classification in Mental Retardation. Am J Ment Defic [Suppl], 1961
6. Harris SE, Cherry DB: Childhood progressive muscular dystrophy and the role of physical therapy. Phys Ther 54:4-12, 1974
7. Tecklin SJ, Holsclaw DW: Cystic fibrosis and the role of the physical therapist in its management. Phys Ther 53:386-394, 1973
8. Witengier M: An adaptic playground for physically handicapped children. Phys Ther 50:821-826, 1970
9. Cronis S, Gleeson AW: Orthopedic screening of school children in Delaware. Phys Ther 54:1080-1083, 1974
10. Ethun CA: Physical therapy for the mentally retarded. Phys Ther 46:1226-1230, 1966
11. DeHaven GE: Is selective hearing an occupational hazard in physical therapy. Phys Ther 54:1301-1305, 1974
12. Odel SJ, Greer JG, Anderson RM: The family of the severely retarded individual. In Anderson RM, Greer JG (eds): Educating the Severely and Profoundly Retarded. Baltimore, University Park Press, 1976, pp 251-261
13. Barsch RH: The Parent of the Handicapped Child. Springfield, IL, Charles C Thomas, Publisher, 1968
14. Roos P: Parents and families of the mentally retarded. In Kauffman JM, Payne JS (eds): Mental Retardation: Introduction and Personal Perspectives. Columbus, Charles E. Merrill Publishing Co, 1975
15. Farber B: Family Organization and Crisis: Maintenance of Integration in Families with a Severely Retarded Child. Lafayette, IN, Child Development Publications of the Society for Research in Child Development, 1960
16. Bayley N: The California Infant Scale of Motor Development. Berkeley, University of California Press, 1936
17. Gesell A, Amatruda C: Developmental Diagnosis. New York, Paul B. Hoeber, Inc, 1949
18. Fiorentino M: Reflex Testing Methods for Evaluating CNS Development. Springfield, IL, Charles C Thomas, Publisher, 1963
19. Bobath K, Bobath B: The facilitation of normal postural reactions and movements in the treatment of cerebral palsy. Physiotherapy 57:246-262, 1964
20. Hoskins TA, Squires JE: Developmental assessment: A test for gross motor and reflex development. Phys Ther 53:117-125, 1973
21. Pearson PH, Williams CE(eds): Physical Therapy Services in the Developmental Disabilities. Springfield, IL, Charles C Thomas, Publisher, 1972
22. Finnie N: Handling the Young Cerebral Palsied Child at Home. New York, E.P. Dutton and Co, 1970
23. Cliff S, Gray J, Nymann C: A Therapist's Guide for Formulating a Developmental Test for Parents of Special Children. El Paso, Guynes Publishing Co, 1974
24. Bobath B: The very early treatment of cerebral palsy. Dev Med Child Neurol 9:373-390, 1967
25. Bobath B: Motor development: Its effect on general development and application to the treatment of cerebral palsy. Physiotherapy 57:516-523, 1971
26. Bobath B: The treatment of neuromuscular disorders by improving patterns of coordination. Physiotherapy 55:18-22, 1969
27. Bobath K, Bobath B: An analysis of the development of standing and walking patterns in patients with cerebral palsy. Physiotherapy 48:144-153, 1962
28. Stockmeyer SA: An interpretation of the approach of Rood to the treatment of neuromuscular dysfunction. Am J Phys Med 46:900-956, 1967
29. Perry C: Principles and techniques of the Brunnstrom approach to the treatment of hemiplegia. Am J Phys Med 46:789-812, 1967
30. Voss DE: Proprioceptive neuromuscular facilitation. Am J Phys Med 46:838-898, 1967
31. Voss DE: Proprioceptive neuromuscular facilitation: The PNF approach. In Pearson PH, Williams CE (eds): Physical Therapy Services in the Developmental Disabilities. Springfield, IL, Charles C Thomas, Publisher, 1972, pp 223-282
32. Cratty BJ: Improving the physical fitness of retardates. In Pearson PH, Williams CE (eds): Physical Therapy Service in the Developmental Disabilities. Springfield, IL, Charles C Thomas, Publisher 1972, pp 383-452
33. Kephart N: The Slow Learner in the Classroom. Columbus, Charles C. Merrill Publishing Co, 1960
34. Ayres JS: Occupational therapy for motor disorders resulting from impairment of the central nervous system. Rehabil Lit 21:302-320, 1960
35. Nawas MM, Braun SH: The use of operant techniques for modifying the behavior of the severely and profoundly retarded, part II. In Anderson RM, Greer JG (eds): Educating the Severely and Profoundly Retarded. Baltimore, University Park Press, 1976, pp 81-96
36. O'Brien F, Azrin N, Bugle C: Training profoundly retarded children to stop crawling. J Appl Behav Anal 5:127-139, 1972
37. Azrin N, Schaeffer R, Wesolowski M: A rapid method of teaching profoundly retarded persons to dress by a reinforcement-guidance method. Ment Retard 14:29-33, 1976
38. Azrin NH, Armstrong PM: The "mini-meal": A method of teaching eating skills to the profoundly retarded. Ment Retard 11:9-13, 1973
39. Roos P: Human rights and behavior modification. Ment Retard 12:3-6, 1974
40. Kazdin A: Issues in behavior modification with mentally retarded persons. Am J Ment Defic 78:34-40, 1973
41. Westervelt VD, Luiselli JK: Establishing standing and walking behavior in a physically handicapped, retarded child. Phys Ther 54:761-765, 1975
42. Griffin JW: Education integration in physical therapy: a study of teachers of therapeutic exercise. Phys Ther 53:402-414, 1973
43. Campbell SK: Facilitation of cognitive and motor development in infants with central nervous system dysfunction. Phys Ther 54:346-353, 1974
44. Campbell SK, Wilson JN: Planning infant learning programs. Phys Ther 56:1347-1357, 1976
45. Marx M: Integrating physical therapy into a cerebral palsy early education program. Phys Ther 53:512-514, 1973
46. Connolly B, Russell F: Interdisciplinary early intervention program. Phys Ther 56:155-158, 1976
47. Gilbert C: Wheelchair insert for hip and trunk support for children with cerebral palsy. Phys Ther 54:254-255, 1974
48. Wilbur S: Foam rubber sidelying support for children with cerebral palsy. Phys Ther 55:1345, 1975

Preparation of Physical Therapists for Employment in Public Schools

A New Approach

SUE E. McLAURIN

Physical therapists are providing services increasingly to children in public school environments because of justified needs as mandated, in part, by Public Law 94-142. Many of these therapists have attained competencies for such employment by participating in short courses or through professional experiences, self-study, and related didactic instruction. A course designed to prepare physical therapists for employment in a public school setting was offered to graduate pediatric students in the Division of Physical Therapy at the University of North Carolina in Chapel Hill. Specific content areas included in-depth knowledge of the public school system, interdisciplinary programming, and continuing education for public school teachers. Teaching units and observation sessions are outlined. Recommendations are offered for developing similar courses that can be incorporated into a graduate pediatric curriculum and are beneficial for preparing physical therapists for public school settings.

Key Words: *Education, graduate; Education, special; Physical therapy.*

President Gerald Ford signed the Education of All Handicapped Children Act (Public Law 94-142) on November 25, 1975. The scope of the law was far reaching, and the law therefore was most appropriately called the "Bill of Rights" for handicapped children. The purpose of Public Law 94-142 was to "assure that all handicapped children have available to them . . . a free appropriate public education which emphasizes special education and related services designed to meet their unique needs . . . ."[1] The term "related services" included, but was not limited to, transportation and supportive services such as speech pathology and audiology, psychological services, and physical and occupational therapy.

The passage of Public Law 94-142 has served as an impetus for the delivery of physical therapy services in educational environments. This monumental legislation outlines laws, policies, and procedures governing public school education and mandates a new and expanded role for physical therapists.

Historically, physical therapy services have been a viable component of public education for exceptional children. These services, however, were primarily provided in a self-contained facility to a select number of mentally or physically handicapped children.[2-7] Since the passage of Public Law 94-142, the focus of physical therapy services has had to shift from a medical orientation to an education orientation.[8-11] Now physical therapists are called on not only to use their professional skills for assessing the physical dysfunction of children, but also for assisting in the interdisciplinary planning and implementing of appropriate services to augment the education of handicapped children. These services are an integral part of the individualized education plan (IEP). The physical therapist, along with other members of the school-based committee, develops the IEP and involves the parents in the evaluation process. Composition of the school-based committee generally includes the principal, the referring teacher, the chairperson of exceptional children's programs, the teacher of exceptional children, the physical therapist or occupational therapist or both, the psychologist, the guidance counselor, the speech and language clinician, and the physical education teacher. Specific techniques germane to physical therapy and appropriate for the IEP are development and reflex testing, posture and gait evaluation, and joint range of motion and muscle strength assessment. In addition, the physical therapist serves as a consultant to the public school staff regarding the use of adequate space and equipment for exceptional children; the elimination of architectural barriers; the appropriateness of adaptive physical education activities; and staff development activities for linking families with community resources, appropriate classroom placement for children, and long-range planning for specific needs of each child. The change in service focus of therapists in public schools is consistent with American Physical Therapy Association policy on physical therapy practice in educational environments. The policy states that "physical therapists contribute unique administrative, consultative, management, and teaching skills that help modify the educational environment so that exceptional children may benefit from their educational environment."[12]

Similarly, Public Law 94-142 had a significant influence on people in the education sector. For the first time, personnel of many education agencies became aware of physical therapy as a related service. Other educators, although familiar with the direct medical service provided by the physical therapist, were not comfortable with the implication of the law that expanded the responsibilities of the physical therapist to include development of individualized education programs, consultation to classroom teachers and other appropriate school personnel, in-service education for management of exceptional children in the classroom, involvement with long-range programming, and recommendations of special place-

Mrs. McLaurin is Physical Therapy Consultant, Developmental Disabilities, North Carolina Division of Health Services, Raleigh, NC 27602 and Adjunct Assistant Professor, Division of Physical Therapy, University of North Carolina School of Medicine, Chapel Hill, NC 27514 (USA).

This article was submitted April 27, 1982; was with the author for revision 62 weeks; and was accepted December 15, 1983.

ment for select students.[13] Many education administrators were additionally concerned about the legal and financial ramifications of the expanded role of the physical therapist. Concurrently, physical therapists were put in a position where they had to become familiar with the skills and responsibilities of the classroom educator and school administrators and with the organization and operation of the school system. In other words, members of both professional groups have been confronted with their own changing roles, the other profession's role changes, and the change in role relationships caused by the new law's expansion of the physical therapist's responsibilities. Professional associations and government agencies responded by preparing guidelines and policies for the implementation of Public Law 94-142. The APTA issued a booklet that provided guidelines for physical therapy practice in educational environments.[12] Moreover, published guidelines for the practice of physical therapy in public schools were disseminated in several states,[14–16] and other states are in the process of preparing policies.

The purpose of this article is to describe a model of professional preparation that was designed for graduate pediatric physical therapy students who were interested in employment or had been employed in public schools. The model is a graduate course that was offered in the Pediatric Specialty Track of the Division of Physical Therapy at the University of North Carolina—Chapel Hill. The content, in essence, provides a broad perspective for the practice of physical therapy in educational settings.

MODEL

An advanced program of studies that is specifically geared to prepare physical therapists for a new and expanded role is one way to meet the needs of practicing physical therapists. For this end, I designed a graduate course entitled "Physical Therapists in Educational Enviroments." The primary goal of the course was to provide physical therapists with a fundamental core of knowledge regarding the history, structure, and services of public schools; the influence of federal, state, and local legislation on public education; the services for exceptional children in public schools; and the role of physical therapists in public education and the implications for exceptional or handicapped children. The intent was to provide information that would serve as a preamble for understanding the everchanging public school arena. The general goal was to prepare physical therapists for employment in public schools who were 1) knowledgeable about public education and its implications for exceptional children; 2) able to plan and organize effective and efficient physical therapy programs while considering the roles of other professionals in public schools; and 3) able to consult with school personnel and to train and supervise them in specific physical therapy management techniques to help an exceptional child benefit from special education. Specific content areas addressed were increased knowledge of the public school setting, interdisciplinary programming as it relates to the IEP, and continuing education for teachers of regular and exceptional children. Each of these areas are discussed in turn.

Course Goals

Knowledge of public school setting. First, I chose a knowledge base germane to physical therapists because physical therapists are obliged to remain abreast of current implications and factual information that relate to public education of the handicapped. The course gave an overview of the history of public education and current education practices to acquaint physical therapists with the relationships of their role to past and current education issues, such as equal education opportunity, zero reject, least restrictive environment, and due process. This knowledge would enable them to use administration and management skills in deciding the most appropriate methods for long-range planning for handicapped children and in establishing policies and procedures for physical therapy services, fiscal management, program monitoring and evaluation, and development of community linkages. The physical therapists' general and specific knowledge of the public school setting would enable them to determine the functions or programs that would be most feasible and desirable for a given public school.

Interdisciplinary programming. Second, because the team approach to serving the education needs of the handicapped child is mandated, physical therapists must have a working knowledge of the roles of other professionals in the school environment and how their roles relate to the province of physical therapy. The course delineated the roles of public school administrators, such as superintendents, supervisors, or principals of regular and exceptional children's programs. The students also became cognizant of the roles of psychologists, special educators, regular educators, guidance counselors, speech and language clinicians, and physical educators. The instructor taught effective communication skills for interacting with school personnel.

The information on learning environments for exceptional children included resource rooms, part-time special classes, self-contained special classes, special day schools, hospital and homebound services, and residential settings. Programming for exceptional children involved recommendations from all disciplines and was based on professional exchanges among individuals. These recommendations would effect appropriate placement in the least restrictive environment for exceptional children.

Continuing education for teachers. Finally, my personal experiences have demonstrated an ongoing need to help regular and special education teachers manage the handicapped child in the classroom. I instructed the students in effective strategies for assessing continuing education needs of regular and special education teachers. Other areas of instruction focused on the value of planning continuing education programs for teachers that were related to the specific perceived needs of the teachers. Topics that have proven to be of interest to teachers are information on medical terminology, handling and positioning of disabled students, classroom engineering and adaptation, building and transportation accessibility and safety, and a host of related subjects that would complement the teacher-directed educational activities.

Course Structure

Once I determined course goals, I outlined the following strategies for instruction: organizing the course, identifying and sequencing objectives, establishing the target group, developing and sequencing units of instruction, developing and selecting effective teaching methods and materials, sequencing the manner of instruction, and assessing the performance of learners. The course objectives derived from the goals were as follows:

1. The learner will identify and interpret federal, state, and local issues that affect public education.
2. The learner will propose appropriate methods for implementing physical therapy services, modify services when applicable, and present options for future physical therapy services based on tenuous funding.
3. The learner will develop models for the delivery of physical therapy services to local school systems, which take into consideration consultation and communication skills and changes in public laws and public policies.
4. The learner will develop models for providing continuing education for school personnel.
5. The learner will evaluate present programs by assessing several approaches to service delivery, reviewing research relating to the implementation of services, and assessing attitudes of school personnel.

The course content was sequenced as follows.

Unit I. Factors of public education: history, structure, and services of public school environments; history of federal, state, and local government roles in public education; public education funding; structure of public school systems; and state and local public school service.

Unit II. Impact of laws, policies, and guidelines on educational personnel and handicapped children: federal, state, and local laws; federal, state, and local policies; federal, state, and local guidelines; and public laws and policies relating to handicapped children.

Unit III. Overview of current issues and topics relating to the education of handicapped children: identifying handicapped children, noting current services, programming for handicapped children, and relating historical issues to current delivery of services.

Unit IV. Expanded role of the physical therapist in public schools: models for service delivery, organization of services, and implementation of services.

Unit V. Future trends for delivery of physical therapy services to handicapped children: legislative considerations, manpower, and public attitudes.

Unit VI. Consultative skills: communicating with teachers, communicating with school administrators, and communicating with parents.

Teaching methods included lecture, conference, and demonstration. The lecture and conference methods were implemented in the university setting, and the demonstration method was performed in the public school setting.

Students augmented their didactic experience by participating in scheduled observation sessions in public elementary schools. I scheduled a total of five observation sessions.

1. Orientation and observation of the total school operation.
2. Observation and participation in a school-based committee meeting.
3. Orientation and observation at the central administrative office (offices of superintendent, assistant superintendent, director of exceptional children's program, and supervisors).
4. Observation noting specific characteristics of the classroom atmosphere in a designated classroom.
5. Presentation of in-service training for regular and special education teachers.

Sessions 1 and 2 were included in Unit I and sessions 3, 4, and 5 were in conjunction with Unit VI.

I developed a formal agreement between the Division of Physical Therapy and the Chapel Hill-Carrboro Public School System to provide on-site experiences for students to complement their instructional units and broaden their perception of public school procedures and personnel. Because the Chapel Hill-Carrboro Public School System has limited physical therapy services, the students had an opportunity to do a needs assessment in the school environment and to make recommendations or suggestions to school administrators regarding physical therapy services.

According to the terms of the agreement, the Chapel Hill-Carrboro Public School System would promote an educational environment in which students would heighten their

1. Cognizance of the roles of educational personnel by observing and participating in school-related activities that have an influence on exceptional children.
2. Knowledge of practical implications of Public Law 94-142 by becoming involved in the identification, referral, screening, assessment, and placement processing in special education programs.
3. Ability to access varied and expanded services that would be in compliance with special education and related service rules and regulations.

The Division of Physical Therapy would provide experienced physical therapists who would

1. Observe handicapped children and education personnel in the educational environment.
2. Provide informal information regarding handicapping conditions.
3. Perform informal needs asessment for projection of present and future needs of the Chapel Hill-Carrboro Public School System.
4. Provide in-service training for personnel in the educational environment.
5. Promote understanding of the role of the physical therapist in the educational environment.
6. Consult with administrators to intensify the appropriate use of therapists in educational environments.

Implementation of the Model

Two students enrolled in the graduate course. Both students possessed the requisite pediatric experience; one in a public school and the other in a pediatric rehabilitation center that provided contractural services to the public school system by direct treatment to a select number of referred students. The physical therapy students were enrolled full-time in the pediatric speciality track in the Physical Therapy Division. The course was implemented through lecture sessions at the university and observations in public schools. The students fulfilled the learning objectives by developing a model of physical therapy services in a public school, presenting a staff development activity of an aspect of the physical therapist's role, and assessing the public school's physical therapy needs and services.

Lecture sessions for physical therapy students were given once a week for two-hour blocks. Public school observation sessions were scheduled during the latter half of the semester and lasted for two hours each session. The rationale for scheduling the observation sessions for the second half of the semester was to provide the physical therapy students with the necessary knowledge before they entered their practical experiences. Observation sessions varied from school to school. The principal in one school directed the observation sessions and involved other school staff in designated sessions. The principal of the second school met with the physical therapy student but participated less in subsequent sessions.

The lecture and observation sessions heightened the physical therapy students' understanding of the impact of federal, state, and local laws and policies on public school education. The students were able to discuss these laws and policies as they related to their on-site experiences. The students also showed increased awareness of various educators' roles and noted particular differences in the leadership styles of the principals. The students were able to observe strengths, weaknesses, and constraints of the two schools and relate them to a therapeutic model, which the class developed during the lecture sessions. The students also prepared a questionnaire for an in-service training.

The in-service training activity was scheduled during a teacher workday at one of the schools; the physical therapy student assigned to that school presented the topic. This topic was selected from the results of the questionnaire that was developed by the physical therapy student and distributed to teachers in the school. The in-service activity at the second school was not implemented because of previous scheduled events, inadequate communication, and time constraints. As an alternative, the physical therapy student and I met informally with the director of exceptional children's programs and other special education teachers from throughout the local education agency to discuss issues relating to physical therapists' roles in public schools.

The students discussed existing physical therapy services and long-range needs of the school system during the scheduled class sessions. At one of the schools, physical therapy services were provided on a weekly basis by contractural arrangement. The physical therapy students discussed this method of service delivery and determined that this model was grossly inadequate to meet the expressed needs by some of the school personnel. This model also precluded much needed communication and interaction between the therapist and regular or special educators.

Although I provided a planned class schedule, arranging continuity between the class sessions and observation sessions at all times was difficult. Class discussions centered around behaviors observed in the public schools as much as possible. Overall, the students became familiar with the ambience of a public school and the roles of personnel employed there.

As the course developed, I discovered some issues that should have been considered. Based on the students' course evaluation and my observations, I developed the following recommendations for constructing similar courses:

1. Closer communication and interaction between the course instructor and pertinent school personnel.
2. More definitive guidelines for observation sessions.
3. Increased semester hour credit for courses with subsequent contact hours.
4. Increased participation in the classroom to facilitate more teacher-therapist interaction.
5. Collaboration with a physical therapist who is providing services for the school.
6. Establishment of rapport with the school principal to provide assurance of program implementation.

CONCLUSION

I recommend a course to prepare physical therapists for employment in public schools in the graduate pediatric curriculum. Many therapists who are currently employed in public schools would probably benefit from a more comprehensive level of instruction in lieu of short continuing education courses.

A follow-up of one of the students enrolled in the course revealed propitious comments. The student who is currently employed in a pediatric setting stated that the knowledge on laws and policies that she gained from the course was especially helpful to her when talking with parents about services for their children. She also found useful the information on development of a needs assessment and medical and educational service models. The direct involvement with the public school and the in-service training component for educators were desirable professional experiences for her.

Physical therapists have become a viable aspect of education for exceptional children. To meet the increasing demands of an expanded role, a systematic comprehensive approach to educating pediatric physical therapists is warranted.

Acknowledgment. I thank Dr. Ruth Mitchell for her advice and assistance on this manuscript.

REFERENCES

1. Education for all handicapped children act (Public Law 94-142): Rules and regulations for implementation of Part B. Federal Register, August 23, 1977
2. Ethun CA: Physical therapy for the mentally retarded: Why? How? And by whom? Phys Ther 46:1226–1230, 1966
3. Semans S: Principles of treatment in cerebral palsy. Phys Ther 46:715–720, 1966
4. Connolly BH, Anderson RM: Severely handicapped children in the public schools: A new frontier for the physical therapist. Phys Ther 58:433–438, 1978
5. Harris SE, Cherry DB: Childhood progressive muscular dystrophy and the role of physical therapy. Phys Ther 54:4–12, 1974
6. Bleck EE: Integrating the physically handicapped child. J Sch Health 49:141–146, 1979
7. Volkoman CS: Integrating the physically disabled student into the elementary school. Education 99:25–30, 1978
8. Mitchell MM, Lindsey D: A model for establishing occupational therapy and physical therapy services in the public school. Am J Occup Ther 33:361–364, 1979
9. Kalish RA, Presseller S: Physical and occupational therapy. J Sch Health 50:265–267, 1980
10. Sellers JS: Professional cooperation in public school physical therapy. Phys Ther 60:1159–1161, 1980
11. Levangie PK: Public school physical therapists: Role definition and educational needs. Phys Ther 60:774–779, 1980
12. Physical Therapy Practice in Educational Environments: Policies, Guidelines, and Background Information. Washington, DC, American Physical Therapy Association, 1980
13. Cecconi CMP, Rothenberg SP: Model instructional program for mainstreaming handicapped children. Phys Ther 60:1022–1025, 1980.
14. Litton FW, Vernon L, Griffin HC: Occupational therapists and physical therapists: Vital members in the rehabilitation and educational process of disabled students. J Rehabil 48:65–67, 1982
15. Guidelines: Physical Therapy Services in North Carolina's Educational Environments. Raleigh, NC, Division for Exceptional Children, Department of Public Instruction, 1980
16. Vernon L, Poulton S: Guidelines: Occupational Therapy and Physical Therapy in the Schools. Baton Rouge, LA, Louisiana State Department of Education, 1980